Handbook of Research on Mathematical Modeling for Smart Healthcare Systems

Debabrata Samanta
CHRIST University (Deemed), India

Debabrata Singh
Siksha 'O' Anusandhan (Deemed), India

A volume in the Advances in Healthcare
Information Systems and Administration (AHISA)
Book Series

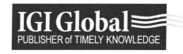

Published in the United States of America by
    IGI Global
    Medical Information Science Reference (an imprint of IGI Global)
    701 E. Chocolate Avenue
    Hershey PA, USA 17033
    Tel: 717-533-8845
    Fax: 717-533-8661
    E-mail: cust@igi-global.com
    Web site: http://www.igi-global.com

Library of Congress Cataloging-in-Publication Data

Names: Samanta, Debabrata, 1987- editor.
Title: Handbook of research on mathematical modeling for smart healthcare
   systems / Debabrata Samanta and Debabrata Singh, editors.
Description: Hershey, PA : Engineering Science Reference, an imprint of IGI
   Global, [2022] | Includes bibliographical references and index. |
   Summary: "As the market for Intelligent System technologies continue to
   grow in healthcare systems, this book recognizes the nature and
   manifestation of this environment, and develops a corresponding pathway
   to holistic Intelligent Computing methodology that helps to serve the
   healthcare system and increase the effectiveness as well as efficiency
   of health care providers"-- Provided by publisher.
Identifiers: LCCN 2022001278 (print) | LCCN 2022001279 (ebook) | ISBN
   9781668445808 (h/c) | ISBN 9781668445822 (ebook)
Subjects: LCSH: Medical technology--Mathematical models. | Medical
   innovations--Mathematical models.
Classification: LCC R855.3 .M385 2022 (print) | LCC R855.3 (ebook) | DDC
   610.285--dc23/eng/20220224
LC record available at https://lccn.loc.gov/2022001278
LC ebook record available at https://lccn.loc.gov/2022001279

This book is published in the IGI Global book series Advances in Healthcare Information Systems and Administration (AHISA) (ISSN: 2328-1243; eISSN: 2328-126X)

British Cataloguing in Publication Data
A Cataloguing in Publication record for this book is available from the British Library.

For electronic access to this publication, please contact: eresources@igi-global.com.

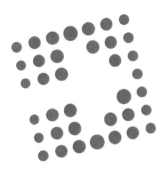

Advances in Healthcare Information Systems and Administration (AHISA) Book Series

Anastasius Moumtzoglou
Hellenic Society for Quality & Safety in Healthcare and P. & A. Kyriakou Children's Hospital, Greece

ISSN:2328-1243
EISSN:2328-126X

MISSION

The **Advances in Healthcare Information Systems and Administration (AHISA) Book Series** aims to provide a channel for international researchers to progress the field of study on technology and its implications on healthcare and health information systems. With the growing focus on healthcare and the importance of enhancing this industry to tend to the expanding population, the book series seeks to accelerate the awareness of technological advancements of health information systems and expand awareness and implementation.

Driven by advancing technologies and their clinical applications, the emerging field of health information systems and informatics is still searching for coherent directing frameworks to advance health care and clinical practices and research. Conducting research in these areas is both promising and challenging due to a host of factors, including rapidly evolving technologies and their application complexity. At the same time, organizational issues, including technology adoption, diffusion and acceptance as well as cost benefits and cost effectiveness of advancing health information systems and informatics applications as innovative forms of investment in healthcare are gaining attention as well. **AHISA** addresses these concepts and critical issues.

COVERAGE

- Medical Informatics
- Pharmaceutical and Home Healthcare Informatics
- E-Health and M-Health
- Measurements and Impact of HISA on Public and Social Policy
- Role of informatics specialists
- Telemedicine
- IS in Healthcare
- Management of Emerging Health Care Technologies
- Rehabilitative Technologies
- IT Applications in Health Organizations and Practices

IGI Global is currently accepting manuscripts for publication within this series. To submit a proposal for a volume in this series, please contact our Acquisition Editors at Acquisitions@igi-global.com or visit: http://www.igi-global.com/publish/.

Titles in this Series

For a list of additional titles in this series, please visit: www.igi-global.com/book-series

Handbook of Research on Healthcare Standards, Policies, and Reform
Ubaldo Comite (University "Giustino Fortunato" Benevento, Italy)
Medical Information Science Reference • © 2022 • 408pp • H/C (ISBN: 9781799888680) • US $435.00

Handbook of Research on Complexities, Management, and Governance in Healthcare
Ubaldo Comite (University "Giustino Fortunato" Benevento, Italy)
Medical Information Science Reference • © 2022 • 410pp • H/C (ISBN: 9781668460443) • US $425.00

Digital Identity in the New Era of Personalized Medicine
Ingrid Vasiliu-Feltes (University of Miami, USA) and Indira Mysore (Bloqcube Inc., USA)
Medical Information Science Reference • © 2022 • 315pp • H/C (ISBN: 9781799889663) • US $295.00

Building Resilient Healthcare Systems With ICTs
Patrick Ndayizigamiye (University of Johannesburg, South Africa) and Macire Kante (University of Johannesburg, South Africa)
Medical Information Science Reference • © 2022 • 298pp • H/C (ISBN: 9781799889151) • US $295.00

Approaches and Applications of Deep Learning in Virtual Medical Care
Noor Zaman (Taylor's University, Malaysia) Loveleen Gaur (Amity University, Noida, India) and Mamoona Humayun (Jouf University, Saudi Arabia)
Medical Information Science Reference • © 2022 • 293pp • H/C (ISBN: 9781799889298) • US $295.00

Prospects of Blockchain Technology for Accelerating Scientific Advancement in Healthcare
Malaya Dutta Borah (National Institute of Technology (NIT), India) Peng Zhang (Belmont University, USA) and Ganesh Chandra Deka (Ministry of Skill Development and Entrepreneurship, Government of India, India)
Medical Information Science Reference • © 2022 • 289pp • H/C (ISBN: 9781799896067) • US $285.00

Quality of Healthcare in the Aftermath of the COVID-19 Pandemic
Anastasius Moumtzoglou (P&A Kyriakou Children's Hospital, Greece)
Medical Information Science Reference • © 2022 • 403pp • H/C (ISBN: 9781799891987) • US $325.00

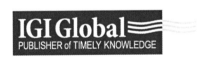

701 East Chocolate Avenue, Hershey, PA 17033, USA
Tel: 717-533-8845 x100 • Fax: 717-533-8661
E-Mail: cust@igi-global.com • www.igi-global.com

To my parents, Mr. Dulal Chandra Samanta and Mrs. Ambujini Samanta; my elder sister, Mrs. Tanus-ree Samanta; brother-in-law, Mr. Soumendra Jana; and daughter, Ms. Aditri Samanta.
Debabrata Samanta

To my parents, Mr. Achyutananda Singh and Mrs. Parbati Singh; wife, Mrs. Swarnaprava Nath; daughter, Devjani Singh; and son, Tatwadarshi Singh, for their love and inspiration.
Debabrata Singh

Editorial Advisory Board

List of Contributors

Acharya, Milu / *Institute of Technical Education and Research, India*............................ 121

Apat, Hemant Kumar / *National Institute of Technology, Rourkela, India* 383

Bajpai, Shreeya / *CHRIST University (Deemed), India* 409

Balasamy, K. / *Bannari Amman Institute of Technology, India*.. 86

Bhatnagar, Vaibhav / *Manipal University Jaipur, India*... 353

Biswal, Anil Kumar / *School of Computer Science, National Institute of Science and Technology (Autonomous), Berhampur, India* 247

Chandra Poonia, Ramesh / *CHRIST University (Deemed), India* 338

Choudhury, Subhashree / *Siksha 'O' Anusandhan (Deemed), India*................................. 180

Dahal, Rajshree / *CHRIST University (Deemed), India*.. 32, 306

Dash, Rajashree / *Department of Computer Science and Engineering, Institute of Technical Education and Research (ITER), Siksha 'O' Anusandhan (Deemed), Bhubaneswar, India* 12

Dash, Rasmita / *Department of Computer Science and Engineering, Institute of Technical Education and Research (ITER), Siksha 'O' Anusandhan (Deemed), Bhubaneswar, India* 12

Dhavale, Sunita Vikrant / *Defence Institute of Advanced Technology, India* 143

Garnayak, Mamata / *Centurion University of Technology and Management, India* 180

Gautam, Anjali / *Vellore Institute of Technology, India* 279

Goswami, Mausumi / *CHRIST University (Deemed), India*... 228

Gupta, Ritwika Das / *CHRIST University (Deemed), India* 32

Islam, Noman / *Iqra University, Pakistan*... 52

Jena, Rasmita / *Udayanath College of Science and Technology (Autonomous), India* 247

Jhansi Lekha, Veeramachaneni / *Vellore Institute of Technology, India*............................ 279

Komalasari, Rita / *Yarsi University, Indonesia*.. 374

Krishnan, Vivin / *CHRIST University (Deemed), India*... 154

Kumar, Ankit / *GLA University, Mathura, India* 353

Kumari, Anisha / *Department of Computer Science and Engineering, National Institute of Technology, Rourkela, India*.. 203

M. P., Karthikeyan / *School of Computer Science and IT, Bengaluru, India* 325

M., Senbagavalli / *Alliance College of Engineering and Design, Alliance University, India*.............. 1

M., Vanitha Archana / *Department of Mathematics, PSG College of Arts and Science, Coimbatore, India*.. 325

Mandala, Jyothi / *CHRIST University (Deemed), India* 110

Mansoor, Nijatullah / *CHRIST University (Deemed), India*.. 338

Manzar, Syed Babar / *NED University, Pakistan* 52

Maram, Balajee / *Chitkara University Institute of Engineering and Technology, Chitkara University, India* 110

Mohanty, Arup Kumar / *Siksha 'O' Anusandhan (Deemed), India* 180

Mohanty, Sagarika / *National Institute of Technology, Rourkela, India* 383

Muloor, Kiran / *LTI, India* 409

Muloor, Kiran Hemanthraj / *LTI, India* 306

Murugan, Karthik Chelakkara / *CHRIST University (Deemed), India* 228

Natarajan, Karthika / *Vellore Institute of Technology, India* 279

Nayak, Rashmiranjan / *National Institute of Technology, Rourkela, India* 383

P., Priyadharshini / *Department of Mathematics, PSG College of Arts and Science, Coimbatore, India* 325

Patra, Manoj Kumar / *National Institute of Technology, Rourkela, India* 261

Poonia, Ramesh Chandra / *CHRIST University (Deemed), India* 353

R., Ganeshan / *VIT Bhopal University, India* 110

Raja, Linesh / *Manipal University Jaipur, India* 353

Rautray, Rasmita / *Department of Computer Science and Engineering, Institute of Technical Education and Research (ITER), Siksha 'O' Anusandhan (Deemed), Bhubaneswar, India* 12

Renuka Devi, K. / *Dr. Mahalingam college of Engineering and Technology, India* 86

S. K., Manju bargavi / *Jain University (Deemed), India* 1

Sahoo, Bibhudatta / *Department of Computer Science and Engineering, National Institute of Technology, Rourkela, India* 203, 261, 383

Sahoo, Sipra / *Siksha 'O' Anusandhan (Deemed), India* 180

Sahoo, Swagatika / *Institute of Technical Education and Research, India* 121

Sahu, Somesh Kumar / *LTI, India* 306, 409

Samanta, Debabrata / *CHRIST University (Deemed), India* 32, 228, 338

Shabbir, Muhammad Hammad / *NED University, Pakistan* 52

Singh, Debabrata / *Institute of Technical Education and Research (ITER), Siksha 'O' Anusandhan (Deemed), India* 247

Somisetty, Pravalika / *Vellore Institute of Technology, India* 279

Sukumaran, Sreeja Cherillath / *CHRIST University (Deemed), India* 154

Syed, Darakhshan / *Iqra University, Pakistan* 52

T., Daniya / *GMR Institute of Technology, India* 110

Taunk, Apurv / *Siksha 'O' Anusandhan (Deemed), India* 180

Turuk, Ashok Kumar / *National Institute of Technology, Rourkela, India* 261

Venigalla, Ramya / *Vellore Institute of Technology, India* 279

Table of Contents

Preface.. xxv

Acknowledgment xxxii

Chapter 1
Artificial Intelligence and Medical Information Modeling.. 1
    Manju bargavi S. K., Jain University (Deemed), India
    Senbagavalli M., Alliance College of Engineering and Design, Alliance University, India

Chapter 2
Utility of Binary Cuckoo Search Approach for Microarray Data Analysis: A Dimensionality
Reduction Approach 12
    Rasmita Dash, Department of Computer Science and Engineering, Institute of Technical
        Education and Research (ITER), Siksha 'O' Anusandhan (Deemed), Bhubaneswar, India
    Rajashree Dash, Department of Computer Science and Engineering, Institute of Technical
        Education and Research (ITER), Siksha 'O' Anusandhan (Deemed), Bhubaneswar, India
    Rasmita Rautray, Department of Computer Science and Engineering, Institute of Technical
        Education and Research (ITER), Siksha 'O' Anusandhan (Deemed), Bhubaneswar, India

Chapter 3
Mathematical Model for Image Processing Using Graph Theory 32
    Rajshree Dahal, CHRIST University (Deemed), India
    Ritwika Das Gupta, CHRIST University (Deemed), India
    Debabrata Samanta, CHRIST University (Deemed), India

Chapter 4
Applications of Big Data in Smart Health Systems... 52
    Darakhshan Syed, Iqra University, Pakistan
    Noman Islam, Iqra University, Pakistan
    Muhammad Hammad Shabbir, NED University, Pakistan
    Syed Babar Manzar, NED University, Pakistan

Chapter 5

Securing Clinical Information Through Multimedia Watermarking Techniques 86
    K. Renuka Devi, Dr. Mahalingam college of Engineering and Technology, India
    K. Balasamy, Bannari Amman Institute of Technology, India

Chapter 6

IoT and Artificial Intelligence for Healthcare Informatics: Evolving Technologies 110
    Jyothi Mandala, CHRIST University (Deemed), India
    Ganeshan R., VIT Bhopal University, India
    Balajee Maram, Chitkara University Institute of Engineering and Technology, Chitkara
        University, India
    Daniya T., GMR Institute of Technology, India

Chapter 7

Intuitionistic Fuzzy Deteriorating Inventory Models With Controllable Carbon Emissions and
Shortages 121
    Swagatika Sahoo, Institute of Technical Education and Research, India
    Milu Acharya, Institute of Technical Education and Research, India

Chapter 8

AI-Driven COVID-19 Patient Screening With Design Thinking Approach- C3IA Tool: A Case
Study 143
    Sunita Vikrant Dhavale, Defence Institute of Advanced Technology, India

Chapter 9

Risk-Based Authentication: A Survey 154
    Vivin Krishnan, CHRIST University (Deemed), India
    Sreeja Cherillath Sukumaran, CHRIST University (Deemed), India

Chapter 10

Prediction of COVID-19 Active, Recovered, and Death Cases Using Artificial Neural Network
and Grey Wolf Optimization 180
    Arup Kumar Mohanty, Siksha 'O' Anusandhan (Deemed), India
    Sipra Sahoo, Siksha 'O' Anusandhan (Deemed), India
    Apurv Taunk, Siksha 'O' Anusandhan (Deemed), India
    Mamata Garnayak, Centurion University of Technology and Management, India
    Subhashree Choudhury, Siksha 'O' Anusandhan (Deemed), India

Chapter 11

Serverless Architecture for Healthcare Management Systems 203
    Anisha Kumari, Department of Computer Science and Engineering, National Institute of
        Technology, Rourkela, India
    Bibhudatta Sahoo, Department of Computer Science and Engineering, National Institute of
        Technology, Rourkela, India

Chapter 12
An Approach on Image Steganography Based on the Least Significant Bit Algorithm.....................228
  Karthik Chelakkara Murugan, CHRIST University (Deemed), India
  Debabrata Samanta, CHRIST University (Deemed), India
  Mausumi Goswami, CHRIST University (Deemed), India

Chapter 13
A Novel Approach for an IoT-Based U-Healthcare System 247
  Rasmita Jena, Udayanath College of Science and Technology (Autonomous), India
  Anil Kumar Biswal, School of Computer Science, National Institute of Science and
    Technology (Autonomous), Berhampur, India
  Debabrata Singh, Institute of Technical Education and Research (ITER), Siksha 'O'
    Anusandhan (Deemed), India

Chapter 14
Smart Healthcare System Using Containerized Internet of Medical Things......................261
  Manoj Kumar Patra, National Institute of Technology, Rourkela, India
  Bibhudatta Sahoo, National Institute of Technology, Rourkela, India
  Ashok Kumar Turuk, National Institute of Technology, Rourkela, India

Chapter 15
Medical Information Modeling for Diabetes Based on Logistic Regression......................279
  Karthika Natarajan, Vellore Institute of Technology, India
  Anjali Gautam, Vellore Institute of Technology, India
  Pravalika Somisetty, Vellore Institute of Technology, India
  Ramya Venigalla, Vellore Institute of Technology, India
  Veeramachaneni Jhansi Lekha, Vellore Institute of Technology, India

Chapter 16
Understanding of the Exploratory Graph Theoretical Approach for Data Analysis With
Supervised and Unsupervised Learning 306
  Kiran Hemanthraj Muloor, LTI, India
  Somesh Kumar Sahu, LTI, India
  Rajshree Dahal, CHRIST University (Deemed), India

Chapter 17
Technological Interventions for Biological Fluid Flow Analysis 325
  Priyadharshini P., Department of Mathematics, PSG College of Arts and Science,
    Coimbatore, India
  Vanitha Archana M., Department of Mathematics, PSG College of Arts and Science,
    Coimbatore, India
  Karthikeyan M. P., School of Computer Science and IT, Bengaluru, India

Chapter 18
Predictive Analysis of Diabetes Using Machine Learning Algorithms 338
  Nijatullah Mansoor, CHRIST University (Deemed), India
  Ramesh Chandra Poonia, CHRIST University (Deemed), India
  Debabrata Samanta, CHRIST University (Deemed), India

Chapter 19
Face Recognition System for Medical Information Modeling Using Machine Learning 353
  Ramesh Chandra Poonia, CHRIST University (Deemed), India
  Linesh Raja, Manipal University Jaipur, India
  Ankit Kumar, GLA University, Mathura, India
  Vaibhav Bhatnagar, Manipal University Jaipur, India

Chapter 20
A Social Ecological Model (SEM) to Manage Methadone Programmes in Prisons 374
  Rita Komalasari, Yarsi University, Indonesia

Chapter 21
Application Placement in Fog-Enabled Internet of Things (IoT) Healthcare System Using Body
Sensor Networks 383
  Hemant Kumar Apat, National Institute of Technology, Rourkela, India
  Rashmiranjan Nayak, National Institute of Technology, Rourkela, India
  Bibhudatta Sahoo, National Institute of Technology, Rourkela, India
  Sagarika Mohanty, National Institute of Technology, Rourkela, India

Chapter 22
Scaling Up of Software Development With Algorithm-Based Agile Methodologies 409
  Somesh Kumar Sahu, LTI, India
  Kiran Muloor, LTI, India
  Shreeya Bajpai, CHRIST University (Deemed), India

Compilation of References 439

About the Contributors 495

Index 501

Detailed Table of Contents

Preface xxv

Acknowledgment xxxii

Chapter 1
Artificial Intelligence and Medical Information Modeling 1
    Manju bargavi S. K., Jain University (Deemed), India
    Senbagavalli M., Alliance College of Engineering and Design, Alliance University, India

Artificial intelligence (AI) is the imitation of human cognitive abilities. It's changing the way people think about medical services, thanks to increased access to medical information and rapid advancements in examination techniques. We look at the current state of AI in medical services and speculate on its future. Artificial intelligence can be used to analyse various types of medical data (structured and unstructured). AI approaches for structured data machine learning methods, such as the old-style support vector machine and neural network, as well as modern deep learning, and regular language processing for unstructured data are among the most well-known AI tactics. Finding and treatment suggestions, patient commitment and adherence, and managerial exercises are all important classifications of utilizations. Malignant growth, nervous system science, and cardiology, for example, are some of the major disease areas that use AI devices. Many government institutions and government organizations are working to adapt smart city concepts and implementation of applications based on data techniques. It would not only streamline the process but it will have a bigger impact on citizen's lives. The smart city component comprises smart education, health, transportation, energy, environments, finance and other sub-domains alongside these. In recent times, big data analytics has been the driving factor to enhance smart city applications and likewise smart health. Evolution of digitalization has been the primary source of evolving smart health components to another level. This paper reviews applications of smart health to enhance smart cities and compare challenges, opportunities and open issues to dig down. This review reveals that there are still many opportunities left for utilizing big data for smart health.

Chapter 2
Utility of Binary Cuckoo Search Approach for Microarray Data Analysis: A Dimensionality
Reduction Approach 12

Rasmita Dash, Department of Computer Science and Engineering, Institute of Technical
Education and Research (ITER), Siksha 'O' Anusandhan (Deemed), Bhubaneswar, India
Rajashree Dash, Department of Computer Science and Engineering, Institute of Technical
Education and Research (ITER), Siksha 'O' Anusandhan (Deemed), Bhubaneswar, India
Rasmita Rautray, Department of Computer Science and Engineering, Institute of Technical
Education and Research (ITER), Siksha 'O' Anusandhan (Deemed), Bhubaneswar, India

In the recent literature, many metaheuristic approaches have been developed to examine, interpret, and analyze high-dimensional data. However, there is always a requirement to design a more productive and cost-effective technique. Many of the authors have acknowledged the capability of the Cuckoo search approach. Inspired by the blooming application of the Cuckoo search algorithm (CSA), the author has proposed a binary cuckoo search algorithm (BCSA) for gene selection and classification of microarray data. With the objective of optimizing gene subset and classification results, BCSA has been implemented. BCSA is optimized using a support vector machine (SVM) classifier and a significant gene set is extracted. This experimental study has been conducted over five microarray datasets. The superiority of this gene subset is shown using a few other classifiers such as k-nearest neighbor and artificial neural network. The model performance is also compared with a few other metaheuristic approaches such as particle swarm optimization, genetic algorithm, artificial bee colony algorithm, and differential evolution.

Chapter 3
Mathematical Model for Image Processing Using Graph Theory 32

Rajshree Dahal, CHRIST University (Deemed), India
Ritwika Das Gupta, CHRIST University (Deemed), India
Debabrata Samanta, CHRIST University (Deemed), India

Image segmentation being an important aspect of computer systems, graph theory provides the most elemental way of representing various parts of an image into mathematical structures. There are many applications of image segmentations that includes face recognition systems, remote sensing, detecting images sent by satellites, optometry, medical image reading and many more. Bi-partite graphs are useful in determination of cuts in the segmentation process. These structures are analysed by considering each vertex as pixel and each weight is some aspect of dissimilarity for two vertices connected by an edge with weights. This makes the problem-solving part very flexible and their computation becomes really easy and fast. The problem is usually parted into small subgraphs that are bound under some continuous forms of graphs like spanning trees, cut vertices or edges, shortest paths graphs and so on. The cluster formation is proved to one of most commonly used method in image segmentation.

Chapter 4
Applications of Big Data in Smart Health Systems 52

Darakhshan Syed, Iqra University, Pakistan
Noman Islam, Iqra University, Pakistan
Muhammad Hammad Shabbir, NED University, Pakistan
Syed Babar Manzar, NED University, Pakistan

Many government institutions and government organizations are working to adapt smart city concepts and implementation of applications based on data techniques. It would not only streamline the process but it will have a bigger impact on citizen's lives. The smart city component comprises smart education, health, transportation, energy, environments, finance and other subdomains alongside these. In recent times, big data analytics has been the driving factor to enhance smart city applications and likewise smart health. Evolution of digitalization has been the primary source of evolving smart health components to another level. This paper reviews applications of smart health to enhance smart cities and compare challenges, opportunities and open issues to dig down. This review reveals that there are still many opportunities left for utilizing big data for smart health.

Chapter 5
Securing Clinical Information Through Multimedia Watermarking Techniques 86
    K. Renuka Devi, Dr. Mahalingam college of Engineering and Technology, India
    K. Balasamy, Bannari Amman Institute of Technology, India

Today, in this technological world, the information available can be easily get copied, manipulated as well as broadcasted among different channels or networks. So, there is a need to protect the information which is available across different networks. In the case of medical field, the reliability and authenticity of the E-medical data is one of the serious concerns. The patient's data without the knowledge of the user might be utilized by the intruders. Those medical data is highly valuable for the purpose of diagnosis, treatment etc., Due to increase in the usage of internet, improved communications, Copyright protection, content authentication, identity theft, and ownership identification are considered to be the bottleneck issues for content proprietor. To resolve those issues, we focused on the study of watermarking technology which is used to improve the security of the data and protects the information from unauthorized access of clinical data. The term watermarking was first introduced and utilized by Andrew Tirkel and Charles Osborne in 1992, where they used this technique to hide the data using the images to preserve the privacy of the data. Watermarking is an emerging technique where the data has been protected by embedding code that it cannot be removed. Multimedia watermarking plays a predominant role in preserving the information from unauthorized access. This technique has been utilized in various areas for preserving data like medical/healthcare, Education, voting systems etc., Watermarking technique is highly utilized for security of various digital media such as text, audio, video and image. This chapter aims to provide the detailed review of various watermarking techniques, its applications for security purposes and the e-verification of medical information.

Chapter 6
IoT and Artificial Intelligence for Healthcare Informatics: Evolving Technologies 110
    Jyothi Mandala, CHRIST University (Deemed), India
    Ganeshan R., VIT Bhopal University, India
    Balajee Maram, Chitkara University Institute of Engineering and Technology, Chitkara
        University, India
    Daniya T., GMR Institute of Technology, India

Most of the IT industries (VMware, Google, Microsoft, etc.) significant research areas are remote healthcare systems which provide easily deployable and ubiquitous healthcare systems in the recent developments. Such systems are providing a platform with the infrastructure as a fully automatic and ubiquitous for sharing the applications and medical information. In remote healthcare systems, user's confidence is improved with providing the patients' data privacy and communication security. Basic idea about health care informatics is described in introduction part. Internet of Things (IoT) in health care systems, Devices and Mobile apps for healthcare and its challenges to medical fields are analyzed in second part. The combination of Healthcare with artificial intelligence (AI) and IoT technology will create a user-friendly application and developed healthcare by solving the issues of healthcare system and providing more security to personal and medical information of patients. A brief discussion of Artificial intelligence in healthcare is provided in part third section of the research. Both the critical and prior circumstances also, the applications of healthcare systems are worked along with the further developments in those applications. The real-time data is collected from IoT and AI devices regarding person's condition and uses the previous records as reference.

Chapter 7

Intuitionistic Fuzzy Deteriorating Inventory Models With Controllable Carbon Emissions and

Shortages... 121
Swagatika Sahoo, Institute of Technical Education and Research, India
Milu Acharya, Institute of Technical Education and Research, India

Nowadays, Global warming, which has its effect on climate change, has turned out to be a delicate topic, and several countries are making an effort to regulate emissions through certain investments in green technology (GT). Mostly, the issue with the emissions is the outcome of inventory management. In view of this, a fuzzy inventory models with time dependent power demand and controllable carbon emissions are formulated. This includes green technology investment involving two-warehouses to reduce emissions from CO_2, during the shipping of goods from the own warehouse to the rented warehouse and finally to the consumers. Further, a constant and Weibull deterioration rates are taken for the goods in rented and own warehouse respectively. Finally, the optimum values of the total average cost, cycle length and GT are obtained. A numerical example is provided to illustrate the models, and the behavior of the total cost function is shown graphically.

Chapter 8

AI-Driven COVID-19 Patient Screening With Design Thinking Approach- C3IA Tool: A Case

Study 143
Sunita Vikrant Dhavale, Defence Institute of Advanced Technology, India

Soon after the covid-19 pandemic was declared, government took major steps in supporting various research organizations and higher education institutes to accelerate artificial Intelligence (AI) based research in tackling global health crisis response and healthcare management. In response, AI proved to be crucial technology in building next-generation epidemic preparedness along with a resilient recovery. While developing AI based healthcare product solutions, one should apply human-centric design thinking principles to capture user emotions, thoughts along with their data privacy concerns. In this book chapter, we will discuss a brief literature review on AI driven COVID-19 patient screening technologies along with their pros and cons. Next, we will discuss need of human centric design thinking in AI driven solutions. Next, in this study, a novel C3IA (CNN based COVID-19 Chest Image Analysis) tool for automatic COVID-19 detection with multi-class classification (COVID/Normal/Pneumonia) using raw chest X-Ray images is proposed. We implemented two-stream CNN architecture with two pre-trained VGG-16 models which incorporates both segmented and un-segmented image features. The trained model is tested on more than 500 Indian patient X-Ray image dataset and confirmed accuracy of 99% in detecting COVID signatures. Further, in this work, we discuss how design thinking approach is followed in various stages while developing the product to provide a user friendly efficient real time COVID-19 Chest X-Ray Image Analysis for common citizen.

Chapter 9
Risk-Based Authentication: A Survey 154
Vivin Krishnan, CHRIST University (Deemed), India
Sreeja Cherillath Sukumaran, CHRIST University (Deemed), India

The rapid adoption of the internet has heralded the era of connected devices and services. Applications and systems are now designed to be internet-centric. The bulk of financial transactions, communications and even healthcare data are transmitted online. Internet-of-Things (IoT) are being used extensively across domains. With the increasing volume of digital and online traffic, the risk window grows as well. Evolving threat vectors have prompted the need for Multi-factor authentication (MFA) systems that utilize multiple modalities to strengthen security. However, with enterprises opting for Bring-your-own-device (BYOD) and the expansion of IoT applications, static MFA proves insufficient. This brings in the need for Risk-based Authentication (RBA) that follows an adaptive and continuous authentication methodology. With contextual attributes of the user factored in to arrive at the risk profile, RBA is more robust. With multiple authentication modalities that are chosen as per risk, RBA can withstand multiple attacks. The potential of RBA is why NIST, US and NCSC, UK have recommended its use. This paper covers the existing categories of authentication systems, available authentication methodologies, the use of multi-factor authentication and existing systems. The need for Risk-based authentication, with an analysis of current RBA methodologies, their future outlook and challenges are covered.

Chapter 10
Prediction of COVID-19 Active, Recovered, and Death Cases Using Artificial Neural Network
and Grey Wolf Optimization 180
Arup Kumar Mohanty, Siksha 'O' Anusandhan (Deemed), India
Sipra Sahoo, Siksha 'O' Anusandhan (Deemed), India
Apurv Taunk, Siksha 'O' Anusandhan (Deemed), India
Mamata Garnayak, Centurion University of Technology and Management, India
Subhashree Choudhury, Siksha 'O' Anusandhan (Deemed), India

The 2019 novel coronavirus was declared a global pandemic by the World Health Organization (WHO) on March 11th, 2020. The world is stressed out because of this disease's high infectiousness and transmission mode. A predictive model of the COVID-19 outbreak is developed for India using state-of-the-art neural network models. The article evaluates the key features to predict the patterns, potential infection rate, and death of the present COVID-19 outbreak in India. In this paper, machine learning methods such as Artificial Neural network (ANN) optimized by a bio-inspired optimization algorithm that is Grey Wolf Optimization (GWO), and Particle Swarm Optimization (PSO) have been implemented for the prediction of infection rate and mortality rate for the 5 days, 15 days, and 30 days ahead. The prediction of various parameters obtained by the proposed approach is effective within a certain specific range and would be a useful tool for administration and healthcare providers.

Chapter 11
Serverless Architecture for Healthcare Management Systems 203
    Anisha Kumari, Department of Computer Science and Engineering, National Institute of
      Technology, Rourkela, India
    Bibhudatta Sahoo, Department of Computer Science and Engineering, National Institute of
      Technology, Rourkela, India

Serverless computing is emerging cloud service architecture in recent years for executing distributed applications, where services are provided based on a pay-as-you-go basis. It allows the developers to deploy and run their applications without worrying about the underlying architecture. Serverless architecture has been popular due to its cost-effective policies, auto-scaling, independent and simplified code deployment. The healthcare service can be made available as a serverless application that consists of distributed cloud services achieving the various requirements in healthcare industry. The services offered may be made available on premise on a cloud infrastructure to users and health service providers. This chapter presents a novel model for serverless architecture for health care systems, where the services are provided as functional units to various stake holders of healthcare system. Two case studies related to healthcare systems which has been adopted serverless framework are discussed.

Chapter 12
An Approach on Image Steganography Based on the Least Significant Bit Algorithm 228
    Karthik Chelakkara Murugan, CHRIST University (Deemed), India
    Debabrata Samanta, CHRIST University (Deemed), India
    Mausumi Goswami, CHRIST University (Deemed), India

Steganography is the practice of communication by covering information within other information mediums. The goal of Steganography is to hide information in such a way that it remains hidden so that it looks normal from a commoner's perspective. It has been prevalent since ancient times, with the first use dating back to 440 BC in Greece. The etymology of Steganography is a combination of the Greek words: steganos, "covered", and graphia, "writing". The modern usage of Steganography, termed Digital Steganography, hides information in files stored on a computer. A standard steganography algorithm has three essential components: Carrier, Message, and Key. Carrier is the file that carries the message and an optional key to add a layer of authentication. Researchers have implemented Steganography utilizing different carriers, for example, image, audio and text. The carrier may or may not have any relation with the confidential information. Image Steganography is a type of Steganography that deals with hiding a message in an image file. The image, as a result, ends up with noise. This noise may lead to distortion and inconsistency in the images. Noise can be made less apparent by using a larger sized image. This project deals with the study of Image Steganography, a literature review of a research paper involving steganography detection in SNS messaging applications with a description of the research, and implementation of Image Steganography for uncompressed image files, using the Least Significant Bit algorithm.

Chapter 13
A Novel Approach for an IoT-Based U-Healthcare System 247
    Rasmita Jena, Udayanath College of Science and Technology (Autonomous), India
    Anil Kumar Biswal, School of Computer Science, National Institute of Science and
        Technology (Autonomous), Berhampur, India
    Debabrata Singh, Institute of Technical Education and Research (ITER), Siksha 'O'
        Anusandhan (Deemed), India

Among the living organisms, the most important metabolic process is health, or what we can say as the power of living and the basic right to get quality health care. In the coming era, the internet will play an important role in monitoring and executing the issues related to the health system of humans through automated sensor response using IoT. IoT connects device to device, things to things, as well as the human body to the network system through the sensors. It can be used to monitor human health-related issues like sugar level, blood pressure level, fever and keep track of a patient's pulse rate and any disease that may be harmful to human life. Today, due to a lack of resources in the world, people are facing many problems related to health. Hence, in wireless Body Area Network (WBAN), a body sensor can monitor the human body to gather a patient's body parameters and store the sensitive data in the cloud using the Arduino Uno. Cloud computing manages authentication, privacy, security, and data management by encrypting data at the source and decrypting it at the destination with a unique key. This paper presents details of the Ubiquitous Health (U-Health) care system and a proposed model and a novel platform for wearable technology to measure the patient's heart rate and any chronic disease without the intervention of human-to-human and human-to-computer systems.

Chapter 14
Smart Healthcare System Using Containerized Internet of Medical Things 261
    Manoj Kumar Patra, National Institute of Technology, Rourkela, India
    Bibhudatta Sahoo, National Institute of Technology, Rourkela, India
    Ashok Kumar Turuk, National Institute of Technology, Rourkela, India

There has been a rapid development of healthcare systems in recent times. The main objective of the intelligent healthcare system is to manage, monitor intelligently, and respond to the requirement of the medical ecosystem. In a smart healthcare system, access to different healthcare services and delivery of those services are done by adopting various technologies. Information and Communication Technology (ICT) has greatly influenced today's healthcare system. The term smart healthcare system comes to the fore because of the integration and application of technologies such as the Internet of Medical Things(IoMT), Cloud computing, Edge Computing, Containerization, Big Data, Artificial Intelligence, etc. In a smart healthcare system, several medical devices are equipped for collection and management of medical data, remote patient monitoring, tracking health status and location of patients, and monitoring and controlling medical devices to act according to the patients' suitability. In the Internet of Medical Things, several medical devices and applications are connected using networking technology and continuously produce a massive amount of data. The IoMT allows analyzing, managing, storing, and transmitting those data, making IoMT a connected healthcare infrastructure. This chapter presents a containerized edge computing architecture for smart healthcare systems using IoMT. The proposed architecture used containers at the edge for timely and fast medical service provisioning in the smart healthcare system. The architecture explains how cloud, edge, and IoMT can be integrated and how containers can be used to provide medical service. Finally, we look ahead and evaluate the future prospects of smart healthcare.

Chapter 15

Medical Information Modeling for Diabetes Based on Logistic Regression..................................... 279

Karthika Natarajan, Vellore Institute of Technology, India

Anjali Gautam, Vellore Institute of Technology, India

Pravalika Somisetty, Vellore Institute of Technology, India

Ramya Venigalla, Vellore Institute of Technology, India

Veeramachaneni Jhansi Lekha, Vellore Institute of Technology, India

In this digital health technology world, many health applications are being developed. Artificial Intelligence (AI) plays an important role for such important. Popular AI techniques include ML for handling structured and unstructured data. Machine learning detects health issues by studying many health records and data of the patients, hence increasing the efficiency of detection of chronic diseases in the medical field. Medical Information Modeling is to predict the medical needs in future and is a representation of a complex system into a simplified representation. Diabetes is one of the major diseases in the world population. It is a chronic disease associated with abnormally high levels of the glucose in the Blood. Gestational diabetes is a temporary condition associated with pregnancy. Several parameters are considered for the study i.e., Age, BMI, Insulin levels, BP, number of pregnancies, glucose levels, etc. Results can be obtained by using machine learning approaches like Logistic Regression, Naive Bayes.

Chapter 16

Understanding of the Exploratory Graph Theoretical Approach for Data Analysis With
Supervised and Unsupervised Learning 306

Kiran Hemanthraj Muloor, LTI, India

Somesh Kumar Sahu, LTI, India

Rajshree Dahal, CHRIST University (Deemed), India

Information is a vital part of optimizing the effectiveness, profitability, and dynamic abilities of organizations of all sizes, which leads to expanded deals, profits, and benefits. Currently, organizations deal with immense datasets, but owning a lot of data doesn't boost the business unless ventures investigate the available data and drive authoritative development. It is possible to automate exploratory data analysis to save a lot of time and effort, since we no longer need to write code for each visualization and statistical analysis. Automation of the process generates a report that includes all the visualization and data analysis as well. During the past decade, many systems have been developed to facilitate EDA, which is known as a challenging task that requires deep analytical skills, expertise, and domain knowledge. Specifically, advances in machine learning have created exciting opportunities not only to facilitate EDA, but to fully automate it. The EDA process generally takes a lot of time since it requires analyzing and visualizing various graphs and plots to determine what type of data we are dealing with, by using AI technologies, we can reduce the amount of time and effort required for EDA. We propose an end-to-end framework architecture, followed by an initial implementation of each component. Comparing the training data with the test data can be done by creating a comparison report.

Chapter 17
Technological Interventions for Biological Fluid Flow Analysis 325

    Priyadharshini P., Department of Mathematics, PSG College of Arts and Science,
       Coimbatore, India
    Vanitha Archana M., Department of Mathematics, PSG College of Arts and Science,
       Coimbatore, India
    Karthikeyan M. P., School of Computer Science and IT, Bengaluru, India

The thermal and mechanical effects of human tissues and physics that governs biological processes has been developed by applying fundamental engineering principles in the investigation of numerous heat and mass transfer applications in biology and medicine. An incompressible magnetohydrodynamic nanofluid flow passing over a stretched surface along with the effect of viscous dissipation is analyzed numerically. In order to create a nonlinear transformed model in terms of ordinary differential equations, suitable similarity transformations are used and solved by employing a Mathematica algorithm. Furthermore, a minimal case comparison standard has been provided to validate the current methodology. The machine learning method is built supervised through a very important parameter. Simulations and machine learning approaches could work together to reveal new and fortunate prospects in computational science and engineering problems. The performance of the parameters in terms of heat and mass transfer is presented with an aid of graph to demonstrate the applicability of the current model.

Chapter 18
Predictive Analysis of Diabetes Using Machine Learning Algorithms 338

    Nijatullah Mansoor, CHRIST University (Deemed), India
    Ramesh Chandra Poonia, CHRIST University (Deemed), India
    Debabrata Samanta, CHRIST University (Deemed), India

Diabetes is a very harmful disease that causes high blood sugar levels and occurs when the blood glucose level is high. Diabetes causes numerous diseases in humans: congestive heart failure, kidney, stroke, kidney, eye problems, dental, nerve damage, and foot problems. With the recent development in the Machine learning concept, it is easy to analyze and predict whether a person is diabetic or not. This research mainly focuses on using several prediction algorithms of machine learning. The algorithms used in this research are: k-nearest neighbour, logistic regression, SVM (Support Vector Machine), Gaussian naive Bayes, Decision tree, Multilayer Perceptron, Random Forest, XGBoost, AdaBoost. Among these algorithms, the XGBoost performed better than the other algorithms achieving an accuracy of 90%, and the f1_score, Jaccard score 91%, 86% respectively. The primary goal of this research is to apply numerous machine learning algorithms on diabetic datasets, analyze their results, and select the best one that performs well.

Chapter 19
Face Recognition System for Medical Information Modeling Using Machine Learning 353

    Ramesh Chandra Poonia, CHRIST University (Deemed), India
    Linesh Raja, Manipal University Jaipur, India
    Ankit Kumar, GLA University, Mathura, India
    Vaibhav Bhatnagar, Manipal University Jaipur, India

Face-recognition systems must be capable of identifying patient faces in an uncontrollable situation. Facial detection is a distinct problem from facial recognition in that it needs to report the location and size of all of the faces in a given image, which is not possible with face recognition. There are numerous changes in the images of the same face, which makes it a difficult problem to solve because of their general likeness in appearance. Face recognition is a very difficult procedure to do in an uncontrolled environment, since the lighting and angle of the face, as well as the quality of the image to be recognized, all have a considerable influence on the outcome of the process. This chapter provides information regarding the various face recognition machine learning models. The performance of the models is compared on the basis of values derived for FAR, FRR, TSR and ERR.

Chapter 20
A Social Ecological Model (SEM) to Manage Methadone Programmes in Prisons 374
    Rita Komalasari, Yarsi University, Indonesia

This chapter presents findings for managing methadone programs in prisons. For the first time, the findings presented in this paper contribute to socio-cultural and ecological approaches to solving problems, as well as providing policy alternatives for managing methadone programs in prisons. The Social Ecological Model (SEM) is used in this research to examine the interaction of public policy, community, institutional, interpersonal, and intrapersonal elements. The findings presented in this paper will have an impact on efforts to improve organizational, interpersonal, and intrapersonal factors.

Chapter 21
Application Placement in Fog-Enabled Internet of Things (IoT) Healthcare System Using Body
Sensor Networks 383
    Hemant Kumar Apat, National Institute of Technology, Rourkela, India
    Rashmiranjan Nayak, National Institute of Technology, Rourkela, India
    Bibhudatta Sahoo, National Institute of Technology, Rourkela, India
    Sagarika Mohanty, National Institute of Technology, Rourkela, India

The advancement of internet technology along with the high adoption rate of various IoT devices with various emergent IoT applications, has put stringent Quality of Service (QoS) and Quality of Experience (QoE) requirements on the service provider. The existing IoT-Cloud model cannot effectively and efficiently cater to the QoS and QoE requirements of these IoT applications effectively and efficiently due to low bandwidth and high propagation delay between the IoT device layer to the cloud data center. In order to meet the stringent requirement of healthcare IoT applications, Fog Computing has been used as an extension of cloud computing to provide multiple IoT services to the end-user at the close vicinity of the IoT devices. Fog computing paradigm is used as a service provider capable to execute various IoT services through hardware and software virtualization in a distributed and heterogeneous manner to execute different IoT applications at the edge of the network. The request generated by the respective IoT devices are mostly random in nature, and the objective of these applications varies dynamically; hence finding the optimal fog resources for the processing and execution is a challenge. In order to find the optimal mapping between the IoT applications and Fog resource, different resource allocation policy has been studied like resource scheduling, task scheduling, task placement, etc. In this article, we have formulated an optimization model for multiple healthcare IoT application placement problems in Fog computing architecture.

Chapter 22
Scaling Up of Software Development With Algorithm-Based Agile Methodologies 409
Somesh Kumar Sahu, LTI, India
Kiran Muloor, LTI, India
Shreeya Bajpai, CHRIST University (Deemed), India

Nowadays, the organization spends a significant part of its investment on operations and implementing any project. Project managers often face challenges regarding project management. Project managers face many challenges that get in the way of completing tasks, including poor communication. Setting backs and failures must be constantly analyzed and applied. Agile project management involves managing software development projects iteratively under continuous release cycles and incorporating customer feedback at each stage. Data science is not about getting accurate models or high-quality, clean data but rather defining feasible problems and developing reasonable measurements of solutions that require quick decisions since every day is different. People get the notion that Agile is a new type of approach that has recently evolved. There are many buzzwords in our technology and software development age, such as continuous delivery and software development. As the 1990s progressed, several software teams changed how they approached planning and delivering their products. The organizations recognized that their conventional project management approaches emphasized long-term planning. With a quickly changing environment and ongoing pressure to keep up with innovations, better and more efficient procedures were required to remain competitive.

Compilation of References 439

About the Contributors 495

Index 501

Preface

Artificial intelligence and machine learning are now available in most healthcare computing platforms. As is generally known, today's dominant technology is smart-based self-analyzed automated systems. The Intelligent System technology market is booming. In the future Smart Intelligent Systems will pave the path for advanced integrated systems that will maintain global economies safe and successful. Intelligent systems comprise not only intelligent gadgets, but also interconnected groups of them, such as networks and other bigger systems. As a result, it's necessary to understand the nature and manifestations of this environment in order to design a path to holistic Intelligent Computing approach that can benefit the healthcare system. Intelligent computing, ubiquitous computing, and ambient intelligence are terms that are being used in a variety of health-care applications. Intelligent is expected to improve traditional health care because of its omnipresent and unobtrusive analytical, diagnostic, supporting, information, and documentary features. Pervasive computing's features, including as remote, automated patient monitoring and diagnostics, could help to accelerate the shift to home care and improve patient self-care and independence. Intelligent computing is projected to improve the effectiveness and efficiency of health care professionals by providing automatic activity documentation, process management, and the right information in specific work settings. This book serves as a platform for presenting the application of novel solutions to difficult health-care problems.

Chapter 1 focuses Artificial intelligence (AI) is a computer programme that mimics human cognitive abilities. Increased availability to medical knowledge and quick developments in examination procedures are affecting people's perceptions of medical services. We examine AI's current state in medical services and forecast its future. Various sorts of medical data can be analysed using artificial intelligence (structured and unstructured). Among the most well-known AI tactics are structured data machine learning methods such as the old-style support vector machine and neural network, as well as current deep learning and regular language processing for unstructured data. The categories of utilizations include finding and treatment suggestions, patient commitment and adherence, and managerial exercises. Some of the primary disease fields that use AI devices include malignant growth, nervous system science, and cardiology, to name a few. Many government entities and organisations are attempting to adapt smart city principles and the installation of data-driven applications. It will not only speed up the process, but it will also have a greater influence on the lives of citizens. Along with this, the smart city component includes smart education, health, transportation, energy, the environment, finance, and other subdomains. In recent years, big data analytics has been a driving force behind the advancement of smart city and smart health applications. The fundamental source of progressing smart health components to the next level has been the evolution of digitalization. This study compares difficulties, possibilities, and outstanding concerns to explore deeper into smart health applications for smart cities. This analysis demonstrates that there are still plenty of potential to use big data for smart health.

Chapter 2 deep dives plan too many metaheuristic ways to examining, interpreting, and analysing high-dimensional data have been established in recent literature. However, there is always the need to devise a more efficient and cost-effective method. The Cuckoo search technique has been acknowledged by a number of authors. The author has developed a binary cuckoo search method (BCSA) for gene selection and categorization of microarray data, which is inspired by the growing application of the Cuckoo search algorithm (CSA). BCSA was implemented with the goal of improving gene subset and classification outcomes. A significant gene set is extracted after BCSA is optimised using a support vector machine (SVM) classifier. Five microarray datasets were used in this experiment. Other classifiers, such as k-nearest neighbour and artificial neural network, are used to demonstrate the superiority of this gene subset. Particle swarm optimization, genetic algorithm, artificial bee colony algorithm, and differential evolution are some of the other metaheuristic methodologies compared to the model's performance.

Chapter 3 intends graph theory provides the most fundamental means of encoding multiple components of a picture into mathematical structures, which is significant in computer systems. Face recognition systems, remote sensing, recognising images supplied by satellites, optometry, medical image reading, and many other applications use image segmentation. Cuts in the segmentation process can be determined using bi-partite graphs. Each vertex is treated as a pixel, and each weight represents a different element of dissimilarity for two vertices connected by a weighted connection. This gives the problem-solving part a lot more flexibility, and it makes computing them a lot easier and faster. Typically, the problem is divided into small subgraphs bound by continuous graphs such as spanning trees, cut vertices or edges, shortest routes graphs, and so on. Cluster generation has been proven to be one of the most widely utilised picture segmentation methods.

In Chapter 4, many government entities and organisations are attempting to adapt smart city principles and the installation of data-driven applications. It will not only speed up the process, but it will also have a greater influence on the lives of citizens. Along with this, the smart city component includes smart education, health, transportation, energy, the environment, finance, and other subdomains. In recent years, big data analytics has been a driving force behind the advancement of smart city and smart health applications. The fundamental source of progressing smart health components to the next level has been the evolution of digitalization. This study compares difficulties, possibilities, and outstanding concerns to explore deeper into smart health applications for smart cities. This examination demonstrates that there are still several potential for data utilisation.

In today's electronic environment, information can be quickly copied, modified, and broadcast through multiple channels or networks. As a result, information that is available across several networks must be protected. In the medical industry, one of the major concerns is the dependability and validity of E-medical data. The data of the patient could be used by attackers without the user's awareness. These medical records are extremely valuable for diagnosis, therapy, and other purposes. Copyright protection, content authentication, identity theft, and ownership identification are regarded bottleneck challenges for content proprietors as a result of increased internet usage and enhanced communications. To address these difficulties, we concentrated on the research of watermarking technology, which is used to increase data security and secure healthcare data from unauthorised access. Andrew Tirkel and Charles Osborne coined the term watermarking in 1992, and they used it to disguise data using graphics in order to protect data privacy. Watermarking is a new technology in which data is safeguarded by embedding code that makes it impossible to delete. Multimedia watermarking is an important tool for protecting data from illegal access. This method has been used to preserve data in a variety of fields, including medical/healthcare, education, voting systems, and so on. The process of watermarking is widely used to secure various digital media. This chapter attempts to provide a comprehensive overview of various watermarking techniques, as well as their applications for security and e-verification of medical data in this Chapter 5.

In recent advancements, most of the IT industries' key research topics have been remote healthcare systems, which enable easily deployable and ubiquitous healthcare solutions. Such systems provide a platform with architecture that is fully automated and ubiquitous for sharing medical information and applications. Users' confidence in remote healthcare systems is boosted by ensuring patient data privacy and communication security. In the introduction section, the basic concept of health care informatics is discussed. The second chapter examines the Internet of Things (IoT) in health-care systems, devices, and mobile apps for healthcare, as well as the challenges it poses to medical fields. By combining health-care with artificial intelligence (AI) and Internet of Things (IoT) technology, a user-friendly application and developed healthcare will be created, eliminating healthcare system challenges and offering more protection to patients' personal and medical information. The final section of the chapter includes a brief examination of artificial intelligence in healthcare. Both essential and preceding situations are considered, as are the applications of healthcare systems, as well as future changes in those applications. Real-time data about a person's state is collected through IoT and AI devices, and past records are used as a reference in Chapter 6.

In Chapter 7, Global warming, which causes climate change, has been a sensitive topic in recent years, and numerous nations are attempting to restrict emissions through investments in green technologies (GT). The majority of the emissions problem stems from inventory management. In light of this, we developed fuzzy inventory models with time-dependent power demand and regulated carbon emissions. This comprises an investment in green technology involving two warehouses to reduce emissions during the shipping of goods from the own warehouse to the rented warehouse, and lastly to the consumers. Furthermore, for items in rented and own warehouses, constant and Weibull deterioration rates are used. Finally, the best total average cost, cycle length, and GT values are found. The models are illustrated with a numerical example, and the behaviour of the total cost function is visually depicted.

Chapter 8 takes soon after the covid-19 pandemic was announced, the government took significant steps to support various research groups and higher education institutions in their efforts to expedite artificial intelligence (AI)-based research in global health crisis response and healthcare management. As a result, AI has shown to be a critical technology in developing next-generation epidemic preparedness and recovery. When creating AI-based healthcare product solutions, human-centric design thinking approaches should be used to capture user emotions, thoughts, and data privacy concerns. We will address a brief literature analysis of AI-driven COVID-19 patient screening methods, as well as their benefits and drawbacks, in this book chapter. The importance of human-centric design thinking in AI-driven solutions will be discussed next. Then, using raw chest X-Ray pictures, a novel C3IA (CNN based COVID-19 Chest Image Analysis) method is developed for automatic COVID-19 identification with multi-class classification (COVID/Normal/Pneumonia). With two pre-trained VGG-16 models, we constructed a two-stream CNN architecture that integrates both segmented and un-segmented image information. The trained model was evaluated on a dataset of over 500 Indian patient X-Ray images and found to be 99 percent accurate in detecting COVID signatures. In addition, we highlight how design thinking is used in various stages of product development to deliver a user-friendly, efficient real-time COVID-19 Chest X-Ray Image Analysis for ordinary citizens.

Chapter 9 throws the internet's increasing popularity has ushered in a new era of connected devices and services. Internet-centric applications and systems are increasingly the norm. The majority of financial transactions, communications, and even health-related information are now done online. The Internet of Things (IoT) is widely employed in many fields. As the volume of digital and online traffic grows, so does the danger window. Multi-factor authentication (MFA) systems that use many modalities to increase security have become necessary as threat vectors have evolved. However, with the adoption of Bring-your-own-device (BYOD) policies and the growth of IoT applications, static MFA is no longer sufficient. As a result, Risk-based Authentication (RBA) with an adaptive and continuous authentication mechanism is required. RBA is more robust when the user's contextual factors are taken into account when calculating the risk profile. RBA can withstand various attacks by using different authentication modalities that are chosen based on risk. The potential of RBA is why it has been endorsed by NIST in the United States and NCSC in the United Kingdom. This chapter discusses the many types of authentication systems, authentication algorithms, multi-factor authentication, and existing solutions. The need for risk-based authentication is discussed, along with an examination of present RBA approaches, their future prospects, and problems.

In Chapter 10, On March 11th, 2020, the World Health Organization (WHO) proclaimed the 2019 new coronavirus a worldwide pandemic. Because of the disease's high infectiousness and mechanism of dissemination, the entire world is concerned. Using cutting-edge neural network models, a COVID-19 outbreak prediction model for India has been constructed. The essay assesses the major characteristics that can be used to predict the patterns, infection rate, and death rate of the current COVID-19 outbreak in India. In this report, machine learning approaches such as Artificial Neural Networks (ANN) optimised by Grey Wolf Optimization (GWO), a bio-inspired optimization algorithm, and Particle Swarm Optimization (PSO) were used to forecast infection rates and mortality rates for the next 5 days, 15 days, and 30 days. The proposed approach's prediction of numerous parameters is effective within a defined range and would be a useful tool for administration and healthcare professionals.

Chapter 11 focuses in recent years, serverless computing has emerged as cloud service architecture for executing distributed applications, with services supplied on a pay-as-you-go basis. It enables developers to deploy and run their apps without having to worry about the architecture. Because of its cost-effective policies, auto-scaling, and autonomous and simpler code deployment, serverless architecture has become popular. The healthcare service can be made available as a serverless application made out of distributed cloud services that meet the industry's diverse needs. Users and health care professionals may be able to access the services via on-premise or cloud infrastructure. This chapter introduces a new serverless architecture approach for health-care systems, in which services are delivered as functional units to multiple stakeholders. Two case studies of healthcare systems that have implemented the serverless framework are discussed.

Chapter 12 deep dives plan to Steganography is the process of hiding information within other information channels in order to communicate. Steganography's purpose is to conceal information in such a way that it remains concealed and appears normal to the average person. It has been around since ancient times, with the first recorded use in Greece in 440 BC. Steganography is derived from the Greek terms steganos, which means "covered," and graphia, which means "writing." Digital Steganography is a modern version of Steganography that hides information in computer files. Carrier, Message, and Key are the three main components of a conventional steganography algorithm. The carrier file contains the message as well as an optional key for authentication. Researchers have used several carriers, including as picture, audio, and text, to develop Steganography. The confidential information may or may not be related to the carrier. Steganography that involves hiding a message in an image file is known as picture steganography. As a result, noise appears in the image. This noise could cause picture distortion and inconsistencies. Using a bigger image size reduces the visibility of noise. This project focuses on Picture Steganography, including a literature evaluation of a research chapter on steganography detection in SNS messaging systems, as well as implementation of Image Steganography for uncompressed image files using the Least Significant Bit technique.

Chapter 13 intends Health, or what we can call the power of life and the essential right to get adequate health care, is the most crucial metabolic process among living beings. The internet will play a key role in monitoring and executing issues relating to human health systems in the coming period, thanks to automated sensor responses enabled by IoT. Through sensors, the Internet of Things connects devices to devices, things to things, and the human body to the network system. It can be used to track human health-related issues such as blood sugar levels, blood pressure levels, temperature, and a patient's pulse rate, as well as any ailment that could be life-threatening. People today face numerous health issues as a result of a global shortage of resources. As a result, a body sensor may monitor the human body to gather a patient's body parameters and store the sensitive data in the cloud using the Arduino Uno in a wireless Body Area Network (WBAN). By encrypting data at the source and decrypting it with a unique key at the destination, cloud computing manages authentication, privacy, security, and data management. This chapter describes the Ubiquitous Health (U-Health) care system, as well as a proposed model and a unique platform for wearable technology that may measure a patient's heart rate and any chronic disease without the use of human-to-human or human-to-computer systems.

In Chapter 14, in recent years, healthcare systems have advanced at a breakneck pace. The basic goal of an intelligent healthcare system is to manage, monitor, and respond intelligently to the needs of the medical environment. In a smart healthcare system, numerous technologies are used to provide access to various healthcare services and to deliver those services. Today's healthcare system has been profoundly influenced by information and communication technology (ICT). The integration and implementation of technologies such as the Internet of Medical Things (IoMT), Cloud computing, Edge computing, Containerization, Big Data, Artificial Intelligence, and others has given rise to the phrase smart healthcare system. Several medical devices are installed in a smart healthcare system for collecting and managing medical data, remote patient monitoring, tracking patients' health state and location, and monitoring and controlling medical devices to behave according to the patients' appropriateness. Several medical equipment and apps are connected via networking technologies to produce a large amount of data in the Internet of Medical Things. IoMT is a connected healthcare infrastructure that enables for data analysis, management, storage, and transmission. This chapter describes a containerized edge computing architecture for IoMT-based smart healthcare systems. In the smart healthcare system, the suggested design uses containers at the edge to provide timely and quick medical service provisioning.

Many health applications are being developed in this digital health technology world. Artificial Intelligence (AI) plays a significant part in this. ML is a popular AI technique for dealing with organised and unstructured data. Machine learning diagnoses health issues by analysing a large number of patient health records and data, boosting the efficiency of chronic disease identification in the medical industry. Medical Information Modeling is a representation of a complicated system into a simplified representation that is used to predict future medical demands. Diabetes is one of the most common diseases in the world. It is a chronic condition characterised by unusually high blood glucose levels. Gestational diabetes is a disease that occurs during pregnancy in this Chapter 15.

Organizations of all sizes can improve their efficacy, profitability, and dynamic skills by using information, which leads to more deals, profits, and benefits. Organizations now deal with massive datasets, but having a lot of data won't help your firm grow unless you study the data and drive authoritative development. Exploratory data analysis can be automated to save time and effort by eliminating the need to create code for each visualisation and statistical analysis. The procedure is automated, which results in a report that includes all of the graphics and data analysis. Many solutions have been developed over the last decade to aid EDA, which is known as a difficult endeavour requiring deep analytical abilities, expertise, and domain knowledge. Machine learning improvements, in particular, have opened up tantalising possibilities for not only facilitating EDA but also entirely automating it. Because the EDA process necessitates evaluating and visualising multiple graphs and plots to establish what type of data we are dealing with, we may reduce the amount of time and effort required by employing AI technology. An end-to-end framework architecture is proposed, followed by an initial implementation of each component. Creating a comparison report allows you to compare the training and test data in Chapter 16.

In Chapter 17, the thermal and mechanical impacts of human tissues, as well as the physics that drives biological processes, have been established through the application of fundamental engineering principles to a variety of heat and mass transfer applications in biology and medicine. The influence of viscous dissipation on an incompressible magneto hydrodynamic nanofluid flow travelling through a stretched surface is numerically studied. Appropriate similarity transformations are performed and solved using a Mathematica approach to construct a nonlinear transformed model in terms of ordinary differential equations. In addition, to validate the current methodology, a minimal case comparison criterion has been provided. A highly significant parameter is used to supervise the machine learning method. Simulations and machine learning techniques may be combined to show new and promising possibilities in computational science and engineering challenges. To demonstrate the applicability of the existing model, the performance of the parameters in terms of heat and mass transport is presented using a graph.

Chapter 18 takes Diabetes is a dangerous disease that produces high blood sugar levels and develops when the glucose level in the blood is too high. In humans, diabetes causes a variety of ailments, including congestive heart failure, kidney failure, stroke, kidney, eye, tooth, nerve, and foot disorders. It is now simple to assess and forecast if a person is diabetic or not thanks to recent advances in the Machine Learning concept. This study focuses on the utilisation of numerous machine learning prediction methods. K-nearest neighbour, logistic regression, SVM (Support Vector Machine), Gaussian naive Bayes, Decision tree, Multilayer Perceptron, Random Forest, XGBoost, AdaBoost are the techniques utilised in this study. The XGBoost algorithm outperformed the others, obtaining a 90 percent accuracy rate.

Chapter 19 throws in an unpredictable situation, face-recognition algorithms must be capable of identifying patient faces. Facial detection differs from facial recognition in that it requires reporting the location and size of all of the faces in a picture, which is impossible with face recognition. Because of their overall likeness in look, there are countless alterations in the photographs of the same face, making it a challenging challenge to address. Face identification is a difficult technique to do in an uncontrolled setting since the lighting, perspective, and quality of the image to be recognised all have a significant impact on the process' outcome. The numerous facial recognition machine learning models are discussed in this chapter. The models' performance is compared using the numbers calculated for FAR, FRR, TSR, and ERR.

In Chapter 20, the insights for managing methadone programmes in prisons are presented in this chapter. The data reported in this research add for the first time to socio-cultural and ecological approaches to problem solving, as well as policy choices for administering methadone programmes in prisons. The interaction of public policy, community, institutional, interpersonal, and intrapersonal components is examined in this study using the Social Ecological Model (SEM). The conclusions of this chapter will influence efforts to improve organisational, interpersonal, and intrapersonal aspects.

Chapter 21 focuses the rapid growth of internet technology, together with the widespread adoption of various IoT devices and emerging IoT applications, has imposed strict Quality of Service (QoS) and Quality of Experience (QoE) standards on service providers. Due to low bandwidth and high propagation latency between the IoT device layer and the cloud data centre, the traditional IoT-Cloud model cannot effectively and efficiently cater to the QoS and QoE needs of modern IoT applications. Fog Computing has been utilised as an extension of cloud computing to give many IoT services to the end-user in close proximity to the IoT devices in order to meet the strict requirements of healthcare IoT applications. The fog computing paradigm is employed as a service provider capable of executing multiple IoT services via hardware and software virtualization in a distributed and heterogeneous way at the network's edge. The requests issued by the corresponding IoT devices are usually random in character, and the goal of these applications changes on a regular basis; hence, determining the best fog resources for processing and execution is difficult. Different resource allocation policies, such as resource scheduling, job scheduling, task placement, and so on, have been researched in order to discover the appropriate mapping between IoT applications and Fog resource. We present an optimization approach for numerous healthcare IoT application placement difficulties in Fog computing architecture in this study.

Chapter 22 deep dives plan to currently, the organisation spends a large portion of its budget on operations and project implementation. Project managers are frequently confronted with difficulties in project management. Poor communication is one of the many obstacles that project managers confront in accomplishing projects. Failures and setbacks must be continually evaluated and applied. Agile project management entails iteratively managing software development projects with continuous release cycles and taking customer feedback into account at each level. Data science is about establishing doable challenges and developing reasonable measurements of solutions that require quick decisions because every day is different. People have the impression that Agile is a new strategy that has only recently emerged. In today's technology and software development world, phrases like continuous delivery and software development abound. Several software teams modified how they planned and delivered their products as the 1990s proceeded. Traditional project management systems emphasised long-term planning, which the organisations understood. To stay competitive in a rapidly changing world with constant pressure to keep up with advancements, better and more efficient methods were required.

Debabrata Samanta
CHRIST University (Deemed), India

Debabrata Singh
Siksha 'O' Anusandhan (Deemed), India

Acknowledgment

We express our great pleasure, sincere thanks, and gratitude to the people who significantly helped, contributed and supported to the completion of this book entitled with *Handbook of Research on Mathematical Modeling for Smart Healthcare Systems*. Our sincere thanks to Fr. Benny Thomas, Professor, Department of Computer Science and Engineering, CHRIST (Deemed to be University), Bengaluru, Karnataka India, and Siddhartha Bhattacharyya,, Principal, Rajnagar Mahavidyalaya, Rajnagar, Birbhum, India for their continuous support, advice and cordial guidance from the beginning to the completion of this book.

We would also like to express our honest appreciation to our colleagues at CHRIST (Deemed to be University), Bengaluru, Karnataka India and Siksha 'O' Anusandhan (SOA) Deemed to be University, Bhubaneswar, Odisha, India for their guidance and support.

We also thank all the authors who have contributed some chapters to this book. This book would not have been possible without their contribution.

We are also very thankful to the reviewers for reviewing the book chapters. This book would not have been possible without their continuous support and commitment towards completing the chapters' review on time.

To complete this book, all the publishing team members at IGI Global extended their king cooperation, timely response, expert comments, guidance, and we are very thankful to them.

Finally, we sincerely express our special and heartfelt respect, gratitude, and gratefulness to our family members and parents for their endless support and blessings.

Chapter 1
Artificial Intelligence and Medical Information Modeling

Manju bargavi S. K.
Jain University (Deemed), India

Senbagavalli M.
 https://orcid.org/0000-0003-3806-8257
Alliance College of Engineering and Design, Alliance University, India

ABSTRACT

Artificial intelligence (AI) is the imitation of human cognitive abilities. It's changing the way people think about medical services, thanks to increased access to medical information and rapid advancements in examination techniques. The authors look at the current state of AI in medical services and speculate on its future. Artificial intelligence can be used to analyse various types of medical data (structured and unstructured). AI approaches for structured data machine learning methods, such as the old-style support vector machine and neural network, as well as modern deep learning, and regular language processing for unstructured data are among the most well-known AI tactics. Finding and treatment suggestions, patient commitment and adherence, and managerial exercises are all important classifications of utilizations. Malignant growth, nervous system science, and cardiology, for example, are some of the major disease areas that use AI devices.

INTRODUCTION

The purpose of this chapter is to debate current state-of-the-art intelligent healthcare systems, with a focus on major areas such as portable and smart phone gadgets for patient monitoring, machine learning for diagnosis of diseases, and assistive structures, such as social robots established for the adaptable living situation. Remote surveillance systems can provide individual and worldwide sensing on a variety of scales. Sensing is divided into three categories: personal, group, and social sensing. Real time tracking systems are built for a single personal and are generally concentrated on gathering and examining personal information. Monitoring users' exercise habits, assessing activity levels, and identifying symp-

DOI: 10.4018/978-1-6684-4580-8.ch001

toms associated with psychiatric problems are all common instances. Although the data generated is intended solely for the user's use, it is normal to share it with medical professionals. FitBit, Google Glass and the Nike+ FuelBand are all intelligent personal monitoring devices. Individuals who participate in health monitoring and share a similar hobby, problem, or aim create a group. In social networks or related groups, where information can be openly distributed or else with information secrecy, collective monitoring systems might be popular.

Patient monitoring applications, such as contests based on specific goals such as running distance, weight loss, calorie consumption, and so on, are common examples. Community or population monitoring refers to when a lot of people participate in health and activity monitoring. Crowd modelling and monitoring entails community-wide data analytics for the greater good. However, it entails collaboration between people who do not trust one another, emphasising the necessity for confidentiality protection and possibly minimal user engagement. Measuring the transmission of diseases over an area, looking for certain medical disorders, and so on are examples of population monitoring. Although the influence of scale on monitoring applications is being investigated, numerous research questions including intelligence sharing, data rights, data synthesis, protection and confidentiality, methods of data mining, delivering valuable opinion, and so on stay unanswered. This chapter discusses the major constraints and opportunities in the gathering, modelling, and processing of medical data in the framework of mortal health and behaviour monitoring. Section I contains an introduction to AI, Section II contains a review of medical information modelling using AI, Section III contains information on the impact of AI medical models on society, and Section IV contains information on the benefits and applications of AI in healthcare systems. Conclusion and references were the subject of Sections V and VI.

Figure 1. Architecture of smart health care monitoring system

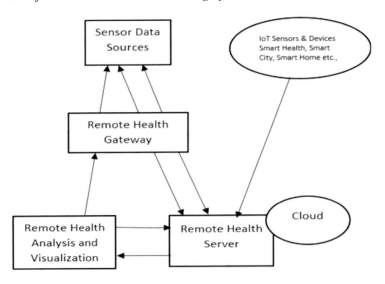

Figure 1. depicts the different stages of the overall architecture of the health care monitoring system. Four different stages are there in this monitoring system, which includes 1. sensor data collection and feature extraction. 2. Remote Health server 3. Remote Health Gateway 4. Remote Health Analysis and Visualization. In the first phase, data collection can be done by using various resources like physical,

virtual, and social sensors, smart phones, smart watches, and bracelets, etc, and user generated content on social media. Once the data collection process is done, then local processing and analytics must happen. This phase ends with some health mobile applications. The same sensed or collected data, events, and data from IoT sensors and devices are to be loaded into the server for further discovery. Personal request and response information can be shared between mobile applications and health servers via remote health gateway. In the second phase of this monitoring system, processing, analysis, and mining of streaming or stored sensing data takes place on a remote health server that is associated with the cloud environment. Storing, filtering, and aggregation operations can be done in a cluster or cloud. The third stage of this system is remote health analytics and visualization. Personal health services and notifications can be shared at this stage on the mobile applications. The Health Analytics or Visualization phase can send a query to a remote server, and the server can respond with analytics knowledge.

RELATED WORK ON MEDICAL INFORMATION MODELING USING AI

(Miltiadis et al., 2021; Muhammad et al., 2020) proposed in this section that digging prominent references within the reference network is a further rational technique of judging the effectiveness of science investigation, and that the overall number of citations obtained by an article is not a good indicator of quality. We add 980 tagged references to a current state-of-the-art database. Then we calculated 14 characteristics and used various machine learning models to analyze them. With the random forest classification method, we were able to acquire an operating characteristic of 50.95 and an area under the precision recall curve (AUCPR) of 0.85. (Li et al., 2021) proposed that the mining prominent references within the contexts (e.g. is a more rational technique of judging the effectiveness of science investigation, and that the overall number of references obtained by an article is not a reliable indicator of quality. We add 980 tagged references to a current state-of-the-art database. Then we calculated 14 characteristics and used various machine learning models to analyze them. With the random forest classification method, we were able to acquire an operating characteristic of 50.95 and an area under the precision recall curve (AUCPR) of 0.85. (Muhammad et al., 2021) This paper provides a detailed overview of heterogeneous clinical signal fusion strategies developed for intelligent healthcare applications.

(Sookhak et al., 2021) This study presents a comprehensive overview of province block-chain-based admission control approaches in the health sector, which serves as foundation for cataloguing current and upcoming advances in the accessibility control field. A particular horticulture of blockchain founded access management techniques is also offered towards emphasise the essential protection needs for designing a distributed access control scheme and to detect the security vulnerabilities with existing methods. This paper also intends to compare and contrast traditional control systems, as well as identify some significant and unresolved difficulties and obstacles as potential future possibilities. (Bhatia, 2021) The project focuses on using IoMT Technology to remotely monitor the health of household pets in their home surroundings. Over a cloud - centric platform FogBus, domestic healthiness is examined for susceptibility in the medium living situation and pervasive behaviors. A time series data granulation is also created, as well as the Probability of Health Vulnerability (PoHV) for evaluating the animal's physical condition seriousness. For real-time animal healthcare research, the Temporal Sensitivity Measure (TSM) is created, which is visualised applying the Self Organized Mapping (SOM) Technique.

(Wang et al., 2021) Without the use of an online reservation centre, the suggested protocol can achieve mutual authentication scheme agreement while also meeting security and privacy criteria. The suggested technique reduces user computational complexity overhead by moving partial calculation workloads to the server. Furthermore, the proposed method uses authentication scheme public key cryptography to address certificate management and key exchange issues. According to a performance analysis, the concept saves 9.9 percent of the computing operating cost just on source constrained station, making it ideal for reduced IoT applications in smart healthcare. (Muhammad et al., 2020) This paper examines several sample public datasets that have been used to evaluate the performance of WCE methodologies and procedures. Finally, the much more significant part of this study is the discovery of various research patterns and outstanding concerns in various WCE domains, with a focus on suggestions for future research for good healthcare and personalization.

(Chauhan et al., 2021) Seven criteria for a healthcare monitoring garbage disposal injected with resource efficiency characteristics to reclaim revenue from disposable ones are defined and evaluated in this study utilizing the decision making trial and evaluation laboratory technique. A fundamental model have being applied to select the criteria centered on their significance and net reason and impact associations. Major factors responsible for a smart health monitoring garbage disposal are (i) digitally associated healthcare facilities, trash discarding firms, and contamination prevention panel, and (ii) delivering a contamination prevention committee's opinion apps to the community as well as additional users. Finally, this research presents a fundamental link prototype between the interconnected handlers of industry 4.0 and life cycle assessment, which may be used to design a smart bio - medical waste disposal approach that integrates cyclical economy grows.

(Shahzad et al., 2021) Many current IoH Matters research and innovation have been conducted in a disjointed combined with autonomous manner, resulting in remedies and recommendations for a range of diseases, medical supplies, and remote support administration. (Jahan et al., 2021) Present a decentralized information capability method for a cooperative healthcare monitoring system that ensures the security and compatibility of clinical documentation through cooperative work. In the suggested approach, clinics exchange patient information in a reorganized ledger while using a differentially private method to ensure data privacy. The suggested system's feasibility is demonstrated by the results of the experiments analysis and data accuracy employing an AI model.

(Ray & Chaudhuri, 2021; Wang, 2020) The material evaluated was described in this review study in terms of methods, forms, behaviors, and procedures. The chosen publications' analysis and evaluation procedures are reviewed, and the essay concludes with a review of the conclusions. This article provides a scholarly evaluation of current predictive methods for healthcare solutions. The ambiguity between analytical techniques and machine learning has been resolved. Even when the identical dataset is used, the predictions of existing forecasting methods differ, according to a review of related literature. Predictive models are also necessary, and new methods must be developed. (Chen et al., 2021) proposed Holistic Big Data Integrated Artificial Intelligent Modeling (HBDIAIM) in this research as a way to enhance the safety and confidentiality of information management interfaces in different smart cities. A divergent evolutionary algorithm is implemented in HBDIAIM in order to provide suitable protection for the secret data admin console in smart city applications.

(Aazam et al., 2021) Targeted on the how a machine learning-based methodology can be leveraged to do is provide different forms of intelligent and impulsive healthcare (oHealth). For the medical and security situations they examined, they used k-nearest neighbours (kNN), support vector machine (SVM) and naïve Bayes (NB) classification techniques on actual data. The observed empirical results shed light on machine learning-based task outsourcing in edge computing. (Yang et al., 2021) For assessing SHMS portfolios in a commodity surroundings, they presented a hybrid explanatory research three-phased

Multi-criteria Decision-making (MCDM) model by combining the Decision-Making Trial and Evaluation Laboratory Model (DEMATEL) approach, this same Analytic Network Process (ANP), as well as Zero-One Goal Programming (ZOGP). The findings showed that the major driver for SHMS development is the Financial Subsidies Policy, and the Medical Device and Drug Management System (MDMS) and Medical Data Informational Network (MDIS) are the best SHMS portfolios for approach weights and restricted possessions. The proposed hybrid decision model can help SHMS portfolios be more reliable.

(Ketu & Mishra, 2021; Rathi et al., 2021) This article also looks into security difficulties, specific security, and threat taxonomies in relation to IoHT confidentiality structures from the standpoint of smart healthcare. This study proposed a low AI facilitated Internet of Things and edge calculating based medical answer that is flexible, reactive, and dependable when treating patients. The system includes data collecting, computation, and analytics at edge nodes, as well as persistent storing and retrieving at edge data centres. Patients are scheduled and supplies are provided in real time by the edge nodes and border controller. (Lu & Sinnott, 2020) Security mechanisms is been designed to safeguard e-health clients and health datasets; yet, smart healthcare systems need structured standards and execution. When it comes to security and privacy, smart medical systems have special requirements. (Taiwo & Ezugwu, 2020) Patients can be remotely controlled from their houses using the suggested solution, and they can also live a more pleasant life by using some functions of smart home control equipment on their handsets. Patients in self-quarantine can utilise the digital stage to report everyday physical health problems and difficulties to clinicians using their cell devices, which is the most meaningful impacts.

(Nasr et al., 2021) Furthermore, this article highlights software integration designs that are critical for developing smart healthcare systems by effortlessly combining the benefits of tools in AI and data analytics. The created structures mentioned emphasis on top of numerous aspects: each established framework's contributions, the entire working technique, performance as outputs, and comparative strengths and limits. (Mishra et al., 2021) Concrete action in designated research, technologies, and managerial segments, notably population health, patients' health, knowledge assortment, and governmental support, has considerable capacity to strengthen the worldwide retort to COVID-19. Implementing such approaches would result in more accurate diagnosis and control mechanisms, as well as a healthier society. (Sarosh et al., 2021) Clinical photographs about patients could be used to identify specific medical disorders via data analysis. Many interconnected innovations are being deployed to modify healthcare systems in COVID-19 outbreak. The confidentiality of health check data is involved in the management of an organized health solution. Hyperchaotic formula, and Deoxyribonucleic Acid (DNA) encoding, established on the linear system, we offer security architecture.

IMPACT OF ARTIFICIAL INTELLIGENCE AND MEDICAL INFORMATION MODELLING ON SOCIETY

All things considered, it is widely assumed that AI tools would complement and improve human work rather than supplanting the work done by doctors and other medical service providers. Computer-based intelligence is ready to assist medical services faculty with a variety of tasks, including regulatory work procedures, clinical documentation, and patient effort, as well as more specialised jobs like image analysis, clinical device robotization, and patient monitoring.

Despite a few roadblocks, Artificial Intelligence (AI) is being used in the medical care framework. Specialists essentially center around the area of significant three illnesses: cardiovascular sickness, sensory system infection, and perilous malignant growth too. In cardiology, the future applications of the AI framework for detecting heart diseases with the help of cardiovascular images were discussed. Heart stroke is a characteristic and regularly blending infection that affects more than 500 million individuals from one side of the planet to the other. It is the most driving reason for death in world. It has additionally high clinical costs across the world almost about US$ 689 billion, which brings genuine hardship to patient families. As a result, research on expectations and clinical therapy for stroke has a huge impact.

Artificial Intelligence (AI) approaches are now being applied in a growing number of stroke-related studies. In stroke-related situations, AI systems can help in three areas: before the best time for infection estimation and examination, recovery, and despite end assumption and discovering evaluation. Approximately 85 percent of the time, stroke is caused by cerebral localised necrosis, or blockages in the vessel. Only a few people may be able to recognise pre-stroke signs and get the help they need. The development of a development detecting gadget made it feasible to predict early strokes. PCA and hereditary fuzzy limited state machine are the most commonly used AI methods for model design. The astonishing technique has to do with a patient's sense of human activity and the beginning of the stroke detection phase.

In an ideal world, the ordinary model would be incredibly distinctive in relation to the patient's development, and a sensible model that identifies blow would be able to animate and assess clinical action and put it into practise right away. In response, a wearable device was proposed for social occasion information for typical and neurotic strides for stroke computation. SVM and hidden Markov models can exclude and reproduce the data, and this calculation can correctly put together 91% of the records to the specified gathering. Neuro-imaging methods such as CT sweep and MRI are also essential for infection assessment in some cases of stroke identification. For human-capable actual injury elucidation, this effect is comparable. In a multisculpt mind MRI, a 3D CNN focused on an injured fracture.

Complete mental images were used as information in SVM, which worked as a more solid foundation than traditional radiology-based technique. A stroke therapy model was proposed for studying perform core value, clinical preliminaries, and meta-investigation with Bayesian rule organisation to further improve the clinical outcome making strategy of thrombolysis (tPA) mending. The model included 56 different types of components and three options for examining, fixing, and successfully estimating the cycle. The subgroup used a connection tree to determine an appropriate thrombolysis (tPA) dose based on the patient's individual characteristics, considering the patient's recovery viability and the risk of dying. There are a few factors that can influence stroke detection and disorder mortality. When compared to traditional methods, AI techniques yield better results in terms of progressing estimation activity. To improve and maintain clinical evaluation methodology, a model was presented for predicting a three-month healing outcome by looking at physiological considerations for the first 48 hours after a stroke with computed degeneration.

Through intensive front stroke and back stroke intra-blood vessel treatment, a data set of 107 patient's clinical data was seen. SVM and artificial neural organisation were used to inspect the data, which resulted in an estimation accuracy of above 70%. The control impact in mind arterio-venous anomaly happy with endo-vascular embolization was determined using AI systems. While a typical degeneration examination portrayal could only achieve a 43 percent accuracy rate, this method's effort is greatly improved, with a precision of 97.5 percent. To compute a 30-day mortality test, an optimal calculation was used, which yielded more exact results than traditional approaches.

Similarly, SVM was utilized to work out the stroke mortality by means of release. Also, the use of the manufactured option oversampling system was proposed to diminish the stroke impact computation bias contemplated among class disparity between a few datasets. Mind pictures were analyzed for working out the impact of stroke fix. CT filter information were analyzed through AI method for assessing the cerebral edema through hemispheric infraction. In comparison to traditional procedures, arbitrary backwoods was designed to automatically sense the cerebrospinal fluids (CSF) and check the progressions in the CT output, which is more precise and capable.

Wounds blackmailed from appealing reverberation imaging and the fix impact through Gaussian strategy relapse process were investigated as part of a relationship. The model was used to figure out the problem of cognitive damage during a stroke and the best way to recover at the right moment. In the Arteries Cardio DL procedure, artificial intelligence (AI) is used to make changed and inconsistent ventricle divisions visible on traditional MRI heart imagesA man-made reasoning (AI) strategy was produced for fixing the guideline of body development in quadriplegia patients with sensory system infection. Farina et al. came across the control of the disconnected man–machine edge, which uses delivery timings for the spinal engine neurons to regulate the upper appendage prosthesis. By a twofold dazed approval study, IBM Watson for cancer conclusion can be a steady AI for disease determination from start to finish.

Skin disease subgroups were identified by examining a clinical image. The applications of these three types of disorders are not entirely unexpected. These three infections are known to cause death in the head; as a result, identifying the stages of the illness early on is critical in preventing the patient's condition from worsening. Furthermore, the investigation gauges on electrophysiology (EP) or electronic clinical record, imaging, and hereditary can all be tentatively reached, and this is the significant force of the man-made reasoning method. Aside from the three major diseases, an Artificial Intelligence (AI) framework has been used to examine visual picture data for diagnosing acquired waterfall infections in another disease. The retinal fundus pictures identified a referable diabetic retinopathy.

MAN-MADE BRAINPOWER APPLICATIONS IN MEDICAL CARE

Artificial Intelligence in present day medication and average region has been a generally forthcoming intriguing issue in current years. Although the use of artificial intelligence in modern medicine has a lot of promise, there are concerns about losing the "human touch" in such a crucial and individual-driven job. Man-made reasoning in current medication signifies to the act of man-made brainpower instruments and customized systems in the recognizable proof and fix of patients who need care. Simultaneously as investigation and fix might seem like unobtrusive stages, there are various other fortuitous methods that happen sought after for a patient assign appropriately taken to consideration, for example,

- Collecting data from patient talks and performing checks
- Using a few reasons for data information to develop a precise identifiable proof
- Using a few reasons for data information to determine a precise recognisable proof
- Characterizing a material fix method
- Organizing and controlling the chose fix method
- Patient noticing
- Recovery, continuation courses of action

Figure 2. Source: 2019 AI global funding report, CB Insights

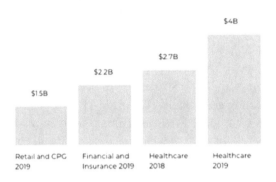

Various decisions have been made regarding the most beneficial usage of AI in medical treatment. The key areas, according to Forbes in 2018, will be managerial job processes, image examination, automated a medical procedure, menial assistance, and clinical decision support. Similar locations were mentioned in a 2018 Accenture report, which included addressed linked machines, dose blunder reduction, and network safety. According to a 2019 McKinsey report, major areas associated with intellectual widgets, focused on and tailored medication, improved mechanics assisted a medical treatment, and electroceuticals are among the most important.

Artificial Intelligence(AI) in medical services offered an assortment of medical care data results that man-made brainpower (AI) has analyzed and audited the main sorts of illnesses that man-made consciousness (AI) has organized. AI (ML) and regular language handling are two significant gatherings of man-made consciousness (AI) gadgets. Two of the most well-known traditional techniques for AI (ML) are available: neural organisation and SVM. An average artificial intelligence (AI) framework should include an AI (ML) component for leading ordered data such as EP information, images, and hereditary data, as well as a Natural Language Processing (NLP) module for allowing unstructured works. The confusing calculation needs to be taught during the medical services results prior to the framework that can support the doctors for illness investigation and treatment strategies. This technique focuses on how PC-based evaluation tactics, which are housed under the same roof as Artificial Intelligence (AI), might aid in the advancement of the health and therapeutic fields.

EXISTING INSTANCES OF AI IN REAL LIFE

There are now numerous instances of AI showing up inside daily existence applications. A genuine illustration of this is the Nest gadgets for home robotization, utilizing AI to decide individual inclinations and changes for our ordinary necessities.

Google Assistant on your cell phone is another model, providing clients with supportive "without a moment to spare" data dependent on what it finds out with regards to your inclinations and past client conduct.

Self-driving vehicles – popularised by Tesla – are one more illustration of AI in real life.

These models utilize various parts of AI to empower innovation to be coordinated in various applications. It is critical to comprehend the distinction between these terms and how they apply to various applications.

CONCLUSION

Artificial Intelligence is one of the greatest disruptors of our age and can possibly be a tremendous resource for clinical gadget organizations in later years. Like with most problematic advances, there are numerous potential entanglements that could forestall the fruitful execution of AI inside the business. The quantity of advantages for computerized reasoning in medical care is immense; regardless of whether that be decreasing the dependence of human information, accelerating the medication improvement interaction, or making medical services less expensive and available to a scope of various populaces. For computerized reasoning to be an achievement in any industry, savvy calculations need unfiltered admittance to a scope of informational indexes. This is quite difficult for the medical services and clinical gadget industry, as guidelines, for example, HIPAA make it trying to share information while staying consistent with laws and guidelines. Regardless of such difficulties, AI keeps on advancing as medical organizations center around extending their computerized capacities. As clinicians, medical services experts and patients begin to become mindful of the advantages related with AI, advancement in the field will keep, making man-made consciousness in medical care less expensive and more open to patients around the world.

REFERENCES

Aazam, M., Zeadally, S., & Flushing, E. F. (2021). Task offloading in edge computing for machine learning-based smart healthcare. *Computer Networks*, *191*, 108019. doi:10.1016/j.comnet.2021.108019

Bhatia. (2021). Fog Computing-inspired Smart Home Framework for Predictive Veterinary Healthcare. *Microprocessors and Microsystems*, *78*, 10322.

Chauhan, A., Jakhar, S. K., & Chauhan, C. (2021). The interplay of circular economy with industry 4.0 enabled smart city drivers of healthcare waste disposal. *Journal of Cleaner Production*, *279*, 123854. doi:10.1016/j.jclepro.2020.123854 PMID:32863607

Chen, J., Ramanathan, L., & Alazab, M. (2021). Holistic big data integrated artificial intelligent modeling to improve privacy and security in data management of smart cities. *Microprocessors and Microsystems*, *81*, 103722. doi:10.1016/j.micpro.2020.103722

Jahan, N., Rashid, I. B., & Al Numan, O. (2021). Collaborative AI in Smart Healthcare System. *International IEEE Conference on Automation, Control and Mechatronics for Industry 4.0 (ACMI)*.

Ketu, S., & Mishra, P. K. (2021). Internet of Healthcare Things: A contemporary survey. *Journal of Network and Computer Applications*, *192*, 103179. doi:10.1016/j.jnca.2021.103179

Li, J., Dai, J., Issakhov, A., Almojil, S. F., & Souri, A. (2021). Towards decision support systems for energy management in the smart industry and Internet of Things. *Computers & Industrial Engineering*, *161*, 107671. doi:10.1016/j.cie.2021.107671

Lu, & Sinnott. (2020). *Security and privacy solutions for smart healthcare systems.* Innovation in Health Informatics A Smart Healthcare Primer Next Gen Tech Driven Personalized Med&Smart Healthcare.

Miltiadis, Visvizi, Sarirete, & Chui. (2021). Preface: Artificial intelligence and big data analytics for smart healthcare: A digital transformation of healthcare primer. *Artificial Intelligence and Big Data Analytics for Smart Healthcare.*

Mishra, A., Basumallick, S., Lu, A., Chiu, H., Shah, M. A., Shukla, Y., & Tiwari, A. (2021). The healthier healthcare management models for COVID-19. *Journal of Infection and Public Health, 14*(7), 927–937. doi:10.1016/j.jiph.2021.05.014 PMID:34119847

Muhammad, G., Alshehri, F., Karray, F., Saddik, A. E., Alsulaiman, M., & Falk, T. H. (2021). A comprehensive survey on multimodal medical signals fusion for smart healthcare systems. *Information Fusion, 76,* 355–375. doi:10.1016/j.inffus.2021.06.007

Muhammad, K., Khan, S., Kumar, N., Del Ser, J., & Mirjalili, S. (2020). Vision-based personalized Wireless Capsule Endoscopy for smart healthcare: Taxonomy, literature review, opportunities and challenges. *Future Generation Computer Systems, 113,* 266–280. doi:10.1016/j.future.2020.06.048

Nasr, Islam, Shehata, Karray, & Quintana. (2021). Smart Healthcare in the Age of AI: Recent Advances, Challenges, and Future Prospects. In *Computers and Society.* Cornell University.

Rathi, Rajput, Mishra, Grover, Tiwari, Jaiswal, & Hossain. (2021). An edge AI-enabled IoT healthcare monitoring system for smart cities. *Computers & Electrical Engineering, 96*(B).

Ray, A., & Chaudhuri, A. K. (2021). Smart healthcare disease diagnosis and patient management: Innovation, improvement and skill development. *Machine Learning with Applications, 3,* 100011. doi:10.1016/j.mlwa.2020.100011

Sarosh, P., Parah, S. A., Bhat, G. M., & Muhammad, K. (2021). A Security Management Framework for Big Data in Smart Healthcare. *Big Data Research, 25,* 100225. doi:10.1016/j.bdr.2021.100225

Shahzad, S. K., Ahmed, D., Naqvi, M. R., Mushtaq, M. T., Iqbal, M. W., & Munir, F. (2021). Ontology Driven Smart Health Service Integration. *Computer Methods and Programs in Biomedicine, 207,* 106146. doi:10.1016/j.cmpb.2021.106146 PMID:34020375

Sookhak, M., Jabbarpour, M. R., Safa, N. S., & Yu, F. R. (2021). Blockchain and smart contract for access control in healthcare: A survey, issues and challenges, and open issues. *Journal of Network and Computer Applications, 178,* 102950. doi:10.1016/j.jnca.2020.102950

Taiwo, O., & Ezugwu, A. E. (2020). Smart healthcare support for remote patient monitoring during covid-19 quarantine. *Informatics in Medicine Unlocked, 20,* 100428. doi:10.1016/j.imu.2020.100428 PMID:32953970

Wang. (2020). GuardHealth: Blockchain empowered secure data management and Graph Convolutional Network enabled anomaly detection in smart healthcare. *Journal of Parallel and Distributed Computing, 142*(August), 1–12.

Wang, W., Huang, H., Xiao, F., Li, Q., Xue, L., & Jiang, J. (2021). Computation-transferable authenticated key agreement protocol for smart healthcare. *Journal of Systems Architecture*, *118*, 102215. doi:10.1016/j.sysarc.2021.102215

Yang, Hsu, & Wu. (2021). A hybrid multiple-criteria decision portfolio with the resource constraints model of a smart healthcare management system for public medical centers. *Socio-Economic Planning Sciences*, 101073.

Chapter 2
Utility of Binary Cuckoo Search Approach for Microarray Data Analysis:
A Dimensionality Reduction Approach

Rasmita Dash

Department of Computer Science and Engineering, Institute of Technical Education and Research (ITER), Siksha 'O' Anusandhan (Deemed), Bhubaneswar, India

Rajashree Dash

Department of Computer Science and Engineering, Institute of Technical Education and Research (ITER), Siksha 'O' Anusandhan (Deemed), Bhubaneswar, India

Rasmita Rautray

Department of Computer Science and Engineering, Institute of Technical Education and Research (ITER), Siksha 'O' Anusandhan (Deemed), Bhubaneswar, India

ABSTRACT

In the recent literature, many metaheuristic approaches has been developed to examine, interpret, and analyze high dimensional data. However, there is always a requirement to design a more productive and cost-effective technique. Many of the authors have acknowledged the capability of cuckoo search approach. Inspired from the blooming application of cuckoo search algorithm (CSA), the authors have proposed a binary cuckoo search algorithm (BCSA) for gene selection and classification of microarray data. With the objective of optimizing gene subset and classification result, BCSA has been implemented. BCSA is optimized using support vector machine (SVM) classifier, and significant gene set is extracted. This experimental study has been conducted over five microarray datasets. Superiority of this gene subset is shown using a few other classifiers such as k-nearest neighbor and artificial neural network. The model performance is also compared with a few other metaheuristic approaches such as particle swarm optimization, genetic algorithm, artificial bee colony algorithm, and differential evolution.

DOI: 10.4018/978-1-6684-4580-8.ch002

INTRODUCTION

There are many applications where high-dimensional data is very common. Geographical data (Chung et al., 2018; Frew et al., 2017), data in computer vision(Feng, Leung, & Eckersley, 2020; Kamoona, & Patra, 2019; Sreenivasan, Havlicek, & Deshpande, 2014),gene expression data(Dash, 2018; Dash, 2017; Dash, Dash, & Rautray, 2019), data set in eCommerce application(Robinson, 2017; Hartley, 2009; Chakkaravarthy, Sangeetha, & Vaidehi, 2019),tomography imaging data(Moodley et al., 2013; Imbriaco, 2011; Lin et al., 2004), ECG(Jayashree, & Kumar, 2019; Berkaya et al., 2018; Chawla, 2011) data etc are all falls into these categories. However, researchers are facing a lot of problems for mining these data. This is due to the fact that i) its curse of dimensionality ii) difficulty in extracting information from the huge space (Sert et al., 2019; Aneiros et al., 2019; Zhou, Zhai, & Pantelous, 2020).

Microarray gene expression data is an imbalanced data i.e. number of observation is within the range of hundreds whereasthe number of genes are hundreds to tens of thousands. Numbers of samples are so less that building a model becomes difficult to learn the characteristics of these data(Dash, & Misra, 2016; Dash, & Misra, 2018). Further numbers of attributes are too high that distinguishing significant and insignificant attributes becomes critical and cost effective.

Many existing algorithms are there for these data analysis. However with the dimension, complexity of these algorithms grows exponentially.With increasing dimensionality, these algorithms soon become computationally intractable and therefore inapplicable in many real applications.

In the past few years many metaheuristic approaches have been developed as a solution to many exponentially increasing complex non-linear optimization problems. These algorithms have many source of inspiration(Hussain et al., 2019; Bianchi et al., 2009; Dokeroglu et al., 2019). Many of them are inspired from behavior of swarm such as Particle Swarm Optimization, Ant Colony System, Artificial Bee Colony, Firefly Algorithm, Cat Swarm Optimization Algorithm etc(Mavrovouniotis, Li, & Yang, 2017; AlRashidi, & El-Hawary, 2008). Some of them are based on nature of evolution such as Genetic algorithm, Differential evolution, Evolutionary Programming etc(Slowik, & Kwasnicka, 2018; Jain, Singh, & Rani, 2018). Considering every technical problem as an optimization problem, Quantum computing (based on quantum mechanics) based Genetic algorithm was proposed as the first physics based algorithm. There after many other algorithms were proposed such as Gravitational search, Simulating Annealing, Harmony search etc. Other categories of algorithms are Bio-inspired approaches inspired from biological sources(Chiroma et al., 2017; Pazhaniraja et al., 2017). All these metaheuristic approaches don't have relationship with the problem need to be optimized. Due to which successfully many metaheuristic approaches are developed to solve a variety of optimization problem.

Inspired from successful application of metaheuristic approaches in many application zones, this research work is directed towards Cuckoo search. Cuckoo Search (CS) is one of the successful metaheuristic approach developed by Yang and Deb (Dash, & Misra, 2016). It is a swarm based optimization technique inspired from the behavior of bird cuckoo. Cuckoo search, its variants and much hybridization are heavily used in current research areas for different categories of optimization process (Shehab, Khader, & Al-Betar, 2017; Mareli, & Twala, 2018; Rautray et al., 2019; Cruz-Duarte et al., 2017; Sarangi et al., 2018; Bibiks et al., 2018). Influenced from its vast application, in this research a binary version of Cuckoo search for feature selection is used for the first time.

To handle the dimensional complexities of gene expression data, this research works in two phases. Assuming that in one phase complete insignificant features can't be eliminated, in the 1st phase top ranked 500 features contributing to the class level are extracted. In the second stage a binary version of cuckoo search algorithm is implemented to extract the most significant features. The algorithm is experimented through multiple simulations, multiple runs and multiple iterations with the hope of getting optimal result.

For this research work, content of each section and subsection discussion is as follows.Section1 discusses high dimensional data, issues in handling theses data, probable solution using metaheuristic algorithms, motivation towards Cuckoo search and a brief description of considered problem statement and proposed solution. Motivation of using Cuckoo search is further cleared with its vast application in unbounded research application through much hybridization in section 2.Basic cuckoo search approach and it working principle is presented through a flow diagram in section 3. The proposed work and its working principle are presented in presented in section 4. The overall experimental setup is shown through section and subsection of 5. In section 6 result analysis is done through a comparative study and followed with a concluding remark in section 7. Following table 1 provides details about description of Cuckoo search with few variants and its application areas

Table 1. Description of Cuckoo search with a few variants and its application areas

Sl.no.	Traditional / Variants of CS	Application area	Reference
1	Multi-objective Cuckoo Search	Electrical machines and transformers	Coelho et al., 2013
2	Improved Binary Cuckoo Search	Electric power generation system	Zhao et al., 2018
3	Extended Cuckoo Search	Motion tracking	Zhang et al, 2018
4	Traditional	Magnetic flux leakage signal	Han et al., 2016
5	hybrid Cuckoo Search	Internet of Things	Jiang et al., 2016
6	efficient Cuckoo Search	Fault diagnosis	Li, Ma, & Yang, 2017
7	Improved Cuckoo Search Algorithm	Monopulse Antennas	Suresh et al., 2017
8	adaptive Cuckoo Search algorithm	Satellite images	Wei, & Yu, 2018
9	hybrid Cuckoo Search	Chaotic system	Sun et al., 2017
10	Hierarchical Cuckoo Search	Wireless communication systems	Osman, & Baki, 2018
11	Traditional	Auto industry	Chitara et al., 2018
12	Traditional	multimachine power systems	Suresh et al., 2018
13	Adaptive Cuckoo Search	Wiener Filter	Zhao et al., 2018
14	Modified cuckoo search	Power dispatch	Sun et al., 2018
15	hybrid cuckoo search	Concentric circular antenna array	Yang, & Deb, 2014

PREVIOUS KNOWLEDGE

As compare to other metaheuristic approaches, Cuckoo search technique has already shown its position. Up to now there are many applications of Cuckoo search using traditional Cuckoo search as well as with its many variants. Few of its applications are highlighted in Table.1. A detailed description of each approach is as follows.

In this paper (Coelho et al., 2013), for correct hysteretic material simulation, and improved multiobjective cuckoo search-based approach is implemented. In this process a lot many parametersneed to be considered, hence multiobjective optimization is a suitable solution strategy. So in this work Duffing's oscillator based improved multi-objective cuckoo search is applied to optimize the parameters of Jiles-Atherton vector hysteresis model. In an electric power system unit commitment problems are nonlinear mixed-integer optimization problem. Here total cost generation required to be minimized in the optimization problem. For this work, (Zhao et al., 2018), the author has proposed a binary version cuckoo search approach called improved cuckoo search algorithm. In this work (Zhang et al, 2018) author has proposed an extended cuckoo search based Kernelised correlation filter(KCF) tracker. In the first phase cuckoo search has been extended using simplex method. There after based on the ECS method with Gaussian distribution, a hybrid motion model is introduced for KCF framework. Prediction of defect dimension is an inverse problem in magnetic flux leakage signal in which after getting the effects its cause is detected. Paper (Han et al., 2016), estimates the defects combining the optimization approach of cuckoo search and particle filter. Inspired from the significant implementation of cuckoo search approach for high dimensional problems

In this paper (Jiang et al., 2016) author has employed Support vector machine(SVM) for dynamic error prediction of sensor. However for proper estimation, parameter value of SVM needs to be chosen carefully. In this regard cuckoo search algorithm is used for parameter optimization of SVM. For radar tracking monopulse antennas play an important role. In paper (Li, Ma, & Yang, 2017) improved cuckoo search is used to perform monopulse antennas. The improvisation of cuckoo search is done to balance the exploration and exploitation level of this algorithm.

In the recent scenario, there are many practical applications of satellite images, however proper enhanced methods are required to improve the contrast of scene. In this regard optimization methods are used. In this paper (Suresh et al., 2017) a novel adaptive cuckoo search approach is used for satellite image enhancement. Here a self adaptive Levy flight operation is implemented to make the algorithm adaptive.

Parameter estimation is a nonlinear problem as it leads to estimation of more than one parameter and it is solved using multiobjective optimization techniques. In this work (Wei, & Yu, 2018), a hybrid cuckoo search approach is implemented to estimate the parameters of chaotic systems. The hybridization work is inspired from differential evolution, based on which mutation operation is implemented. Further opposition based learning is used to initialize population in each generation. Generation of high dimensional space is a complex nonlinear problem and it is difficult to solve. One such problem is Beampattern sidelobe (SL) suppressing especially for large-scale antenna array. In (Sun et al., 2017), author has applied hierarchical cuckoo search approach for sidelobe reduction. In this approach the population is utilized in hierarchical levels. An automated transfer line balancing problem is solved by (Osman, & Baki, 2018) using cuckoo search approach. The transfer line produces cylinder heads at a high volume incorporates identical machines that can be operated under different cutting conditions. Selection of relevant cutting conditions affects the productivity and cost of transfer lines. Considering this work as an optimization problem cuckoo search is implemented.

In 2018 Chitara et.al., explored Cuckoo search algorithm for power system stabilizer designing for multimachine power systems. Performance of cuckoo search is compared with few other state-of-art metaheuristic approaches such as genetic algorithm, particle swarm optimization and harmony search algorithm. Finally cuckoo search based optimizer has shown its superiority as compared to other designed approaches. In satellite image, noise reduction is required to improve the visualization capability of an image. A 2D finite-impulse response Wiener filter driven by the adaptive cuckoo search algorithm is proposed for noise reduction in Multispectral satellite images. These images are contaminated with the Gaussian noise ofdifferentvariance levels (Suresh et al., 2017) and issues were well handled using adaptive cuckoo search approach. A non-convex, non-continuous or nonlinear solution space called aseconomic dispatch problems is solved using cuckoo search approach (Zhao et al., 2018). However, the searching capability of cuckoo search is improved incorporating a self adaptive approach. In this work the new solution space is generated through an improved lambda iteration strategy. In a paper (Sun et al., 2017), an improved discrete cuckoo search algorithm is adopted to suppress the maximum sidelobe level of large-scale concentric circular antenna array.

Inspired by the vast adoption of cuckoo search swarm optimization technique through its baseline approach, improvisation form andmany hybridization forms, author has tried to introducebinary version of cuckoo search technique for feature selection in high dimensional datasets. As cuckoo search is quite successful in high dimensional search space analysis, this study designed a gene selection technique in microarray datasets though a variant of cuckoo search.

BASICS OF CUCKOO SEARCH (CS)

Algorithm Cuckoo Search
Random initialization of n host nests
While (! Termination Condition) **do**
Random generation of a cuckoo
Fitness evaluation of cuckoo, F.
Random selection of a nest among n nests, j
If $F_i > F_j$
Replace the new solution with j
Abandon a fraction (Pa) of worse nest & build new ones.
Keep & rank the best current nests
Return the best nest

Cuckoo search (CS) is one of latest and widely used swarm intelligence based meta-heuristic algorithm. CS algorithm is inspired by the kind of bird species called the cuckoo. Cuckoos are fascinating birds because of their aggressive reproduction strategy and beautiful sounds which they can make (Yang, & Deb, 2014). The adult cuckoos lay their eggs in the nests of other host birds or species (Rautray, & Balabantaray, 2018). The egg in the nest represents a solution, and one egg can be laid by each cuckoo that represents new and possibly better solution. The standard CS algorithm can be characterized by three idealized rules: i) laying one egg by each cuckoo in a random nest represents a solution sets, ii) the nests containing the best eggs will take over to the next generation, iii) an alien egg can be discovered by a host bird with a probability (P_a) for the fixed number of available nests. If this condition satisfies, either the egg can be discarded or abandon the nest by the host, and built a new nest elsewhere.

For easy implementation, CS algorithm can be used each nest with a single egg. In such situation there is no difference between nest, egg or cuckoo. The nest corresponds to an egg represents one cuckoo. In some complicated cases, the algorithm can be extended to each nest with multiple eggs that represents a set of solutions.

In this algorithm each egg in the nest represents a candidate solution. Thus the cuckoo egg may represent a global best solution. Let for current iteration t, the ith cuckoo is represented as x_i^t. For the next new generation the same cuckoo x_i^{t+1} is updated using equation-1.

$$x_i^{t+1} = x_i^t + \alpha \otimes L\acute{e}vy(\lambda)$$ (1)

Where α is step size, which should be proportional to scale of optimization problem (i.e. $\alpha > 0$), $\otimes$ is entry wise move during multiplication and Lévy(λ) is random numbers drawn fromLévy distribution. A flow diagram for the working principle of cuckoo search algorithm is shown in Fig.1.

Figure 1. Flow diagram of Cuckoo search technique

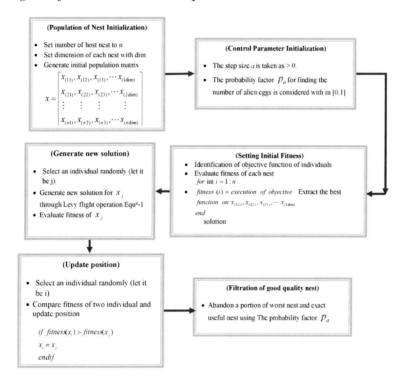

SIGNIFICANT GENE EXTRACTION APPROACH: PROPOSED WORK

In section 2 of this research work, we have highlighted the potentiality of Cuckoo search through its implementation in various application areas. Taking this inspiration, a binary version of Cuckoo search is designed to extract the relevant information from the dataset in terms of its significant features. In detail steps of the feature selection process are shown in Fig.2. This is an investigation carried over high dimensional gene expression datasets. These data are highly noisy, as it contains relevant information along with some irrelevant content.

On the other hand, Cuckoo search is a wrapper technique. Trying to learn these techniques with such data most of the time misleads from its objective. Thus, somewhat data refinement is required prior to work with the wrapper techniques. So, an initial refinement process is essential to be implemented.

This approach works in two phases. Basically, all these gene expression data are defined with high dimensional space which is quite stressful for analyses. These data contain a large list of gene values and most of them are noisy. Thus, identifying the noise-free genes from such a pool of genes is very difficult.

Figure 2. Significant gene set extraction using BCSA approach

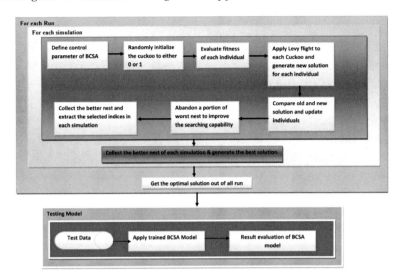

Thus, to make this analysis an effective one, in this work metaheuristic based cuckoo search approach is designed. Cuckoo search is a learning technique, when the original data is applied, it misleads the model from its objective. Therefore, we have tried to come up with a solution, in which feature selection is applied in two steps assuming that in one step complete noise reduction may not be possible. Thus, our approach works in the following way.

In the initial stage of preprocessing procedure, for proper analysis of data, the gene values are brought to a range of [0, 1]. Then first level of feature extraction is done by reducing noise. In this level the proportion of noisy and noise free genes are evaluated using signal-to-noise ratio. The output is sorted in descending order and high valued genes are taken out. In this work top 500 genes are extracted.

After the first stage of reduction, the dataset is scale down. Further this dataset with 500 genes are again too high to learn a model as it may distract from its destiny. Therefore in the second stage noise is further minimized using cuckoo search based metaheuristic approach. Designing a binary version of cuckoo search algorithm, the author has suggested a wrapper based noise reduction technique. Significant features are extracted optimizing the classifier performance. Thus, an efficient classifier is also plays a major role to reduce the data complexity though noise reduction. From many literatures (Dash, & Misra, 2016) it has been clearly observed that support vector machine is one of the efficient classifiers for analyzing a dataset. Therefore,binary cuckoo search and SVM based a feature selection and classification model is designed to extract the significant features though optimizing the classification performance.

As the performance of a model depends on both metaheuristic technique as well as classifier combination, for the comparative analysis different metaheuristic technique and classifier combinations are handled. All these analyses are carried out at different level using 4 performance measures such as accuracy, sensitivity, precision and gmean.

Steps of Proposed Cuckoo Search-Based Feature Selection Algorithm

Step 1: Collect gene expression data values.
Step 2: Conduct data pre-processing using the min-max data normalization technique.

Step 3: Apply initial screening process to select top 500 genes.

Step 4: Apply parameter initialization of Cuckoo search approach such as number of host nest (NHN), step constant α_{SC}, standard normal variable u and v, the control factor of Levy flight operation β_{cp} and probability of getting exotic eggs pc

Step 5: For each nest $ns_i \in 1,2,3, L \ NHN>$ and,

For each dimension $d_j \in <1,2,3, L \ dim>$,
    Initialize the variable randomly with 0 or 1.

Step 6: Iterate the steps from 7 to 12 t times, $t \in <1.2.3L, T$, where T is maximum number of iteration

Step 7: Initialize fitness value *Fit* and global fitness Fit_{global} to 0

Step 8: For each nest $ns_i \in 1,2,3, L \ NHN>$, figure out the fitness of each nest considering classification accuracy as evaluation criteria and store it in $Fit_{current}$.

Step 9: If ($Fit_{current} > Fit$) then update then update *Fit* i.e. $Fit = Fit_{current}$, and update the index of nest i.e. $ns_i = ns_i^t$

Step 10: Estimate the maximum fitness value and store it in Fit_{max}.

Step 11: If ($Fit_{max} > Fit_{global}$) then update Fit_{global} by $Fit_{global} = Fit_{max}$, and update index wrt Fit_{global} and store it in $index_{global}$

Step 12: Discard the worst nest wrt p_c and construct the solution space by applying Levy for the next generation.

Step 13: Generate the optimal solution with the selected features depending on index values.

ENVIRONMENTAL SET UP FOR THE EXPERIMENTAL VALIDATION

In the following subsections, a detail experimental analysis is presented to prove efficacy of proposed model. The experimental set up is done in the following way.

Data Set Description

In this work 5 microarray gene expression data are examined. The detail description of each dataset is presented in Table.2.

The principal characteristic of gene expression dataset is high dimensional in nature. These are imbalanced dataset in the sense that number of observations is too small as compare to number of attributes. Mostly the samples are within 200 and genes are in the range of thousands and sometimes it goes beyond ten thousands. Thus knowledge extraction becomes complex. To handle these data, metaheuristic approaches are used to learn a model.

Data Preprocessing with Initial Feature Selection Process

In this approach, two level of feature extraction is implemented. As most of the features are noisy, extraction in one level may not lead to an optimal solution. Further, learning a model taking both relevant and irrelevant information may deviate the result from the expected result.

Table 2. Class division and number of features in microarray datasets

Sl.No	Dataset	Number of observations		Number of features
1	Leukemia (David, 2002)	38		7129
		27	11	
2	AllAml (Golub et al., 1999)	44		7129
		29	15	
3	ADCALung (Gordon, 2002)	149		12533
		15	134	
4	CNS (Singh, 2002)	60		7129
		39	21	
5	Prostate (Ash, 2000)	102		12600
		52	50	

In the raw data, the feature values are scaled to a small value to very large. This range also varies depending on the dataset. Interpretation of such data becomes difficult for a training algorithm. For example if distance function is used in training process, then highly distant feature may dominate other. Similarly if the feature values are quite uniform, then the algorithm may converge fast. Therefore it is required to bring the feature value to a specified range and this process is called as data normalization. Thus in the preprocessing stage implementing min-max normalization technique as in equation-1 data value is brought to a range of [0-1] using equation-2.

$$Feature_{normalised\,value} = \frac{Feature_{original\,value} - Feature_{min(original\,value\,in\,the\,series)}}{Feature_{max(original\,value\,in\,the\,series)} - Feature_{min(original\,value\,in\,the\,series)}} \quad (2)$$

Further in the preprocessing stage two level of feature extraction is carried out. In the 1st level of feature extraction, noisy features are dropped out. In this stage, contribution of each feature towards level of knowledge is evaluated. In this regard for each feature, level of signal with respect to level of noise is calculated. The highly contributing features are those features whose are in the higher order of estimation those are extracted. However in this level it is difficult to predict how many feature may finally considered for obtaining the desire objective. Thus the number of feature in the initial stage is restricted to 500.

Implementation of Proposed BCSA

Now the original dataset is reduced to 90% and in the reduced dataset hardly few features are insignificant. In the second stage binary version of CS algorithm is implemented to extract the most significant feature. First cross validation approach is used to break the entire data into many folds. Thereafter data is divided for training as well as testing purpose.

Here 10 runs are considered to extract the most significant feature. In each run there are 10 simulations and in every simulation CS algorithm is iterated for 1000 times. For each run, the global optimal solution is obtained comparing all simulation in terms of feature indices. Finally output of each run is compared and superior solution is picked up.

Classifier Used for the Proposed Work

In this experimental work, three classifiers are used such as artificial neural network (ANN), k-Nearest Neighbor (KNN), and support vector machine (SVM), out of which SVM is used select the optimal feature subset and rest two are used to validate the model.

KNN classifier is considered as the simplest classifier since only one parameter i.e. k value = number of neighbour is required to be optimized (Dash, 2018). As per this approach, the entire test sample moves to the nearest k neighbour classes with respect to the nearest distance. For the distance calculation Euclidian distance measure or any other distance measure can be used.

Here ANN is a single layer feed forward neural network. Final reduced dataset(obtained using BCSA) in terms of different feature value is the number of input layer neuron. The middle (hidden) layer consists of 8 neurons and output layer with 1 neuron (Han et al., 2016). Activation function is linear in input layer and sigmoidal in hidden and output layer respectively.

Different variation of Support vector machines are widely accepted for high dimensional data classification. It has several advantages such as adequate generalization of new objects and a representation that depends on few parameters. For a particular model it does not get stuck at local optimum for any objective function (Dash, 2017; Dash, & Misra, 2017; Demšar, 2006). For binary classification problem SVM is highly effective and here we have used quadratic SVM for performance measurement. Thus SVM is considered as a classification model to train the network for BCSA.

SIMULATION RESULT ANALYSIS

Result of all simulation is presented in terms of three performance metrics such as accuracy, sensitivity and specificity. Again for its depth study, each performance measure is analyzed in terms of three values such as best, mean and standard deviation. For all the dataset, result is presented from Table.3 to Table.7 keeping in objective of getting the optimal result out of all 10 runs. For each run, the entire process of simulation is discussed in subsection 5.3 and shown in Fig.1.

Table 3 shows the simulation result on Leukemia dataset. The model is trained in order to minimize the classification error, thus considering mean accuracy, performance of model is evaluated. In the 8th run proposed model shows better result with mean accuracy 80%.

Table.4 shows the performance result of proposed approach on the AllAml dataset. Here all the simulations are independent. The model is designed in such a way that for all runs executions don't depend on its previous execution. Thus for AllAml dataset, the optimal result is produced at 4th run with mean accuracy 97%.

Binary cuckoo search-based feature selection and classification approach is implemented for AD-CALung dataset in Table.5. In 6th run the performance result is optimal with 98% mean accuracy.

The result evaluation of CNS dataset by BCSA is presented in Table 6. Considering a minimum number of significant features performance is evaluated. This simulation shows at 4th run, the performance of BCSA is optimal with 90% mean accuracy.

Table 3. Result evaluation and feature generation on Leukemia dataset

No.of Run	Accuracy			Sensitivity			Specificity		
	mean	Best	Std	mean	Best	Std	mean	Best	Std
1	0.78	0.81	0.03	0.63	0.88	0.15	0.78	0.88	0.03
2	0.75	0.84	0.04	0.35	0.92	0.36	0.75	0.84	0.06
3	0.73	0.84	0.04	0.16	0.86	0.29	0.73	0.86	0.05
4	0.76	0.83	0.04	0.47	0.83	0.32	0.76	0.84	0.05
5	0.71	0.71	0.00	0.00	0.00	0.00	0.71	0.71	0.00
6	0.78	0.83	0.02	0.67	0.97	0.12	0.78	0.91	0.04
7	0.78	0.81	0.02	0.66	0.96	0.10	0.78	0.89	0.03
8	**0.80**	**0.88**	**0.04**	**0.69**	**0.88**	**0.09**	**0.80**	**0.92**	**0.04**
9	0.77	0.82	0.02	0.65	0.98	0.10	0.77	0.93	0.03
10	0.76	0.81	0.04	0.50	0.95	0.32	0.76	0.84	0.05

Table 4. Result evaluation and feature generation on AllAml dataset

No.of Run	Accuracy			Sensitivity			Specificity		
	mean	Best	Std	mean	Best	Std	mean	Best	Std
1	0.95	0.97	0.01	0.96	0.96	0.00	0.95	0.94	0.11
2	0.90	0.92	0.01	0.92	0.96	0.03	0.90	0.85	0.06
3	0.95	0.95	0.00	0.93	0.93	0.00	0.95	0.98	0.15
4	**0.97**	**0.97**	**0.01**	**0.97**	**1.00**	**0.01**	**0.97**	**0.98**	**0.08**
5	0.89	0.89	0.00	0.88	0.90	0.01	0.89	0.98	0.13
6	0.92	0.92	0.00	0.98	1.00	0.03	0.92	0.87	0.07
7	0.95	0.97	0.01	0.97	0.99	0.01	0.95	1.00	0.12
8	0.93	0.95	0.01	0.93	0.93	0.01	0.93	0.98	0.16
9	0.95	0.97	0.03	0.93	0.96	0.03	0.95	0.96	0.11
10	0.94	0.95	0.01	0.96	0.96	0.00	0.94	0.80	0.06

For Prostate dataset, performance of BCSA is presented in Table 7. Here performance is high with mean accuracy 96% in 9th run.

Thereafter this research work using BCSA is compared with few other metaheuristic approaches such binary version of genetic algorithm (BinaryGA), differential evolution (BinaryDE), artificial bee colony algorithm (BinaryABC) and particle swarm optimization (BinaryPSO). To avoid biasing with respect to single classifier, this analysis is further extended using few other classifiers such as k-nearest neighbor (KNN) and artificial neural network(ANN).

The performance measures used for this analysis are accuracy, specificity, sensitivity and gmean and the best classification performance result is presented to choose the optimal classifier.

Table 5. Result evaluation and feature generation on ADCALung dataset

Dataset- ADCALung									
No.of Run	**Accuracy**			**Sensitivity**			**Specificity**		
	mean	**Best**	**Std**	**mean**	**Best**	**Std**	**mean**	**Best**	**Std**
1	0.97	0.97	0.00	0.97	0.97	0.00	0.97	0.98	0.08
2	0.95	0.96	0.00	0.96	0.98	0.01	0.95	0.89	0.14
3	0.95	0.95	0.00	0.95	0.95	0.00	0.95	1.00	0.13
4	0.97	0.97	0.00	0.97	0.98	0.01	0.97	0.99	0.08
5	0.95	0.95	0.00	0.95	0.96	0.00	0.95	0.95	0.20
6	**0.98**	**0.99**	**0.00**	**0.98**	**0.99**	**0.00**	**0.98**	**0.99**	**0.08**
7	0.97	0.97	0.00	0.97	0.98	0.00	0.97	0.91	0.07
8	0.97	0.97	0.00	0.97	0.98	0.01	0.97	0.96	0.10
9	0.97	0.97	0.00	0.97	0.98	0.00	0.97	1.00	0.15
10	0.97	0.97	0.00	0.96	0.96	0.00	0.97	0.99	0.12

Table .Result evaluation and feature generation on CNS dataset

Dataset- CNS									
No.of Run	**Accuracy**			**Sensitivity**			**Specificity**		
	mean	**Best**	**Std**	**mean**	**Best**	**Std**	**mean**	**Best**	**Std**
1	0.87	0.95	0.04	0.95	0.98	0.01	0.87	0.83	0.15
2	0.86	0.93	0.04	0.96	0.98	0.01	0.86	0.81	0.15
3	0.90	0.90	0.00	0.90	0.90	0.00	0.90	0.89	0.05
4	**0.90**	**0.91**	**0.00**	**0.90**	**0.91**	**0.00**	**0.90**	**0.86**	**0.06**
5	0.89	0.90	0.02	0.89	0.89	0.03	0.89	0.87	0.04
6	0.83	0.84	0.00	0.80	0.85	0.02	0.83	0.83	0.03
7	0.81	0.82	0.01	0.80	0.85	0.05	0.81	0.83	0.03
8	0.83	0.86	0.01	0.76	0.80	0.02	0.83	0.89	0.05
9	0.78	0.80	0.01	0.70	0.73	0.02	0.78	0.84	0.03
10	0.83	0.84	0.01	0.79	0.79	0.01	0.83	0.86	0.04

Table 8 to Table 12 shows the classification result of all the classifiers. Further a deeper level of analysis is carried out and shown in Table 13.

Leukemia dataset is analyzed in Table 8. The high performance with respect to different classifier and performance measures are highlighted. There are 12 outputs of each individual approach. Out of which 10 times proposed BCSA shows highest result, and thus rest of the techniques are not comparable.

For AllAml dataset, the result is presented in table 9.Here also proposed BCSA shows its superiority over others. With respect to KNN and SVM, most of the time performance is high. However, when ANN is used there is no such marginal difference in performance as compared to other techniques.

Table 7. Result evaluation and feature generation on Prostate dataset

No.of Run	Accuracy			Sensitivity			Specificity		
	mean	Best	Std	mean	Best	Std	mean	Best	Std
1	0.92	0.94	0.01	0.85	0.88	0.03	0.92	0.98	0.02
2	0.95	0.95	0.00	0.91	0.92	0.00	0.95	1.00	0.04
3	0.92	0.93	0.01	0.84	0.89	0.02	0.92	0.95	0.04
4	0.94	0.95	0.01	0.90	0.90	0.00	0.94	0.96	0.03
5	0.93	0.96	0.01	0.88	0.94	0.03	0.93	0.96	0.03
6	0.89	0.89	0.01	0.85	0.85	0.01	0.89	0.88	0.03
7	0.87	0.88	0.01	0.87	0.93	0.08	0.87	0.88	0.03
8	0.92	0.94	0.01	0.85	0.88	0.03	0.92	0.98	0.02
9	**0.96**	**0.96**	**0.01**	**0.90**	**0.91**	**0.03**	**0.96**	**0.96**	**0.04**
10	0.92	0.94	0.01	0.85	0.88	0.03	0.92	0.98	0.02

Dataset- Prostate

Table 8. Comparative result of proposed approach with few considered Metaheuristic approaches on Leukemia dataset

Feature Selection Approaches	Types of Classifier											
	KNN				ANN				SVM			
	Acc	Sen	Spec	Gmn	Acc	Sen	Spec	Gmn	Acc	Sen	Spec	Gmn
Proposed Technique	**100**	**100**	**100**	**100**	**100**	**100**	**100**	94.72	**88.56**	**88.32**	**92.00**	95.42
BinaryPSO	99.32	100	96.94	97.37	**100**	97.37	96.94	97.16	83.89	77.82	81.83	94.77
BinaryABC	92.10	98.00	98.00	94.9	94.85	94.9	**100**	94.77	86.13	83.7	86.13	**96.94**
BinaryGA	92.31	98.87	98.10	97.37	**100**	97.37	96.94	96.54	87.78	78.82	83.79	94.90
BinaryDE	0.96	100	96.94	97.37	**100**	97.37	96.94	**97.37**	87.78	78.82	83.79	94.85

Leukemia Dataset

Table 9. Comparative result of proposed approach with few considered Metaheuristic approaches on AllAml dataset

Feature Selection Approaches	Types of Classifier											
	KNN				ANN				SVM			
	Acc	Sen	Spec	Gmn	Acc	Sen	Spec	Gmn	Acc	Sen	Spec	Gmn
Proposed Technique	**99.44**	99.25	**99.44**	94.81	97.09	96.30	96.55	96.43	**97.00**	**100.0**	**98.00**	94.81
BinaryPSO	99.11	**99.52**	99.11	94.77	99.11	97.13	**97.01**	94.21	93.09	95.3	92.60	94.77
BinaryABC	97.09	96.30	96.55	96.27	97.44	96.87	96.59	**100.00**	91.08	94.13	91.74	96.27
BinaryGA	98.43	97.54	97.73	97.08	**99.34**	**97.33**	96.55	96.38	94.31	96.61	94.56	97.08
BinaryDE	96.94	97.37	95.64	**97.12**	97.79	96.71	96.82	96.43	95.10	91.35	90.78	**97.12**

AllAml Dataset

In Table 10, the performance of the learning technique for ADCALung dataset is presented. It is observed that more than 50% of the time BCSA shows its superiority.

Table 11 presents the performance of the learning technique on CNS data. It shows that most of the models are comparable specially BinaryPSO, BinaryABC and BCSA.

The result analysis of the Prostate dataset is presented in Table 12. Here also proposed BCSA is showing a better result as compared to other learning techniques.

Finally, in Table.13, a summary of each classifier's performance is shown. It shows the number of times a particular technique shows the highest performance in %. It is clearly observed that, BCSA is superior as compared to other techniques.

Table 10. Comparative result of the proposed approach with few considered Metaheuristic approaches on ADCALung dataset

ADCALung Dataset												
Feature Selection Approaches	**Types of Classifier**											
	KNN				**ANN**				**SVM**			
	Acc	**Sen**	**Spec**	**Gmn**	**Acc**	**Sen**	**Spec**	**Gmn**	**Acc**	**Sen**	**Spec**	**Gmn**
Proposed Technique	**98.66**	**98.39**	**98.53**	94.72	99.44	99.25	99.44	**96.94**	**99.00**	**99.12**	**99.34**	97.37
BinaryPSO	97.09	96.3	96.55	97.16	99.11	**99.52**	99.11	94.90	97.37	97.37	96.34	96.54
BinaryABC	98.43	97.54	97.73	94.77	96.94	97.37	95.64	94.85	95.25	97.37	95.25	97.37
BinaryGA	97.09	96.3	96.55	96.54	**100.0**	94.90	**100.0**	94.74	92.88	94.74	92.88	**98.37**
BinaryDE	98.43	97.54	97.73	**97.37**	98.43	97.54	97.73	95.53	94.94	97.37	94.94	96.49

Table 11. Comparative result of the proposed approach with few considered metaheuristic approaches on CNS dataset

CNS Dataset												
Feature Selection Approaches	**Types of Classifier**											
	KNN				**ANN**				**SVM**			
	Acc	**Sen**	**Spec**	**Gmn**	**Acc**	**Sen**	**Spec**	**Gmn**	**Acc**	**Sen**	**Spec**	**Gmn**
Proposed Technique	85.65	86.67	81.05	85.91	85.65	86.82	**89.74**	88.89	**91.00**	**91.00**	86.00	**89.90**
BinaryPSO	83.79	**87.78**	78.09	**91.91**	83.79	87.18	85.98	86.57	88.33	82.78	**92.86**	84.62
BinaryABC	**86.59**	87.22	**88.10**	88.45	**86.59**	84.05	85.86	**89.47**	86.11	83.89	92.31	85.00
BinaryGA	82.84	86.67	76.80	86.67	82.84	**89.12**	87.58	86.79	83.89	88.33	87.41	81.82
BinaryDE	82.96	83.89	78.81	81.52	82.96	87.18	**89.74**	87.76	86.11	88.33	88.24	**89.90**

Table 12. Comparative results of the proposed approach with few considered Metaheuristic approaches on the Prostate dataset

Prostate Dataset												
Feature Selection Approaches	Types of Classifier											
	KNN				ANN				SVM			
	Acc	Sen	Spec	Gmn	Acc	Sen	Spec	Gmn	Acc	Sen	Spec	Gmn
Proposed Technique	**94.46**	**98.25**	**95.24**	83.94	91.14	92.98	88.44	84.42	**96.00**	91.00	**96.00**	88.23
BinaryPSO	90.81	92.98	85.93	**88.79**	90.97	92.40	86.97	**95.00**	94.46	89.08	92.00	90.40
BinaryABC	89.13	89.47	81.82	85.93	**92.46**	92.98	**89.63**	94.32	90.81	91.14	90.79	**91.28**
BinaryGA	89.20	92.98	90.00	83.09	92.00	92.98	86.36	88.27	89.13	90.97	87.35	89.71
BinaryDE	89.08	91.23	82.61	86.36	90.79	**93.57**	85.51	90.32	89.20	**92.46**	90.80	88.23

Table 13. Overall performance analysis of considered classification approaches (in %)

Datasets					
Feature Selection Approaches	Leukemia	AllAml	ADCALung	CNS	Prostate
Proposed Technique	91.66	41.66	58.33	33.33	41.66
BinaryPSO	8.33	16.66	8.33	25.00	16.66
BinaryABC	-	8.33	8.33	33.33	25.00
BinaryGA	-	16.66	25.00	8.33	-
BinaryDE	8.33	16.66	8.33	16.66	16.66

CONCLUSION

Inspired from successful application of many metaheuristic approaches and especially Cuckoo search algorithm, in this research work a feature selection and classification model is designed. This implementation is a binary version of the cuckoo search approach, to decide whether to consider a feature or discard it. This evaluation is done with respect to the classification outcome. Thus selected features with better classification results are assumed to be significant. A comparative study is also presented with a few other binary versions of metaheuristic approaches such as PSO, DE, GA and ABC. Result analysis is conducted considering 5 performance measures such as accuracy, specificity, sensitivity and gmean. Ultimately for all considered high dimension gene expression datasets, BCSA shows its superiority.

REFERENCES

Alizadeh, A. A., Eisen, M. B., Davis, R. E., Ma, C., Lossos, I. S., Rosenwald, A., Boldrick, J. C., Sabet, H., Tran, T., Yu, X., Powell, J. I., Yang, L., Marti, G. E., Moore, T., Hudson, J. Jr, Lu, L., Lewis, D. B., Tibshirani, R., Sherlock, G., ... Staudt, L. M. (2000). Distinct types of diffuse large B-cell lymphoma identified by gene expression profiling. *Nature*, *403*(6769), 503–511. doi:10.1038/35000501 PMID:10676951

AlRashidi, M. R., & El-Hawary, M. E. (2008). A survey of particle swarm optimization applications in electric power systems. *IEEE Transactions on Evolutionary Computation*, *13*(4), 913–918. doi:10.1109/TEVC.2006.880326

Aneiros, G., Cao, R., Fraiman, R., Genest, C., & Vieu, P. (2019). Recent advances in functional data analysis and high-dimensional statistics. *Journal of Multivariate Analysis*, *170*, 3–9. doi:10.1016/j.jmva.2018.11.007

Beer, D. G., Kardia, S. L. R., Huang, C.-C., Giordano, T. J., Levin, A. M., Misek, D. E., Lin, L., Chen, G., Gharib, T. G., Thomas, D. G., Lizyness, M. L., Kuick, R., Hayasaka, S., Taylor, J. M. G., Iannettoni, M. D., Orringer, M. B., & Hanash, S. (2002). Gene-expression Profiles Predict Survival of Patients with Lung Adenocarcinoma. *Nature Medicine*, *8*(8), 816–823. doi:10.1038/nm733 PMID:12118244

Berkaya, S. K., Uysal, A. K., Gunal, E. S., Ergin, S., Gunal, S., & Gulmezoglu, M. B. (2018). A survey on ECG analysis. *Biomedical Signal Processing and Control*, *43*, 216–235. doi:10.1016/j.bspc.2018.03.003

Bianchi, L., Dorigo, M., Gambardella, L. M., & Gutjahr, W. J. (2009). A survey on metaheuristics for stochastic combinatorial optimization. *Natural Computing*, *8*(2), 239–287. doi:10.100711047-008-9098-4

Bibiks, K., Hu, Y. F., Li, J. P., Pillai, P., & Smith, A. (2018). Improved discrete cuckoo search for the resource-constrained project scheduling problem. *Applied Soft Computing*, *69*, 493–503. doi:10.1016/j.asoc.2018.04.047

Chakkaravarthy, S. S., Sangeetha, D., & Vaidehi, V. (2019). A survey on malware analysis and mitigation techniques. *Computer Science Review*, *32*, 1–23. doi:10.1016/j.cosrev.2019.01.002

Chawla, M. P. S. (2011). PCA and ICA processing methods for removal of artifacts and noise in electrocardiograms: A survey and comparison. *Applied Soft Computing*, *11*(2), 2216–2226. doi:10.1016/j.asoc.2010.08.001

Chiroma, H., Herawan, T., Fister, I. Jr, Fister, I., Abdulkareem, S., Shuib, L., Hamza, M. F., Saadi, Y., & Abubakar, A. (2017). Bio-inspired computation: Recent development on the modifications of the cuckoo search algorithm. *Applied Soft Computing*, *61*, 149–173. doi:10.1016/j.asoc.2017.07.053

Chitara, D., Niazi, K. R., Swarnkar, A., & Gupta, N. (2018). Cuckoo search optimization algorithm for designing of multimachine power system stabilizer. *IEEE Transactions on Industry Applications*, *54*(4), 3056–3065. doi:10.1109/TIA.2018.2811725

Chung, I. M., Kim, J. K., Lee, K. J., Park, S. K., Lee, J. H., Son, N. Y., Jin, Y.-I., & Kim, S. H. (2018). Geographic authentication of Asian rice (Oryza sativa L.) using multi-elemental and stable isotopic data combined with multivariate analysis. *Food Chemistry*, *240*, 840–849. doi:10.1016/j.foodchem.2017.08.023 PMID:28946350

Coelho, L. S., Guerra, F., Batistela, N. J., & Leite, J. V. (2013). Multiobjective cuckoo search algorithm based on Duffing's oscillator applied to Jiles-Atherton vector hysteresis parameters estimation. *IEEE Transactions on Magnetics*, *49*(5), 1745–1748. doi:10.1109/TMAG.2013.2243907

Cruz-Duarte, J. M., Garcia-Perez, A., Amaya-Contreras, I. M., Correa-Cely, C. R., Romero-Troncoso, R. J., & Avina-Cervantes, J. G. (2017). Design of microelectronic cooling systems using a thermodynamic optimization strategy based on cuckoo search. *IEEE Transactions on Components, Packaging, and Manufacturing Technology*, *7*(11), 1804–1812. doi:10.1109/TCPMT.2017.2706305

Dash, R. (2017). A two stage grading approach for feature selection and classification of microarray data using Pareto based feature ranking techniques: A case study. *Journal of King Saud University-Computer and Information Sciences*.

Dash, R. (2018). An adaptive harmony search approach for gene selection and classification of high dimensional medical data. *Journal of King Saud University-Computer and Information Sciences*.

Dash, R., Dash, R., & Rautray, R. (2019). An evolutionary framework based microarray gene selection and classification approach using binary shuffled frog leaping algorithm. *Journal of King Saud University-Computer and Information Sciences*.

Dash, R., & Misra, B. (2017). Gene selection and classification of microarray data: A Pareto DE approach. *Intelligent Decision Technologies*, *11*(1), 93–107. doi:10.3233/IDT-160280

Dash, R., & Misra, B. B. (2016). Pipelining the ranking techniques for microarray data classification: A case study. *Applied Soft Computing*, *48*, 298–316. doi:10.1016/j.asoc.2016.07.006

Dash, R., & Misra, B. B. (2018). Performance analysis of clustering techniques over microarray data: A case study. *Physica A*, *493*, 162–176. doi:10.1016/j.physa.2017.10.032

Demšar, J. (2006). Statistical comparisons of classifiers over multiple data sets. *Journal of Machine Learning Research*, *7*(Jan), 1–30.

Dokeroglu, T., Sevinc, E., Kucukyilmaz, T., & Cosar, A. (2019). A survey on new generation meta-heuristic algorithms. *Computers & Industrial Engineering*, *137*, 106040. doi:10.1016/j.cie.2019.106040

Feng, M. Q., Leung, R. Y., & Eckersley, C. M. (2020). Non-Contact vehicle Weigh-in-Motion using computer vision. *Measurement*, *153*, 107415. doi:10.1016/j.measurement.2019.107415

Frew, R., Higgs, G., Harding, J., & Langford, M. (2017). Investigating geospatial data usability from a health geography perspective using sensitivity analysis: The example of potential accessibility to primary healthcare. *Journal of Transport & Health*, *6*, 128–142. doi:10.1016/j.jth.2017.03.013

Golub, T. R., Slonim, D. K., Tamayo, P., Huard, C., Gaasenbeek, M., Mesirov, J. P., Coller, H., Loh, M. L., Downing, J. R., Caligiuri, M., Bloomfield, C. D., & Lander, E. S. (1999). Molecular classification of cancer: class discovery and class prediction by gene expression monitoring. *Science, 286*(5439), 531-7.

Gordon, G. J. (2002). Translation of Microarray Data into Clinically Relevant Cancer Diagnostic Tests Using Gege Expression Ratios in Lung Cancer And Mesothelioma. *Cancer Research, 62*, 4963–4967. PMID:12208747

Han, W., Xu, J., Zhou, M., Tian, G., Wang, P., Shen, X., & Hou, E. (2016). Cuckoo search and particle filter-based inversing approach to estimating defects via magnetic flux leakage signals. *IEEE Transactions on Magnetics*, *52*(4), 1–11. doi:10.1109/TMAG.2015.2498119

Hartley, D. (2009). Secure ecommerce web application design principles, beyond PCI DSS. *Computer Fraud & Security*, *6*(6), 13–17. doi:10.1016/S1361-3723(09)70074-0

Hussain, K., Salleh, M. N. M., Cheng, S., & Shi, Y. (2019). Metaheuristic research: A comprehensive survey. *Artificial Intelligence Review*, *52*(4), 2191–2233. doi:10.100710462-017-9605-z

Imbriaco, M., Iodice, D., Erra, P., Terlizzi, A., Di Carlo, R., Di Vito, C., & Imbimbo, C. (2011). Squamous cell carcinoma within a horseshoe kidney with associated renal stones detected by computed tomograpy and magnetic resonance imaging. *Urology*, *78*(1), 54–55. doi:10.1016/j.urology.2010.06.006 PMID:20801492

Jain, M., Singh, V., & Rani, A. (2018). A novel nature-inspired algorithm for optimization: Squirrel search algorithm. *Swarm and Evolutionary Computation*.

Jayashree, J., & Kumar, S. A. (2019). Evolutionary correlated gravitational search algorithm (ECGS) with genetic optimized Hopfield neural network (GHNN)–A hybrid expert system for diagnosis of diabetes. *Measurement*, *145*, 551–558. doi:10.1016/j.measurement.2018.12.083

Jiang, M., Luo, J., Jiang, D., Xiong, J., Song, H., & Shen, J. (2016). A cuckoo search-support vector machine model for predicting dynamic measurement errors of sensors. *IEEE Access: Practical Innovations, Open Solutions*, *4*, 5030–5037. doi:10.1109/ACCESS.2016.2605041

Kamoona, A. M., & Patra, J. C. (2019). A novel enhanced cuckoo search algorithm for contrast enhancement of gray scale images. *Applied Soft Computing*, *85*, 105749. doi:10.1016/j.asoc.2019.105749

Li, X., Ma, S., & Yang, G. (2017). Synthesis of Difference Patterns for Monopulse Antennas by an Improved Cuckoo Search Algorithm. *IEEE Antennas and Wireless Propagation Letters*, *16*, 141–144. doi:10.1109/LAWP.2016.2640998

Lin, A., Foroozan, R., Carrier, D., & Yen, M. T. (2004). Diagnosis of metastatic carcinoma to the cavernous sinus by computed tomograpy–guided fine-needle aspiration. *American Journal of Ophthalmology*, *138*(5), 864–866. doi:10.1016/j.ajo.2004.05.036 PMID:15531326

Mareli, M., & Twala, B. (2018). An adaptive Cuckoo search algorithm for optimisation. *Applied Computing and Informatics, 14*(2), 107-115.

Mavrovouniotis, M., Li, C., & Yang, S. (2017). A survey of swarm intelligence for dynamic optimization: Algorithms and applications. *Swarm and Evolutionary Computation*, *33*, 1–17. doi:10.1016/j.swevo.2016.12.005

Moodley, S., Schoenhagen, P., Gillinov, A. M., Mihaljevic, T., Flamm, S. D., Griffin, B. P., & Desai, M. Y. (2013). Preoperative multidetector computed tomograpy angiography for planning of minimally invasive robotic mitral valve surgery: Impact on decision making. *The Journal of Thoracic and Cardiovascular Surgery*, *146*(2), 262–268. doi:10.1016/j.jtcvs.2012.06.052 PMID:22841167

Osman, H., & Baki, M. F. (2018). A Cuckoo Search Algorithm to Solve Transfer Line Balancing Problems With Different Cutting Conditions. *IEEE Transactions on Engineering Management, 65*(3), 505–518. doi:10.1109/TEM.2018.2797223

Pazhaniraja, N., Paul, P. V., Roja, G., Shanmugapriya, K., & Sonali, B. (2017, March). A study on recent bio-inspired optimization algorithms. In *2017 Fourth International Conference on Signal Processing, Communication and Networking (ICSCN)* (pp. 1-6). IEEE. 10.1109/ICSCN.2017.8085674

Rautray, R., & Balabantaray, R. C. (2018). An evolutionary framework for multi document summarization using Cuckoo search approach: MDSCSA. *Applied Computing and Informatics, 14*(2), 134-144.

Rautray, R., Balabantaray, R. C., Dash, R., & Dash, R. (2019). CSMDSE-Cuckoo Search Based Multi Document Summary Extractor: Cuckoo Search Based Summary Extractor. *International Journal of Cognitive Informatics and Natural Intelligence, 13*(4), 56–70. doi:10.4018/IJCINI.2019100103

Robinson, C. (2017). Disclosure of personal data in ecommerce: A cross-national comparison of Estonia and the United States. *Telematics and Informatics, 34*(2), 569–582. doi:10.1016/j.tele.2016.09.006

Sarangi, S. K., Panda, R., Das, P. K., & Abraham, A. (2018). Design of optimal high pass and band stop FIR filters using adaptive Cuckoo search algorithm. *Engineering Applications of Artificial Intelligence, 70*, 67–80. doi:10.1016/j.engappai.2018.01.005

Sert, O. C., Şahin, S. D., Özyer, T., & Alhajj, R. (2019). Analysis and prediction in sparse and high dimensional text data: The case of Dow Jones stock market. *Physica A*, 123752.

Shehab, M., Khader, A. T., & Al-Betar, M. A. (2017). A survey on applications and variants of the cuckoo search algorithm. *Applied Soft Computing, 61*, 1041–1059. doi:10.1016/j.asoc.2017.02.034

Singh, D., Febbo, P. G., Ross, K., Jackson, D. G., Manola, J., Ladd, C., Tamayo, P., Renshaw, A. A., D'Amico, A. V., Richie, J. P., Lander, E. S., Loda, M., Kantoff, P. W., Golub, T. R., & Sellers, W. R. (2002). Gene Expression Correlates of Clinical Prostate Cancer Behavior. *Cancer Cell, 1*(2), 203–209. doi:10.1016/S1535-6108(02)00030-2 PMID:12086878

Slowik, A., & Kwasnicka, H. (2018). Nature Inspired Methods and Their Industry Applications—Swarm Intelligence Algorithms. *IEEE Transactions on Industrial Informatics, 14*(3), 1004–1015. doi:10.1109/TII.2017.2786782

Sreenivasan, K. R., Havlicek, M., & Deshpande, G. (2014). Nonparametric hemodynamic deconvolution of FMRI using homomorphic filtering. *IEEE Transactions on Medical Imaging, 34*(5), 1155–1163. doi:10.1109/TMI.2014.2379914 PMID:25531878

Sun, G., Liu, Y., Chen, Z., Liang, S., Wang, A., & Zhang, Y. (2018). Radiation Beam Pattern Synthesis of Concentric Circular Antenna Arrays Using Hybrid Approach Based on Cuckoo Search. *IEEE Transactions on Antennas and Propagation, 66*(9), 4563–4576. doi:10.1109/TAP.2018.2846771

Sun, G., Liu, Y., Li, J., Zhang, Y., & Wang, A. (2017). Sidelobe reduction of large-scale antenna array for 5G beamforming via hierarchical cuckoo search. *Electronics Letters, 53*(16), 1158–1160. doi:10.1049/el.2016.4768

Suresh, S., Lal, S., Chen, C., & Celik, T. (2018). Multispectral Satellite Image Denoising via Adaptive Cuckoo Search-Based Wiener Filter. *IEEE Transactions on Geoscience and Remote Sensing*, *56*(8), 4334–4345. doi:10.1109/TGRS.2018.2815281

Suresh, S., Lal, S., Reddy, C. S., & Kiran, M. S. (2017). A novel adaptive cuckoo search algorithm for contrast enhancement of satellite images. *IEEE Journal of Selected Topics in Applied Earth Observations and Remote Sensing*, *10*(8), 3665–3676. doi:10.1109/JSTARS.2017.2699200

Wei, J., & Yu, Y. (2018). An effective hybrid cuckoo search algorithm for unknown parameters and time delays estimation of chaotic systems. *IEEE Access: Practical Innovations, Open Solutions*, *6*, 6560–6571. doi:10.1109/ACCESS.2017.2738006

Yang, X.-S., & Deb, S. (2014). Cuckoo search: Recent advances and applications. *Neural Computing & Applications*, *24*(1), 169–174. doi:10.100700521-013-1367-1

Zhang, H., Zhang, X., Wang, Y., Qian, X., & Wang, Y. (2018). Extended cuckoo search-based kernel correlation filter for abrupt motion tracking. *IET Computer Vision*, *12*(6), 763–769. doi:10.1049/iet-cvi.2017.0554

Zhao, J., Liu, S., Zhou, M., Guo, X., & Qi, L. (2018). An Improved Binary Cuckoo Search Algorithm for Solving Unit Commitment Problems: Methodological Description. *IEEE Access: Practical Innovations, Open Solutions*, *6*, 43535–43545. doi:10.1109/ACCESS.2018.2861319

Zhao, J., Liu, S., Zhou, M., Guo, X., & Qi, L. (2018). Modified cuckoo search algorithm to solve economic power dispatch optimization problems. *IEEE/CAA Journal of Automatica Sinica, 5*(4), 794-806.

Zhou, J., Zhai, L., & Pantelous, A. A. (2020). Market segmentation using high-dimensional sparse consumers data. *Expert Systems with Applications*, *145*, 113136. doi:10.1016/j.eswa.2019.113136

Chapter 3
Mathematical Model for Image Processing Using Graph Theory

Rajshree Dahal
CHRIST University (Deemed), India

Ritwika Das Gupta
CHRIST University (Deemed), India

Debabrata Samanta
https://orcid.org/0000-0003-4118-2480
CHRIST University (Deemed), India

ABSTRACT

Image segmentation being an important aspect of computer systems, graph theory provides the most elemental way of representing various parts of an image into mathematical structures. There are many applications of image segmentations including face recognition systems, remote sensing, detecting images sent by satellites, optometry, medical image reading, and many more. Bi-partite graphs are useful in determination of cuts in the segmentation process. These structures are analysed by considering each vertex as pixel, and each weight is some aspect of dissimilarity for two vertices connected by an edge with weights. This makes the problem-solving part very flexible, and their computation becomes easy and fast. The problem is usually parted into small subgraphs that are bound under some continuous forms of graphs like spanning trees, cut vertices or edges, shortest paths graphs, and so on. The cluster formation is proved to be one of most commonly used methods in image segmentation.

INTRODUCTION

Image Segmentation is a traditional and important concept that is studied under the field of computer science. It is mainly concerned with breaking up of an image into many tiny subsets that are disjoint structures and each one of these subsets represent an important aspect of the image. The quality of segmentation obtained is highly valuable to whole process of image processing as it have lot of influence

DOI: 10.4018/978-1-6684-4580-8.ch003

to the total extraction and consecutive steps. A lot of research activities have been taking place in this field in computer science background and still there is lot of scope for its further development. Many famous works in this field have been completed with amazing results in medical background, preconisation, tracking and reconstruction. From the initial stage the basic idea behind image segmentation has been the cluster formations of the data. In 1938 gestalt theory expressed this idea in a distinct manner by identifying a group of principles for example likeness, closeness and continuity that clarifies the idea of man-made awareness system. This theory has been the base of many research work conducted in image segmentation since then in the hope that significant clusters could imitate some the local or universal aspects of an image. Image intensity and colour has been the main focus during the initial research activities like that of Robert edge detector method, Canny edge detector method or the Sobel edge detector method. More over some work has been done due to thresholding process for differentiation of objects and background as many distinct structures has been seen in them. The PDE based methods or partial differentiation-based methods gives segmentation considering the constant change occurring in curves in space minimizing the energy to obtain a required segmentation. Breaking up of regions and assimilation of region is also another popular method which uses iterations to obtain a particular regularity condition. Although rigorous research has been conducted in image and video segmentation and numerous algorithms and methods are established: Thresholding, Edge detection, Region growing methods, clustering methods, and compression-based methods, Watershed transformations, Morphically methods, Graph partitioning methods etc. but in general there exists no segmentation algorithm which can be commonly applied on all the domains. (Chen and L. Pan et al. 2018)

The main step is pre-processing of the image that removes the variety of instabilities of the image including noise by filtration and particular noise removing procedures. Further, the obtained image is partitioned or segmented by the algorithms available for image segmentation. The most problematic stage of image segmentation is the processing stage followed by the structure extraction process. These structures are further used in organisation of images. Some of the application of image processing is in areas like OCR, recognition of face and finger print, biometric, image detection by satellites, image analysis in medical field and so on.

A flowchart of various step included in image processing step is summarized in Figure 1 below:

Figure 1. Flowchart of image processing method

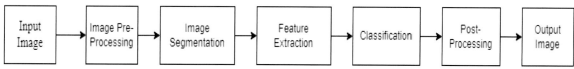

The various segmentation techniques and their subdivisions are summarized in Figure 2 below:

The following table 1 gives a brief description of the various Image Segmentation methods along with their advantage and disadvantage.

Figure 2. Flowchart of segmentation techniques and sub-techniques

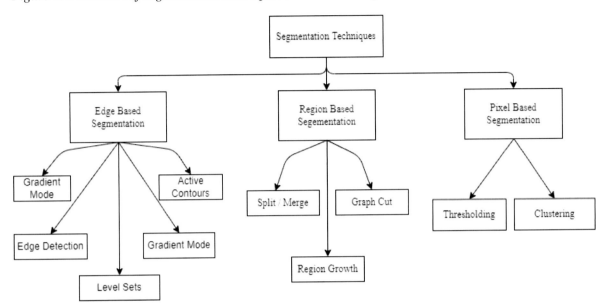

Table 1. A comparative study of various available image segmentation methods

Segmentation Technique	Description	Advantage	Disadvantage
Pixel-based segmentation	A digital image is broken down into multiple segments or groups of pixels, also known as super pixels.	Can deal with complex images.	It requires a manual interaction and also cannot be used in case of non-interactive applications.
Edge-based Segmentation	It is based on the concept of discontinuity identification.	Gives a better output if images have a good contrast between objects.	It depends on the peaks of image and spatial ideas of images are not taken into consideration.
Region-based Segmentation	It is based on graph segmentation ideas that break images into homogenous graphs.	Gives a better similarity identification and is prone to noise.	It is one of the expensive methods on the basis of time and memory consumption.
Thresholding Method	Based on the peaks of histogram for the threshold value of image.	Simple method without any requirement of prior knowledge.	Depends on the peaks of histogram.
Watershed Method	It works on the concepts on topological ideas.	Gives stable results and boundaries that are obtained are continuous	Calculation complexity.
Clustering Method	Divides the image into homogenous clusters.	It is highly useful in real life problem due to the use of fuzzy graphs in this method.	The membership function identification is critical.
PDE-based Segmentation	It's working is based on partial differential equations.	It is a fast and time efficient method.	It is computationally complex.
ANN-based Segmentation	It makes use the simulation in decision making.	Complex programs are almost null.	Training requires more time.

GRAPH THEORETIC APPROACH TO IMAGE PROCESSING

If G is a graph represented as the set G=(V,E) then, V represents the set of vertices and E is the edge set. This set of edges may or may not be ordered. If G is ordered then the edge set E of G is representing directed graph and if it is unordered then the set of edges E represents an undirected graph. Usually, a dot represents the vertex and links or arcs represent the edges. If two vertices say x and y are connected by an edge say e then we represent it as $e_{x,y}$ and if $e_{x,y} \in E$ then these two vertices x and y are called adjacent vertices. We may represent the group of all vertices adjacent to a particular vertex u by $\aleph(u)$. Another aspect that we may come across is edges having particular weights that are some real values, we may represent it as $w(e)$ where $e \in E$. As per the requirement of the topic, we can consider the weight value as measure of attraction or length of the link among two vertices. To consider weight value as attraction measure, we take two vertices that are adjacent to each other and bound very closely if the weight value is more. Moreover, to consider the edge value as length value we check the bond between the adjacent vertices to be as much low as possible. A path of graph G is an alternating sequence of vertices and edges, $\mu = e_1 v_1 e_2 v_2 \ldots e_n v_n$ for all $n \in [1, k-1]$. Also, two vertices x and y are connected in a graph G if and only if $\exists$ a unique path between them starting at x and ending at y. The link between two vertices x and y in G may be represented by x~y in G. If every pair of vertices in a graph is connected, then we may say that graph is connected else it is disconnected. (G. Cheung, E. Magli et al. 2018)

If we have two graphs G and K then K is called as a sub graph of G if and only if $V(K) \subseteq V(G)$ and $E(K) \subseteq E(G)$. Also, if K is a connected subgraph of G and x~y in G for x belongs to K and y does not belong to K then we say that K is a connected component of the graph G shown in Figure 3.

Figure 3. 4x4 pixel in 2D, 4-connected graph showing pixel adjacency and 8-connected graph showing pixel adjacency

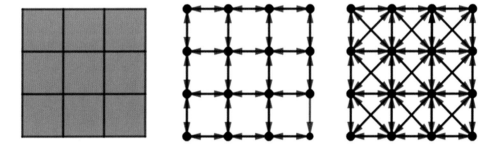

As stated earlier in image processing method using graphs, we function using the adjacency graphs of pixel which includes the set of vertices as set elements of the image and edge set is mostly based on the relation of these elements of image. Generally, we may define edge set E as for pairs of vertices x and y such that:

$$\Delta(x, y) \leq \varnothing \qquad (1)$$

Where Δ is the distance between x and y vertices and $\varnothing$ is some constant. This relation was given by Euclid and is termed as the Euclidean relation of adjacency. While dealing with two dimensional images, pixels are tested in a regular network of Cartesian form with $\varnothing = 1$ and obtaining a connected graph of size 4 and $\varnothing = \sqrt{2}$ gives connected graph of size 8. Whereas in three-dimensional image $\varnothing = 1$ and obtaining a connected graph of size 6 and $\varnothing = \sqrt{3}$ gives connected graph of size 26. This has been shown in the Figure 4 below: (J. Mu et al. 2018)

Figure 4. 3x3x3 voxel volume image, 6-connected graph showing v0xel adjacency

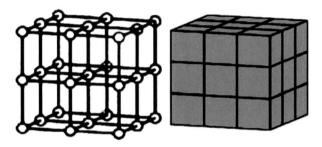

The weights of the edges in an adjacency graph with pixels are mostly selected in order to indicate the content in the image. However, it may or may not be built on ideas of changes in strength or some other aspect underlying in between the elements of image that are adjacent to each other. Sometimes graph structures may also be studied on ideas other than those related to pixel of adjacent graphs. For the segmentation purpose, an image taken is characterised as a graph and the partitioning is what mainly used for breaking up of these graphs into many distinct components that are connected. Vertex labelling or graph cut is the form of representation after undertaking partitioning of a graph. Both these forms of representation are interrelated and opting any one form is only based of choice. Casually, a graph is said to have a vertex labelling if every vertex of the graph is linked to some part of the other set having labels. This set contains vertices indicating some class of object or the background. Similarly, a cut is defined as a set of edges which in case detached from the graph, results in splits of the graph into two or more components that are connected. (B. Chaudhuri et al. 2018)

REGION SEPARATION

In an image a group of connected pixels having similar characteristics is usually termed as a region. The image, object and region are interconnected due to the fact that there may be several objects in an image and several regions in an object that tallies with various portions of the object. To have a proper interpretation and analysis of an image, a proper partitioning of it into objects or its parts is a necessary task. Since there are possibilities of errors during the segmentation, the communication between regions and objects may not be perfect therefore towards the end of interpretation methods precise knowledge of the object is taken into account. The most important step in image segmentation is to patent the different regions of different objects clearly which achieved by image partitioning thorough the characterisation of the gray value of the pixel in an image. We know that gray values are the values given to the elements array that an image is made up of. In an image array, the pixels or gray values are the observations of that particular index and qualities like the membership of a region are resultant of gray values. (B. Chaudhuri et al. 2018)

The two methods of image partitioning are segmentation on the basis of region and using edge detection method for boundary approximation. The main idea in the segmentation of an image on the basis of region is grouping the pixels of a corresponding object and then marking them to show their similarity in regards of their region. This is called the segmentation process. Similarity between the pixels and their three-dimensional closeness are the two most important aspects of this process which can be achieved by checking the modifications in the gray value in a region and firmness in the region respectively. However, these tasks may not reliable for all types of images. Hence, we can opt for other segmentation techniques that include grouping the pixels and then matching them on the basis of knowledge of their domain. Thresholding and labelling methods are quite convenient to use in most of the simple situations. The method segmentation of an image obtained by partitioning an image into pixel lying near the boundary region considers the adjacent pixels as edges. These edge pixels on the boundary and adjacent neighbours on the other side may have varying gray values and this difference is used to find the region boundary. The principle is that both segmentation on the basis of region and edge detection method should provide identical outcomes. Extracting out the regions can also be done using algorithms like region filling algorithm but over the year region segmentation and edge detection method has been the most effective one.

Let us consider the set of pixels in an image as *I* and a homogeneity predicate as P. We find a partition set *S* of this set *I* in n number of regions R_j.

$$\bigcup_{j=1}^{n} R_j = I \tag{2}$$

The homogeneity predicated and partition of the image set has the property as:

$$P(R_j) = \text{True} \tag{3}$$

And that two regions that are adjacent cannot be merged into one:

$$P\left(R_j \bigcup R_k\right) = False \tag{4}$$

The gray value image conversion into binary image is best partition method in the image segmentation process. Thresholding algorithms to obtain binary image can X. Chen and L. Pan, be simplified into a greater number of levels. The approach for the algorithms should not be directly from the gray value but from the knowledge-based facts of its characters. (X. Chen and L. Pan et al. 2018)

SIMILAR INDEX VALUE IDENTIFICATION

Although many techniques and algorithms have been provided already for the segmentation of an image but they can prove to be very tedious at times when the image is complex. Hence an easier way of computing this could be beneficial for our work. The similarity between segments of an image can be put to use to derive a mathematical method their computation. We denote this similarity index as η denotes the relationship between the pixel and its neighbourhood that describes the similarity in relationship for each pixel and its neighbour. The division of the range of η into various sub ranges in order to categorise those pixels that have same region. The output after segmentizing an image is usually in the system of a set of regions that as a whole is the complete image or may be as a set curve pulled out from the image. Some characteristics for example colour, strength or quality of each of the pixels in a region is alike while adjacent regions may have distinctive dissimilarity. In order to have a clear view of the similarity or dissimilarity of pixels it is highly recommended to have proper measure that would automatically segment the image shown in Figure 5.

Figure 5. Graph cuts and labelling

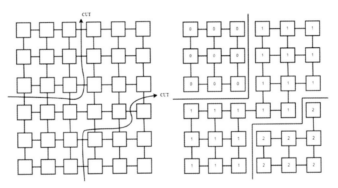

One of such ways of determination could be the approach from local intensity value. However, this may have the limitation of considering only a few numbers of points, too many pixels having similar intensity value, sensitivity to noise or light etc. Hence, it is the need of the hour to have a better and reliable approach for this task. Comparison between central pixel and neighbouring locals could be of help.

Let us consider the following 5x5 pixel window.

Box 1.

$Z_{2,-2}$	$Z_{2,-1}$	$Z_{2,0}$	$Z_{2,1}$	$Z_{2,2}$
$Z_{1,-2}$	$Z_{1,-1}$	$Z_{1,0}$	$Z_{1,1}$	$Z_{1,2}$
$Z_{0,-2}$	$Z_{0,-1}$	$Z_{0,0}$	$Z_{0,1}$	$Z_{0,2}$
$Z_{1,-2}$	$Z_{1,-1}$	$Z_{1,0}$	$Z_{1,1}$	$Z_{1,2}$
$Z_{2,-2}$	$Z_{2,-1}$	$Z_{2,0}$	$Z_{2,1}$	$Z_{2,2}$

The task is to obtain the similarity index η of the central pixel $z_{0,0}$ and its neighbouring pixels as follows:

$$\eta = \frac{f(\theta)}{f(z_{0,0})} \tag{5}$$

where $f(z_{0,0})$ is the gray level intensity of the pixel $z_{0,0}$ and $f(\theta)$ is the weighted mean value of the neighbourhoods of the central pixel $z_{0,0}$ that can be given as below:

$$f(\theta) = \frac{\sum_{j=1,k=1}^{5,5} \phi_{jk} f(x_{jk})}{\sum_{j=1,k=1}^{5,5} \phi_{jk}} \tag{6}$$

Here, ϕ_{jk} is a certain constant.

In equation (1) if $f(z_{0,0})=0$ then it may be adapted as:

$$\eta = \frac{f(\theta)}{f(z_{0,0})+1} \tag{7}$$

In order to consider small gaps or errors that may arise we can add a constant say A as well such as:

$$\eta = \frac{f(\theta)-A}{f(z_{0,0})+1} \tag{8}$$

This value of η considers the difference between level of similarity by compassion between central pixel and its neighbouring pixels. Our approach of image segmentation is through the idea of finding such similarities or dissimilarities of pixels in the same regions on the basis of colour, light, quality or other alike factors.

MINIMAL SPANNING TREE BASED METHOD

The method of segmentation by considering a spanning tree which is minimal or in short *MST* is a very common concept in the ground of graph theory where the tree considered as tree that is spanning of a graph G is defined by $T=(V,E^*)$ and $E^* \subseteq E$. A graph G may possess many different trees that are spanning trees and among these spanning trees the minimal spanning tree is the one that has the least weights among all the spanning trees[13,20]. Many different algorithms are available to find the MST and one very common example is the Prim's Algorithm where iterations of boundary edges are repeated having the least weight of edge. Image Segmentations that are built on the basics of MST are usually connected to clustering methods in graph theory. In this method outcomes after applying the MST are in the form of an adjacency graphs in undirected form. A neighbourhood system is provided and edges with weights are given between two neighbours are presented only if they satisfy the given neighbourhood law. Then, the removal of edges is carried out to obtain selective common subgraphs to complete the clustering. The gestalt principles of similarity in between vertices of a graph are what mainly concentrated on by this clustering process. In the initial days, the image segmentation taken up under MST was fully based on the intrinsic connection of MST as well as cluster form. The base of this connection instinctively lies in the fact that MST contains edges of spanning trees with minimal sum of weights and approves the link of the vertices having most similarity to each other. Further, the MST binds these vertices as well as moves through the tiny dissimilarities between various clusters. This task highly time taking and complicated when it comes to those clusters having large variations inside it. In real world complex picture, many a times the insight of valid clusters having different densities so it is usually expected to take into account the different between two clusters as well as inside a cluster. The MST based segmentation taken into consideration the gestalt law but there lacks exact computation of the definition for quantitative results. Partitioning images hierarchically using MST gives us subdivision in different balances grounded on the rule that maximum alike pixel must remain combined in ordered manner and those not similar should be kept apart. Agraph having partitions with the greatest change between nearby sub-graphs are created by breaking the MST at the maximum weights of edge. Improvements to MST-based algorithms, such as the recursive MST method, have also been proposed. Subdivision is created by partition of one graph parts in each iteration. As a result, the method can result in a final division with a predetermined number of sub-graphs. The method appears to be inefficient in this form.

A new MST-based method has been presented that takes advantage of both differences between sub-graphs and alterations within a sub-graph. The division is combined with a section amalgamation procedure to obtain consequences that meet certain total properties. Adaptive thresholding is the main to this procedure's success. Unlike single linkage clustering, where the threshold is set by a constant A, the threshold here is flexible and depends on the size of the clusters. If the connectivity between two components is lesser than the greatest edge in also of the sections' MST plus this verge, they can be merged. The merging criterion's formal definition is:

$$|e'| = \min\left(Int\left(B_1\right) + \frac{A}{|B_1|}, Int\left(B_2\right)\frac{A}{|B_2|} \right) \tag{9}$$

where A is the constant, $|B_1|$ and $|B_2|$ are sizes of components B_1 and B_2. The Int (B) is the highest edge width in the MST of B. $|e'|$ is the edge of lowest weight value connecting components B_1 and B_2.

The method is delicate to edges in flat areas and less delicate to places with substantial inconsistency, as shown by this equation. The segmentation results produced with this technique are shown in Figure 2. The two photos have regions with considerable variances or varying levels of information, yet the segmentation results keep the majority of perceptually relevant structures without biasing the size of regions. We can see from the explanation above that MST-based algorithms clearly specify cluster structures in the background of graphs with edge weights. These procedures can naturally organise pixels articulated by subordinate properties like strength, colour, or surface. The algorithms, on the other hand, are heavily reliant on the premise that labelling of pixels within the similar section is reliable. When pixels fit in to multiple article programs, this isn't always the case. As a result, this class of algorithms is frequently utilised as a starting point for further high-level applications. MST frequently creates a division by breaking it at the maximum weight of edges, allowing for the creation of a second region by cutting the tree again. This means that MST uses hierarchical segmentation, which allows any over-segmentation to be converted into higher-level counterparts without losing the cluster feature (P. Salembier et al. 2019). Figure 6 shows Output with Minimal Spanning Tree Based Method.

Figure 6. Output with minimal spanning tree based method

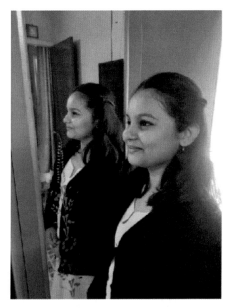
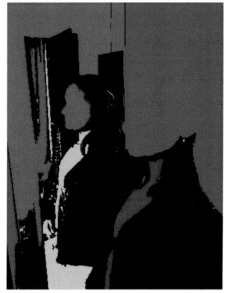
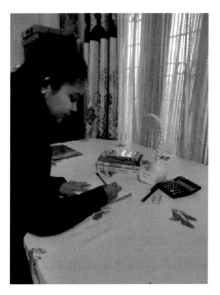
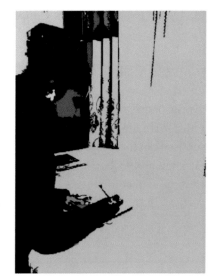

GRAPH WITH COST FUNCTIONS

Minimal Cost Methods

In 1990, Wu and Leahy proposed using cut of graphs for picture subdivision for the primary time. Graph cut, like MST, is a concept that is clearly well-defined on a graph with edge weight. Graph cut built approaches are distinct from earlier approaches in that they give a broad basis for ideal splitting the graph altogether. This has the benefit of allowing multiple cost functions to be defined for different applications using a pure specification of sectioned objects. The graph cut in the preceding equation allows us to define graph partitioning in a straightforward and relevant way: reduction of the cut makes vertices in distinct sets unlike. However, in order to solve a real-world graph divisor problem, vertices in the identical set must be comparable. Existing graph cut approaches investigate these two constraints, attempting to meet one or both of them.

Wu and Leahy minimised a cost function, minimal cut, that was defined exactly in the manner of the equation above. The greatest flow between two vertices is same as the value of the least cut of s/t, which can be computed proficiently, according to the Ford–Fulkerson theorem. Many writers have also described a more general scenario in which the Gomory–Hu technique is used to identify a $\Bbbk$ -partition of graph G, which is equivalent to "identifying the greatest flow between $\Bbbk$ -pairs of vertices". Let us consider two vertices x and y such that *x~y* in G that is ∃ more than one or at least one path in G starting from x ending at y. We consider a function which allocates a value say cost to each and every path of the graph. In these paths we consider at least one path for which the we assign a value is the minimal. We try to find the least cost path values existing between the various sets of vertices. The minimum cost value of the path may be considered as remoteness of the linkage between the various sets of vertices. This concept is of high value in many fields of research. In cases where the graphs used practically in image processing, total number of links between each pair is rather huge and the solution searching process for an optimal solution may be very tiresome. Hence, we have existing algorithms for this purpose. (W. Huang et al. 2019)

Method of Normalized Cut

The slight cut idea is instinctive for illustrating the gestalt principle; yet, the situation favours small components. To solve this difficulty, consider requiring that each separate set be "fairly huge". Numerous studies have been carried out to lecture this issue, resulting in a variety of normalised objective functions.

Shi offer a well-known objective function in terms of normalised cut to prevent this artificial bias (Ncut). The total weight considered over thevol (.)is the entire link from vertices in a set (e.g., A) to entire set of the vertices in the graph, are used to calculate the graph cut. Figure 7 shows Output with Normalized Cut.

Figure 7. Output with normalized cut

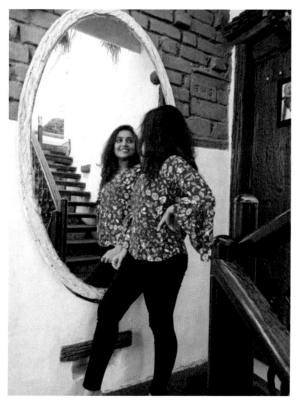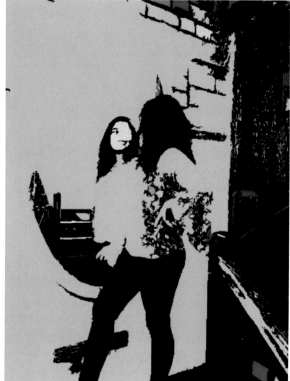

Officially, we represent $vol(A) = \sum_{v_i \in A, v_j \in V} w(v_i, v_j)$ where $w(v_i, v_j)$ represents the weights for firm image quantity amongst binary vertices linked by an edge. The we can define Ncut cost function as:

$$Ncut(A,B) = \frac{cut(A,B)}{vol(A)} + \frac{cut(A,B)}{vol(B)} \tag{10}$$

$$Ncut(A,B) = \frac{\sum_{(x_i > 0, x_j < 0)} -w(v_i, v_j) x_i x_j}{\sum_{x_i > 0} d_i} + \frac{\sum_{(x_i \langle 0, x_j \rangle 0)} -w(v_i, v_j) x_i x_j}{\sum_{x_i < 0} d_i} \tag{11}$$

where x_i is the pointer variable. We have $x_i = 1$ if vertex v_i is in A and $x_i = -1$ if not. Also, $d_i = \sum_j w(v_i, v_j)$ shows the total number of connections from v_i to all the other vertices. As a matter of fact, the above definition instructs that the partitions having set vertices that are smaller in size would not possess value of Ncut that are small which implies that the least cut prejudice is avoided. The value of minimization in above equation can be presented as a general eigen value problem which is a very commonly studied concept in graph theory dealing with spectral analysis. Rewriting the Ncut problem taking into account its matrix transformation, we have

$$\min Ncut(A, B) = \min_z \frac{z^T (D - W) z}{z^T D z} \tag{12}$$

with respect to $z(i) \in \{1, -b\}, b = \sum_{x_i > 0} d_i / \sum_{x_i < 0} d_i$ and $z^T D 1 = 0$ where D represents the degree matrix and W represents adjacency matrices of G. Also, we may obtain the Laplacian of G given by relating these two matrices as: $L = D - W$. Here, $-b$ is the fraction of links from vertex v_i to other vertices internally located and externally located of the same set. The easier version of optimizing the equation is by removing the distinctness and allowing z to take random values from real numbers. Rayleigh-Ritz proved that the eigenvectors that are consistent to the next least overall eigenvalue of a matrix of L is the required solution in actual values to this stress-free form of the equation. Applying a common thresholding method on these eigenvectors gives us the segmentation of the graph. Another method to find the partitions with multiple classes may be obtained by a process of iteration of bipartition on the graph until the required stage of solution is obtained. The problems exist not only in segmenting the image but also in clustering of graphs usually called as graph cut. Few of the cut functions including ratio cut or Min-Max cut problems gives us variety of graphs in Laplacian form in clustering process. Such methods are a solution to minimal cut principle thus giving a stable partitioning. Another type clustering idea is by spectral method that usually out does all other existing methods due to efficiency and simplification in concepts. Some approaches have been given on image segmentation by combining the internal and border area information. The fraction of the cost of outer boundary and internal ideas are reduced by some graph partition algorithms.

Furthermore, there exists some the cases where the internal and border area information arecombined and ratio of outer border cost and inner profit is reduced with the help of partitions to present an algorithm. Let G is the graph with a directed path say P and this path is a cycle beginning and end at the same vertex say u. Then, the cost of this path cost($\mathcal{P}$) defined the total distance of the border area and mass, weight($\mathcal{P}$) shows the rate of a piece of the area. We may define the graph cut cost function as:

$$Region(A, B) = \frac{cost(\mathcal{P})}{weight(\mathcal{P})} \tag{13}$$

Also, the mean cut defines the weight on the edge of a graph and accordingly formulated as:

$$MeanCut(A, B) = \frac{cut(A, B|weight(x, y))}{cut(A, B \mid 1)} \tag{14}$$

Here, *cut(A,B|weight(x,y))* is the cut *(A,B)* with respect to weight of x and y and *cut(A,B|1)* defines *cut(A,B)* compared to the edge weights value 1.

The ratio cut gives the region cuts due to iterative segmentations and formulated as:

$$RatioCut(A,B) = \frac{cut_1(A,B)}{cut_2(A,B)} \tag{15}$$

IMPROVISED NORMAL CUTS METHOD

The improvisation in the normalised cuts methods is in terms of processing of the colour images. The given image or picture is represented in the form of a graph that has weights replacing points by vertices. These weights are representations of edges in the graph that has alike measures for example as that of distance between two points evaluated by some system of measurement. In some of the methods we consider every collection and pick every element from them which in turn is expected to be broken into clusters that associates with the vertex of the graph. Moreover, each pair of vertices are formed by a fraction of edges and weights that resembles a degree of similar elements. Next the edges in the graph are cut in a way such that all the associated elements come under one set. For a supreme condition, the coefficients of the edges having weights in the components internally must be bigger with respect to the coefficients of associating edges. A cluster is obtained from every component and weight coefficients generally measures the similarity criteria which may be an approach through colour or intensity. The basic idea for this method is that we break or cut associated components such that for individual group the cutting cost is much lower when equated to the common similarity criteria.

Let us consider a weighted graph V having components A and B. Then, formula may be presented as:

$$Ncut(A,B) = \frac{cut(A,B)}{associate(A,V)} + \frac{cut(A,B)}{associated(B,V)} \tag{16}$$

$$Ncut(A,B) = 2 - \left(\frac{associate(A,A)}{associate(A,V)} + \frac{associate(B,B)}{associated(B,V)} \right) \tag{17}$$

Here cut(A,B) represents the total of weighted amounts of edges for graph V such that one of the endpoints is in A and next is B and associate(A,V) is sum total of the weighting amounts:

$$cut(A,B) = \sum_{u \in A, v \in B} w(u,v)$$

$$associate(A,V) = \sum_{u \in A, t \in B} w(u,t) \tag{18}$$

In case, where the cut of the components obtained is having smaller edges with lower weight amounts then this parameter is smaller. Now we obtain the minimization to this problem as below:

$$min_x Ncut(x) = \left(\frac{min_z(z^T)(D-W)z}{(z^T)(D)} \right) \tag{19}$$

With the help of the conditions $z(i) \in \{1, -b\}, b = \sum_{x_i>0} d_i / \sum_{x_i<0} d_i$ and $z^T D1=0$ and x as the vector of indication. Here, we have $x_i=1$ if the given vertex is inside of A and otherwise it is taken as -1. As usual W is the matrix of weights $W(i,j)=w(i,j)$ and D is the matrix of diagonals.

$$b = \frac{\sum_{x_i>0} d_i}{\sum_{x_i<0} d_i} \tag{20}$$

In conditions where, $y \in \Re$ where $\Re$ is Rayleigh Quotient then the equation reduces to an eigenvalue problem:

$$(D - W)_z = \lambda D_z \tag{21}$$

Summarizing the steps according to the above three equations:

1. Firstly, in a precise manner mention the graph and its matrix of weights for the given image.
2. The smallest eigen value vectors are solved in the second and third equation.
3. If itis required, we may break the areas into small sub parts of regions in a recursive manner. We then check for the existence of borderline or boundary line in every pair of pixels. In conditions where there is boundaries present, the strength is same as that of the gradient of image which may be used in calculation of coefficient of weights of the boundary

$$w_{edge} = \frac{-f^2}{e^{2\sigma^2}} \tag{22}$$

where σ symbolises 10% the strength of the boundary.

The factor of weight is given by,

$$w = w_{edge} w_{colour} \tag{23}$$

Here the closeness in the shades is used for identification as the vital alterations in the shades show the variation of items. Such shades present also in the smaller parts of the given image. If the alterations are highly noticeable in the shades, then, the factor of weights is increased by a factor of 0.01.Following table 2 has comparative study of types of cuts.

Table 2. Comparative study of types of cuts

Type of cuts	Formulation	Area considered
Minimal cut	$$Mincut(A,B) = \sum_{u \in A, v \in B} weight(u,v)$$	Areas with shorter boundary
Ncut	$$Ncut(A,B) = \frac{\sum_{(x_i > 0, x_j < 0)} - w(v_i, v_j) x_i x_j}{\sum_{x_i > 0} d_i} + \frac{\sum_{(x_i \langle 0, x_j \rangle 0)} - w(v_i, v_j) x_i x_j}{\sum_{x_i < 0} d_i}$$	Partitions with equal weights
Region	$$Region(A,B) = \frac{cost(\mathcal{P})}{weight(\mathcal{P})}$$	Boundary with smooth surface
Mean Cut	$$MeanCut(A,B) = \frac{cut(A,B|weight(x,y))}{cur(A,B\,|\,1)}$$	Overall area
Ratio cut	$$RatioCut(A,B) = \frac{cut_1(A,B)}{cut_2(A,B)}$$	Overall area

METHOD OF GRAPH CUTS

The method of cuts of graph in obtaining the interactive image segmentation is one of the vastly used techniques in current years. The main aim of this technique is to obtain an item with lesser amount of connectivity between users. Although many methods are available but there is still scope for some additional ideas for achieving a perfectly segmented image. Graph cut method one such idea that gains a lot of priority in this field. This method is useful due to the fact that it helps in reduction of energy function that contains the data which are generally obtained using colouring possibilities in internal and external area and a three-dimensional coherence as well. The three-dimensional coherent terms used is the extent of the borderline that is controlled using the distinction in image. Hence the minimization or reduction of energy with this gain more partiality in terms of short borderline. This occurrence is sometimes refereed to as the "shrinking bias". It may not be wrong to state that by the Graph cut methods it may be complex to obtain segmentations of image having sleek and extended structures(Z. Tang et al. 2018).

In graph theoretical approach, we may state that the graph cut helps in obtaining the grade of variation between two parts or components. A cut of a graph is the set of edges that is subdivided into two disjoint sets X and Y. This gives us the segmentation in terms of graph cuts the value of which may be given as:

$$Cut(x,y) = \sum_{x \in X, y \in Y} w(x,y) \tag{24}$$

Here, x and y are the vertices that belongs to the two components of X and Y. This presents the algorithm of segmentation for the given framework which is autonomous to the characters used and boosts the precision and firmness depending on the parameters of various images taken into consideration. The task in such a partitioning of graphs is to select such a subset of the original set of vertices in way that these subsets undertake only those spanning edges that is minimal and also abides by a particular cardinality condition. The applications of graph partitions into sets can been seen in various fields like solution of linear systems including sparse matrix, parallel processing as well as VLSI design of circuit and image segmentation.

Figure 8. Graph

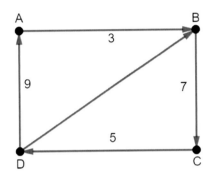

Above Figure graph shows:

1. the vertices A, B,C and D which are the nodes,
2. edges are links between two vertices with direction,
3. the path is sequence of vertices linked by edges
4. Cycle or Loop: A-B-C-D-A
5. Length of path
6. Diameter length of largest path.

CONCLUSION

Graph based image segmentation is the most commonly used method for image segmentation due to the advantage that it gives the clearest arrangement of the elements of the image into mathematically strong format and aids the construction of problems that are efficiently computable. In the recent years, many practical applications in fields like medical analysis, video observations and image extraction have been thoroughly advantaged by this particular method of segmentation. The use of image processing in medical field is generally for the extraction of a particular tissue or organ that is to be studied. Even though today there are numerous methods formulated specifically for medical image partitioning but the method of graph cut on s/t models provides both region and borderline information. This enables to have a collaborative supervision from the operator without any initialization of past prototype of objects. Hence, this makes the graph cut based method as the most approved among all other method in medical field. Expressing the problems through graphs gives a spontaneous system for obtaining solutions with strong mathematical base. Partitioning of medical elements is done by extractions of outlines as paths having shortest lengths on the weighted graphs. For the better integration of object-based ideas and highly accurate segmentation the user interface method is vigorously taken up. Dijkstra's algorithm is used to obtain all accessible paths having minimum cost from one point to all other points in the image in live-wire method of image segmentation. After these methods got popularised, several proposals were made for improvement of regarding alterations such as the live lanes and live wires of the fly which would minimize the search area among graph categories. Modifications made for live wire in the form of three-dimensional medical image analysis and some cross methods that uses combinations of graphs for theoretical approach are also available in many articles. Contour models have also evolved for contour withdrawal from two end points by finding the paths of the least length of graphs having weights. Moreover, outlines of proofs producing the results for the discovery of boundary in a model of contour is correspondent with the Riemann space least distance calculation. Integrations of past knowledge of space has also been studied vastly for the shape models of statistics or global shape of study. These graph methods give the least path problem solutions more correct manner unlike those obtained by approximating the values by solving the partial differential equations in such contour models. By the use of aptly defined graphs in these methods, the computational preciseness and time for searching are suitable for the medical requests.

REFERENCES

Ahmed, S. (2012). Applications of Graph Coloring in Modern Computer Science. *International Journal of Computer and Information Technology*, *3*(2), 1–7.

Allani, O., Zghal, H. B., Mellouli, N., & Akdag, H. (2016). A knowledge-based image retrieval system integrating semantic and visual features. *Procedia Computer Science*, *96*, 1428–1436.

An, J., Zhang, X., Zhou, H., Feng, J., & Jiao, L. (2018, July). Patch Tensor-Based Sparse and Low-Rank Graph for Hyperspectral Images Dimensionality Reduction. *IEEE Journal of Selected Topics in Applied Earth Observations and Remote Sensing*, *11*(7), 2513–2527. doi:10.1109/JSTARS.2018.2833886

Benchamardimath, B., & Hegadi, R. (2012). *Graph Theoretical Approaches for Image Segmentation*. Academic Press.

Bin, X., Jiajun, B., Chen, C., Wang, C., Cai, D., & He, X. (2013). EMR: A scalable graph-based ranking model for content-based image retrieval. *IEEE Transactions on Knowledge and Data Engineering*, *27*(1), 102–114.

Boykov, Y., & Funka-Lea, G. (2006). Graph Cuts and Efficient N-D Image Segmentation. *International Journal of Computer Vision*, *70*, 109–131. https://doi.org/10.1007/s11263-006-7934-5

Chaudhuri, B., Demir, B., Chaudhuri, S., & Bruzzone, L. (2018, February). Multilabel Remote Sensing Image Retrieval Using a Semisupervised Graph-Theoretic Method. *IEEE Transactions on Geoscience and Remote Sensing*, *56*(2), 1144–1158. doi:10.1109/TGRS.2017.2760909

Chen, X., & Pan, L. (2018). A Survey of Graph Cuts/Graph Search Based Medical Image Segmentation. *IEEE Reviews in Biomedical Engineering*, *11*, 112–124. doi:10.1109/RBME.2018.2798701 PMID:29994356

Cheung, G., Magli, E., Tanaka, Y., & Ng, M. K. (2018, May). Graph Spectral Image Processing. *Proceedings of the IEEE*, *106*(5), 907–930. doi:10.1109/JPROC.2018.2799702

Dickinson, S., Pelillo, M., & Zabih, R. (2001). Introduction to the special section on graph algorithms in computer vision. Pattern Analysis and Machine Intelligence. *IEEE Transactions on.*, *23*, 1049–1052. doi:10.1109/TPAMI.2001.954597

Fracastoro, G., Thanou, D., & Frossard, P. (2020). Graph Transform Optimization with Application to Image Compression. *IEEE Transactions on Image Processing*, *29*, 419–432. doi:10.1109/TIP.2019.2932853 PMID:31403414

Gowda, & Shashidhara, Ramesha, & Kumar. (2021). Recent advances in graph theory and its applications. *Advances in Mathematics: Scientific Journal.*, *10*, 1407–1412. doi:10.37418/amsj.10.3.29

Hernández-Gracidas, C., & Enrique Sucar, L., & Montes-y Gómez, M. (2009). Modeling spatial relations for image retrieval by conceptual graphs. *Proceedings of the First Chilean Workshop on Pattern Recognition.*

Huang, W., Bolton, T. A. W., Medaglia, J. D., Bassett, D. S., Ribeiro, A., & Van De Ville, D. (2018, May). A Graph Signal Processing Perspective on Functional Brain Imaging. *Proceedings of the IEEE*, *106*(5), 868–885. doi:10.1109/JPROC.2018.2798928

Li, C.-Y., & Hsu, C.-T. (2008). Image retrieval with relevance feedback based on graph-theoretic region correspondence estimation. *IEEE Transactions on Multimedia*, *10*(3), 447–456.

Li, M., Wang, X., Gao, K., & Zhang, S. (2017). A Survey on Information Diffusion in Online Social Networks. *Models and Methods. Information*, *8*, 118.

Majeed, A., & Rauf, I. (2020). Graph Theory: A Comprehensive Survey about Graph Theory Applications in Computer Science and Social Networks. *Inventions, 5*, 10. doi:10.3390/inventions5010010

Malmberg, F., Lindblad, J., Sladoje, N., & Nyström, I. (2010). A graph-based framework for subpixel image segmentation. *Theoretical Computer Science*. Advance online publication. doi:10.1016/j.tcs.2010.11.030

Mu, J., Xiong, R., Fan, X., Liu, D., Wu, F., & Gao, W. (2020). Graph-Based Non-Convex Low-Rank Regularization for Image Compression Artifact Reduction. *IEEE Transactions on Image Processing*, *29*, 5374–5385. doi:10.1109/TIP.2020.2975931 PMID:32149688

Pranav, P., & Chirag, P. (2013, December). Various Graphs and Their Applications in Real World. *International Journal of Engineering Research & Technology (Ahmedabad)*, *2*(12).

Rajan, M. A., Girish Chandra, M., & Lokanatha, C. (2008). Concepts of Graph Theory Relevant to Ad-hoc Networks. *International Journal of Computers, Communications & Control*, *3*, 465–469.

Salembier, P., & Garrido, L. (2000). Binary Partition Tree as an Efficient Representation for Image Processing, Segmentation, and Information Retrieval. *IEEE Transactions on Image Processing*, *9*, 561–576.

Salembier, P., Liesegang, S., & López-Martínez, C. (2019, May). Ship Detection in SAR Images Based on Maxtree Representation and Graph Signal Processing. *IEEE Transactions on Geoscience and Remote Sensing*, *57*(5), 2709–2724. doi:10.1109/TGRS.2018.2876603

Sanchez, V., & Hernández-Cabronero, M. (2018, October). Graph-Based Rate Control in Pathology Imaging with Lossless Region of Interest Coding. *IEEE Transactions on Medical Imaging*, *37*(10), 2211–2223. doi:10.1109/TMI.2018.2824819 PMID:29993629

Shi, J., & Malik, J. (2000). Normalized cuts and image segmentation. *IEEE Transactions on Pattern Analysis and Machine Intelligence*, *22*, 888–905.

Shrinivas, Vetrivel, Santhakumaran, & Elango. (2010). Applications of graph theory in computer science an overview. *International Journal of Engineering Science and Technology*, 2.

Sravanthi, K. (2014). Applications of Graph Labeling in Communication Networks. *Oriental Journal of Computer Science and Technology*, *7*(1), 139–145.

Tang, Z., Yap, P.-T., & Shen, D. (2019, August). A New Image Similarity Metric for Improving Deformation Consistency in Graph-Based Groupwise Image Registration. *IEEE Transactions on Biomedical Engineering*, *66*(8), 2192–2199. doi:10.1109/TBME.2018.2885436 PMID:30530309

Tosuni, B. (2015). Graph Theory in Computer Science - An Overview. *International Journal of Academic Research and Reflection*, *3*(4).

Xu & Uberbacher. (1997). 2D image segmentation using minimum spanning trees. *Image and Vision Computing*, *15*, 47-57.

Chapter 4
Applications of Big Data in Smart Health Systems

Darakhshan Syed
Iqra University, Pakistan

Noman Islam
Iqra University, Pakistan

Muhammad Hammad Shabbir
NED University, Pakistan

Syed Babar Manzar
NED University, Pakistan

ABSTRACT

Many government institutions and government organizations are working to adapt smart city concepts and implementation of applications based on data techniques. It would not only streamline the process, but it will have a bigger impact on citizen's lives. The smart city component comprises smart education, health, transportation, energy, environments, finance, and other subdomains alongside these. In recent times, big data analytics has been the driving factor to enhance smart city applications and likewise smart health. Evolution of digitalization has been the primary source of evolving smart health components to another level. This chapter reviews applications of smart health to enhance smart cities and compare challenges, opportunities, and open issues to dig down. This review reveals that there are still many opportunities left for utilizing big data for smart health.

INTRODUCTION

Today's modern epoch is developed on the concept of digitization. Conventional medicine, which has biotechnology at its foundation, has started get digitalized and information-based as science and innovative ideas have advanced. In addition, smart treatment has been developed, embracing a new phase of digital technologies. Smart healthcare is more than just a technical progress; it is a multi-level transformation.

DOI: 10.4018/978-1-6684-4580-8.ch004

Mediatized improvements i.e. from illnesses to patient-centered services), informatization development modifications i.e. from physician to hospital and medical digitalization), changes in treating patients i.e. from public to personalized administration), and improvements in the preventive and therapeutic principle are all examples of this transformation. These developments are focused on addressing people's specific requirements while improve the effectiveness of medical treatment, considerably enhancing the medicinal and health experiences, and representing modern medication's potential development trajectory in the near future.

Smart health has been the main concern over the years for not only one country or continent but for the whole world. Smart health is not only effective for healthcare entities but will also have a huge contribution on the evolvement of smart city(Al Nuaimi, E et al.2015). Government and other non-health care entities can also benefit with this health care model. It's not only about advancement of technology but a combination of many powerful technologies that have emerged as a whole new world in no time. All of these robust technologies along with big data have converted medical science into healthcare science. Things are now expanding from smart healthcare to smart hospitals with digitized systems, automated operations, more powerful equipment, remote patients tracking, advanced training and many more. These changes will also create a huge impact on individual users, doctors, medical authorities, research institutes. Individual users will have quick access to health care without having to wait for the availability of a doctor. Patients have transparency over the process. Doctors on the other hand balance their workload with the help of robotics. Financial documents and supply chain management can be managed using blockchain and have a sheer transparency. Remote tracking of patients can be done with combination of IoT, Big Data and Cloud Computing using wearable devices and transmission of data on cloud servers will be saved and available to doctors on finger tips. Remote treatment and real time care facilities will be available using 5G. Virtual simulation of doctors training and surgery can be done using virtual reality and augmented reality. Robotics has also been playing a huge role in automating predefined tasks and providing food, medicines, taking temperatures etc. to avoid human interaction.

Advancement of technologies has been the main factor behind smart healthcare but it's not being served like a piece of cake. Fig 1 shows the various sources of big data in smart health systems. There are multiple challenges and requirements that need to be overcome. Secure pipelines needed to deploy to tackle hackers attack. Data storage and scalability needs to tackle using Big Data. Predefined systems inclusion in robots to avoid errors and severe problems. Data transparency, data security, knowledge sharing, overpopulation are all the other factors that needed to be dealt with (See Figure 1). This paper has been divided into multiple segments involving all the aspects of smart health. Origin of health care has been explained then all the deriving technologies behind smart health have been explained with possible use cases. Then the next segment describes the benefits and opportunities from smart health to all the entities. In the next section requirements which are prerequisite for implementing smart health has been described. After that this paper focuses on challenges that are being faced by different sectors either individual or composite. In the end this paper concludes smart healthcare. Figure 1 shows Sources of big data in smart health systems

Figure 1. Sources of big data in smart health systems

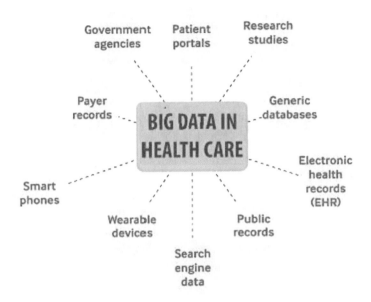

CONCEPT OF SMART HEALTHCARE

The healthcare profession is no longer an outcast, untouched by the wonders of current technology advancements. With technical breakthroughs and the intersection of computer science, electronics, and associated technologies, it is now feasible to develop a smart healthcare system in which all medical organizations are linked and can interact with one another. The present trends in the health industry support this viewpoint. Smart Health care systems are becoming a reality thanks to technology solutions like Artificial Intelligence and Robotics, Machine Learning, Internet of Things and Cloud computing etc. (Tripathi, G et al. 2020). Standard healthcare operations have been transformed into smart medical services as cognitive intelligence technologies, communication services, and the Internet of Medical Things have advanced. Many elderly people do require ongoing virtual care supervision. Intelligent healthcare platforms necessitate the collection, transmission, and manipulation of enormous amounts of multimodal clinical information generated by various detectors and healthcare products, which is difficult and may render some remote patient monitoring technologies impossible. Moving cognitive computing to the edge of network is a potential approach for enabling efficient and comfortable remote management. To allow smart health services with optimal real-time and cost-effective remote patient monitoring, it is critical to implement economical edge-based categorization and data reduction algorithms (Abdellatif, A.A. et al.,2019).

"Smart Planet" proposed by IBM (Armonk, NY, USA) was the driving factor behind smart health care. Smart health care was not the sole proprietor for smart planet. There were other components like smart grid, smart transportation smart energy, smart factory and others etc. (Zeinab, et aL.Elmustafa, 2017). Smart Planet tends to provide enormous benefits and infrastructure that uses modern sensors to get information, process it and advance computers and cloud computing (Martin, J.L et al., 2010). Smart Health care systems can be achieved in many ways and can use wearable devices, IoT, cloud computing, mobile internet, 5G and other mediums in order to connect people, institutions and different entities to make life smarter in an intelligent manner. It also encourages health care related entities to carry out smart health operations in effectible way. Apart from health care entities it also benefited for government and insurance companies to manage health care programs through it. Government welfare agencies can scrutinize financial applications from data provided across the country. Likewise insurance companies can create effective packages for particular disease or for specific age. In short it is a top notch information gathering ecosystem in the medical arena. (Gong, F., et al., 2013).

KEY TECHNOLOGIES OF SMART HEALTHCARE

Lack of technologies and expertise has always been a concern in the health care sector (Tripathi, A.et al.,2018). Indeed technology was still a concern for healthcare professionals until 2018 according to American Medical Association. Lack of visibility in technology was preventing the officials from implementing it in their organizations. Digital technologies will also equalize and stabilize relationships between patients and medical professionals. Consequently these technologies will not only be effective in providing quality treatment but also create room for medical authorities and hospitals to accommodate more applications at a time and provide real time treatment. It will also provide cheaper, inexpensive, real-time and effective solutions for critical disease. By each passing year, health technologies will also be widely used in all aspects of health care. From a patient's perspective they can seek medical help with the help of virtual assistants; Patient's data will be transmitted and analyzed on regular intervals using wearable devices, sensors and other IoT devices. From a doctor's point of view clinical decisions can be made from advanced algorithms using decision support systems, Surgeries can be made through human made robots, From hospitals point of view remote treatments through 5G can make patients' experience more enhanced (Farahani, B. et al., 2018). Frequent use of these technologies will save thousands of lives and better experience for all the entities of the health sector either doctors, patients or hospitals. It will drastically reduce risk of medical procedures and effective utilization of resources and more hassle free processes for patients. From the perspective of scientific research institutions, Manual drug screening can be replaced by machine learning techniques to find suitable subjects with help of big data (Tian, S. et al., 2019).

The Internet of Medical Services is a radical idea that changes the healthcare industry and the variety of medical technologies that use IoT to make more money at some point in the near future. The researcher can track a user's behaviors using data collected with the use of portable, naturally occurring substances, and integrated sensors, mobile characteristics, and gadget user activity. With more information, state-of-the-art as well as AI or Deep Learning (DL)-based algorithms can be used to indicate their health status. To ensure performance improvement, flexibility, and enable non-safety as well as delay-based IoT areas, traditional cloud technology that depends on structures for large data processing for the purpose of evolutionary analysis is used (Mansour, R.F., et al., 2021).

Now the future of health care is shaping in front of us with implementation of digital technologies such as Artificial Intelligence, Virtual Reality, Augmented Reality, Robotics, Nanotechnology, 5G, Cloud Computing, IoT, Blockchain, Big Data etc.Figure 2 shows the key technologies of smart health.

Figure 2. Key technologies of smart health (Hanine, M et al., 2018)

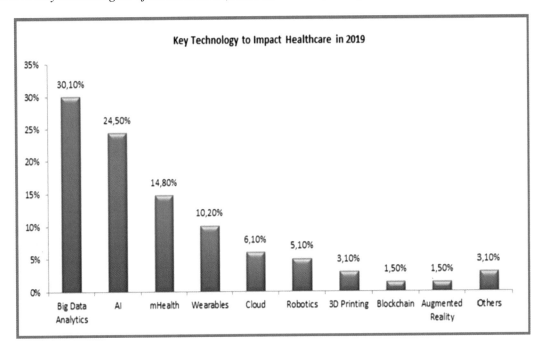

Artificial Intelligence (AI)

AI and associated innovations are becoming more common in economic and social development, and they're starting to show up in healthcare. Many elements of care coordination, as well as administrative operations inside providers, payers, and pharmaceutical companies, could be transformed by these solutions (Davenport, T et al., 2019). AI engines can mitigate risk factors and streamline the life of doctors, patients and hospitals by performing predefined tasks in no time and fraction of a cost. In 2015 it was analyzed that 10% of overall USA death was due to error and incorrect diagnosis of disease. Decision support systems can be made to automate diagnosis of disease. Identify patients at high risk and require immediate treatments.

Apart from robotics AI in healthcare depends vastly on life saving information using mass datasets. Lots of time consuming work can be automated by analyzing data and allows health care tools to perform automated tasks. The most common form of machine learning is predicting medicine treatment like what type of treatment will be suitable to a patient on the basis of various parameters and past records. A handful of studies have already shown that AI can operate as well as or superior than humans at crucial healthcare activities like medical diagnostics. Algorithms are already surpassing radiologists in terms of detecting dangerous tumors and advising investigators on how to build cohorts for expensive clinical trials. However, we anticipate it will be several years before AI surpasses humans in large medical business sectors for a variety of purposes.

Natural language processing mainly refers to communication between computer and humans in terms of voice and text. NLP involves reading on human written language (Gobinda, G.C et al., 2003), precinct human spoken words and translates one language into another. It is mainly based on deep neural networks which is sub domain of machine learning(Dam, S et al., 2018)and in health care it can help automate or aligned clinical reports of the patient (Belgacem, A et al.,2018).

In the early 1980s, knowledge - based systems based on special collections of 'if-then' logic were the leading AI technique, and they were widely exploited economically at the time. They were extensively used in healthcare for 'clinical decision assistance' reasons over the last few decades and are still actively used today. Many electronic medical systems companies now include a set of guidelines with their software.

In addition to AI, Robotic process automation is a type of technology that automates organized technological operations for administrative reasons, such as those incorporating information systems, as though they were performed by a person following a script or set of rules. They are low-cost, simple to program, and explicit in their activities as compared to other methods of AI. Process automation is a term that refers to computer programs running on servers rather than robots. To behave as a semi-intelligent user of information platforms, it uses a combination of procedure, business requirements, and 'presentation layer' connectivity. They're utilized in healthcare to automate procedures including prior authorization, patient information updates, and invoicing. They could be used to retrieve information from, for example, faxed images and feed it into transaction processing systems when paired with other technologies such as image detection.

The most difficult hurdle for AI in many healthcare fields is guaranteeing its acceptance in daily clinical practice, rather than whether the technology will be competent enough to be beneficial. AI systems must be authorized by authorities, incorporated with Electronic health care systems, standardized to the point where products available to work in the same way, presented to doctors, paid for by public or private payer organizations, and modified in the field in the near future in order for general acceptance to occur. These obstacles will be addressed in the end, but it will require more time than the maturation of the technology.

Text Mining

A significant volume of written and quantitative data about individuals, medications, organizational notes, consultations, doctor remarks, and other topics is stored in healthcare management systems. Electronic health records contain data that can help improve healthcare service effectiveness, promote healthcare research, reduce inaccurate clinical diagnosis and treatment plans, and reduce wasteful healthcare spending. However, the difficulty, complexity, and usage of technical vocabulary of the unorganized textual content that hold the health information vary widely, rendering information finding more difficult. A variety of text mining algorithms can help medical professionals take advantage of a once-in-a-lifetime potential to extract absolutely fundamental from textual data repositories (Pramanik, M.I et al., 2017). Clinical technology and health treatment are two frameworks of text mining in healthcare. A variety of text mining techniques are commonly used for research purposes to examine huge numbers of academic papers in published databases and to study the heterogeneity of health and physiological investigations conducted. Since no academic comes across any new patterns or genomes without prior understanding of them, it's very likely that some traits and interconnections between biological entities go unreported in the contemporary literature because pertinent details is dispersed and no scholar has adequately correlated them.

Investigators have only specialized in a few subcategories due to the human brain's limited capability, whereas text mining tools and procedures provide adequate links between many subcategories for uncovering new learning or forming speculations. Numerous investigations have built comprehensive text-mining systems to address biological research and the diverse needs of consumers. The MedScan tool, for example, is an automated text mining tool that can infer correlations between various biomedical domains. TXTGate is another text mining program that uses information from numerous online biological datasets to do gene-based text characterization and grouping. Text mining-based prediction algorithms have additionally been utilized to provide smart healthcare services, allowing predictive models to autonomously code complex data using text mining categorization and functionality.

Virtual Reality (VR)

Virtual reality is a vigorous evolution technology in the health sector. It's regarded as a wide range of computer-based services that allows the user to gaze around and explore within a presumably realistic or physical environmentU.S. In other regards, virtual reality is a digital depiction of real environments that works on the premise that consumers may experience and engage with a virtual world, perceived or actual. In 2018, there were 171 million unique virtual users around the world, up from 200,000 in 2014. Nowadays, the healthcare sector is adopting virtual reality advancements to improve patient care since it allows different innovations to be learnt in a safe setting. Virtual data can now be leveraged to effectively instruct new clinicians, nurses, rescuers, and other healthcare workers in anatomical, pathologies, first aid, and other healthcare responsibilities. It contributes to the development of trustworthiness without incurring any harm. According to PwC experts in UK, virtual and augmented reality might enhance global GDP by 294 billion dollars by supporting development and skills. The rapid adoption of virtual reality has resulted in considerable price reductions as well as the creation of user-friendly, cordless, light, and economical systems. As a result, it's reasonable to believe that virtual reality isn't just a passing craze (Saab, M.M et al., 2021).

Centers for Disease Control and Prevention (CDC) states that opioids should not only be the only treatment for patients affected with chronic non cancer pain (Dowell, D et al. 2016). For more than two decades researchers and medical professionals are working on virtual reality to conquer anxiety disorder, stress, depression(Wiederhold, B.K et al.,2005), stress disorder and patients suffering from non-cancer chronic pain and affected with severe incidents (Wiederhold, B.K et al., 2014). Virtual reality in healthcare is basically a simulation of a screen where sounds, graphics, motion and environment represent the 3D human made environment which allows the human mind to manipulate and feel the existence of the environment (McGrath, J.L et al.,2018).

Virtual simulation not only helps in patients' treatment but can also be more effective in training and assessment of medical professionals. It simulates surgical operations (Schwid, H.A et al., 1999)and replicates the environment for new professionals to better understand the intensity which in result will improve outcomes and enhanced technical abilities (Dalgarno, B et al., 2010). When implementing this technology all the necessary parameters like duration, pace, level of simulation, standardization, level of learner etc. should be considered to ensure effectiveness of training (Lemheney, A.J et al., 2016). Virtual reality is still in the phase of discussion and unexplored methodology. There are many arguments in favor of virtual reality but all of them are on the basis of theory. More research and vast amount of data is needed to carry out virtual reality experiments in order to teach health care professionals (Fertleman, C et al., 2018). Virtual reality solutions in the health sector were characterized as follows by investigators (Javaid, M et al., 2020):

1. Virtual surgery is a term used to describe a procedure that by utilizing virtual 3D renderings, the specialist may successfully schedule the surgery treatment. It provides a better approach for the medical community to communicate, measure, and evaluate the pressure required to perform. It is the most effective way for modelling surgery treatments since it generates a basic visual that aids in better preparation and practice.

2. The operation's preparation Virtual surgeries can save time and minimize danger for specialists in different locations, and it can be accessed digitally. The surgeon employs immersive glasses in a 3D VE to start communicating with the surgical intervention, and this technology can build a detailed visual of the person during the surgery.

3. Virtual Diagnosis also supports, by minimizing the utilization of magnetic resonant image and computerized radiography scans, virtual reality can give effective medical tools for professionals and clinicians to make correct diagnoses. The procedure of gathering patient data for medical evaluation is made easier by the widely recognized symptoms of infection and signs of disease.

4. Physical treatment can also benefit from virtual reality. The way individuals use virtual reality during physical activity may influence to disparities between patients. When it comes to physical activity, VR therapy is more effective. It's a helpful tool in the treatment of burn injuries who aren't in too much agony.

Robotics

Eventually, robotics were developed. In settings like industries and stores, they conduct pre-defined activities such as lifting, moving, welding, or constructing goods, as well as carrying supplies to hospitals and clinics. Gradually, robots have become more interactive with people and are easier to teach by guiding them through a process. Other AI features are being incorporated in their 'brains,' making them quite intelligent. The same advances in cognition that researchers seen in other areas of Artificial intelligence are likely to be implemented into practical robots in the coming future. Automated robotic systems for surgery, which were first allowed in the United States in 2000, give surgeons 'superpowers,' allowing them to see better, make more accurate and least invasive procedures, stitch injuries, and so on. However, experienced human surgeons continue to make important judgments. Gynecologic surgery, prostate surgery, and head and neck surgical intervention are all common surgical treatments that use robotic surgical intervention.

Robotics is one the most exciting and powerful technology that helps in evolving smart health care. In 2019 many experiments had been performed on robot companions (Luo, F., et al., 2018). Some of them consist of microphone, sensors, cameras to interact with their companions and to treat chronic pain, monitor medications, continuous tracking of health stats like temperature, sugar and others. Along with medical treatment they also help patients with their other features like playing music, talking, stories and keeping indulge with many more things(Patel, A.R et al.,2017).

Robotics has also increased its importance in the past one year due to an epidemic that requires minimum human interaction and isolation of humans to prevent this global disease. These robots can do many predefined work and carry out some common tasks like providing medicines, sterilizing, taking temperatures and many more duties that don't require any brain processing and human interaction. This results in minimizing the risk to life for physicians and physicians actively involved in the management of the COVID-19 epidemic. The aim of this study is to shed light on the importance of medical robotics in general and therefore link its application to the COVID-19 management perspective, so that hospital management can respond to the maximum use of robots (Agarwal, R et al., 2020). Robotics are now adopted in medical settings to assist health personnel and improve the quality of care, in addition to surgical units. During the COVID-19 epidemic, medical facilities began using robots for a far broader range of jobs in order to help decrease pathogen direct exposure. It's become evident that health robots' automation savings and risk minimization give benefit in a lot of different disciplines.

Nanotechnology

Nanotechnology is an emerging domain that encompasses a wide range of products originating in electronics, economics, biochemistry, and biologists. Rapid breakthroughs in science and technology have opened up a blooming new sector of nanotechnology, which has created a slew of new options for medical innovations and illness medication in human health care. Technological solutions intended to interface with the body at cellular scales with a high level of reliability are examples of nanotechnology implementations in medicine and biochemistry.

Inventory of consumer products in 2009, 1015 different products were listed, constituting the basis of nanotechnologies produced by 485 companies around the world (Mapetu, J.P.B et al., 2019). Nanotechnology is advanced technology that deals with atoms, molecules and super molecules. It is basically the evolutionary science of the really small has immense possibilities for quality healthcare, including more appropriate drug delivery, faster and more acute illness diagnosis, and vaccine delivery via aerosol particles and patches. It builds nanoparticles and particles, while performing its function in many areas, it is also used to diagnose diseases in the human body. The applications of nanotechnology relate to small devices which process the human body on a subcellular scale (Sahoo, S et al., 2007). Nanotechnology has a huge impact on healthcare and has defined a new era called nanomedicine (Allhoff, F et al., 2009). It has also created security concerns among professionals and the general public. While it is prudent to study the adverse health effects of the manufacture and use of nanomaterials, with adequate guarantees and standards emanating from nanosafety and toxicity studies, there is no reason to doubt the overriding advantage. Provide nanomedicines (Jain, K.K et al., 2008). The EU Nanomedicine Technology Platform (Arulkumar, V et al., 2021)defines nanomedicine as "the realization of the application of advanced nanotechnologies in healthcare".

The fact that the patients' body does not accept the complete therapeutic dose provided is a serious difficulty in medical advances. Scientists can use nanotechnology to confirm that pharmaceuticals are given to various areas of the body with better accuracy, and the drugs can be made so that the primary ingredient penetrates cell membranes more effectively, lowering the desired amount of dosage.

Gene therapy is a relatively new strategy for treating or preventing genetic abnormalities by fixing flawed genes that cause bacterial growth and delivering fixed genetic traits or replacing incorrect and misleading ones (Sahoo, S et al., 2007). Lab - on - chip industry has expanded to include nanotechnology on a chip. When certain nanotechnology particles are used as identifiers or flags, biological examinations assessing the existence or functioning of specific compounds become faster, more accurate, and more versatile. Cardiovascular illnesses are currently the leading cause of death, sickness, and disabilities. As a result of numerous heart disorders, an increasing number of patients are dying. Nowadays, nanotechnology provides a broad framework in the domain of cardiovascular science by providing instruments to investigate cardiac science's frontiers at the cellular level. Cardiovascular disorders can be efficiently treated with nanotechnology-based techniques. Diagnostics, imaging, and biomedical engineering can all benefit from these techniques.

5G Networks

With an expanding variety of remote services, the extremely fast increasing healthcare business demands a strong communications infrastructure to adequately communicate patients, medical practitioners, medical devices, and others for information exchange. The next evolution of wireless communication, 5th Generation (5G) mobile networks, will undoubtedly boost healthcare and revolutionize the direction of healthcare provision.

Virtual health supervision and intelligent health treatment are strengthening and undergoing a dramatic evolution as the invention of a global communication system accelerates. To facilitate modernized health care, we are currently using the advanced long-term evolution (A-LTE) network. Nonetheless, smart hospitals and health care are not yet fully developed all over the world. The fifth generation (5G) network will raise the standard of smart health care. The needs of a smart hospital, on the other hand, will differ from those of other applications like as education, industry, and the general public. With various small devices interconnected with the sensing devices, the smart hospitals will be interconnected 24 hours a day, seven days a week. To put it another way, the future intelligent hospitals will be built on 5G and the IoT, which will improve the system's accessibility and efficiency.

Smart healthcare industry is steadily growing across the world with the help of digitalization in almost all advanced technologies. 5G has a huge impact on smart health care. Around 100 hospitals from all over the world are working on healthcare use cases such as remote group consultation, remote surgery, emergency rescue, intra hospitals monitoring etc.

Japan has a large number of elderly people i.e. around 30% of its total population is aged more than 60. In Europe there are hundreds of thousands immigrate each passing year and to accommodate all of the citizens Europe needs a significant change in their health care sector. Similarly China's current condition is quite even and at the same time they has a fastest growing population and digital healthcare is the key to address these issues with having 5G on top of it (Arulkumar, V et al., 2021).

5G not only offers high bandwidth but also offers low latency and massive connections to deal with various healthcare cases like (Muteeh, A et al., 2021).

1. *Remote group consultation:*5G supports high bandwidth with a maximum of 8K remote group consultations that allows speed sharing and transfer of medical records like images and high definition videos. This will allow medical professionals to conduct remote consultation from wherever they are instead of physically present.
2. *Remote Ultrasound*: Rural areas have lack of hospitals and furthermore they lack in ultrasound physicians and resources and in need of remote ultrasound with no latency. Remote ultrasound can be performed using 5G with a robotic arm controlled by a physician. This can only be done with a 5G as private lines take lots of money and effort in deploying lines remotely in rural areas or islands. On the other hand Wifi is far from being secure for data transmission with no latency
3. *Remote Emergency Rescue:* In general, 5G can transmit real-time patient information tracked by medical equipment and the location of an ambulance, as well as videos of what's going on inside and outside the car. . This allows doctors in hospitals to remotely arrange group calls and consult doctors remotely in an ambulance.

Some prominent cases along with examples are shown below in Figure 3.

Figure 3. 5G use cases and related examples (Latif, S et al.,2017)

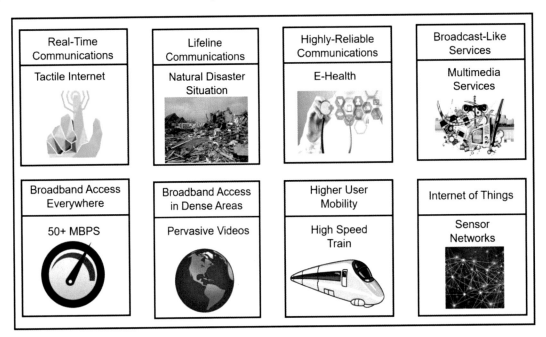

Biomedical robotic–assisted operation has the potential to improve accuracy and aid treatment practitioners in enhancing postoperative results. 5G-enabled telesurgery improves not only the accessibility to marginalized populations, but also the much-needed run-time communication among experts across many facilities. This system, dubbed the Internet of Healthcare Skills (Alliance, N et al., 2014), will indirectly aid in the mutual training and advancement of surgical expertise while reducing costs and time restrictions.

The development of next-generation technology is accelerating due to increased request from carriers, businesses, and consumers. The 5G infrastructure is projected to be unavailable owing to a range of services and capabilities. As a result, a smart hospital centered on 5G networks may not reached the desired latencies. The present cloud architecture, on the other hand, is tailored to the 5G network. The incorporation of other innovations with the 5G network for medical applications will inflate the performance of 5G in health care, is uncertain, and cannot be overlooked. The sixth generation (6G) networking can be adopted to address the challenges of the 5G network, delivering great software and services in all domains. However, if 5G fails to deliver on its promises, the 6G concept will emerge as a reality.

Internet of Things (IoT)

Nowadays IoT is widely used in almost all aspects of daily life. IoT is also gripping command on healthcare sector by providing services and assisting emergency services to patients (Dananjayan, S et al., 2021). IoT refers to the connecting of gazillions of physical devices to gather and transmit data through the Internet. The Internet of Things is made up of a variety of sensors and other application specific. It establishes connectivity between remotely situated objects, portable devices, and other commonly used real devices using wireless transmission mechanisms. The IoT has a big role to play in improving healthcare approaches. To collect patient information, many bodies have various sensors. Internal data is collected via body-implanted sensing devices, while local and external information is collected by the everlasting sensing elements (Rahmani, A.M et al., 2018). Physicians examine the information they acquire in order to forecast sickness. Different machine learning categorization techniques were utilized in the constructed model to categorize the obtained data in order to distinguish between normal and unhealthy patients. Machine learning classifiers can detect the early diagnosis and effectively.

The fact that smartphones have been the crucial part of every one's life and can be connected with various devices and sensors to monitor health of subject (Kishor, A et al., 2021). It can also be used with e health applications like early diagnosis of disease with use of sensors and emergency notifications. This type of surveillance system needs to acquire vast amounts of data from smart equipment's and evaluate this data for utilization of smart healthcare (Wu, T., et al., 2017). It also provides an efficient tracking and monitoring that helps in improvements of people (Chen, X et al., 2018).

There are still many blockers while implementing IoT services in the healthcare sector like all of the sensors and mobile devices have limited battery supply. Frequent charging of these devices have become a burden and source of frustration to the end user and make the end user experience awful (Subramani-yaswamy, V et al., 2019). Also these devices can easily be hacked. There should be a proper security management system with IoT health care (Yang, Y et al., 2017). Also energy consumption for cloud centers is quite high and that makes the cost of cloud computing is quite expensive. Monitoring system acquires cloud computing with very low energy consumption and low latency (Elhoseny, M et al., 2018).

IoT combined with machine learning algorithms could be used for early detection of heart diseases. It involves multi tier architecture for transmitting data from subject to wearable devices and storing that data into cloud based system and regression analysis on predicting early heart disease. This data will also be redirected to health professionals to analyze the data and prescribed solutions according to it (Gupta, V et al., 2018).

Cloud Computing

Cloud computing makes it easy to access shared information and data in a flexible, dynamic, and transparent manner. It relieves consumers of the burden of managing computation on their computers. It allows customers to not only preserve but also retrieve their content and compute over the internet at any time and from any location (Kumar, P.M et al., 2018). Cloud computing is healthcare is used in complex data processing, scalable data centers, resource sharing, parallel computing, data integration with different formats using data lakes and managing security problems (Elmagzoub, M et al., 2021). The health sector is a multifaceted framework that seeks to avert, analyze, and cure infections in order to create a society with fewer health and mental problems. The study discovered a link between information management in the pharmaceutical business and cloud computing systems that could be beneficial for the economy. In many cases, large industries or company organizations require the right implementation of data application services in order to strengthen the client interaction mechanism, which can aid in the firm's success. Cloud computing has the potential to become a significant element of the healthcare business in the near future. The healthcare business is currently facing huge hurdles as a result of the epidemic, and the demand for modern technologies is growing in this domain. The concerns and obstacles that are encountered in terms of information security necessitate an appropriate solution that can improve this service's performance. Furthermore, additional study is needed in this subject to have a better awareness of the concerns and provide appropriate recommendations to address the obstacles (Verma, P et al., 2018).

IoT based data is also stored in cloud servers from different types of sensors. Network latency is a major problem in a remote monitoring system and a solution to network latency must be offered during remote mode processing. A framework called UbeHealth is proposed to analyze network latency and service quality challenges (QoS) that provide better health performance in smart cities (Sharma, D.K et al., 2021).

Blockchain

Data accessibility, provenance, data integrity, auditing, data authenticity, adaptable access, authenticity, privacy, and confidentiality are all major concerns for today's healthcare data warehouses. Furthermore, many present healthcare DBMSs are centralized, posing the potential of ocuring a bottleneck in the event of a catastrophe. Blockchain is a revolutionary decentralized platform that has the ability to completely remodel, reconfigure, and revolutionize the way information is managed in the healthcare industry(Muhammed, T et al., 2018). Bitcoin and cryptocurrency are not the only reasons for the block chain being famous but it also allows to have digital record keeping and a transparent ledger of transactions that is not possible to temper. Although blockchain focus was on financially for a long period of time but now the trend seems to change that other sectors are also incorporating blockchain technology like health care. Block chain technology employs the notion of smart contracts, which define terms of service that are accepted upon by all healthcare participants in the web, eliminating the need for an intermediaries. It cuts down on wasteful administrative expenses. Peer-to-peer platforms, public key encryption, and consensus procedures are the three primary elements that underpin block chain technology. It can aid in the establishment of a smooth data interchange without the need of a middleman, increasing customer trust in telehealth services. It allows doctors to retain extensive patient information, treatment/ procedure histories, and test findings in a decentralized, traceable, and irreversible manner. One of the major roadblocks to blockchain technology's acceptance in telehealthcare platforms is that it may raise costs for individuals who already live in distant places with low facilities.

Table 1 provides the summary of key technologies involved in smart healthcare system. It also highlights the major hurdles before the technology was used, how the technology addressed these challenges and specific needs for further advancement of the domain.

SMART HEALTHCARE SERVICES

Diagnostic and therapeutic research organizations (e.g., hospitals or clinics), provincial health analytical decisions of organizations, and single or family clients are the main types of service goals for smart healthcare. Based on diverse purposes, smart healthcare applications can be categorized into the following categories.

Table 1. Key technologies of smart healthcare

No.	Issue(s) before the technology	Technology	Specific needs / requirements/ further research
1	Deaths occur due to error and incorrect diagnosis of disease	Artificial Intelligence (AI)	Decision support systems knowledge - based systems
2	• The difficulty, complexity, and usage of technical vocabulary of the unorganized textual content that hold the health information vary widely. • rendering information finding more difficult	Text Mining	• Improving healthcare service effectiveness • Promoting healthcare research • Reducing inaccurate clinical diagnosis and treatment plans • Reducing wasteful healthcare spending.
3	• The treatment of patients having burn injuries, cancer, chronic pain etc., who are in too much agony is difficult for both the patient and doctor. • More effective in training and assessment of medical professionals.	Virtual Reality (VR)	• Development of trustworthiness without incurring any harm. • Creation of user-friendly, cordless, light, and economical systems.
4	• Minimum human interaction and isolation of humans to prevent this global disease. • The quality of care surgical units is not effective.	Robotics	• Carrying supplies to hospitals and clinics. • Robots give surgeons 'superpowers,' allowing them to see better, make more accurate and least invasive procedures, stitch injuries, and so on.
5	• There is no proof of either the patient has actually taken the medicine or discard it. • The patients' body does not accept the complete therapeutic dose provided. • Genetic abnormalities	Nanotechnology	• Faster and more acute illness diagnosis. • Confirmation that the pharmaceuticals are given to various areas of the body with better accuracy. • A relatively new strategy for treating or preventing genetic abnormalities by fixing flawed genes that cause bacterial growth and delivering fixed genetic traits or replacing incorrect and misleading ones.
6	• The extremely fast increasing healthcare business demands a strong communications infrastructure.	5G networks	• Adequate communication with patients. • Raising the standard of smart health care. • Smart Hospitals offering remote group consultation, remote surgery, emergency rescue, intra hospitals monitoring etc.
7	• Late diagnosis of severe illnesses. • Lack of up-date regarding the current state of patient.	Internet of Things (IoT)	• Acquiring vast amounts of data from smart equipment's and evaluate this data for utilization of smart healthcare. • An efficient tracking and monitoring that helps in improvements of patients.
8	• Patients are unable to manage their data at the local storage.	Cloud Computing	• Complex data processing, scalable data centers, resource sharing, parallel computing, data integration with different formats using data lakes and managing security problems of patients.
9	• Many present healthcare DBMSs are centralized, posing the potential of occurring a bottleneck in the event of a catastrophe.	Blockchain	• Completely remodeling, reconfiguring, and revolutionizing the way information is managed in the healthcare industry. • Increasing customer trust in telehealth services.

1. Support in the Treatment Plan and Recovery of Patients

The assessment and treatment of chronic illnesses has become much more sophisticated as a result of the use of advances in artificial intelligence, robotic surgery, and augmented reality. It has accomplished specific achievements, such as the identification of hepatitis, bowel cancer, and melanoma, by using artificial intelligence to build the health monitoring system. Artificial intelligence diagnostic results are more accurate than those of researchers and clinicians. Deep learning technologies, notably in pathologies and scanning, are frequently more reliable than trained practitioners. IBM's Watson, an artificial intellectual system that provides an optimal answer using in examination of all medical derived from the literature information, is the most remarkable and significant technology in the category of medical decision assistance technologies. The strategy has a significant impact on diabetic and tumor prognosis. Professionals can use the health monitoring technology to provide expert guidance learning algorithms to enhance diagnostic performance, eliminate delayed and misdiagnosed diagnoses, and ensure that patients get prompt and suitable medical care. Intelligent diagnosis allows for a more precise statement of the patient's health and illness level, which aids in the development of a specific treatment approach, and specialists have endorsed the system.

The treatments on its own will improve in precision. With the use of smart diagnosis, the patient's chemotherapy treatment can be tracked proactively throughout the procedure in tumor radiation, for example. Specialists can improve the chemotherapy program, track the progression of the illness, and reduce the risk of physical surgery (Yaqoob, I et al., 2021). An immersive communication sequence is created between the virtual environment, the actual reality, and individuals by modelling the objective and transferring it to the real life for accurate synchronization. Subversive variations can occur in medical training, study, interaction, and clinical treatment as a result of the introduction of this innovation.

2. Supervision of Health

Chronic conditions have progressively risen to the peak of the human cancer continuum and have formed a discovery since the start of the 21st century. Chronic illnesses have a protracted line of treatment, are irreversible, and are expensive to treat. As a result, disease care monitoring is very critical. The conventional hospital- and physician centered health management approach, on the other hand, seems to be ill equipped to deal appropriately with the growing number of individuals and illnesses(Wu, X et al., 2018). The modern digital medical health supervision approach emphasizes patient self-control. It stresses individual self-monitoring in real time, quick health data reporting, and appropriate medical behavior modification. The advent of surgically implanted smart gadgets, home automation, and smart healthcare information systems linked by IoT technology offers a solution to this issue. 3rd generation wearable/ implantable devices can integrate smart equipment, micro controllers, and wireless components to intelligently sense and supervise different physiological markers of patient populations while minimizing energy consumption, trying to improve comfort, and enabling the data to be merged with health records from other sources. This strategy entails a transition from situation surveillance to continual awareness and care coordination. It decreases the disease's related dangers while making it simpler for healthcare centers to track the human disease prospects of diagnosis.

Aged and disabled people can get help around the house with home automation. Smart home devices are customized apartments and residences that include sensing devices and actuating equipment built into the residential system to analyze the tenants' physical indications and surroundings. Smart houses can also help you live better(Andreu-Perez, J et al., 2015). Smart home devices and health surveillance are the two main functions of smart residences in healthcare. These innovations can assist individuals who really need care lessen their dependency on healthcare professionals and enhance their standard of living at home by providing some simple tasks while gathering health information.

Patients can use applications and a healthcare information portal to self-manage their conditions. The Anxiety Recognition and Relief system, for example, utilizes a smart wearable device to constantly monitor person's body levels of pressure and proactively assist the body in anxiety reduction(Liu, L et al.,2016). It's also feasible to combine healthcare information from numerous mobile devices into a clinical selection assistance system to develop a multilayer health decision - making support platform that can get maximum use of the knowledge for accurate diagnosis of diseases. It can

3. Early Detection of Illness and Vulnerability Assessments

Standard illness danger prognosis relies on medical authorities taking the effort to gather patient data, comparing that data to authorized organization recommendations, and then publicize the prediction findings. This technique has a time delay and does not offer users with correct recommendations. Illness risk prediction is adaptive and tailored in smart healthcare. It allows individuals and clinicians to take part, effectively evaluate their illness risk, and implement customized prevention strategies based on their own surveillance data. The new illness risk predictive algorithm gathers data from wearable devices and smart apps, transfers it to the cloud via a connection, and analyses the results using big data-based algorithms before sending the anticipated results to users via short messaging in real time. These strategies have been demonstrated to work. They assist physicians and patients in making changes to their health behaviors and routines at any moment, as well as strategic decision in developing regional healthcare policies with the goal of lowering illness risk. For instance, in a study designed to prevent hyperglycemia by estimating the postprandial blood glucose reaction, investigators used methodologies that incorporated blood glucose specifications, food patterns, anthropometry, physical exercise, gut microbiome, and other aspects to accurately predict improvements in glycemic index and minimize the chances of diabetes through a personalized diet after tracking the blood glucose feedback of 800 individuals for 46,898 meal options each week (Akmandor, A.O et al., 2017).

4. Hospitals That are Cutting Edge by Smart Monitoring

Local, hospital, and household healthcare are the three major aspects of patient monitoring. To enhance the current patient care practices and add new features, intelligent hospitals rely on data and knowledge technology-based settings, particularly those based on IoT efficiency and automation operations. Smart hospitals provide three categories of services: services for hospital personnel, facilities for patients, and facilities for managers. In hospital management decisions, the needs of these facilities users must be taken into account.

The knowledge infrastructure, which connects electronic devices, smart building, and staff in healthcare administration, uses the Internet of Things to combine numerous electronic systems. This technique can also be used to trace medical tools and physiological specimens, as well as identify and analyze patients in clinics. For drug creation and exchange, inventory control and other operations, intelligent healthcare is also used in the pharmaceutical sector. A different RFID tag can be provided to each patient and the knowledge can be kept in a database that can be constantly monitored and retrieved via mobile devices to enable secure, trustworthy, sustainable, and effective circulation of medical materials through RFID technologies (Redfern, J et al., 2017). In regards of decision, establishing an integrated management software can enable services like allocation of resources, quality assessment, and performance monitoring, as well as lower medical expenses, maximize resource usage, and assist hospitals in determining developmental choices.

Individuals have access to a wide range of activities. These activities includes medical examination platforms physically, online consultations, and doctor-patient contacts. These computerized solutions shorten the time it takes for individuals to receive medical assistance. Patients wait less time and get more personalized care. To summarize, smart hospitals' future developments are collaboration, refining, and increased automation (Franssen, J.et al., 2018).

5. Contributing With Pharmaceutical Research

Pharmaceutical investigation and advancement will become even more exact and efficient with the use of artificial intelligence and machine learning in scientific analysis. Target screening, pharmaceutical discovery, drug testing, and other aspects of the drug research process are all included. In order to uncover efficient strategic points, typical drug objective screening systematically crosses existing medicines with numerous possible target molecules in the individual body. This strategy is not only time-consuming, but it is also frequently neglected. Artificial intelligence-assisted automated testing of medication and focus effects has considerably boosted screening performance. E.g. The Watson approach was used to identify ribonucleic acid-binding enzymes in amyotrophic terminal disease and to perform genomics investigations on malignancies. Furthermore, the artificial intelligence technology can gather real-time data from the external world and can optimize or modify the filtering process whenever required (Chen, Q et al., 2018). The Internet of Things, big data, and intelligent systems are all used in drug studies. First, utilizing artificial intelligence to assess and match a lot of cases that can make it easier to screen for eligibility requirements and identify the most eligible target individuals, reducing time and enhancing target audience targeting. Patients are then constantly monitored employing smart wearable devices to gather more timely and comprehensive information at real time, such as when smart technologies are used to analyze lung diseases clinical studies (Bakkar, N et al., 2018).Involvement of related technologies in the development of the trial protocol can improve patient security and the reliability of research. 40 All data is gathered and consolidated onto the right opportunity so that experts can analyze it.

Table 2 highlights provides the summary of smart healthcare services.

Table 2. Smart healthcare services

No.	Issue(s) before the services	Service	Advantages
1	• Diagnostic results achieved from researchers and clinicians were not accurate. • No precise statement regarding the illness level. • Lack of track in the progression of the illness, and the risk of physical surgery.	Support in the treatment plan and recovery of patients	• Deep learning technologies, notably in pathologies and scanning, are frequently more reliable than trained practitioners. • An immersive communication sequence is created between the virtual environment, the actual reality, and individuals by modelling the objective and transferring it to the real life for accurate synchronization. • Professionals can use the health monitoring technology to provide expert guidance learning algorithms.
2	• Aged and disabled people do not have any help around the house with home automation. • No mechanism for detecting potential dangers for clients.	Supervision of health	• It decreases the disease's related dangers. • Patients can use applications and a healthcare information portal to self-manage their conditions.
3	• Standard illness danger prognosis has issue of time delay and does not offer users with correct recommendations.	Early detection of illness and vulnerability assessments	• Accurate collection of data. • Future predictions becomes more realistic. • Supports strategic decision in developing regional healthcare policies with the goal of lowering illness risk.
4	• Hospitals need smart assistance in determining developmental choices. • No smart solutions to save the time	Hospitals that are cutting edge by smart monitoring	• IoT efficiency and automation operations. • Accurately trace medical tools and physiological specimens. • Computerized solutions reduced the time.
5	• Standard strategies were time-consuming. • Lack of data manipulation techniques.	Contributing with pharmaceutical research	• Real-time data from the external world support to optimize the filtering process. • Target screening, pharmaceutical discovery, drug testing, and other aspects of the drug research process are improved.

BENEFITS AND OPPORTUNITIES FOR SMART HEALTH

Intelligent cities, in principle, are made up of a variety of automated development of smart residences, internet of vehicles, remote surgery, and smart tourism that allow inhabitants to access a variety of advanced services, administer cities, and set in motion beneficial and curative acts. In the framework of healthcare, a smart city can assist doctors in achieving smart health care coverage. A smart town can use smart management technology to assist the digital acquisition, computation, preservation, distribution, and interchange of internal user information such as workforce, social, and other types of data. Furthermore, the basic infrastructure of an intelligent cities can enable the intelligent monitoring and administration of health records, medical equipment and materials, communications networks, and automated supervision and control of healthcare, consequently resolving many serious health risk challenges. Currently, there are many cities that are in a state of development or in competition with smart health cities and are struggling, trying to get out and talk about underdeveloped cities and take advantage of different opportunities. These opportunities also create a range of roles for different industries. Therefore, you can look for possible options by implementing large-scale information scanning in urban applications. Later in this excerpt, we look at a small advantage and gap that can help make the decision to change or redesign a city to become a skilled city. With a given decision, renewed sensitivity, flexibility and organization can be achieved. Despite increased passenger complacency and the enthusiastic organization of standard facilities and resources(Liu, J et al., 2018),(Al-Azzam et al., 2019),(Pal, D et al., 2018),(Ismagilova, E et al., 2020),(Condoluci, M. et al., 2016). Some of the benefits of this beautiful city are related to:

1. Consistent use of resources: Smart health creates a number of opportunities, one of which is resource utilization. As many tools are missing or too expensive, it is too difficult to justify the reasons for a more balanced use of these tools. For example, asset management and geographic data frameworks (GIS) can be valuable from innovative frameworks. The existence of monitoring frameworks will make it easier to identify waste sources and better rotate assets, while controlling costs and reducing the use of energy and common assets. An important part of smart urban applications is also that they are designed for connection and selection of information, which can also facilitate a more coordinated effort for applications and administrations.
2. Higher standard of living: With a given decision, renewed sensitivity, flexibility and organization can be achieved. Despite increased passenger complacency and the enthusiastic organization of standard facilities and resources. Some of the benefits of this beautiful city are related to:
3. Higher standard of openness and clarity: the prerequisite for better wellness programs and particularly sensible eye and application control will lead to higher levels of interoperability and responsiveness. Sharing data and resources is becoming the norm. In addition, it produces simple information for all included. This will increase collaboration and correspondence between components and create more organizations and apps that will further increase the flexibility of the city. One model is the United States government, which has collected and disseminated a wide variety of data, tasks and content directly and directly. This allowed residents and authorities to exchange and use data effectively.

These benefits of cultivation nonetheless require critical levels of sophistication and dedication in terms of smart welfare programs, resources, and people. Opportunities to get these benefits are available; Whatever their needs, commit the resources to further development, better attempts at advancement, and practical use of vast data. It is more than necessary to establish methods to ensure data accuracy, superior type, high security, security and control of data, in the same way as using data documentation rules to provide information. In addition, progress can be extremely helpful when considering organizing and protecting environmental and business assets and basic resources with an increasingly accepted authoritative purpose.

Massive computer programs can serve different parts of a messy city. Provides better experiences for customers and organizations that help associations do better. Improving clinical consideration by improving preventive thinking, instrument finding and treatment organizations, clinical consideration captures the thoughts and thoughts of patients. Transport structures can take unimaginably huge data for updating course and schedules, forced to change requirements and be even more harmless to the biological system.

Sending huge information applications like brilliant wellbeing applications needs the assistance of a nice information and correspondence advancement structure. It maintains sharp metropolitan regions since it gives important plans and besides fascinating courses of action that may not be possible without it. For example, it enables beneficial vehicle orchestrating by giving basic ways to deal with managing their organizations from different fields/zones to lessen transportation costs. Various models join giving better water to the board and improved waste organization by applying headways to sufficiently manage these organizations. For example, wasting the heads fuses waste grouping, evacuation, reusing, and recovery, which would all be able to be beneficially regulated using the plans. More models consolidate new turn of events and essential procedures for the prosperity of designs and better environment; danger the board; prosperity and security; air quality and pollution; general prosperity; ceaseless the suburbs; bio-assortment setback; and energy profitability. All around, a quick city can be made more insightful while utilizing ICT and gigantic data for an impressive part of its applications and organizations.

The inclusion of huge information systems will solve many problems such as: B. Sensing capabilities and equipment. Furthermore, it helps to develop, organize and strengthen collaboration and correspondence between different substances in a dynamic city. This should be possible by creating extensive information networks that serve as a substance for developing synergistic and innovative programs for applications in regions such as education, social protection, energy, legislation, collection, climate and security. It also enables the gradual search for solutions to problems in agriculture, transportation and management groups when applications and facilities are coordinated and data flows efficiently between applications and substances. There are several examples of massive information applications serving vibrant urban communities such as *centralized health system*. With the help of smart health applications, the data become centralized and accessible across the city in the capacity and investigation apparatuses. In keen medical care frameworks, the patient observing gadgets burn-through a shifting measure of energy in various states, i.e., rest, alert, dynamic, and inactive. Therefore, a state-based situation is needed to display the energy utilization of these gadgets to examine their conduct. For this reason, Medium Access Control (Macintosh) and group based directing conventions have been explored in the writing. The Macintosh layer conventions guarantee the activity of these gadgets with negligible obligation cycling. These conventions decrease energy utilization by keeping the transmitter out of gear or rest state. Accordingly, the transmission delay is limited, and simultaneously, the organization throughput and lifetime are augmented. These conventions have a fundamental job in energy preservation as they control the principle wellsprings of energy wastage, i.e., bundle impact, catching, control parcel overhead, and inactive tuning in. Macintosh conventions are named either plan based or dispute based. On account of conflict based conventions, e.g., Transporter Sense Different Access/Crash Evasion (CSMA/CA), the gadgets contend with one another to get to the transmission channels for information correspondence. They are adaptable, and simultaneously, don't force exacting time-synchronization on the asset starving gadgets. Nonetheless, they cause exorbitant overhead and keep the gadgets hanging tight for more than anticipated. The affectability of a patient's imperative signs requires prompt transmission to the medical services workforce. Timetable based conventions, then again, utilizes Time Division Different Access (TDMA) for proficient use of the transmission medium. These conventions diminish crash, catching, and inactive tuning in; nonetheless, they bring about unnecessary looking out for the piece of observing gadgets.

We investigated a few instances of enormous information, the practices, those will be termed as primary advisers that lead a fast growing city practices endeavors. Many made different degrees of progress and most added important segments to improve keen city administrations and applications.

CHALLENGES IN SMART HEALTH SYSTEM

Smart cities face a number of challenges to implement and execute plan and sending of huge data applications for smart metropolitan networks. Splendid metropolitan zones are seen as incredibly amazing and propelling conditions, thusly it is basic to avoid or if nothing else decline the troubles drew in with clever applications plan and improvement for sharp metropolitan networks. There are in like manner a couple of discussions related to the definition, use and benefits of colossal data for splendid metropolitan networks. These relate to open enormous data instruments, steady assessment, accuracy, depiction, cost, and transparency. Such issues can impact the display of clever city applications and organizations relying upon colossal data. Is it possible that data would one say one is of the challenges? How? Here we will address a segment of the basic troubles in using huge data in splendid metropolitan territories.

Origin of Data and its Characteristics

The data comes from different sources in a large number of projects. There are many new data plans, many of which are unstructured. This data must be regulated and described in a coordinated manner using a first-tier information collection system. Much extraordinary data that differs from the recognized data more resolved are the three drawbacks: speed, volume and aggregation. A few more have been added such as authenticity, truthfulness, inconsistency value and variability. The simple attempt to extract these different attributes from large amounts of data leads to complex models and approaches and makes them difficult to control. This is simply because current data mining techniques or programming devices cannot handle the large size and complexity. Some issues can also be viewed later, such as: B. Evaluation design, assessment, mining, data creation, urgency, presentation and hidden colossal data. While smart urban applications are being considered in big data issues, there are drawbacks in several places. On the one hand, collecting data without someone else is hindered by the existence of different sources with different plans and types and by different approaches and access that converge. In addition, thinking about unstructured data makes it difficult to correctly characterize, organize and use applications.

Exchange of Data and Information

Distribution of data and information between different city districts is another test. Every organization, office or city office regularly has its own public or mysterious information store or dissemination community. The vast majority of them are reluctant to share data that could be considered priceless. In addition, some data can be controlled by certain security vulnerabilities that make it difficult to share between different components. The test here is to get straight to the point, not overcome the almost indisputable contrast between social problems and use huge data and secure benefits for the safety of the residents. It adapts to each city on the first level as different regions and initiatives are included. Advanced urban applications need to find ways to counter or reduce controls in order to achieve a constant exchange and exchange of information between different substances. Also when transferring multiple organized data sources between partner workstations, for example certain types of data. B. Temporary geospatial data can be reactivated quickly. In this sense, it is difficult to know the semantics of the data uniformly and to concentrate the new data on the basis of the expressed cycle data and the consistent data. As a result, it will be difficult to create a database for a rated city.

Data Transparency and Quality

The quality of the data looks different in the more central parts of the big news. There are several challenges associated with the idea of data. Data obtained from different people in extraordinary and confidential environments in indisputable information collections is rarely processed in the default settings. Depending on the free support and easy use of the different providers, you will get the data for which a planning gap is identified and, in this sense, it will be more likely that problems of consistency, heterogeneity and uniqueness will arise. Likewise, "there is no complete and complete technique for obtaining and manipulating data somewhere in a data center that is assembled for evaluation." This will bring new challenges such as weak data and reliability. For example, sensor data collected by an untouchable controller without an associated controller may have been created by sensors that are set incorrectly, incorrectly, or have exceeded their lifespan. Likewise, the test can loosen existing research data (given the potential error) and reveal results that can be used by others who may not be thinking about these questions. With this in mind, it's important to constantly relive and relive easy-to-use event data, share and discuss it with all parts of a large city, to ensure residents appreciate and apply practices accurately and maintain consistency.

Cognitive Computing

Since it focuses on how to cope with complicated situations and knowledge ambiguity, cognitive computing is well suited to solving medical problems. Managing with probable knowledge is the fundamental challenge in bioinformatics. New advances in the merging fields of cognitive technology and computer sciences are required to achieve the goal of a smart hospital: While the data's large complexity is sometimes seen as a disadvantage.

Solitude and Security

In any event, when e-health approach can help in alleviating different wellbeing related concerns, yet its ability to get unmatched information can risk the residents' protection. Assurance of protection and security of the framework is an inescapable issue that the examination local area is as yet attempting to change. Security insurance and security is first in around each feature of human existence. By the by, in a keen city setting, it is even of more prominent significance and the reason is on the grounds that the data that is gotten is extremely close to home. From the information or data that is gathered in a keen city, it is conceivable to get information about the propensities for residents, their societal position, other individual data, and even the data identified with their religion. All these individual data factors are very sensitive in nature, and when they are coordinated with the wellbeing data of an individual, the result is much more delicate. Thus, it derives an incredible trouble and a few difficulties that are as yet needed to be considered. Certain endeavors have been led to clarify the idea of the protection of residents and to offer conceivable answers to ensure that protection. Furthermore, different endeavors are contributed towards the security assurance in health, Trust-commendable Wellbeing and Health (Defrost) is one of the delegate projects in this setting. The idea of Defrost means to determine different difficulties and troubles to offer dependable and solid data frameworks for wellbeing and wellbeing. Likewise,

The Essential Medical care IT Progressed Exploration Activities on Security (SHARPS) is another task that points in making upgrades in the establishments, prerequisites, advancement, plan, and sending of security, just as on protection techniques and apparatuses that are utilized for m-wellbeing. Such activities are the exploration needs and challenges with them are overwhelming.

Data Mining Isn't Everything

Making smart regarding health information is not easy, as Yvonne Rogers highlighted out. Smart healthcare has the potential to empower more individuals to manage their own health, resulting in increased awareness and knowledge. However, it presents a slew of moral concerns. Who owns the health information gathered? Who is willing to reveal their personal health information? What happens to the new streams of health data? When creating a smart hospital, all of these concerns must be addressed. These are big problems that aren't easy to solve, and they can be summed as "What comes after data mining?" or, in Tim Menzies' words, "Estimation is fine - but what about enabling the management to make decisions?"

Value

Value is a vulnerable argument that reminds us of the habits that public experts use to influence people in the use of blueprints. For example, use an energy saving system that controls public power to use new structures, fragments or functions to select and record information. This is encouraged to create a strong energy in the leader's structure; In any case, the operation is also too expensive. If such an effort is not carried out correctly from the beginning, it can create a major problem, generate huge costs and affect the city in hostile ways. For example, testing a practical traffic light and construction signs costs a lot. These tests incur enormous resource costs, e.g. Ex. B. On models with heavy loads, while shipping and testing installation. Therefore, exorbitant hardware and programming must be exchanged to continue emergency development, city recognition and smart applications.

Overpopulation Issue

Population has a direct impact on the challenges faced by a developing city. People have influence and are touched by smart apps. In particular, the size of the city's general population has an extraordinary impact on the size of the huge amounts of data. In addition, the construction of the general population increases the size of the data provided quickly and can become very large. This is a big problem, as rapid improvement will lead to stagnation, pollution and the spread of social irregularities, as opposed to widespread urbanization that poses a combination of certain contingent financial and social problems that are generally at risk. Monetary and natural justice of metropolitan areas. Along these lines, beautiful urban applications must scale quickly and reduce the ability to handle the created volume and huge data aggregation to avoid such problems. Ultimately, the goal is to build and deploy crisp urban applications fast enough to generate and manage huge data. Rapid development is beautiful for best results.

Perspective, judgment, disturbance, and inconsistent data are all prevalent characteristics of medical information. Some neural network algorithms have previously been applied in machine learning to handle these tough challenges. Traditional healthcare strategies are constrained by the extremely complicated characteristics of medical information, but neural network-based machine learning approaches can contribute significantly to the health care environment because they can adequately integrate the ambiguous qualities of human rationalization with the habitual comprehensiveness, accurate and consistent logic, and great information processing of computers. We may claim, based on current research and practice, that effective use of machine learning methodologies, tools, and strategies can support healthcare organizations in providing a wide range of opportunities to facilitate and improve health treatment.

In short, some compete with large urban applications based on large amounts of data. These challenges have different effects and recommendations for such applications and locations, fluctuate in difficult situations, and are varied. Also, different applications have different data usage requirements. For example, the semaphore requires quick responses from the application to logically control traffic. Naturally viable applications may have the option of processing multiple assigned responses because all decisions are considered over long periods of time. Trade, publishing, research, dynamics, and the right responses are a problem; however, the degree of importance varies depending on the application. Obtaining gradual responses depends largely on how we deal with the problems discussed above. Table 3 highlights the major challenges associated with smart health systems.

REQUIREMENTS

This section covers the key segments needed to plan and execute keen city applications using the information parts. Information assortment and catching from sensors, clients, electronic information peruses and numerous others represent the principal issue to deal with as the volume quickly develops. Putting away, coordinating and preparing this information to produce helpful outcomes in the following issue. On a very basic level, to have viable arrangements, it is needed to choose various plan and advancement needs in an arranged way, for instance adaptable plan, snappy sending, accomplishing more intensive sense, more thorough interconnections, and more knowledge. To additionally muddle the issues, taking care of interconnected correspondence frameworks to get to logical data in savvy city applications and actual spaces to help great dynamic cycles expects regard for different parts of network, security and protection.

Table 3. Challenges of smart health system

No.	Challenge	Issue(s) associated specified with the challenge
1	Origin of Data and its characteristics	• Multiple data plans are used. • Many of data plans are unstructured. • Difficult to correctly characterize and organize. • Speed of data. • Volume of data. • Aggregation of data. • Complex models are difficult to control. • Convergence is difficult.
2	Exchange of Data and Information	• Reluctance in sharing data. • Security vulnerabilities. • Difficult to know the semantics of the data uniformly. • Difficult to maintain consistency in data.
3	Data Transparency and Quality	• Data obtained from confidential environments in indisputable. • Weak data and reliability. • Incomplete research data is another potential error. • Applying data accurately is difficult.
4	Cognitive Computing	• Managing the patient's information. • Complex environment.
5	Solitude and Security	• Origin of data. • Societal position of patient. • Getting data while maintaining the integrity of data is challenging.
6	Data Mining Isn't Everything	• Marinating the obtained data • Proper evaluation of the gathered data.
7	Value	• Creating energy. • Tests requires enormous energy. • Smart applications needs to be optimal.
8	Overpopulation Issue	• Management of huge data set. • Slow development. • Effective use of machine learning is required. • Use of tool for evaluation in case of massive data.

The use of large information to shrewd urban communities in terms of health departments can be grouped into two sorts, disconnected huge information applications and constant huge information applications. Ongoing huge information applications are distinctive on the grounds that they depend on immediate information and quick investigation to show up at a choice or activity inside a short and unmistakable course of events. As a rule, if a choice can't be made inside that course of events, it gets pointless. Accordingly, it is critical to settle on all information essential for such choice accessible in a convenient style and that the investigation is done in a quick and solid manner. Therefore, constant large information applications ordinarily need higher mechanical prerequisites. Large information applications for savvy cities arranged in territories like energy, traffic, schooling, and medical services are considered disconnected. Be that as it may, those expected to give intuitive activities, upgrades and controls for wise applications are constant applications.

Smart city applications such as health applications have been implemented from big data concept, it is important to address a few necessities that originate from the exceptional idea of shrewd city needs and enormous information attributes. In this segment we endeavor to examine a few of these prerequisites to give an overall rule to the plan and improvement endeavors. These necessities are distinguished depending on the kind of large information applications and the difficulties of executing these applications for keen urban areas. A portion of these necessities are mechanical while others are identified with residents' mindfulness and governments' jobs. Besides, a portion of these prerequisites are the one of the basic entities and apply to any enormous information application, although the rest are explicit to the extraordinary necessities of keen city conditions.

Optimize and Manage Big Data

The advantages of smart health applications is that they produce enormous volumes of information in an assortment of arrangements and from numerous areas like traffic, energy, instruction, and medical care, and assembling. This information is created and gathered in monstrous sums and consistently, hence offering ongoing perspective on what's going on in the city whenever. To guarantee appropriate and helpful usage of this information in brilliant city applications, it is essential to have reasonable and viable large information the board devices set up. Large information the executives incorporate advancement and execution of designs, game plans, practices and procedures that properly manage the full data lifecycle needs all through its usage in splendid city applications. As the data comes from different sources with different plans, there is a necessity for bleeding edge data the board includes that will prompt be perceiving the various organizations and wellsprings of information, organizing, overseeing, grouping, and controlling every one of these kinds and constructions. Large information the executives for savvy city applications ought to likewise give versatile dealing with monstrous information to help disconnected applications just as low dormancy handling to serve viably continuous applications. The ideas, methods, and difficulties of huge information the board are examined further in and.

Big Data Processing Platforms

Smart health applications in big data for the developing cities need to perform information investigation that normally require immense handling ability such as scalability and reliability. This prompts the requirement for versatile and dependable programming and equipment stages. The product stages for shrewd urban areas should offer elite registering capacities, be streamlined for the equipment being utilized, is steady and dependable for the diverse information concentrated applications being executed, underpins stream handling, gives an undeniable degrees of issue strength, and is upheld by a very much prepared and able group and seller. There are diverse accessible programming stages for enormous information investigation like many big data platforms which give the stream handling needed by ongoing huge information applications like astute transportations in a savvy city. These stages function admirably on group frameworks that can give a ground-breaking and versatile equipment stage to meet the necessities of enormous information applications for shrewd urban communities. Huge information can be additionally handled on the Cloud utilizing both huge information stages as an Assistance and Framework as a Help. This will assuage the application proprietors from the Burden of getting committed stages, which is generally expensive and permit them to utilize all around tried profoundly dependable stages provided by the Cloud specialist organizations.

Well Established Network Infrastructure

For the smart health applications or any other department, big data must be needed for the developing city. Most of the big data applications related to health for developing cities require smart networks that connect their components such as different EMRs. The established current columns, separated, and accumulated occasions can be moved to a concentrated handling to convey the middle of the road preparing focuses in the keen organization for pre-preparing or for additional sifting and collection prior to being moved to the fundamental dynamic unit. The unified methodology is acceptable if the current created occasions are not enormous and there are no constraints on the organization assets used to move these occasions. The conveyed approach is more reasonable for tremendous occasions to such an extent that it is wasteful and some of the time difficult to move all the created occasions to a solitary area inside satisfactory execution and time limits. Sifting and collection will be significant for this situation particularly for savvy urban communities as it will help decrease the measure of production and accelerate information preparation. This should be possible at the occasion sources and the middle of the road focuses utilizing an open-circle or a shut circle approach. In open-circle approach separating and accumulation arrangements are pre-characterized while in shut circle approach sifting and total strategies are intuitively characterized dependent on the recent developments and choices, current framework and organization assets, or outer keen city application arrangements. In the two methodologies, occasion sifting and conglomeration ought to be managed without trading off the uprightness, exactness and rightness of the information being accumulated. This is imperative to protect the nature of the dynamic interaction in the continuous huge information applications.

Advanced Algorithms

The standard and optimized algorithms that are implemented in the development of regular health applications may not be adequateto manage health applications that are used in big data because of many dependable reasons and also because of their one of a kind prerequisites and squeezing with velocity handling. For instance, most accessible information mining calculations are not truly reasonable for large information mining applications as their plan depends on restricted and very much characterized informational indexes. Huge information applications for savvy urban communities should actualize progressed and more refined calculations to manage large information productively. A portion of these calculations should be intended for continuous application while others can be intended for cluster or disconnected handling. These calculations should be advanced to deal with high information volumes, huge assortment of information types, time requirements on dynamic cycles, and circulated parts across different geological areas. Likewise, these calculations need to work successfully across heterogeneous conditions and be fit for overseeing and working in profoundly powerful conditions.

Use of Latest Technology

Big data smart health applications include enormous scope of heterogeneous frameworks and information, it is beneficial to adhere to the norm for planning and executing such arrangements. This will add adaptability for redesigning, keeping up, and include many application highlights for brilliant urban communities. What's more, this will encourage the combination among shrewd city parts and huge information segments. Moreover, it is essential to set standard guidelines for latest applications to accomplish a simple mix between the accessible keen city framework and climate and the presented enormous information applications. This can be accomplished by playing out a full investigation of the public authority substances, partner, and the framework to survey the status to be important for a future keen city. In light of such examination guidelines, the latest models of plan and rules can be created for large information applications improvement for the keen city.

Reliability and Security

With the rapid advancement of e-health, an increasing number of states have made significant advancement in the improvement of electronic medical assistance. The general tendencies are the digitization of diagnostic instruments and the structuralization of electronic health information. The increasing rise of medical information will further learn the benefits of mining medical data, while also delivering comfort to individuals. Clearly, figuring out how to securely store such a great amount of information is a challenge that needs to be addressed immediately. Furthermore, the unique nature of medical data necessitates a high level of privacy protection. This emphasizes the significance of developing a secure method to protect data security.For the smart health applications, the data first collected then processed contains many sensitive and private information. Guarantee that all innovation and applications segments incorporate and keep up adequate degrees of security and protection systems. There are many EMR and other medical record systems that keep the records of the patients, they are also considered as private and confidential. Either a developing city gives numerous positive benefits to its occupants, it likewise represents a few dangers to their security, prosperity and protection by depending intensely on their information. The chance of unlawful access or malignant assaults to such foundations can prompt cataclysmic outcomes influencing the city framework, its administration elements and its inhabitants. Huge information applications fashioners and engineers should incorporate security and protection arrangements and strategies as an indispensable piece of the plan and execution of the application.

Recognition for Better Citizen

In the fast growing cities, the citizens must be well informed of how to access and use the smart health applications for a developed city conveniently. Their dynamic interest in giving data identified the various issues with the shrewd city, in this case the application will help in improving the nature of gathered information and the presentation of the applications. Subsequently, more compelling choices can be produced using gathered large information to upgrade distinctive savvy city parts. Another significant perspective in resident mindfulness is their insight and practice of good wellbeing, security and protection rehearses. Satisfactory preparing and mindfulness crusades should be done to ensure that individuals know and are equipped for securing their own information and climate.

Government Role

The role of governing bodies for the developing cities either for the smart health sector or any other department should set up core values of receptiveness, straightforwardness, investment, and coordinated effort to keep the trade and stream of large information leveled out. Governments assume a fundamental part in a shrewd city; subsequently, it is needed to have progressed frameworks to oversee huge information gathered and utilized by government elements. Furthermore, the public authority should survey and recalibrate data and information arrangements as vital by zeroing in on protection, information reuse, information exactness, information access, chronicling, and conservation. In this manner, it should have very much characterized information to guarantee educated use regarding the datasets. To adequately uphold huge information applications, brilliant regional governments should adjust the valuable employment of information against people's security worries by tending to a portion of the principal ideas of protection laws. This incorporates characterizing "actually recognizable data", and the job of individual control.

Alongside these overall non-useful prerequisites for huge information applications, every application will likewise have its own arrangement of useful for the operational necessities. These necessities are assembled and investigated when the application is used for advancement in the shrewd city. Together the two arrangements of prerequisites ought to completely characterize all the vital necessities and assets to effectively configuration, create, test and send the necessary application. As the various prerequisites for enormous information shrewd city applications are accumulated, it very well might be additionally useful to utilize recreations to help improve and anticipate the results of such applications. Reproduction strategies offer an alternate more reasonable perspective on how the applications may act and what the normal results will be. This methodology diminishes a framework's expense in the usage and testing stages and in upgrading the necessary assets for the venture. Instances of such strategies are quickened time recreations of traffic streams permit the framework to be dynamic and adaptable just as decreasing the expense of executing traffic signals and signals.

CONCLUSION

Smart health comprises many advanced technologies consequently has a broad and vast future ahead. Many startups, research institutions and health institutions have already started working on it to make the whole process pipeline as smooth as possible. Similarly all the advanced technologies have a greater impact on smart healthcare. From the doctors point of view. Life cycle of smart healthcare has also some challenges and requirements that need to be addressed with the passage of time.Smart healthcare will also contribute to a smart city which will help in connecting administrations and healthcare officials with citizens in a much adequate way. There are still many challenges and hurdles that need to be overcome on a timely basis. Smart healthcare is gaining momentum on each passing day and creating opportunities and exploring new ideas like robotics impact on COVID 19 as well as many other things growing up on the IoT and AI side with the combination of big data and cloud computing, considering the fact that 5G presence with all of these technologies will take it to next layer.

However individual users will be facilitated with highly effective procedures on fingertips in a more secure manner. Hospitals can streamline their process, with evolution of IoT they can automate their processes instead of highly depending on humans. Research institutions can reduce their cost, time saving research and maintain accuracy.

All of these advancements raise huge hopes for the future: Smart configurations will be able to follow our health autonomously and, to some extent, will relocate the center of treatment away from clinician's premises, easing the financial burden on already overburdened medical centers and bringing the precautionary component to the forefront. There has been a definite paradigm shift away from explicitly assessing your health vitals and toward devices that blend into the surroundings and track key metrics. Second, customers are extremely interested in being their own health administrators and taking an active role in their health.

REFERENCES

Abdellatif, A. A. (2019). Edge-based compression and classification for smart healthcare systems: Concept, implementation and evaluation. *Expert Systems with Applications*, *117*, 1–14. doi:10.1016/j.eswa.2018.09.019

Agarwal, R., Baghel, N., & Khan, M. A. (2020). Load balancing in cloud computing using mutation based particle swarm optimization. In *2020 International Conference on Contemporary Computing and Applications (IC3A)*. IEEE.

Akmandor, A. O., & Jha, N. K. (2017). Keep the stress away with SoDA: Stress detection and alleviation system. *IEEE Transactions on Multi-Scale Computing Systems*, *3*(4), 269–282.

Al-Azzam, M. K., Alazzam, M. B., & Al-Manasra, M. K. (2019). MHealth for decision making support: A case study of EHealth in the public sector. *International Journal of Advanced Computer Science and Applications*, *10*(5), 381–387.

Al Nuaimi, E., Al Neyadi, H., Mohamed, N., & Al-Jaroodi, J. (2015). Applications of big data to smart cities. *Journal of Internet Services and Applications*, *6*(1), 1–15. doi:10.118613174-015-0041-5

Allhoff, F. (2009). The coming era of nanomedicine. *The American Journal of Bioethics*, *9*(10), 3–11.

Alliance, N. (2014). *5g white paper-executive version*. White Paper.

Andreu-Perez, J. (2015). From wearable sensors to smart implants--toward pervasive and personalized healthcare. *IEEE Transactions on Biomedical Engineering*, *62*(12), 2750–2762.

Arulkumar, V., & Bhalaji, N. (2021). Performance analysis of nature inspired load balancing algorithm in cloud environment. *Journal of Ambient Intelligence and Humanized Computing*, *12*(3), 3735–3742.

Bakkar, N. (2018). Artificial intelligence in neurodegenerative disease research: Use of IBM Watson to identify additional RNA-binding proteins altered in amyotrophic lateral sclerosis. *Acta Neuropathologica*, *135*(2), 227–247.

Belgacem, A., Beghdad-Bey, K., & Nacer, H. (2018). Task scheduling in cloud computing environment: A comprehensive analysis. In *International Conference on Computer Science and its Applications*. Springer.

Chen, Q., & Lu, Y. (2018). Construction and application effect evaluation of integrated management platform of intelligent hospital based on big data analysis. *Chin. Med. Herald.*, *15*(35), 161–164.

Chen, X., Ma, M., & Liu, A. (2018). Dynamic power management and adaptive packet size selection for IoT in e-Healthcare. *Computers & Electrical Engineering*, *65*, 357–375.

Condoluci, M. (2016). Enabling the IoT machine age with 5G: Machine-type multicast services for innovative real-time applications. *IEEE Access: Practical Innovations, Open Solutions*, *4*, 5555–5569.

Dalgarno, B., & Lee, M. J. (2010). What are the learning affordances of 3-D virtual environments? *British Journal of Educational Technology, 41*(1), 10–32.

Dam, S. (2018). An ant-colony-based meta-heuristic approach for load balancing in cloud computing. In *Applied Computational Intelligence and Soft Computing in Engineering* (pp. 204–232). IGI Global.

Dananjayan & Raj. (2021). 5G in healthcare: How fast will be the transformation? *Irish Journal of Medical Science, 190*(2), 497-501.

Davenport & Kalakota. (2019). The potential for artificial intelligence in healthcare. *Future Healthcare Journal, 6*(2), 94.

Dowell, D., Haegerich, T. M., & Chou, R. (2016). CDC guideline for prescribing opioids for chronic pain—United States, 2016. *Journal of the American Medical Association, 315*(15), 1624–1645.

Elhoseny, M. (2018). Secure medical data transmission model for IoT-based healthcare systems. *IEEE Access: Practical Innovations, Open Solutions, 6*, 20596–20608.

Elmagzoub, M. (2021). A Survey of Swarm Intelligence Based Load Balancing Techniques in Cloud Computing Environment. *Electronics (Basel), 10*(21), 2718.

Farahani, B., Firouzi, F., Chang, V., Badaroglu, M., Constant, N., & Mankodiya, K. (2018). Towards fog-driven IoT eHealth: Promises and challenges of IoT in medicine and healthcare. *Future Generation Computer Systems, 78*, 659–676. doi:10.1016/j.future.2017.04.036

Fertleman, C. (2018). A discussion of virtual reality as a new tool for training healthcare professionals. *Frontiers in Public Health, 6*, 44.

Franssen, J., Pagnozzi, J., & Arrillaga, G.-P. (2018). RFID Technology for Management and Tracking: e-Health Applications. *Sensors (Basel), 18*(8).

Gobinda, G. C. (2003). Natural language processing. *Annual Review of Information Science & Technology, 37*, 51–89.

Gong, F., & ... . (2013). Primary exploration in establishment of China's intelligent medical treatment. *Modern Hospital Management, 11*(2), 28–29.

Gupta, V. (2018). An energy efficient fog-cloud based architecture for healthcare. *Journal of Statistics and Management Systems, 21*(4), 529–537.

Hanine, M. (2018). QoS in the Cloud Computing: A Load Balancing Approach Using Simulated Annealing Algorithm. In *International Conference on Big Data, Cloud and Applications*. Springer.

Ismagilova, E. (2020). Security, privacy and risks within smart cities: Literature review and development of a smart city interaction framework. *Information Systems Frontiers*, 1–22.

Jain, K. K. (2008). Nanomedicine: Application of nanobiotechnology in medical practice. *Medical Principles and Practice, 17*(2), 89–101.

Javaid, M., & Haleem, A. (2020). Virtual reality applications toward medical field. *Clinical Epidemiology and Global Health*, 8(2), 600–605.

Kishor, A., & Chakraborty, C. (2021). Artificial intelligence and internet of things based healthcare 4.0 monitoring system. *Wireless Personal Communications*, 1–17.

Kumar, P. M., & Gandhi, U. D. (2018). A novel three-tier Internet of Things architecture with machine learning algorithm for early detection of heart diseases. *Computers & Electrical Engineering*, 65, 222–235.

Latif, S. (2017). How 5g wireless (and concomitant technologies) will revolutionize healthcare? *Future Internet*, 9(4), 93.

Lemheney, A. J. (2016). Developing virtual reality simulations for office-based medical emergencies. *Journal of Virtual Worlds Research*, 9(1).

Liu, J., & Liu, Y. (2018). Application of computer molecular simulation technology and artificial intelligence in drug development. *Technol. Innov. Appl.*, 2, 46–47.

Liu, L. (2016). Smart homes and home health monitoring technologies for older adults: A systematic review. *International Journal of Medical Informatics*, 91, 44–59.

Luo, F. (2018). An improved particle swarm optimization algorithm based on adaptive weight for task scheduling in cloud computing. *Proceedings of the 2nd International Conference on Computer Science and Application Engineering*.

Mansour, R. F., Amraoui, A. E., Nouaouri, I., Diaz, V. G., Gupta, D., & Kumar, S. (2021). Artificial Intelligence and Internet of Things Enabled Disease Diagnosis Model for Smart Healthcare Systems. *IEEE Access: Practical Innovations, Open Solutions*, 9, 45137–45146. doi:10.1109/ACCESS.2021.3066365

Mapetu, J. P. B., Chen, Z., & Kong, L. (2019). Low-time complexity and low-cost binary particle swarm optimization algorithm for task scheduling and load balancing in cloud computing. *Applied Intelligence*, 49(9), 3308–3330.

Martin, J. L., Varilly, H., Cohn, J., & Wightwick, G. R. (2010). Preface: Technologies for a smarter planet. *IBM Journal of Research and Development*, 54(4), 1–2. doi:10.1147/JRD.2010.2051498

McGrath, J. L. (2018). Using virtual reality simulation environments to assess competence for emergency medicine learners. *Academic Emergency Medicine*, 25(2), 186–195.

Muhammed, T. (2018). UbeHealth: A personalized ubiquitous cloud and edge-enabled networked healthcare system for smart cities. *IEEE Access: Practical Innovations, Open Solutions*, 6, 32258–32285.

Muteeh, A., Sardaraz, M., & Tahir, M. (2021). MrLBA: Multi-resource load balancing algorithm for cloud computing using ant colony optimization. *Cluster Computing*, 1–11.

Pal, D., Triyason, T., & Padungweang, P. (2018). Big data in smart-cities: Current research and challenges. *Indonesian Journal of Electrical Engineering and Informatics*, 6(4), 351–360.

Patel, A. R. (2017). Vitality of robotics in healthcare industry: an Internet of Things (IoT) perspective. In *Internet of Things and Big Data Technologies for Next Generation Healthcare* (pp. 91–109). Springer.

Pramanik, M. I. (2017). Smart health: Big data enabled health paradigm within smart cities. *Expert Systems with Applications, 87,* 370–383.

Rahmani, A. M. (2018). Exploiting smart e-Health gateways at the edge of healthcare Internet-of-Things: A fog computing approach. *Future Generation Computer Systems, 78,* 641–658.

Redfern, J. (2017). Smart health and innovation: Facilitating health-related behaviour change. *The Proceedings of the Nutrition Society, 76*(3), 328–332.

Saab, M. M. (2021). Nursing students' views of using virtual reality in healthcare: A qualitative study. *Journal of Clinical Nursing.*

Sahoo, S., Parveen, S., & Panda, J. (2007). The present and future of nanotechnology in human health care. *Nanomedicine; Nanotechnology, Biology, and Medicine, 3*(1), 20–31.

Schwid, H. A. (1999). Use of a computerized advanced cardiac life support simulator improves retention of advanced cardiac life support guidelines better than a textbook review. *Critical Care Medicine, 27*(4), 821–824.

Sharma, D. K. (2021). The aspect of vast data management problem in healthcare sector and implementation of cloud computing technique. *Materials Today: Proceedings.*

Subramaniyaswamy, V. (2019). An ontology-driven personalized food recommendation in IoT-based healthcare system. *The Journal of Supercomputing, 75*(6), 3184–3216.

Tian, S., Yang, W., Grange, J. M. L., Wang, P., Huang, W., & Ye, Z. (2019). Smart healthcare: Making medical care more intelligent. *Global Health Journal, 3*(3), 62–65. doi:10.1016/j.glohj.2019.07.001

Tripathi, A., Shukla, S., & Arora, D. (2018). A hybrid optimization approach for load balancing in cloud computing. In *Advances in Computer and Computational Sciences* (pp. 197–206). Springer. doi:10.1007/978-981-10-3773-3_19

Tripathi, G., Ahad, M. A., & Paiva, S. (2020). S2HS-A blockchain based approach for smart healthcare system. In *Healthcare.* Elsevier.

Verma, P., Sood, S. K., & Kalra, S. (2018). Cloud-centric IoT based student healthcare monitoring framework. *Journal of Ambient Intelligence and Humanized Computing, 9*(5), 1293–1309.

Wiederhold, B. K. (2014). Special issue on virtual reality and pain. Cyberpsychology Behavior and Social Networking, 17(6).

Wiederhold, B. K., & Wiederhold, M. D. (2005). *Virtual reality therapy for anxiety disorders: Advances in evaluation and treatment.* American Psychological Association.

Wu, T. (2017). An autonomous wireless body area network implementation towards IoT connected healthcare applications. *IEEE Access: Practical Innovations, Open Solutions, 5,* 11413–11422.

Wu, X. (2018). Mixed reality technology launches in orthopedic surgery for comprehensive preoperative management of complicated cervical fractures. *Surgical Innovation, 25*(4), 421–422.

Yang, Y., Liu, X., & Deng, R. H. (2017). Lightweight break-glass access control system for healthcare Internet-of-Things. *IEEE Transactions on Industrial Informatics*, *14*(8), 3610–3617.

Yaqoob, I. (2021). Blockchain for healthcare data management: Opportunities, challenges, and future recommendations. *Neural Computing & Applications*, 1–16.

Zeinab, K. A. M., & Elmustafa, S. A. A. (2017). Internet of things applications, challenges and related future technologies. *World Scientific News*, *2*(67), 126–148.

Chapter 5
Securing Clinical Information Through Multimedia Watermarking Techniques

K. Renuka Devi

Dr. Mahalingam college of Engineering and Technology, India

K. Balasamy

(iD) https://orcid.org/0000-0003-0973-5698

Bannari Amman Institute of Technology, India

ABSTRACT

Today, in this technological world, the information available can be easily copied, manipulated, as well as broadcasted among different channels, which should be protected. In the case of the medical field, the reliability and authenticity of e-medical data is one of the serious concerns. The patient's data without the knowledge of user might be utilized by the intruders. Medical data is highly valuable for the purpose of diagnosis and treatment. Due to increase in the usage of internet, copyright protection, content authentication, and identity theft are considered to be the bottleneck issues for content proprietors. To resolve those issues, the authors focused on the study of watermarking technology, which is used to improve the security of data and protect information from unauthorized access. Multimedia watermarking plays a predominant role in preserving the information from unauthorized access. This chapter aims to provide the detailed review of various watermarking techniques, their applications for security purposes, and the e-verification of medical information.

INTRODUCTION

Digital data is a combination of several contents such as audio, video, image, text etc., and those digital data will be transmitted in large content over the internet. Networks acts as a driver for the growing trend of those digital content (Sanjay Kumar et al., 2020). So, the data or information which is available over the network are prone to attacks and can be easily accessed by the intruders. Nowadays, the protection

DOI: 10.4018/978-1-6684-4580-8.ch005

for image centric data is one of the utmost tasks where the images are tampered generally by the image processing software (Hurrah et al., 2019). So, the watermarking technique plays a significant role in protecting our content. The watermarking technique which we develop should have high computational efficiency. There are several multimedia editing software and different protecting methods like cryptography and Steganographic Techniques are available. But these techniques are less fortified to protect these digital contents. Therefore, digital watermarking scheme are utilized to secure those digital entities and so this method is evolving rapidly (Dixit et al., 2017). The watermarking technique has been utilized in various fields for securing the data like database systems, for protection of IP address etc., To make the watermarking techniques distinguished from other technique, it should satisfy some of the requirements pertains such as capacity, robustness/security, and imperceptibility (Chin-Feng Lee et al., 2018).

The conditions in which watermarking apply to several digital data like:

1. The watermark data rate should be high.
2. Watermark must stay inside the host data in order to maintain robustness.
3. It should not be removable.
4. The watermark must be private and accessible to the outside party in which they must be authorized.

THE CONCEPT OF WATERMARKING

Watermarking is a concept of modifying the content of specific information by embedding information about the data which is predominant to the user. There are two important characteristics of watermarking (Baljit Kaur et al., 2017).

- The information/ data should not make any modifications to the host environment.
- The information/ data should associate to the host environment.

The Watermarking technique also includes a subset of information hidden which is not associated with the host environment (for instance: by covert communications). However, specific authors describe this situation as information hiding (Umair Khadam et al., 2016).

The Watermarking technique consists of two definite modules:

- The module which embeds the information/ data to the host environment.
- The module which reveal the given piece of information hosts a watermark and eventually retrieves the delivered information.

Based on the above module definitions and the characteristics of embedded information, the watermarking methodology is utilized for several kinds of applications for protecting the multitude of vital information from the intruders (Kamaruddin et al., 2018; Sowmya et al., 2021).

Generally, the concept of watermarking technique includes two phases (Raniyah Wazirali et al., 2021) which is illustrated in Figure 1:

1. Embedding phase
2. Extraction phase

Figure 1. Watermarking technique - concept

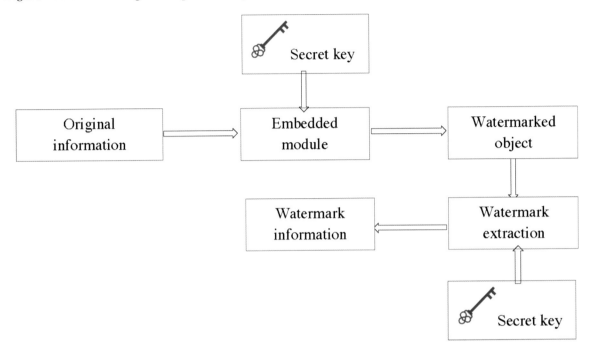

The original information was incorporated to the embedded module, where this process allows the users to include watermarked information to their digital data. It utilizes a secret key for inserting the secret data to the original information (Manivannan et al., 2017; Podilchuk et al., 2001; Haiming et al., 2018). This process which is mainly utilized for authentication of data, copyright protection etc., The embedding a watermark has been illustrated by equation 1.

$$X = s(1 + \alpha W) \tag{1}$$

Where,

S corresponds to the original host signal,

X corresponds to the Watermarked signal,

W corresponds to the watermark consisting of a random, Gaussian distributed sequence,

α is a scaling factor.

This step produces the Watermarked object as a result which is utilized in the next phase called Watermark extraction, where this phase is used to extract the data from the watermarked object (Manivannan et al., 2017; Podilchuk et al., 2001; Haiming et al., 2018). This phase uses the same secret key which is used by the embedding phase for extracting the data from the watermarked object. Figure 1 shows more details about Watermarking technique - concept. This has been illustrated by equation 2.

$$sim\left(W, \widehat{W}\right) = \frac{\widehat{W}.W}{\sqrt{\widehat{W}.\widehat{W}}} \tag{2}$$

Where,

$\widehat{W}$ corresponds to the extracted watermark from the received, possibly distorted signal Y,

W corresponds to the watermark consisting of a random, Gaussian distributed sequence.

Classification

The different watermarking techniques has been classified based on document's type such as text, audio, video, and image(Qasim et al., 2017). These techniques are divided into different categories in order to improve the transparency and robustness of the original information (Tahera Akhtar Laskar et al., 2013). The watermarking methodology is often classified based on three distinct classes which is illustrated in Figure 2 –

1. Multimedia based
2. Characteristic based
3. Application based

Figure 2. Watermarking – classification

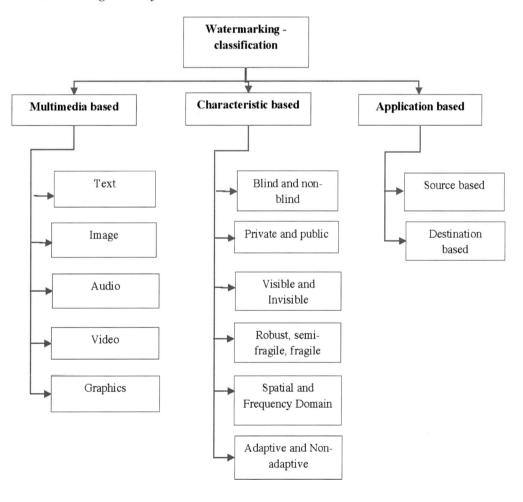

MULTIMEDIA BASED

There are different kinds of watermark classification for multimedia which is shown in Figure 3. This includes (Raniyah Wazirali et al., 2021),

1. Text watermarking
2. Image watermarking
3. Video watermarking
4. Graphic watermarking

Figure 3. Types of multimedia based watermarking

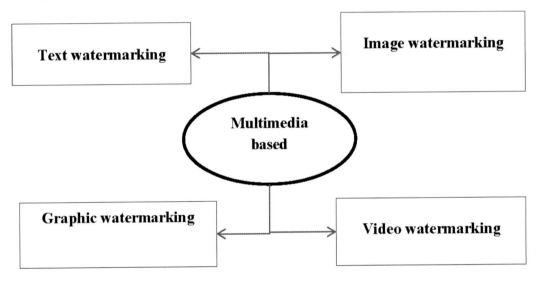

Text Watermarking

The data in the form of text consists of different entities such as word, sentence, paragraph etc., The syntax and semantics included here is important in the transformation to incorporate digital watermark into the text.

The utilization of internet has been increased rapidly due to the transfer of information and accessibility over the digital world. Among all other watermarking techniques, text composes of more complex and demanding method where this watermarking technique can be administered. This technique comprises of multiplicity of tasks, therefore this has been lead to finite research scope in this field (Kamaruddin et al., 2018).

The contents of digital text includes various entities in the form of articles, webpages etc., These entities whenever gets uploaded, they may get vulnerable to different kinds of attacks and copying, as a result their security and protection becomes an influential matter. Because of insufficient techniques in processing of those digital contexts, the protection of those content becomes difficult. The protection of the above said digital text depends on the effectiveness of watermarking methods and techniques. The sample image for text watermarking has been shown in Figure 4.

Figure 4. Text watermarking – sample image

Text Watermark
For Blogger

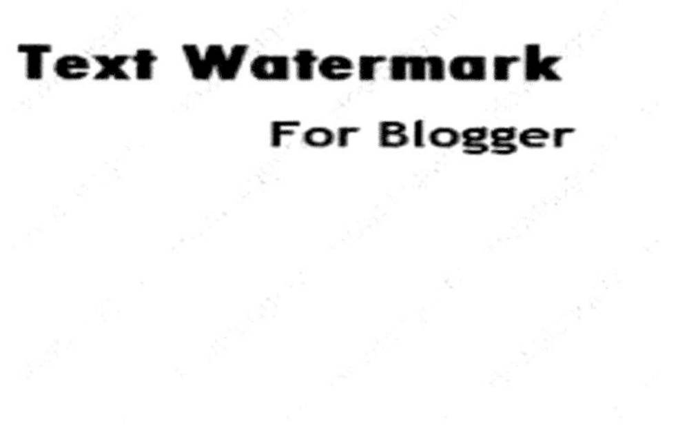

Image Watermarking

In this methodology, the ownership of the hidden information has been enhanced by embedding it into cover media (Vaidya et al., 2017; Savakar et al., 2019). One of the bottlenecks in protecting information is the copyright abuse of the digital content. There are several properties which make the watermarking technique most significant is that robustness, security, imperceptibility, complexity, and verification (Jobin Abraham, 2011).

Those embedded watermarked information consists of string of bits which incorporates the proprietor's name or image of specific symbol(Lalit Kumar Saini et al., 2014).

The watermarked information by image should be undetectable by the intruders (Altaa et al., 2012; Thapa et al., 2011; Dhiman et al., 2016). The protection of information by algorithms should make the data highly secure and it shouldn't be known by the attackers (Akhtar et al., 2016). Even though the watermark is detectable, it shouldn't be breakable by the intruders. The image watermarking technique plays a crucial role in protecting the user's data at utmost concern (Mohammad Abdullatif et al., 2013; Shweta Wadhera et al., 2021). The sample image for image watermarking has been shown in Figure 5.

Figure 5. Image watermarking – sample image

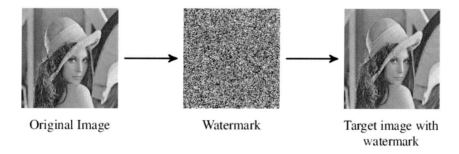

Original Image   Watermark   Target image with watermark

Video Watermarking

Digital video watermarking is a methodology of incorporating the video signal into the original data. Those incorporated data is mainly used for identification of owner's copyright (Jayamalar et al., 2010).

There are several video watermarking techniques have been developed. Those techniques have been used to incorporate watermark in order to maintain the video's accuracy. This method is utilized for prohibiting the exploitation of the digital contents by embedding watermarks in the video sequence for the purpose of protecting the contents from illegal copying and manipulation identification (Shahid et al., 2018). To identify manipulation, exploitation of digital contents, illegal copying, ownership problems, a variety of strong and fragile video watermarking techniques have been developed. Those techniques will be suitable for compressing and uncompressing information by employing Fourier, DCT, DWT, Fractal transforms (Kumar et al., 2020). The video watermarking techniques should meet the challenges such as frame averaging, frame swapping, statistical analysis, lossy compressions and find the solutions for them. The sample image for video watermarking has been shown in Figure 6.

The video watermarking techniques are classified into various techniques such as:

- Spatial domain
- Frequency domain
- Format-specific

Figure 6. Video watermarking – sample image

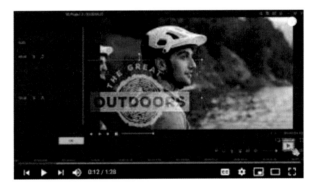

Spatial Domain

Spatial domain is a technique which mainly concentrated on altering the pixel values of randomly selected images (Mishra et al., 2018). This algorithm will incorporate the raw data into pixels of image directly (Kumar et al., 2016). The algorithm under spatial domain includes LSB, Patchwork, texture mapping coding, etc.,

Least Significant Bit (LSB)

LSB is one of the simplest methodology for implementation. During this process, a watermark bit has been embedded to the LSB of each pixel. During extraction or detection method, the final bit of each pixel has been used to convey the watermark (Kumar et al., 2016). Even though the watermark has been cropped, it is possible to retrieve the needed data. Its because the data has been embedded n number of times. This methodology is highly sensitive to noise, so that it cannot be used for practical utilization but this is not so robust.

- **Benefits of LSB:**
  - Simple to implement.
  - Complexity for computation of LSB is very less for both embedding and extraction technique.
  - Quality of image is less.
- **Drawbacks of LSB:**
  - Not very robust.
  - Techniques like cropping, shuffling will degrade the watermark which is embedded.
  - Has noise sensitivity.

Patchwork Technique

The Patchwork algorithm incorporates information into the brightness of pixels by altering the image's statistical qualities. This technique utilizes the pair of points which is chosen randomly. The pixel points are named as (a_i, b_i) and the difference between those two points have been calculated and it equals zero was centered at Gaussian distribution. The pixel point a_i has been incremented by one and another pixel point b_i has been decremented by one (Abraham et al., 2019). In the above said scenario, the distribution center only will get changed but the image's brightness will remain unchanged. With the aim of withstanding the attack of compression and filtering, this technique enlarges those pixels to a pair of blocks. As a result of this, the brightness will get increased in one block and brightness will get reduced in the corresponding block.

- **Benefits:**
  While comparing with LSB, patchwork technique is highly robust against different kinds of attacks.

- **Drawbacks:**
  Information which is hidden will be less while comparing with other techniques.

Texture Mapping Coding

It is a technique where the watermark has been concealed under the texture part of the image. It will be useful which contains some text part in the image where the data will get hidden under the random pattern of the image(Abraham et al., 2019). From this it is clear this methodology will be suitable for images with variety of textures.

- **Benefits:**
  - The information has been incorporated in the part of random pattern of the image.
- **Drawbacks:**
  - It will be suitable for the areas which have more number of texture images.
  - This requires human intervention.

Frequency Domain

Frequency domain is also known as transform domain. It is due to the fact that some values are modified from their original values. The commonly utilized methods of frequency domain technique includes Discrete Cosine Transform (DCT), Discrete Fourier Transform (DFT), Discrete Wavelet Transform (DWT), and Discrete Hadamard Transform (DHT) (Namita Tiwari et al., 2017).

Discrete Cosine Transform (DCT)

Discrete Cosine Transform is considered to be one of the widely used methodology in digital watermarking world. While comparing frequency domain with spatial domain, this technique is highly robust and it is one of the biggest advantage of it (Liu et al., 2017). It is robust against basic image processing functionalities such as low pass filtering, blurring etc., In the other case this technique is not so robust against some attacks such as scaling, rotation etc., So, the transform domain techniques are hard to implement due to the large value of its computational complexity. The Discrete Cosine Transform of two dimensional image is outlined in equation 3,

$$C = \{g(i,j), i,j = 0,1,\ldots,M-1\} \tag{3}$$

Where,

g is an input image,

g(i,j) is the intensity of the pixel.

- **Benefits:**
    - In DCT transformation, the watermark is hidden into the coefficient of high as well as middle frequency, as a result of this, the visibility of image will not get affected and it won't be removed by any of the intruders (Moosazadeh et al., 2019).
- **Drawbacks:**
    - During the process of quantization, some higher frequency component gets suppressed.
    - DCT transformation won't work for under scaling attacks.

Discrete Fourier Transform (DFT)

Discrete Fourier Transform is one of the technique for transformation which converts the continuous functions into the component of frequencies. In general, the image's Fourier transformation have such complex values and this leads to the image's magnitude and phase representation (Fares et al., 2020). The Discrete Fourier Transform of two dimensional image f(u,v) of size MxN is outlined in equation 4,

$$F\left(x,y\right) = \sum_{u=0}^{M-1}\sum_{v=0}^{N-1} f\left(u,v\right).e^{\frac{-j2\pi ux}{M}}.e^{\frac{-j2\pi vy}{N}} \tag{4}$$

Where,

u = 0,1,2….M-1 and

v = 0,1,2,….N-1

F(u,v) is the value of image at (u,v),

F(x,y) is the coefficient of DFT at (x,y).

- **Benefits:**
    - DFT technique has been unchanged to rotation, scaling, and translation. So that it is easy to recover from geometric distortion.

- **Drawbacks:**
  - The implementation of DFT is complex while comparing with other methods.
  - The cost of computation is also high.

Discrete Wavelet Transform (DWT)

Discrete Wavelet Transform (DWT) is based on tiny waves which is called as minimum duration and wavelet of variable frequency. In this technique, the decomposition of image has been varied into three different directions such as horizontal, vertical and diagonal. The decomposition process in DWT is explained as follows: initially the image has been subdivided in the form of four wavelets such as LL, LH, HL, and HH. L denotes low pass filter and H denotes high pass filter. The first filter (either H or L) denotes in horizontal direction and the second filter (either H or L) denotes in vertical direction (Anand et al., 2020). DWT is largely seen in different domains such as image compression, image processing etc.,

- **Benefits:**
  - DWT is highly robust to cropping.
  - The ratio of compression is also high.
  - It has multi resolution property.
- **Drawbacks:**
  - The cost of computation is high.
  - The time for performing compression is also high.
  - Noise is present which is adjacent to the image's edges.

Discrete Hadamard Transform (DHT)

Discrete Hadamard Transform (DHT) is a kind of non-sinusoidal transformation and this technique is based on Hadamard matrix. Hadamard matrix is a square matrix whose entries are +1 or -1 as well as their rows are mutually orthogonal. This technique utilizes minimum number of coefficients while comparing with other techniques (Elham Moeinaddini et al., 2015). The following relation has been satisfied by the Discrete Hadamard Transformation which is given in equation 5:

$$HH^T = 1 \tag{5}$$

Where,
H=NxN, Hadamard matrix,
I= Identity matrix.

- **Benefits:**
  - The cost of computation is less.
  - The real values used here are +1 or -1.
  - It is more efficient methodology.
- **Drawbacks:**
  - While comparing with other techniques, it is less complex then other transformation technique but it is more complex than spatial domain methodology.

Format-Specific

In video watermarking scheme, format specific can be based on specific formats like MPEG-2 and MPEG-4 based techniques. Namita Tiwari and Sharmila proposed a watermarking feature which is based on MPEG-4 (Namita Tiwari et al., 2017). They proposed a method based on scrambling technique which adopts spread spectrum watermarking technique based on the requirements of MPEG-4 (Vassaux et al., 2002). The above algorithm can be utilized embedding and detection techniques without modifying the watermarking algorithm. To reduce the time complexity of video processing, the formats which is based on MPEG-1, MPEG-2 and MPEG-4 structures are highly involved in combining watermarking and compression methodologies.

- **Drawbacks:**
  - ○ MPEG based formatting structures are highly vulnerable to re-compression technique with different kinds of parameters.

Graphic Watermarking

Text watermarking has been implemented based on the classification of position and method of embedded watermark. There are few restrictions in familiarities of language. So, a new classification methodology has been introduced based on Chinese characters (Liu et al., 2014). The graphic watermarking technique has been divided into various levels based on position embedded, pixel, line, etymon, character, row, paragraph, page, and chapter which is shown in Figure 7. Each level consists of specific number of upper levels based on definite rule (Agarwal et al., 2015). The pixel composed of text graphics units. Any kind of text composed of multitude of pixels. The chapter consists of higher order of text (Shukla et al., 2016). For each level, there are various kinds of embedding methodologies, which includes varying the grey scale value, substituting font with similar other font, modifying the variance between etymon of words (Agrawal et al., 2003). The sample image for graphic watermarking has been shown in Figure 8.

The characteristic for each level includes:

- Self-characteristics,
- Similarity and
- Structural feature.

SECURING OF MEDICAL DATA

The protection of medical data is one of the important and complex process in healthcare domain. The integrity of the data will be maintained by controlling the access of the database only to the authorized users (Tekieh Mohammad et al., 2015). Techniques like Type-Based Proxy Re-Encryption, and signatures schemes, such as the Bilinear Aggregate Signature Scheme can be utilized to maintain the integrity of the data. A prototype based on secure medical database will be implemented to secure the non-secure medical database. The strong analysis tool is required to handle and analyse those clinical information. However, there might be huge sensitive data to be analyzed as well as several security protocols should be required to analyze those data (Kumar et al., 2018). But the implementation of those security protocols might be provoking. So, it is important to protect both the patient's privacy and allow the analysts to conduct analysis. Those health data can be protected by utilizing the anonymization techniques such as masking and de-identification techniques (Singh et al., 2017). But the usage of those anonymization techniques might result in the loss of quality and it cannot be used for further analysis.

Issues in Securing Healthcare Data

The major reason for security threats and attacks occurs due to inadequate measures taken. Several measures for protection of data includes tools for threat detection, upgraded software applications, security patches etc., (Singh et al., 2013). Healthcare data includes information to be identified such as name, address to sensitive information which includes medical ID numbers, health insurance data and patients' medical histories. In general, the healthcare domain is considered to be one of the weaker one, where the data could be easily get breached (Song et al., 2010). So, the data should be protected in most efficient manner (Ahmed et al., 2016).

Figure 7. Graphic watermarking levels

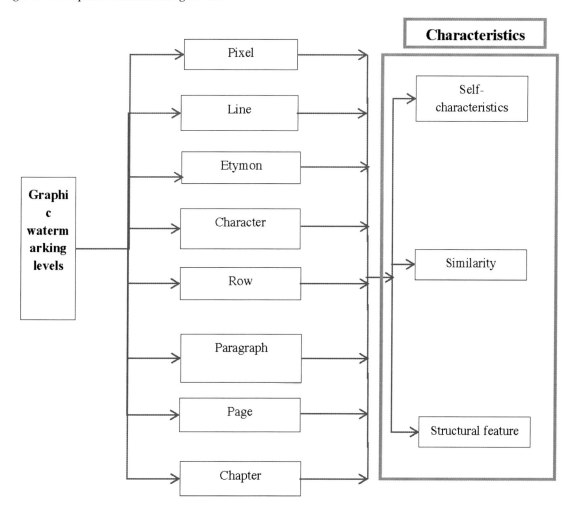

Figure 8. Graphic watermarking – sample image

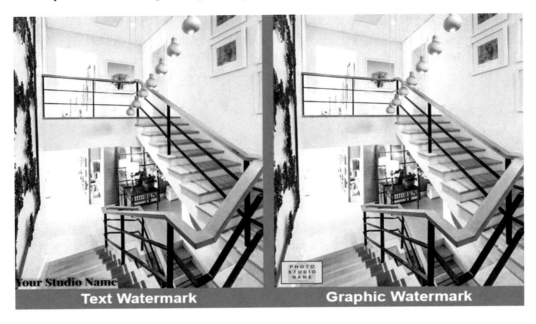

Those sensitive and individual data can be protected by utilizing right measures and techniques. There are several situations which acts as a bottleneck in healthcare domain include:

- Several agents relate to the health arena that is permitted to access the health content but they utilize for unethical ways.
- The external user who is considered to be the real one, access the data but they are actually considered as unauthorized persons.

So, the watermarking technique plays a predominant role in efficient analysis and protection of patient's data from unauthorized access (Singh et al., 2017).

Importance of Watermarking in Healthcare Domain

Watermarking is one of the significant methodologies for protecting the data in healthcare domain. Basically, the healthcare data contains confidential as well as unprotected data which is corresponding to patient's health. The digital watermarking acts as an enhanced tool to address different kinds of issues like improvising the protection and confidentiality of healthcare data, and for systematic retrieval of information (Khaloufi et al., 2018).

The wavelet based watermarking scheme incorporates several watermarks into medical images. Those watermarks convey the authenticated data, patient's personal information, and health reports of those patients. This methodology also embeds the reference watermark for maintaining the integrity of the healthcare image(Sanjay Kumar et al., 2018; Ali et al., 2018). The flow of watermarking in healthcare domain is illustrated in Figure 9.

Figure 9. Process of watermarking in healthcare domain

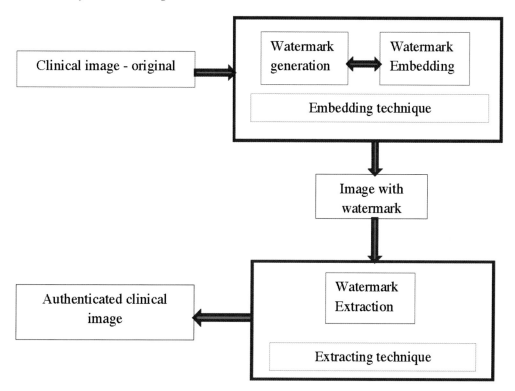

WATERMARKING CRITERIA

The main requirements of watermark which includes **robustness, imperceptibility, Security, Capacity, Verifiability, Computational cost, Fragility** which is illustrated in Figure10. It plays a significant role in the watermarking field to ensure high quality of processed data.

Robustness

Robustness is the ability to detect the watermark after performing some kind of signal processing methodologies which includes spatial filtering, scanning and printing, lossy compression etc., and also include other functionalities such as digital to analog, analog to digital. It is also noted that not all watermarking algorithms doesn't expose the same level of robustness, however they might get failed under stronger attacks (Piva et al., 2002). This kind of watermarking requirement is highly required when copyright information is to be inserted. Robustness is specified when the embedded watermark is not damaged (Agarwal et al., 2019). So, this kind of methodology is highly advantageous for copyright protection(Verma et al., 2015; Tao et al., 2014; Zhang et al., 2010). The robustness is classified into different methodologies:

- Robust
- Fragile
- Semi – fragile

Figure 10. Watermarking requirements

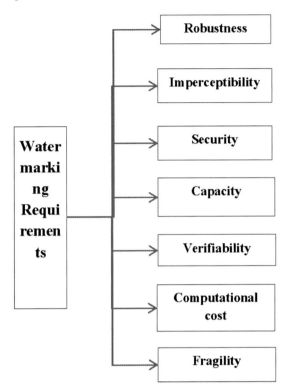

Imperceptibility

Imperceptibility, also called as Invisibility and Fidelity which could be considered as most significant and elegant requirement in system of watermarking where it is invisible to the human eye and it refers to the similarity between original image and watermarked image. The image that is watermarked must be identical to the original image and the watermark that is embedded should be unnoticeable irrespective of contrast in image or brightness (Agarwal et al., 2019). The robustness and Capacity are dependent of each other; the problem is that when imperceptibility has been achieved, the robustness and Capacity will get degraded and vice versa. This requirement has been modulated by increasing the robustness and Capacity of the image. However, the watermark is not always pretend to be invisible, it chose to be visible watermark into that image.

Security

The security requirement specifies that when the watermark has been applied on specified target, it shouldn't be removed. The process of removing the watermark without any worsening condition with respect to host signal will become difficult task. It is the condition to protect the data against several attacks (Zhang et al., 2017). Those attack types will be classified as:

- unauthorized removal,
- unauthorized embedding, and

- unauthorized detection

To protect the data against those attacks, the specific feature must be available for efficient handling of data. For unauthorized removal, the watermarked data should be robust and it shouldn't be removed. For unauthorized embedding, the watermarked data should be fragile or semi-fragile in order to encounter the change that has been resulted. For unauthorized detection, the watermark should be imperceptible. The security feature in watermark plays a vital role to provide ownership, privacy as well as the protection of data.

Capacity

The feature of capacity in watermark requirement indicates the amount of bits that has been incorporated to the original image. The quantity of information that has been incorporated into the watermarked image also called as payload of data (Korus et al., 2014). The volume of the image will get differ depending on the application the watermark that has been created for. The concept of understanding the capacity of the image reveals that there is a limit to the information that has been embedded and moreover, it should satisfy the former requirements such as imperceptibility and robustness.

Verifiability

The feature of verifiability helps to verify the authenticity of the digital contents. By the concept of watermarking methodology, the user can be able to retrieve information regarding the ownership of protected data that has been copyrighted (Alkawaz et al., 2016). It also used to protect the data from unauthenticated copying of digital contents.

Computational Cost

The feature of computational cost for incorporating the watermarked information into the original image and extracting those watermarked content from the embedded image should be minimum. The computational cost which addresses two issues such as the total time that is essential for embedding and extracting the image and the overall embedders and detectors associated with the watermarking technique (Sivasubramanian et al., 2020). In order to receive a significant watermarking result, consistent trade off among the requirements such as robustness and computational complexity should be maintained.

Fragility

The feature of fragility plays an important role in the detection of modification that has been occurred in the original image or host image (Subashini et al., 2013).

WATERMARKING - APPLICATIONS

The watermarking applications could be seen in various areas and the important one are discussed here. Those applications are given in the Figure 11.

Figure 11. Watermarking applications

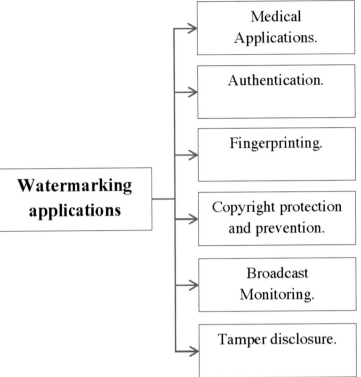

Medical Applications

Medical field is one of the important areas which utilize various data which is highly confidential and sensitive. So, it is considered to be very important to protect those data from illegal usage. The watermarking technology plays a significant role by satisfying several features such as capacity, robustness, privacy and imperceptibility. Based on the results from various reports, a patient might be cured and will get right treatment (Nikolic et al., 2016). A crisis might occur if results of multiple patients get mixed. To improve the authenticity of images, reverse watermarking technique has been utilized. The authentication feature improves the integrity of the image, and to maintain the quality, the feature of reflection has been utilized.

Authentication

Today in this technological world, the process for modifying the data content has become simple and easy by the utilization of different kind of multimedia editing programs. For the purpose of making the content summarized, digital signature plays an important part in it. The modification of content will be indicated by denoting a gap in the content and as well as the signature also gets changed (Lee et al., 2019). The watermarking methodology plays a vital role in maintaining the authentication of data (Priya et al., 2017).

Fingerprinting

Fingerprinting is a kind of application which utilizes watermarking technique to safeguard the privacy of the data. For each kind of information obtained from digital entity, a special context of data and information will be incorporated to the content for protecting the legality of the data. The efficiency of the data depends on the watermarking property which is invisible and this feature has been obtained by the content ((Subashini et al., 2013). The significant property of this application is based on tracing copies from illegally published data (Kumar et al., 2018).

Copyright Protection and Prevention

Copyright protection is a kind of application where watermarking technique has been implemented significantly. The ownership of specific data will be determined by the application of it. Based on the utilization of different kind of watermarking algorithms and techniques, the copyright prevention of important documents will get maintained (Ray et al., 2020). The watermark technique will embed a key for permitting copy, which results in bit stream and based on the result, a decision has been made to accept the legal ones and to prohibit the illegal ones (Sherekar et al., 2008).

Broadcast Monitoring

To check the broadcasting feature, a specific watermark has been incorporated into the objects such as audio, video, text and image. In added to that, the copyrighted owner of the data will track the broadcast based on various techniques of communication through mobile, radio or TV. Those information will be distributed by means of internet (Ray et al., 2020). To detect the features of broadcasting, the digital watermarking is decoded and then it is applied. From the above cited technique, the broadcasting has been monitored in order to improve privacy (Taha et al., 2018).

Tamper Disclosure

A large number of data and documents are available across online to be accessed by many users where those documents are prone to various kinds of attacks such as unauthorized access by intruders, redistribution of content and copying of data (Lee et al., 2019). Tamper disclosure is a kind of application that utilizes the watermarking methodology for detecting and identifying the damaged areas in the contents of original documents (Prabhishek Singh et al., 2013).

CONCLUSION

In this paper, we discussed about the brief introduction about multimedia watermarking and how it plays a significant role in protecting the data by embedding some kind of special information. A brief review on watermarking types such as text, image, graphic and video watermarking have been highlighted. This paper also stated about various issues faced by the medical field and how the watermarking techniques plays an important role in protecting those clinical information. In added to that, the requirements or important criteria such as capacity, robustness, Imperceptibility, security, verifiability, computational cost and fragility of watermarking to be satisfied by various kinds of applications are discussed. The utilization of watermarking methodology in various applications such as copyright protection and prevention, authentication, broadcast monitoring, medical field, tamper disclosure in order to ensure the protection of the sensitive information also have been discussed.

REFERENCES

Abdullatif, Akram, Chebil, & Gunawan. (2013). Properties of Digital Image Watermarking. *Proceedings of the IEEE 9th International Colloquium on Signal Processing and its Applications*, 235–240. 10.1109/CSPA.2013.6530048

Abraham, J. (2011). Digital Image Watermarking: An Overview. *National Seminar on Modern Trends in EC & SP*, 36–42.

Abraham, J., & Paul, V. (2019). An imperceptible spatial domain color image watermarking scheme. *Journal of King Saud University-Computer and Information Sciences*, *31*(1), 125–133. doi:10.1016/j.jksuci.2016.12.004

Agarwal, H., Raman, B., & Venkat, I. (2015). Blind reliable invisible watermarking method in wavelet domain for face image watermark. *Multimedia Tools and Applications*, *74*(17), 6897–6935. doi:10.100711042-014-1934-1

Agarwal, N., Singh, A. K., & Singh, P. K. (2019). Survey of robust and imperceptible watermarking. *Multimedia Tools and Applications*, *78*(7), 8603–8633. doi:10.100711042-018-7128-5

Agrawal, R., Haas, P. J., & Kiernan, J. (2003). Watermarking relational data: Framework, algorithms and analysis. *The VLDB Journal-The International Journal on Very Large Data Bases*, *12*(2), 157–169. doi:10.100700778-003-0097-x

Ahmed, F., & Moskowitz, I. S. (2016). A Semi-Reversible Watermark for Medical Image Authentication. *Proceedings of the 1st Transdisciplinary Conference on Distributed Diagnosis and Home Healthcare*, 59–62. 10.1109/DDHH.2006.1624797

Akhtar, Z., & Khan, E. (2016). Identifying high quality jpeg compressed images through exhaustive recompression technique. *Proceedings of the International conference on advances in computing, communications and informatics (ICACCI)*, 652–656. 10.1109/ICACCI.2016.7732120

Ali, Z., Imran, M., Alsulaiman, M., Zia, T., & Shoaib, M. (2018). A zero-watermarking algorithm for privacy protection in biomedical signals. *Future Generation Computer Systems*, *82*, 290–303. doi:10.1016/j.future.2017.12.007

Alkawaz, M. H., Sulong, G., Saba, T., Almazyad, A. S., & Rehman, A. (2016). Concise analysis of current text automation and watermarking approaches. *Security and Communication Networks*, *9*(18), 6365–6378. doi:10.1002ec.1738

Altaa, A. A. J., Sahib, S. B., & Zamani, M. (2012). An Introduction to Image Steganography Techniques. *Proceedings of the 2012 International Conference on Advanced Computer Science Applications and Technologies (ACSAT)*, 122–126. 10.1109/ACSAT.2012.25

Anand, A., & Singh, A. K. (2020). An improved DWT-SVD domain watermarking for medical information security. *Computer Communications*, *152*, 72–80. doi:10.1016/j.comcom.2020.01.038

Dhiman, S., & Singh, O. (2016). Analysis of Visible and Invisible Image Watermarking - A Review. *International Journal of Computers and Applications*, *147*(3), 975–8887. doi:10.5120/ijca2016911055

Dixit, A., & Dixit, R. (2017). A Review on Digital Image Watermarking Techniques. International Journal of Image, Graphics &. *Signal Processing*, *9*(4), 56–66. doi:10.5815/ijigsp.2017.04.07

Fares, K., Amine, K., & Salah, E. (2020). A robust blind color image watermarking based on Fourier transform domain. *Optik (Stuttgart)*, *208*, 164562. Advance online publication. doi:10.1016/j.ijleo.2020.164562

Haiming, L. (2018). Embedding and Extracting Digital Watermark Based on DCT Algorithm. *Journal of Computer and Communications*, *6*(11), 287–298. doi:10.4236/jcc.2018.611026

Hurrah, N. N., Parah, S. A., Loan, N. A., Sheikh, J. A., Elhoseny, M., & Muhammad, K. (2019). Dual watermarking framework for privacy protection and content authentication of multimedia. *Future Generation Computer Systems*, *94*, 654–673. doi:10.1016/j.future.2018.12.036

Jayamalar, T., & Radha, V. (2010). Survey on Digital Video Watermarking Techniques and Attacks on Watermarks. *International Journal of Engineering Science and Technology*, *2*(12), 6963–6967.

Kamaruddin, N. S., Kamsin, A., Por, L. Y., & Rahman, H. (2018). A Review of Text Watermarking: Theory, Methods, and Applications. *IEEE Access: Practical Innovations, Open Solutions*, *6*, 8011–8028. doi:10.1109/ACCESS.2018.2796585

Kaur, B., & Sharma, S. (2017). Digital Watermarking and Security Techniques: A Review. *International Journal of Computer Science and Technology*, *8*(2), 44–47.

Khadam, U., Iqbal, M. M., Azam, M. A., Khalid, S., Rho, S., & Chilamkurti, N. (2016). Digital Watermarking Technique for Text Document Protection Using Data Mining Analysis. *IEEE Access: Practical Innovations, Open Solutions*, *7*, 64955–64965. doi:10.1109/ACCESS.2019.2916674

Khaloufi. (2018). Security model for Big Healthcare Data Lifecycle. *Proceedings of the 8th International Conference on Current and Future Trends of Information and Communication Technologies in Healthcare (ICTH 2018)*, 294–301. 10.1016/j.procs.2018.10.199

Korus, P., Białas, J., & Dziech, A. (2014). A new approach to high-capacity annotation watermarking based on digital fountain codes. *Multimedia Tools and Applications*, *68*(1), 59–77. doi:10.100711042-011-0986-8

Kumar, C., Singh, A. K., & Kumar, P. (2018). A recent survey on image watermarking techniques and its application in e-governance. *Multimedia Tools and Applications*, *77*(3), 3597–3622. doi:10.100711042-017-5222-8

Kumar, S., & Dutta, A. (2016). Performance analysis of spatial domain digital watermarking techniques. *Proceedings of the 2016 IEEE International conference on information communication and embedded systems (ICICES)*, 1–4. 10.1109/ICICES.2016.7518910

Kumar, S., & Singh, B. K. (2018). A Review of Digital Watermarking in HealthCare Domain. *Proceedings of the 3rd International Conference on Computational Systems and Information Technology for Sustainable Solutions (CSITSS)*, 156–159. 10.1109/CSITSS.2018.8768733

Kumar, S., & Singh, B. K. (2018). A Review of Digital Watermarking in HealthCare Domain. *Proceedings of the 3rd IEEE International Conference on Computational Systems and Information Technology for Sustainable Solutions*, 156–159. 10.1109/CSITSS.2018.8768733

Kumar, S., Singh, B. K., & Yadav, M. (2020). A Recent survey on multimedia and database watermarking. *Multimedia Tools and Applications*, *79*(27), 20149–20197. doi:10.100711042-020-08881-y

Kumar, S., Singh, B. K., & Yadav, M. (2020). A Recent Survey on Multimedia and Database Watermarking. *Multimedia Tools and Applications*, *79*(27), 20149–20197. doi:10.100711042-020-08881-y

Laskar & Hemachandran. (2013). Digital image watermarking techniques and its Applications. *International Journal of Engineering Research & Technology (Ahmedabad)*, *2*(3), 1–8.

Lee, C.-F., Shen, J.-J., & Chen, Z.-R. (2018). A Survey of Watermarking-Based Authentication for Digital Image. *Proceedings of the 3rd International Conference on Computer and Communication Systems*, 207–211. 10.1109/CCOMS.2018.8463259

Lee, C. F., Shen, J. J., Chen, Z. R., & Agrawal, S. (2019). Self-Embedding Authentication Watermarking with Effective Tampered Location Detection and High-Quality Image Recovery. *Sensors (Basel)*, *19*(10), 1–18. doi:10.339019102267 PMID:31100886

Liu, S., Pan, Z., & Song, H. (2017). Digital image watermarking method based on DCT and fractal encoding. *IET Image Processing*, *11*(10), 815–821. doi:10.1049/iet-ipr.2016.0862

Liu, X., Zhang, J., Wang, H., Gong, X., & Cheng, Y. (2014). A Novel Text Watermarking Algorithm Based on Graphic Watermarking Framework. *Proceedings of the Ninth International Conference on Broadband and Wireless Computing, Communication and Applications*, 84–88. 10.1109/BWCCA.2014.49

Manivannan, M., & Suseendran, G. (2017). A Review of Watermarking Requirements, Techniques, Documents, Human Perception and Applications for Medical Images. *International Journal of Innovative Research in Applied Sciences and Engineering*, *1*(2), 58–65. doi:10.29027/IJIRASE.v1.i2.2017.58-65

Mishra, A., Rajpal, A., & Bala, R. (2018). Bi-directional extreme learning machine for semi-blind watermarking of compressed images. *Journal of Information Security and Applications*, *38*, 71–84. doi:10.1016/j.jisa.2017.11.008

Moeinaddini, E., & Ghasemkhani, R. (2015). A novel image watermarking scheme using blocks coefficient in DHT domain. *Proceedings of the International Symposium on Artificial Intelligence and Signal Processing (AISP)*, 159–164. 10.1109/AISP.2015.7123512

Mohammad, T., & Bijan, R. (2015). Importance of Data Mining in Healthcare: A Survey. *Proceedings of the IEEE/ACM International Conference on Advances in Social Networks Analysis and Mining*, 1057–1062. 10.1145/2808797.2809367

Moosazadeh, M., & Ekbatanifard, G. (2019). A new DCT-based robust image watermarking method using teaching-learning-based optimization. *Journal of Information Security and Applications, 47*, 28–38. doi:10.1016/j.jisa.2019.04.001

Nikolic, M., Tuba, E., & Tuba, M. (2016). Edge detection in medical ultrasound images using adjusted canny edge detection algorithm. *Proceedings of the 2016 24th Telecommunications Forum (TELFOR),* 1–4. 10.1109/TELFOR.2016.7818878

Piva, A., Bartolini, F., & Barni, M. (2002). Managing copyright in open networks. *IEEE Transactions on Internet Computing, 6*(3), 18–26. doi:10.1109/MIC.2002.1003126

Podilchuk, C. I., & Delp, E. J. (2001). Digital watermarking: Algorithms and applications. *IEEE Signal Processing Magazine, 18*(4), 33–46. doi:10.1109/79.939835

Priya, C. V. L., & Raj, N. R. N. (2017). Digital watermarking scheme for image authentication. *Proceedings of the 2017 IEEE International Conference on Communication and Signal Processing (ICCSP),* 2026–2030. 10.1109/ICCSP.2017.8286758

Qasim, A. F., Meziane, F., & Aspin, R. (2017). Digital watermarking: Applicability for developing trust in medical imaging workflows state of the art review. *Future Generation Computer Systems, 27*, 45–60. doi:10.1016/j.cosrev.2017.11.003

Ray, A., & Roy, S. (2020). Recent trends in image watermarking techniques for copyright protection: A survey. *International Journal of Multimedia Information Retrieval, 9*(4), 249–270. doi:10.100713735-020-00197-9

Saini, L. K., & Shrivastava, V. (2014). A Survey of Digital Watermarking Techniques and its Applications. *International Journal of Computer Science Trends and Technology, 2*(3), 70–73.

Savakar, D. G., & Ghuli, A. (2019). Robust invisible digital image watermarking using hybrid scheme. *Arabian Journal for Science and Engineering, 44*(4), 3995–4008. doi:10.100713369-019-03751-8

Shahid & Kumar. (2018). Digital Video Watermarking: Issues and Challenges. *International Journal of Advanced Research in Computer Engineering and Technology, 7*(4), 400–405.

Sherekar, S., Thakare, V., & Jain, S. (2008). Role of Digital Watermark in e-governance and ecommerce. *International Journal of Computer Science and Network Security, 8*(1), 257–261.

Shukla, D., Tiwari, N., & Dubey, D. (2016). Survey on digital watermarking techniques. International Journal of Signal Processing. *Image Processing and Pattern Recognition, 9*(1), 239–244. doi:10.14257/ijsip.2016.9.1.23

Singh & Chandha. (2013). A Survey of Digital Watermarking Techniques, Applications and Attacks. *International Journal of Engineering and Innovative Technology, 2*(9), 165–175.

Singh, A. K., Kumar, B., Singh, G., & Mohan, A. (2017). *Medical Image Watermarking: Techniques and Applications. Multimedia Systems and Applications.* Springer. doi:10.1007/978-3-319-57699-2

Singh, G. (2017). A review of secure medical image watermarking. *Proceedings of the IEEE International Conference on Power, Control, Signals and Instrumentation Engineering (ICPCSI)*, 3105–3109. 10.1109/ICPCSI.2017.8392297

Singh, P., & Chadha, R. S. (2013). A survey of digital watermarking techniques, applications and attacks. *International Journal of Engineering and Innovative Technology*, *2*(9), 165–175.

Sivasubramanian, N., & Konganathan, G. (2020). A novel semi fragile watermarking technique for tamper detection and recovery using IWT and DCT. *Computing*, *102*(6), 1365–1384. doi:10.100700607-020-00797-7

Song, C., Sudirman, S., Merabti, M., & Llewellyn-Jones, D. (2010). Analysis of digital image watermark attacks. *Proceedings of the 7th IEEE Consumer Communications and Networking Conference*, 1–5. 10.1109/CCNC.2010.5421631

Sowmya, S. (2021). Protection of Data using Image Watermarking Technique. *Global Transitions Proceedings*, *2*(2), 386–391. doi:10.1016/j.gltp.2021.08.035

Subashini, V. J., Poornachandra, S., & Ramakrishnan, M. (2013). A fragile watermarking technique for fingerprint protection. *Proceedings of the IEEE Recent Advances in Intelligent Computational Systems (RAICS)*, 322–326. 10.1109/RAICS.2013.6745495

Taha, T. B., Ngadiran, R., & Ehkan, P. (2018). Adaptive image watermarking algorithm based on an efficient perceptual mapping model. *IEEE Access: Practical Innovations, Open Solutions*, *6*, 66254–66267. doi:10.1109/ACCESS.2018.2878456

Tao, H., Chongmin, L., Mohamad Zain, J., & Abdalla, A. N. (2014). Robust Image Watermarking Theories and Techniques: A Review. *Journal of Applied Research and Technology*, *12*(1), 122–138. doi:10.1016/S1665-6423(14)71612-8

Thapa, M., Sandeep, D., & Meenakshi, A. (2011). Digital Image Watermarking Technique Based on Different Attacks. *International Journal of Advanced Computer Science and Applications*, *2*(4), 14–19. doi:10.14569/IJACSA.2011.020402

Tiwari & Sharmila. (2017). Digital Watermarking Applications, Parameter Measures and Techniques. *International Journal of Computer Science and Network Security*, *17*(3), 184–194.

Vaidya, P., & PVSSR, C. M. (2017). A robust semi-blind watermarking for color images based on multiple decompositions. *Multimedia Tools and Applications*, *76*(24), 25623–25656. doi:10.100711042-017-4355-0

Vassaux, B., Nguyen, P., Baudry, S., Bas, P., & Chassery, J. (2002). Scrambling technique for video object watermarking resisting to mpeg-4. *Proceedings of the Video/Image Processing and Multimedia Communications 4th EURASIP-IEEE Region 8 International Symposium on VIPromCom*, 239–244. 10.1109/VIPROM.2002.1026662

Verma, V. S., & Jha, R. K. (2015). An Overview of Robust Digital Image Watermarking. *IETE Technical Review*, *32*(6), 479–496. doi:10.1080/02564602.2015.1042927

Wadhera, S., Kamra, D., Rajpal, A., Jain, A., & Jain, V. (2021). A Comprehensive Review on Digital Image Watermarking. *Proceedings of the WCNC-2021: Workshop on Computer Networks & Communications*, 126–140.

Wazirali, R., Ahmad, R., Al-Amayreh, A., Al-Madi, M., & Khalifeh, A. (2021). Secure Watermarking Schemes and Their Approaches in the IoT Technology: An Overview. *Electronics (Basel)*, *10*(14), 1–28. doi:10.3390/electronics10141744

Zhang, G., Kou, L., Zhang, L., Liu, C., Da, Q., & Sun, J. (2017). A New Digital Watermarking Method for Data Integrity Protection in the Perception Layer of IoT. *Security and Communication Networks*, *2017*, 1–12. doi:10.1155/2017/3126010

Zhang, Y., Qin, H., & Kong, T. (2010). A novel robust text watermarking for word document. *Proceedings of the 3rd International Congress on Image and Signal Processing*, 38–42. 10.1109/CISP.2010.5648007

Chapter 6
IoT and Artificial Intelligence for Healthcare Informatics:
Evolving Technologies

Jyothi Mandala
CHRIST University (Deemed), India

Ganeshan R.
VIT Bhopal University, India

Balajee Maram
Chitkara University Institute of Engineering and Technology, Chitkara University, India

Daniya T.
ⓘD https://orcid.org/0000-0001-7549-7419
GMR Institute of Technology, India

ABSTRACT

Most of the IT industry's significant research areas are remote healthcare systems that provide easily deployable and ubiquitous healthcare systems in the recent developments. In remote healthcare systems, user confidence is improved with providing the patients data privacy and communication security. The basic idea about healthcare informatics is described in the introduction. Internet of things (IoT) in healthcare systems, devices and mobile apps for healthcare, and its challenges to medical fields are analyzed in the second part. The combination of healthcare with artificial intelligence (AI) and IoT technology will create a user friendly application and developed healthcare by solving the issues of healthcare system and providing more security to personal and medical information of patients. A brief discussion of artificial intelligence in healthcare is provided in the third section of the research. Both the critical and prior circumstances and the applications of healthcare systems are worked along with further developments in those applications.

DOI: 10.4018/978-1-6684-4580-8.ch006

INTRODUCTION

Self-patterned objects are interconnecting the entire world with the help of using the internet for processing its activities (Pablo Pico-Valencia et al, 2020). Each human being around the globe uses the automotives, smart home applications, health services and all smart applications all around the world and these applications are enabled by the IoT devices in recent years (Anas Dawod et al., 2019). Artificial intelligence (AI) applications in healthcare are mainly focused by the researches in medical informatics and as well as academic institutions. According to embedded systems, medical devices are designed (Joan Cabestany et al., 2018). Transforming, refining and computations are the human tasks which are too complex. These tasks are made easy by using IoT or AI enabled devices (RittwikSood et al., 2018). A framework of Machine to Machine communication is called as Internet of Things technology in which the internet facilities provided to the machines (Marco Conoscenti et al., 2017).

Health Informatics

The field of engineering is called as Health informatics in which different techniques or methods are developed for collection, processing and developments of patient's data. From different modalities and sources like medical scans, diagnostic test results and electronic health recordsthe patient's data is collected(K. Navin et al., 2017). Computational techniques are used for solving different problems which are obtained from the health domains (Ching-Kuan Liu et al., 2017).

The combination of multidisciplinary fields is called as Health informatics, and these are computational innovation application development and its designing process which are used for healthcare improvement (Misha Pavel et al., 2015). In software engineering, theoretical computer science, bio-inspired computing, information engineering, information systems, software engineering, information technology, data science, behavior informatics, particular computer engineering and autonomic computing, medicine fields and computing fields combination is involved. The context of library science uses the term informatics in some countries for hospital data management.

Archival Science and Databases in Healthcare

Informatics concepts, health informatics tools and methods are combined with the patent's care knowledge of the Archival clinical informaticians:

1. Assess the health care professional's knowledge needs and information, families of patient's with them also.
2. Evaluation, characterization and clinical processes refining.
3. Clinical decision support systems refining, implementation and its development.
4. Maintain the main role in clinical information systems continuous improvement, evaluation, management, implementation, development, customization and procurement.

Information technology and health care professionals are combined with the Clinicians for developing health informatics tools which enhances the patient care as effective, efficient, safe, equitable and patient-centered. Clinical informaticists called as computer scientists. In clinical informatics, the creation of MD is announced as physician certification by the American Board of Medical Specialties (ABMS) organization with certification of specialist medical degree (MD)in October 2011at United States. In October 2013, American Board of Preventive Medicine (ABPM) offer the clinical informatics subspecialty board certification using first examination with 432 passing candidates for becoming a inaugural class of Diplomats 2014 in clinical informatics. For physicians, there exist Fellowship programs in clinical informatics in order to become a board-certified physician. From any school which is approved by the ABPM, a graduation certificate is required for physicians including with primary residency program completion certificate like Internal Medicine and then those are eligible for licensed practice medicine where their fellowship program is located. 24 months of duration is required for fellowship program and this duration is divided by fellows as didactic method, Informatics rotations, clinical work in their primary specialty and research.

Human existence nature upgradation is requires the actualization by using the permitted progressive answers with innovative changes. The innovative developments are considered by the analysts with wellbeing data identification, assessing and wellbeing related issues managements. Incorporated medical care innovation advancement along with increased efficiency is achieved at medical care framework each level in this manner. The health care industry crucial part is acquired with Long-term care (LTC) facilities and takes care for fastest-growing group of the population. In LTC facilities electronic health records (EHRs) adoption are more popular in health care industry (Ulrich Beez et al., 2015). Specific issues are take care by the Electronic Health (e-Health) application frameworks advancement which are related to the conventional medical care frameworks as pervasive information access, wellbeing controls of powerful patient, checking of distant patient, decentralized electronic-medical care records and quick clinical intercession. By using these frameworks, patient secured information is managed, personal satisfaction is enhanced, results are improved, coordinated effort is increased, e-medical care administrations efficiency is increased and expenses are decreased. In order to share the information securely for health care systems, EHRs are required in between medical drug manufacturers, healthcare organizations, pharmacists, patients, researchers and medical insurance providers. Main challenge of patients' sensitive data is security. A tech industry e-health is considered by the Eisenach which denoted the internet assembly, medical services and systems administration. Therefore clients and partners framework is incredibly benefits. In clinical informatics convergence, Internet security administrations and general security of systems most research area is E-security by which the new innovation advancements are used in identifying the issues, decreasing the expenses.

The combination of the Internet of Things (IoT) with these models, frameworks and gadgets are more popular (Christopher Coelho et al., 2015). Interrelated correspondence advance improvement is synchronized with best usage of IoT, for instance, operational frameworks, industry, business, medical care registering knowledge and etc. In order to make reasonable executions, there is a requirement of strong security and high efficient encompassing e-Health frameworks with all benefits, security data advancement safe and efficient usage. In different areas such as healthcare, society and business are uses the Artificial intelligence (AI) and related technologies widely. By using these techniques, different aspects of patient care, administrative processes and pharmaceutical organizations are transformed. The network of several physical devices is forming the framework of Internet of Things (IoT) in which different sensors, software, electronic devices are embedded and works mainly on collecting and exchanging the data. This impact is most important for the medicine field. Health-related services uses the most of the IoT-related technology as 40% and making more than $117 billion market than any other categories. Healthcare is defined from the medical informatics which is formed from the junction of information technologies and medicine and thus costs are reduced, efficiency of lives increased.

Several studies already exist for disease diagnosis by using artificial intelligence which is already proved as more efficient than humans at performing the healthcare tasks. Most of the radiologists perform the algorithms nowadays for identifying the malignant tumors and for costly clinical trials uses the researcher's guidance in construction of associates. From many years researchers believe that humans were replaced by the artificial intelligence (AI) in medical process domains because of deployment of many reasons. AI in healthcare rapid implementation barriers and automate aspects of care are offered by the artificial intelligence (AI) which is described in this paper.

IOT in the Healthcare Industry

Internet of things technology based devices are widely used in present days of world especially healthcare sector is most impacted. In present days people had received the unsure or unsafe advices from schedule medical appointments or services which are provided through the smart phones without visiting the hospital and avoidance of waiting more time for allotted time for us. Blood pressure (BP) is monitored with the weighing scale connected sensors or devices to the patient, information are represented and life-saving advices are provided to the patient by the real-time diagnostics. IoT is used in preventive care and bed-side patients monitoring along with the usage of personal care solutions in healthcare industry. Some of the sensors are wired by people such as smart watch etc. are identifying the heart rate of person, calculating the number of steps covered by the person in certain time and number of calories burned in exercise. These sensor devices or applications are helps in preventing health issues with great security and changes the lifestyles. The network of several physical devices is forms the framework of Internet of Things (IoT) in which different sensors, software, electronic devices are embedded and works mainly on collecting and exchanging the data. Healthcare is defined from the medical informatics which is formed from the junction of information technologies and medicine and thus costs are reduced, efficiency of lives increased.

IoT devices best examples are wireless insulin pumps and Pacemakers those are work in critical condition of patient and also breaking data situations also these devices are working appropriately in any way. Healthcare IoT systems vulnerabilities are demonstrated by the cyber threat analyst during the conference of Black Hat in 2011. Broken security gaps of analyst who is diabetic causes a insulin pump to respond to a remote control device and monitors the altered values on glucose pump because of wireless signals interception. Even device manufacturers were changed, further reports are shown according to uncovered issues and then regarding wireless device policies of Federal Communication Commission's review is requested by the two members of American congress which done the insufficient action by prompting it.

According to the own firmware and software, IoT devices are accessed with the latest version of anti-malware protections which are improving the performance of device by reducing the attacks. If artificial pancreases and pacemakers are added to these devices which causes the serious damage of adoption of IoT in healthcare systems because of the vulnerabilities in information technology (IT) and these are addressed actively. The key indication of early stages of technology is fully deployed IoT systems lacking. Signal strength issues in hospitals and electromagnetic radiation long term effects on people are the examples of problems which included in this technology. In the healthcare industry adoption of the technology is increased and considered that most important parameter is security. In IoT ecosystem all the devices and sensors are always connected. The adoption of IoT devices with stakeholders then there is no guarantee for authenticity, trust and privacy.

Devices and Mobile Apps for Healthcare

The key parameter related to the data and knowledge about age of information. Customer age is also entered which is used for determining the requirements of customers. One of the business models changing look example is *myTomorrows,* by which the pharma is connected to the customers.

A "health selfie" is created by the apps, devices and new age in this field. For example:

1. *The Myo* is a game motion controller, used for patients or orthopedics who required exercise after a fracture. By using this Myo, angle of movement is measured by doctors and their progress is monitored by the patients itself.
2. Electrocardiogram (ECG) and heart rate is measured with *Zio Patch* and Drug Administration and US Food is approved.
3. Electroceuticals are bioelectrical drugs in which the Glaxo invested as a recent announcement, nerves micro-stimulation is the work of these drugs.
4. A robotic surgery is developed by the J&J with Google and along with this Philips is also joined for working on wearable devices like monitoring the blood pressures.
5. According to sensor technology, Novartis is working with Google (again) and these techniques as blood glucose levels measuring wearable device, smart lens and etc.

The development of pharma is mainly depends on the information of sensors and used in identifying the healthy people from the patients with clinical trials. There is a rapid improvement in sales if once these sensor devices or gadgets are used by the runners and athletes. The pharma industry uses these sensor devices widely not only in monitoring the respiratory rate, electronic cardio gram (ECG), blood pressure and pulse but also in sleep patterns, inflammation as advanced data. More emerged device handling is supported by the number of mobile apps, including with SleepBot and myDario. A program of ranked health is recently announced by the hacking Medicine Institute which evaluates the rank health-focused connected devices and applications. Recently researchers observe wearable devices as smart watch or phone displaying the health information regarding to blood pressure, heart beat and body temperature. By using these devices we are checking the WhatsApp or email. The health condition of elder people is also monitored and this information is transferred to the physicians, tele-carer and family members.

Challenges for MIoT

IoT devices are accessed by the powerful and simple applications from the IoT platforms, and in designing process of mIoT apps, visualization dashboards and analytics applications use the data by the users. 5 key capabilities are mentioned below must be enabled as:

1. Simple connectivity: An efficient connection in between device management functions and devices are done through the good IoT platform, cloud-based services are used in measurement and organizational transformation is achieved.
2. Easy device management: Unplanned outages minimization, low maintenance costs, throughput improvement and better availability of resources are achieved through the enabling of device management.

3. Information ingestion: IoT data is stored and transformed in intelligent manner. The required data is extracted easily by using the APIs bridge which divides the cloud and data. From diverse data sources data is transferred to the platforms and then rich analytics are extracting the required values.

4. Informative analytics: From IoT data huge volumes gain insight uses in the operations optimizations and make better decisions. Current conditions are monitored with the real-time analytics and response is obtained accordingly. Both structured and unstructured data with leverage cognitive analytics used in situation understanding, changing conditions and evaluating the reasons through options. The usage of intuitive dashboard is making it easy and convenient.

5. Reduced risk: A single console generates the isolate incidents and notifications anywhere in the company environment.

Artificial intelligence in healthcare

Edward H. Shortliffe as an American biomedical informatician is establishes the artificial intelligence in healthcare and this field uses the artificial intelligence technology and machine learning techniques for imitating the humans in dealing the complicated healthcare and medical data, interpretation in analysis of healthcare data. According to the input data, approximate conclusions are obtained in the Artificial intelligence which is the ability of computer algorithms. Patient monitoring and care, personalized medicine, drug development, treatment protocol development and diagnosis processes are practices to which the AI programs are applied. The clinical decision support systems are the systems in healthcare sector AI implementation industry focus large part. High efficient solutions and responses are allowed by adapting the machine learning algorithms and huge amount of data collection. Because number of possibilities of big data, healthcare industry uses the big data and this is discovered by the several companies. The market opportunities are investigated by different companies through the areas as those are healthcare industry important points and these are "data assessment, storage, management, and analysis technologies". Healthcare industries with AI algorithms are contributed by the different companies and some of the examples are as follows:

1. IBM's Watson Oncology is in development center for identifying the cancer at Memorial Sloan Kettering. In the treatment of chronic disease Consumer Value Stores (CVS)health is working with the International Business Machines (IBM) on AI applications and drug development connections are discovered by the analysis scientific papers by Johnson & Johnson. AI technology improvement in healthcare industry is explored by the joint project which is conducted by the Rensselaer Polytechnic Institute and IBM in May 2017 and its name as Health Empowerment by Analytics, Learning and Semantics (HEALS).

2. Most effective cancer drug treatment is predicted by the analysis of medical research which is done by the in-cooperation of Knight Cancer Institute of Health & Science University's and Microsoft's Hanover project. Programmable cells development and tumor progression medical image analysis are included in other projects.

3. Several health risks are detected by using the collected data through mobile app by the UK National Health Service on Google's Deep Mind platform. In NHS patient's medical images analysis, National Health Service (NHS) is involved with the second project which is used in cancer cells detection along with the computer version developments.

4. The services of different medical systems are uses the Tencent and these services are as AI-powered diagnostic medical imaging service, AI Medical Innovation System (AIMIS), Tencent Doctorwork and WeChat Intelligent Healthcare.
5. Intel Capital is an Intel's venture capital arm which invests the startup Lumiata and this develops the care options after identifying the risk patients by using AI technology.
6. Deep learning software is developed by the Kheiron Medical for breast cancer detection in mammograms.
7. Deep learning and AI techniques are used in finding the Fractal Analytics for speed up the diagnostic x-rays and improvement in radiology.
8. Neuroprosthetic is next generation of Neuralink which interfaces the number of neural paths in brain. A chip is inserted in place of a chunk of skull in this process by a surgical robot for avoiding the injury.

Types of AI of Relevance to Healthcare

The combination of several technologies is forming the Artificial intelligence. Healthcare industry uses different techniques according to their requirements but particular tasks and processers adoption process is slow. High importance AI technologies to healthcare are described below as:

Machine Learning – Neural Networks and Deep Learning

The attaching process of data to the models and learning process of models with these data uses the statistical method of machine learning. AI most common form is Machine learning, the organizations of 1,100 US managers whose are already purchased the AI and in that 63% of companies uses the machine learning techniques by their employees in their business. Because of different approaches of AI many versions are exists.

Traditional machine learning most common application precision medicine in healthcare – according to the different treatment context and patient features, the prediction of treatment process for making the patient as successful wealthy person. A training dataset is required medicine applications and machine learning techniques for which training dataset is knows the outcome variable called as supervised learning. The neural network is a machine learning complex form – since the 1960s neural network has been available and from several decades, healthcare industry uses this technology in determination of presence of disease in a person and in some categorization applications. Therefore inputs, outputs are having the problems and weights of variables are attached with inputs and outputs. The process of neutral networks is same as the process of neurons signals in brain. Deep learning method is used when the complex problems are raised and the outcomes are predicted with the presence of number of features of neural network models. Today's cloud architectures and graphics processing units fast processing not covers the thousands of hidden features which are exists in these models. Cancerous tissues are identified by using the deep learning technology in healthcare system with the observation of radiology images. The small observations in medically diagnosed images or radiology images which are not been observed or identified by human eye are detected by the Deep learning. Therefore, in the analysis of oncology-oriented images most commonly used techniques are deep learning and radiomics. In diagnosis, greater accuracy outcomes obtained when it uses the combination of these two technologies than other techniques as computer-aided detection or CAD, image analysis using automated tools. Speech recognition uses the

Deep learning techniques in the form of natural language processing (NLP). A deep learning model each feature has less observations with humans in statistical analysis. Therefore, model's outcomes explanation is too difficult for identification of disease.

Natural Language Processing

Since 1950s, human language has been a goal of AI researchers. The language related processes as translation, text analysis and speech recognition applications are included in the Natural language processing (NLP). Semantic and statistical NLP are the two approaches in Natural language processing. According to machine learning techniques, Statistical NLP is processed and has high reorganization accuracy and huge dataset or body language is required to learn the model. Clinical documentation creation, understanding, classification and then research publication is involved in NLP dominant applications in healthcare. Unstructured clinical notes are analyzed by NLP systems on patients, reports are prepared for patient and then interactions are recorded which all those are used in conversational AI.

Rule-Based Expert Systems

Expert systems were the dominant technology according to the 'if-then' rules collections for AI in the 1980s which are used for later periods continuously commercially. These are widely used in healthcare with the employment of 'clinical decision support' which has been used for couple of years. The present day's rules are furnished with the different electronic health record (EHR).

A particular knowledge domain series of rules designing are required in expert systems which use the knowledge engineers, human experts and human experts. These expert systems are easily understood and work efficiently. But in case of large rules, variation is occurred in different rules then this technology is breaks. There is a difficulty in changing the rules for knowledge domain changes and consumes more time for changing. Different approaches are used in this changing process according to machine learning algorithms and data.

Diagnosis and Treatment Applications

Since 1970's, AI has been focused by the disease treatment and diagnosis, when the blood-borne bacterial infections diagnosis use the standard development of MYCIN. Accurate treatment and diagnosis obtained from rule-based systems but, and this system were not adopted for clinical practice. This is because of insufficient or poor medical record systems and clinician workflows, the human diagnosticians are better than these diagnostics.

More recently, media focus the detection of cancer tissues, their treatment and precision medicine which attracted the IBM's Watson. The capabilities of NLP and machine learning techniques combination form the Watson. The early interest of the customers regarding to this technology application is too dull because of realization of addressing the cancer cell is too difficult therefore the combination of these Watson systems with care processes. A group of 'cognitive services' is called the Watson and through the application programming interfaces (APIs), this Watson system is provided, with the inclusion of data-analysis programs based on machine learning, vision, language and speech. According to technical Watson APIs are capable which is feeling by observer, but overly determined objective as cancer treatment. Free 'open source' programs like Google's TensorFlow are suffers from Watson and other proprietary programs which are provided by some vendors.

Healthcare organizations are having some implementation issues with AI bedevil. EHR systems are incorporation with rule-based systems are widely used with the inclusion of NHS, machine learning based more algorithmic systems precision lacking in this method. If there is a change in medical knowledge then the maintenance of rule-based clinical decision support systems is too complicated, explosion of data is not handled by it and take care about proteomic, genomic, metabolic and other 'omic-based' approaches.

On these issues, early startups and Tech firms are working constantly. Health delivery networks are collaborated with Google for designing the prediction models in order to alert the high-risk conditions as heart failure situations of clinicians. Image interpretation algorithms based on artificial intelligence are developed by different startups. Patients with serious cases are identified by the 'clinical success machine' which offered by the Jvion and also identifies the treatment protocols for the need of patient to treat. Therefore clinicians are getting the information about the patient provided by the decision support systems and helps in identifying the best diagnosis with treatment. According to genetic profiles of patient, certain cancer treatment recommendations and diagnosis are focused by different methods. Genetic basis are present in most of the cancers, the increasing amount of those genetic basis such as cancer genetic variants are must be identified by the human clinicians. Roche owns the Flatiron Health and Foundation Medicine which is specialized in this approach.

Patient Engagement and Adherence Applications

Patient appointment and observance has long been seen as the 'last mile' healthcare problem– the final barrier between ineffective and good health outcomes. Most of the patients are take care about their health condition and security of health. Member experience, financial outcomes and utilization are the factors which are addressed by AI and big data increasingly.

A plan of care is developed for improving the patient health condition and this process uses the clinical reports which play an important role by the hospital staff or experienced diagnostics. But in some cases, the patients are not in cooperation with the prescription plan like losing weight, following the treatment plan, filling prescriptions and scheduling a follow-up visit. Therefore this become a major problem to the patients who does not obey all these parameters regarding to the prescribed drugs as recommended and course of treatment. In a survey, more than 300 healthcare executives, clinical leaders less than 50% of their patients are with more than 70% of the respondents and less than 25% of their patients are with 42% of respondents were highly engaged. AI-based technologies with healthcare systems are effectively produce the outcomes even if the patient in a serious condition. Alerting messages are involved in this method to the corresponding respondent and care takers. High efficient solutions and responses are allowed by adapting the machine learning algorithms and huge amount of data collections. Because of number of possibilities of big data, healthcare industry uses the big data and this is discovered by several companies.

'Choice architecture' effective designing is healthcare system another focus in order to mould the patient behavior as strong for fighting with the disease. Biosensors, EHR systems, smart phones, watches, conversational interfaces are providing the information and the comparisons are made in between the effective treatment pathways and patient data for similar associates by the software. Patients, providers, call-centre agents, nurses and care delivery coordinators are getting the information about these recommendations.

Administrative Applications

Healthcare systems have a great many administrative applications. Patient care system is achieving the best efficiencies with the usage of artificial intelligence (AI) comparing it with administrative applications systems but providing the substantial efficiencies. for example, the average US nurse spending more time as 25% of work time on administrative and regulatory activities, so in healthcare system requires these applications. Robotic Process Automation (RPA) technology is used which is more applicable to this objective. Different healthcare applications use these applications in clinical documentation, claims processing, medical records management and revenue cycle management.

Chatbots are experimented in some healthcare organizations for patient tele health, interaction, mental health and wellness. These simple transactions are based on NLP which makes appointments or refilling prescriptions. The language related processes as translation, text analysis and speech recognition applications are included in the Natural language processing (NLP). According to the survey every five in 500 US users are used these chatbots in healthcare whose are expressing their confidential matters regarding health, complex health conditions, their mental stabilities and poor usability.

The Future of AI in Healthcare

In future, best offerings are provided to the healthcare systems by the artificial intelligence (AI). The advancements in care units are must be improved in the form of machine learning which is used in precision medicine development. Early diagnosis of disease and better treatment recommendations are effectively suggested by the AI which will ultimately master that domain as well. Pathology images and most radiology images are examined at some point by a machine but, a better analysis of medical images with rapid advances in AI. Capturing of clinical notes, patient communication is the tasks uses the Speech and text recognition which are already employed. The greatest challenge to AI in these healthcare domains is not whether the technologies will be capable enough to be useful, but rather ensuring their adoption in daily clinical practice. Because of widespread adoption of this technique, regulators are must be approved the AI systems, EHR systems are combined with AI systems, taught to clinicians, paid for public or private payer organizations, similar products work in a similar fashion standardization with sufficient degree and update this field up to time and date. All these challenges are overcome ultimately but taking more time and integration of different techniques with them. As a result, we expect to see limited use of AI in clinical practice within 5 years and more extensive use within 10. On a large scale human clinicians are not replaced by the AI systems by observing the above concepts but, they make more efforts for taking care of patients. Over time, human clinicians may move toward tasks and job designs that draw on uniquely human skills like empathy, persuasion and big-picture integration. Perhaps the only healthcare providers who will lose their jobs over time may be those who refuse to work alongside artificial intelligence.

CONCLUSION

A tremendous impact in medical field is with the technical revolution. The implementation of medical practice is improved by the communication tools and communication systems.An overview of the IoT and AI technologies with healthcare sector facing challenges are provided or elaborated in this paper.

Identified issues preventing solutions are also provided in this paper. In remote healthcare systems, user's confidence is improved with providing the patient's data privacy and communication security. Because of the fast enhancing nature of IoT and AI advancement, a full-fledged technology implementation is healthcare. However, a lot of technology suggestions are grasped by the society and making them as more efficient to take care of elderly people and sick people.

REFERENCES

Beez, U., Humm, B. G., & Walsh, P. (2015). Electronic health records. *2015 International Conference on Computational Science and Computational Intelligence (CSCI).*

Cabestany, J., Rodriguez-Martín, D., Pérez, C., & Sama, A. (2018). Artificial Intelligence Contribution to eHealth applications. *2018 25th International Conference "Mixed Design of Integrated Circuits and System" (MIXDES).* 10.23919/MIXDES.2018.8436743

Coelho, C., Coelho, D., & Wolf, M. (2015). An IoT smart home architecture for long-term care of people with special needs. *2015 IEEE 2nd World Forum on internet of things (WF-IoT).* 10.1109/WF-IoT.2015.7389126

Conoscenti, M., Vetrò, A., & De Martin, J. C. (2017). Peer to Peer for Privacy and Decentralization in the internet of Things. *2017 IEEE/ACM 39th International Conference on Software Engineering Companion (ICSE-C).* 10.1109/ICSE-C.2017.60

Dawod, Georgakopoulos, Jayaraman, & Nirmalathas. (2019). Advancements towards Global IoT devices Discovery and Integration. *2019 IEEE International Congress on Internet of Things (ICIOT).*

Liu, C.-K., Hsu, C.-Y., Yang, F.-Y., Wu, J., Kuo, K., & Lai, P. (2017). Population health management outcomes obtained through a hospital-based and telehealth informatics-enabled telecare service. *2017 IEEE Biomedical Circuits and Systems Conference (BioCAS).* 10.1109/BIOCAS.2017.8325127

Navin, K., Mukesh Krishnan, M. B., Lavanya, S., & Shanthini, A. (2017). A mobile health based smart hybrid epidemic surveillance system to support epidemic control programme in public health informatics. *2017 International Conference on IoT and Application (ICIOT).* 10.1109/ICIOTA.2017.8073606

Pavel, M., Jimison, H. B., Korhonen, I., Gordon, C. M., & Saranummi, N. (2015). Behavioral Informatics and Computational Modeling in Support of Proactive health Management and care. *IEEE Transactions on Biomedical Engineering, 62*(12), 2763–2775. doi:10.1109/TBME.2015.2484286 PMID:26441408

Pico-Valencia, P., Holgado-Terriza, J. A., & Quiñónez-Ku, X. (2020). A Brief Survey of the Main internet Based Approaches. An Outlook from the internet of Things Perspective. *2020 3rd International Conference on Information and Computer Technologies (ICICT).* 10.1109/ICICT50521.2020.00091

Sood, Kaur, Sharma, Mehmuda, & Kumar. (2018). IoT enabled Smart Wearable device – Sukoon. *2018 Fourteenth International Conference on Information Processing (ICINPRO).*

Chapter 7
Intuitionistic Fuzzy Deteriorating Inventory Models With Controllable Carbon Emissions and Shortages

Swagatika Sahoo
Institute of Technical Education and Research, India

Milu Acharya
Institute of Technical Education and Research, India

ABSTRACT

Nowadays, global warming, which has its effect on climate change, has turned out to be a delicate topic, and several countries are making an effort to regulate emissions through certain investments in green technology (GT). Mostly, the issue with the emissions is the outcome of inventory management. In view of this, a fuzzy inventory model with time dependent power demand and controllable carbon emissions is formulated. This includes green technology investment involving two warehouses to reduce emissions from during the shipping of goods from the own warehouse to the rented warehouse and finally to the consumers. Further, constant and Weibull deterioration rates are taken for the goods in rented and own warehouse respectively. Finally, the optimum values of the total average cost, cycle length, and GT are obtained. A numerical example is provided to illustrate the models, and the behaviour of the total cost function is shown graphically.

INTRODUCTION

Greenhouse gases (GHGs) are the major cause of global warming. The emissions from GHGs are "carbon dioxide, methane, and nitrous oxide" Datta (2017). Among these, CO_2 plays a crucial role in the global warming which is responsible for climate change. The main reasons for the emissions are "the burning of fossil fuels for industrialization, transportation, power generation, and deforestation". Hence, it is

DOI: 10.4018/978-1-6684-4580-8.ch007

high time to make the public aware of the consequences of these emissions. Nowadays, most countries are making efforts to lessen their emissions through the implementation of new technologies, effectual inventory control, and judicious managerial decisions.

Particularly for the prevention of climate change, different countries are preparing themselves so that under carbon emission regulation policies they can slow down carbon emissions. That is to say, they are forming legislation to control emissions. Therefore, industries are taking an interest in "greener transportation fleets" (Bae et al. (2011)), "energy-efficient warehousing" (Ilic et al. (2009)), and "environmentally friendly manufacturing processes" (Liu et al. (2012)). In general, the effects of emissions can be reduced by using environmentally friendly raw materials and cleaner energy, implementing new energy-saving technologies and green packaging, and developing energy management plans, among other things. Emissions from transportation and storage processes are mainly controlled by decisions taken for inventory management.

Bonney and Jaber (2011) investigated "the impact of environmentally responsible inventory models". Hua et al. (2011) analysed "a managerial approach to control carbon footprints in an inventory management system under a carbon emission treading mechanism". Bouchery et al. (2012) discussed an inventory model by including "carbon emission regulation policies to implement cost-efficient methods to decrease emissions." Likewise, Benjaafar et al. (2013) have reflected on a model "to reduce its carbon emissions level via changing its production, inventory, warehousing, logistics, and transportation operations". Chen et al. (2013) examines "an environmentally sensitive EOQ model under an emission cap in order to derive analytical results about carbon emission and inventory-related cost".

Taleizadeh et al. (2020) explored "a sustainable economic order quantity (EOQ) for a greenhouse farm." Tiwari et al. (2019) included "carbon emission reductions as the objective in an EOQ model by assuming an unlimited single warehouse and non-instantaneously deteriorating items." Mishra et al. (2020b) established "an EOQ model for non-instantaneously deteriorating items with carbon emissions."

In reality, food products, electronic goods, medicines, agricultural items, etc. either deteriorate or have their expiration dates. So, EOQ/EPQ models without shortage for a constant rate of deterioration, the exponential rate of decay, and other variable rates of deterioration are common in models suggested by Mishra (1975), Ghare and Scharder (1963), Covert and Philip (1973). Again, mathematical models with different rates of deteriorations along with shortages were introduced by Goswami and Chaudhuri (1991), Chakrabati and Chaudhuri (1997) and Sahoo et al. (2019). An EOQ model for Weibull deterioration items with shortages was developed by Skouri et al. (2009). Patro et al. (2017) established "an EOQ model with time dependent Weibull deterioration." Sharmila and Uthayakumar (2016) have developed an inventory model with assumptions were considered to fulfil the optimality.

Covert and Philip, (1973) established "an inventory model for deteriorating items with a Weibull distribution deterioration rate". "An EOQ model for Weibull deterioration items with shortages was developed by Skouri et al. (2009). Patro et al. (2017) established "an EOQ model with time dependent Weibull deterioration." Sharmila and Uthayakumar (2016) have developed an inventory model with three rates of production under stock, with the demand being time dependent and the deterioration rate varying with the shifting of time with shortages. It has been seen that the misfortune rate and expected life time of numerous-products can be presented in terms of Weibull distribution.

Many retailers implement two-warehouses to achieve market stability for their products. The two warehouses are categorized as owned warehouses (OW), with a certain capacity, and rented warehouses (RW), where the excess items can be kept safely. In this situation, initially the purchaser is supplied from the RW, then from the OW, or vice versa. By means of these ideas, Shah and Cardenas-Barron (2015) have proposed "a two-warehouse inventory model where the supplier offered the retailer a discount in cash or a fixed credit period." Jaggi et al. (2015) developed "a deteriorating inventory model with imperfect items under a two-warehouse policy". Tiwari et al. (2016) extended the work of Jaggi et al. (2015) by assuming "a trade credit policy and inflation for non-instantaneously deteriorating products under shortages".

A good number of researchers are involving themselves in doing research with the considerations of inventory models with fuzzy parameters. In their proposed models, either the per unit costs or the parameters involved in the demand functions are taken to be fuzzy to meet the erratic market states, where as in crisp inventory models, all the above-mentioned parameters are identified and have certain values. As in the case of real-life problems, getting a stable market requirement is hard to find. In view of this, some of the researchers active in this area are: Zimmermann ((1978), (1996)), Kaufmann and Gupta (1991), Kacprzyk and Staniewski (1982), Mahata and Goswamy (2009a), Vijayan and Kumaran (2008), Patro et al. (2017, 2017), Sahoo et al. (2020a), Sahoo and Acharya (2021) etc. Triangular, trapezoidal, pentagonal, intuitionistic, cloudy, etc. fuzzy numbers have been used by different researchers, like Uthra et al. (2017) and Sahoo et al. (2020b), in order to determine the optimal order quantity and optimal total cost/profit for different inventory models. Similarly, the methods used for de-fuzzification of results are the signed distance method, Yager's ranking index method, extension of Yager's ranking index method, and generalised intuitionistic fuzzy number (GIFN). Researchers who have played key roles in the use of different de-fuzzification methods are Jaggi (2016), Patro (2017), De et. Al. (2019), Sahoo et al. ((2020), (2021)).

As discussed by Atanassov (1989) that "the generalizations of fuzzy sets theory are considered to be one of Intuitionistic fuzzy set (IFS) theory". All the arithmetic operations on the intuitionistic fuzzy numbers are discussed in (Ponnivalavan and Pathinathan, 2015). Uthra and Shunmugapriya, (2017) have suggested a generalised intuitionistic pentagonal fuzzy number and derived a new ranking formula that suggests both membership and non-membership parts of a fuzzy number.

Newness behind devising of the model: (i) EOQ model for Weibull deteriorating items; (ii) OW and RW are considered (iii) green technology investment cost and carbon emission cost are also introduced; (iv) partial backordering have also taken into consideration; (v) models with fuzzy parameters is presented using generalised intuitionistic fuzzy number for the scale parameter; (vi) ranking technique is used to de-fuzzify total cost. Table-1 focuses on the assumptions introduced in different researchers-

The present work is planned in the following sequence: introduction and literature review, preliminaries, notations and assumptions. Model formulations, numerical examples and sensitivity analysis, and managerial insights, conclusion and future work.

PRELIMINARIES

1. Intuitionistic Fuzzy Sets [Atanasssov, (1989)]

"Let X be the universal set. An Intuitionistic fuzzy set (IFS) M in X is given by

$$M = \left\{ \left(x, \overline{\mu_M}(x), \overline{\gamma_M}(x) \right) : x \in X \right\}$$

where the function $\overline{\mu_M}(x), \overline{\gamma_M}(x)$ respectively are the degree of membership and degree of non-membership of the element $x \in X$ to the set M, which is a subset of X, and for every

$$x \in X, 0 \leq \overline{\mu_M}(x) + \overline{\gamma_M}(x) \leq 1.$$

For each Intuitionistic fuzzy set

$$M = \left\{ \left(x, \overline{\mu_M}(x), \overline{\gamma_M}(x) \right) : x \in X \right\} \text{ in } X, \pi_M(x) = 1 - \overline{\mu_M}(x) - \overline{\gamma_M}(x)$$

is called the hesitancy degree of x to lie in M. If M is a fuzzy set, then $\pi_M(x) = 0$ for all $x \in X$".

Table 1. Review studies discussing inventory models (1=yes; 0=No)

Reference sequence	RW and OW Inventory system	Power demand	Partially backlogged	Green investment	Carbon emission	Intuitionistic fuzzy
Bonney and Jaber (2011)	0	0	0	1	1	0
Hua et al. (2011)	0	0	0	1	1	0
Bouchery et al. (2012)	0	0	0	0	1	0
Benjaafar et al. (2013)	0	0	0	0	1	0
Chen et al. (2013)	0	0	0	0	0	0
Jaggi et al. (2014)	1	0	0	0	0	0
Dye and Yang (2015)	0	0	1	0	1	0
Jaggi et al. (2015)	1	0	0	0	0	0
Datta (2017)	0	0	0	1	1	0
Taleizadeh et al. (2018a)	0	0	1	0	1	0
Tiwari et al. (2019)	1	0	0	0	1	0
Taleizadeh et al. (2020)	0	0	1	0	1	0
Mashud et al. (2021)	1	0	1	1	1	0
This Study	1	1	1	1	1	1

2. Intuitionistic Fuzzy Number [Atanasssov, (1989]

"An IFS $M = \left\{ \left(x, \overline{\mu_M}(x), \overline{\gamma_M}(x) \right) : x \in X \right\}$ of the real line R is called an Intuitionistic fuzzy number if

M is convex for the membership function $\overline{\mu_M}(x)$.

M is concave for the non-membership function $\overline{\gamma_M}(x)$.

M is normal, that is there is some $x_0 \in R$ such that $\overline{\mu_M}(x) = 1, \overline{\gamma_M}(x_0) = 0$ ".

3. Generalized Intuitionistic Pentagonal Fuzzy Number [Uthra et al., 2017]

"Define an Intuitionistic fuzzy number A to be generalized Intuitionistic pentagonal fuzzy number (GIPFN) in the parameter

$$l_1 \leq k_1 \leq l_2 \leq k_2 \leq k_3 \leq k_4 \leq l_4 \leq k_5 \leq l_5$$

denoted by

$$M = \{(k_1, k_2, k_3, k_4, k_5), (l_1, l_2, k_3, l_4, l_5); W_M, V_M\}, 0 \leq W_M, V_M \leq 1$$

if its membership function and non-membership function are as follows."

$$\overline{\mu_M}(x) = \begin{cases} 0 & x < k_1 \\ W_M - \dfrac{W_M(x-k_2)}{k_1-k_2}, & k_1 \leq x \leq k_2 \\ 1 + \dfrac{(W_M-1)(x-k_3)}{k_2-k_3}, & k_2 \leq x \leq k_3 \\ 1 + \dfrac{(W_M-1)(x-k_3)}{k_4-k_3}, & k_3 \leq x \leq k_4 \\ W_M - \dfrac{W_M(x-k_4)}{k_5-k_4}, & k_4 \leq x \leq k_5 \\ 0, & x > k_5 \end{cases}$$

$$\overline{\gamma_M}(x) = \begin{cases} 1 & x < l_1 \\ 1 + \dfrac{(V_M-1)(x-l_1)}{l_2-l_1}, & l_1 \leq x \leq l_2 \\ V_M - \dfrac{V_M(x-l_2)}{k_3-l_2}, & l_2 \leq x \leq k_3 \\ \dfrac{V_A(x-k_3)}{l_4-k_3}, & k_3 \leq x \leq l_4 \\ V_M + \dfrac{(1-V_M)(x-b_4)}{l_5-l_4}, & l_4 \leq x \leq l_5 \\ 1, & x > l_5 \end{cases}$$

Figure 1. For GIPFN

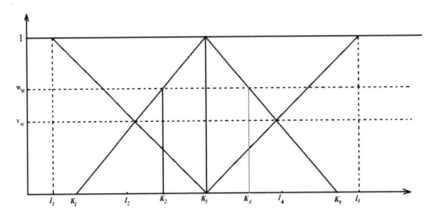

4. The Ranking Formula for Generalized Intuitionistic Pentagonal Fuzzy Numbers (GIPFN) (Uthra et al., 2017)

"The generalized intuitionistic pentagonal fuzzy number M having the centroids C_1, C_2, C_3 corresponding to the triangles MRN and RQP, and the quadrilaterial RNOP." Now, these three centroids form a triangle $C_1 C_2 C_3$ and give a new centroid $_c$. The centroid of these centroids for membership function is

$$C(x_0, y_0) = \left(\frac{(k_1 + 2k_2 + 3k_3 + 2k_4 + k_5)}{9}, \frac{3W_M + 1}{9} \right)$$

And the ranking formula for the function is

$$S(\overline{\mu_M}) = x_0 . y_0 = \left(\frac{(k_1 + 2k_2 + 3k_3 + 2k_4 + k_5)}{9} \right) \times \frac{3W_M + 1}{9} \tag{1}$$

Where the three centroids for the membership part of GIPFN obtained from figure 2 are

$$C_1 = \left(\frac{k_1 + k_2 + k_3}{3}, \frac{W_M}{3} \right); \ C_2 = \left(\frac{k_2 + k_3 + k_4}{3}, \frac{W_M + 1}{3} \right); \ \text{and} \ C_3 = \left(\frac{k_3 + k_4 + k_5}{3}, \frac{W_M}{3} \right)$$

And similarly, the centroid of these centroids of non-membership function is

$$C'(x_0, y_0) = \left(\frac{(l_1 + 2l_2 + 3k_3 + 2l_4 + l_5)}{9}, \frac{3V_M + 5}{9} \right)$$

The ranking formula for the non-membership function is

$$S(\overline{\gamma_M}) = x_0.y_0 = \left(\frac{(l_1 + 2l_2 + 3k_3 + 2l_4 + l_5)}{9}\right) \times \frac{3V_M + 5}{9} \tag{2}$$

As per figure 3, the centroids for the non-membership part of GIPFN are

$$C_1 = \left(\frac{l_1 + l_2 + k_3}{3}, \frac{2 + V_M}{3}\right); \quad C_2 = \left(\frac{l_2 + k_3 + k_4}{3}, \frac{V_M + 1}{3}\right); \quad \text{and } C_3 = \left(\frac{k_3 + l_4 + l_5}{3}, \frac{V_M + 2}{3}\right)$$

From (1) and (2) the rank of M is defined as

$$R(M) = \frac{W_M S(\overline{\mu_M}) + V_M S(\overline{\mu_M})}{W_M + V_M} \tag{3}$$

Figure 2. Graph for membership part of GIPFN

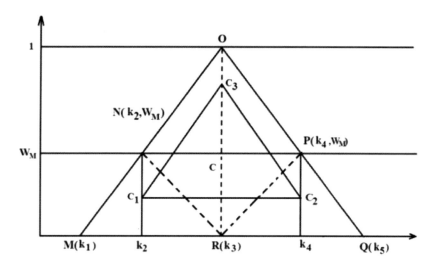

Figure 3. Graph for non-membership part of GIPFN

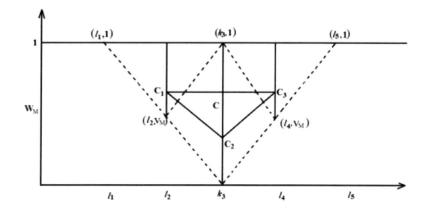

Notations and Assumptions Used in the Models

1. Notations

a. G_c: Investment for green technology
b. T: Time cycle
c. t_1: time period where there is no deterioration
d. t_2: time period where there is deterioration
e. B_o: units of product which satisfy partial back-logged demand
f. w: on-hand inventory level after B_o units are back-logged
g. q: quantity ordered after shortage
h. C_{CC}: cyclic capital cost
i. R_{TC}: slashed shipping cost
j. T_{AC}: total cost (per annum)
k. C_T: per delivery fixed shipping cost
l. s: distance covered from OW to customer via RW.
m. C_V: per delivery variable shipping cost
n. C_f: burning up of fuel when truck is empty
o. C_p: additional fuel required by the truck for transportation of one-ton goods.
p. w_p: weight of goods
q. τ: total trips
r. e_v: emission cost (formed by vehicles)
s. e_t: additional emission cost for shipping of one unit of the product
t. k_0: cost for ordering ($/unit)
u. P_c: purchasing cost ($/unit)
v. F_r: holding cost for RW ($/unit)
w. H_o: holding cost for OW ($/unit)
x. $\mathbf{H} = H_r + H_o$
y. S_c: backorder cost ($/unit)
z. l: lead time
aa. I_p: interest paid
bb. v: purchasing cost for a small part of goods
cc. C_o: capacity of OW

2. Assumptions

The mathematical model is based on the following assumptions:

a. Lead time: constant
b. Replenishment rate: infinite
c. Planning horizon: infinite
d. Shortages: partially backlogged
e. Rate of backlogging: η
f. Demand rate

$$R(t) = \begin{cases} \dfrac{\gamma t^{(1-m)/m}}{mT^{1/m}} & when \ \ I(t) \geq 0 \\ \eta \left(\dfrac{\gamma t^{(1-m)/m}}{mT^{1/m}} \right) & when \ \ I(t) < 0 \end{cases}$$

where γ and m are the scale and shape parameters respectively.

g.   Non-deterioration period: $[0, t_1]$
h.   Deterioration period: $[t_1, t_2]$
i.   Deterioration rate in RW: β (Constant)
j.   Deterioration rate in OW: Weibull ($\theta(t) = \alpha \psi t^{\psi - 1}$ where $0 < \alpha < 1$, $\psi > 0$ are called scale and shape parameter respectively)
k.   Number of prepayment instalments: $n1$ (Constant)
l.   Cyclic capital cost of prepayments: C_{CC}
m.   Green technology Cost: G_c (decision variable)
n.   Amount of carbon emission after G_c is invested: ω
o.   Parameter that changes the capability of green technology to reduce emission: χ
p.   Fraction of the emission reduction by implementing G_c: $f = \omega(1 - e^{\chi G_c})$

Mathematical Model Formulation

A green inventory model is developed with two warehouses, namely rented and owned, by paying the dues in n_1 number of multiple instalments, where the sellers deposit v prior to the shipping of the items. In each time interval $[0, T]$, the lead time is taken to be l. Once all the products are received, the retailer deposits the rest of the purchase cost, i.e., $(1-v)$. Then the retailer keeps part of the products in RW and the rest in OW. As per the unit holding cost is higher in the case of the owned warehouse, the demand is fulfilled from RW first. After the competition of the products from RW, the business starts with OW. In the present model, products are transported by trucks under the consideration of both fixed and variable transportation costs, which includes the carbon emission cost. These emissions are hazardous to all living organisms. To keep CO_2 emissions under control, green technology is used with an appropriate green-technology cost. After the lot $q = w + B_o$ is received, B_o units are expended on the demand that was backlogged, and afterwards, on-hand inventory goes down to w. In this process, y units of products are stocked in OW and the remaining $w - y$ products are placed in RW to fulfil the market demand. The carrying costs of OW and RW satisfy the inequality $H_o > H_r$. In the case of RW, the inventory level decreases because of the constant deterioration α and power demand R(t). The inventory level can go to zero at any time $t = t_1$.

But in case of OW, the stock decreases during $[0, t_1]$, followed by a constant rate of deterioration β, and in the time interval $[t_1, t_2]$, the stock level which is a combined outcome of demand and Weibull rate of deterioration, reduces to zero level at time $t = t_2$. During $[t_2, T]$ shortage arises at a constant rate η.

1. Model: 1 (Crisp Sense)

In case of RW, the differential equation meant for the level of inventory $I_r(t)$ is

$$\frac{dI_r}{dt} + \alpha I_r = -\frac{\gamma t^{\frac{(1-m)}{m}}}{mT^{\frac{1}{m}}}, \quad 0 \le t \le t_1 \tag{4}$$

Using boundary conditions

$$I_r(0) = w - y \text{ and } I_r(t_1)\text{-}0, \tag{5}$$

the solution of equation (4) after eliminating second and higher-degree terms arise in the expansion of the exponential function is

$$I_r(t) = \frac{(1-\alpha t)\gamma}{T^{\frac{1}{m}}} \left[\left(t_1^{\frac{1}{m}} - t^{\frac{1}{m}} \right) + \frac{\alpha}{(n+1)} \left(t_1^{\frac{(m+1)}{m}} - t^{\frac{(m+1)}{m}} \right) \right] \tag{6}$$

Now, substituting the value of $I_r(0) = w - y$ in equation (6), we have

$$w = y + \frac{\gamma}{T^{\frac{1}{m}}} \left[t_1^{\frac{1}{m}} + \frac{\alpha t_1^{\frac{(m+1)}{m}}}{(m+1)} \right] \tag{7}$$

Again, in case of the OW, the inventory level $I_o(t)$ in the time interval $[0,T]$ is identified through the following differential equations:

$$\frac{dI_o}{dt} + \beta I_o = 0, \quad 0 \le t \le t_1 \tag{8}$$

$$\frac{dI_o}{dt} + \lambda \psi t^{\psi-1} I_o = \frac{-\gamma t^{\frac{(1-m)}{m}}}{mT^{\frac{1}{m}}}, \quad t_1 \le t \le t_2 \tag{9}$$

$$\frac{dI_o}{dt} = -\frac{\eta \gamma t^{\frac{(1-m)}{m}}}{mT^{\frac{1}{m}}}, \quad t_2 \le t \le T \tag{10}$$

With

$I_o(0)=y; I_o(t_2)=0; I=o(T)= -R$ (11)

The solution of equation (8) is

$I_o(t)=y(1-\beta t), 0\leq t\leq t1$ (12)

The solution of equation (9) is

$$I_o(t) = \frac{\gamma(1-\lambda t^{\psi})}{T^{\frac{1}{m}}}\left[\left\{t_2^{\frac{1}{m}} - t^{\frac{1}{m}}\right\} + \frac{\lambda}{m\psi+1}\left\{t_2^{\frac{m\psi+1}{m}} - t^{\frac{m\psi+1}{m}}\right\}\right]$$ (13)

The solution of equation (10) is

$$I_0(t) = \frac{\gamma\eta}{T^{\frac{1}{m}}}\left(T^{\frac{1}{m}} - t^{\frac{1}{m}}\right) - R, t_2 \leq t \leq T$$ (14)

As $I_o(t)$ is continuous throughout in the interval $[0,T]$, therefore by the continuity condition at $t=t_2$ we get

$$R = \frac{\gamma\eta}{T^{\frac{1}{m}}}\left(T^{\frac{1}{m}} - t_2^{\frac{1}{m}}\right)$$ (15)

The costs associated to the model:

a.   Ordering cost (k_0) is constant.
b.   Purchasing cost:

$$P_c(y+R) = P_c\left[y + \frac{\gamma}{T^{\frac{1}{m}}}\left[t_1^{\frac{1}{m}} + \frac{\alpha t_1^{\frac{(m+1)}{m}}}{(m+1)}\right] + \frac{\gamma\eta}{T^{\frac{1}{m}}}\left(T^{\frac{1}{m}} - t_2^{\frac{1}{m}}\right)\right]$$ (16)

c.   Holding cost:

$$
\begin{aligned}
-&\approx \frac{H_r\gamma}{T^{\frac{1}{m}}}\left[\frac{t_1^{\frac{m+1}{m}}}{m+1}+\alpha t_1^{\frac{2m+1}{m}}\left(\frac{1}{2(2m+1)}\right)-\frac{\alpha^2(m+1)t_1^{\frac{3m+1}{m}}}{2(3m+1)}\right]+H_o\left[yt_1\left(1-\frac{\alpha t_1}{2}\right)\right] \\
&+\frac{H_o\gamma}{T^{\frac{1}{m}}}\left[\left\{\frac{t_2^{\frac{m+1}{m}}}{m+1}+\frac{\lambda\psi t_2^{\frac{m\psi+m+1}{m}}}{(\psi+1)(m\psi+m+1)}-\lambda t_2^{\frac{2m\psi+m+1}{m}}\left(\frac{(m\psi+1)}{(2m\psi+m+1)(\psi+1)}\right)\right\}\right. \\
&-\left\{t_1\left(t_2^{\frac{1}{m}}-\frac{mt_1^{\frac{1}{m}}}{m+1}+\frac{\lambda t_2^{\frac{m\psi+1}{m}}}{m\psi+1}\right)-\frac{\lambda t_1^{\psi+1}}{\psi+1}\left(t_2^{\frac{1}{m}}+\frac{t_2^{\frac{m\psi+1}{m}}}{m\psi+1}\right)\right. \\
&\left.\left.+\frac{m^2\psi t_1^{\frac{m\psi+m+1}{m}}}{(2m\psi+m+1)(m\psi+1)}+\frac{m\lambda^2 t_1^{\frac{2m\psi+m+1}{m}}}{(2m\psi+m+1)(m\psi+1)}\right\}\right]
\end{aligned}
$$

(17)

d.   Shortage cost:

$$
-S_c\int_{t_2}^{T}I_o(t)dt=\frac{S_c\gamma\eta}{2}(T-t_2)\left(1-\frac{t_2^{\frac{1}{m}}}{T^{\frac{1}{m}}}\right)
$$

(18)

e.   Cyclic capital cost:

$$
C_{CC}=\left(\frac{n_1+1}{2n_1}\right)I_pP_clvq
$$

(19)

It is calculated by the formula mentioned in Mashud et al. (2021).

f.   The shipping cost is the cost is generated from transport cost and carbon emission cost which is given as follows.

$$
T_{RC}=\tau\left[C_T+\left(2sC_fC_V+sC_VC_pw_pq\right)+\left(2se_v+se_tq\right)\times\left(1-\omega\left(1-e^{-\chi G_c}\right)\right)\right]
$$

(20)

g.   The total green technology investment cost is the product G_c and the total cycle length (T):

$$
G_c^{TI}=G_cT
$$

(21)

h. The per cycle total cost is

$$T_{AC} = \frac{1}{T} \left[k_0 + P_c(y+R) + \frac{}{} + S_c + C_{cc} + T_{RC} + G_c^{TI} \right]$$

$$T_{AC} = \frac{1}{T} \left[k_0 + P_c \left[y + \frac{\gamma}{T^{\frac{1}{m}}} \left[t_1^{\frac{1}{m}} + \frac{\alpha t_1^{\frac{(m+1)}{m}}}{(m+1)} \right] + \frac{\gamma\eta}{T^{\frac{1}{m}}} \left(T^{\frac{1}{m}} - t_2^{\frac{1}{m}} \right) \right] + \frac{}{} + \frac{S_c\gamma\eta}{2} (T-t_2) \left(1 - \frac{t_2^{\frac{1}{m}}}{T^{\frac{1}{m}}} \right) \right.$$

$$\left. + \left(\frac{n_1+1}{2n_1} \right) I_p P_c lvq + \tau \left[C_T + \left(2sC_fC_V + sC_VC_pw_pq \right) + \left(2se_v + se_tq \right) \times \left(1 - \omega \left(1 - e^{-\chi G_c} \right) \right) \right] + G_cT \right]$$

(22)

2. Model 2: (Fuzzy Case)

We take γ, the scale parameter, as a GIPFN. Let

$$\bar{\gamma} = \left\{ \left(\bar{\gamma}_1, \bar{\gamma}_2, \bar{\gamma}_3, \bar{\gamma}_4, \bar{\gamma}_5 \right) \left(\bar{\gamma}_1', \bar{\gamma}_2', \bar{\gamma}_3', \bar{\gamma}_4', \bar{\gamma}_5' \right) ; W_{\tilde{\gamma}}, V_{\tilde{\gamma}} \right\}$$

Now, $\tilde{T}_{AC}$ is given by

$$\tilde{T}_{AC} = \frac{1}{T} \left[k_0 + P_c \left[y + \frac{\tilde{\gamma}}{T^{\frac{1}{m}}} \left[t_1^{\frac{1}{m}} + \frac{\alpha t_1^{\frac{(m+1)}{m}}}{(m+1)} \right] + \frac{\tilde{\gamma}\eta}{T^{\frac{1}{m}}} \left(T^{\frac{1}{m}} - t_2^{\frac{1}{m}} \right) \right] + \frac{}{} + \frac{S_c\tilde{\gamma}\eta}{2} (T-t_2) \left(1 - \frac{t_2^{\frac{1}{m}}}{T^{\frac{1}{m}}} \right) \right.$$

$$\left. + \left(\frac{n_1+1}{2n_1} \right) I_p P_c lvq + \tau \left[C_T + \left(2sC_fC_V + sC_VC_pw_pq \right) + \left(2se_v + se_tq \right) \times \left(1 - \omega \left(1 - e^{-\chi G_c} \right) \right) \right] + G_cT \right]$$

$$S(\bar{\mu}_{M_{\tilde{\gamma}}}) = \frac{1}{T} \left[k_0 + P_c \left[y + \frac{S(\overline{\mu_M})}{T^{\frac{1}{m}}} \left[t_1^{\frac{1}{m}} + \frac{\alpha t_1^{\frac{(m+1)}{m}}}{(m+1)} \right] + \frac{S(\overline{\mu_M})\eta}{T^{\frac{1}{m}}} \left(T^{\frac{1}{m}} - t_2^{\frac{1}{m}} \right) \right] + \frac{}{} \right.$$

$$\left. + \frac{S_cS(\overline{\mu_M})\eta}{2} (T-t_2) \left(1 - \frac{t_2^{\frac{1}{m}}}{T^{\frac{1}{m}}} \right) + \left(\frac{n_1+1}{2n_1} \right) I_p P_c lvq \mid \tau \left[C_T + \left(2sC_fC_V + sC_VC_pw_pq \right) \right. \right.$$

$$\left. \left. + \left(2se_v + se_tq \right) \times \left(1 - \omega \left(1 - e^{-\chi G_c} \right) \right) \right] + G_cT \right]$$

$$S(\overline{\gamma}_{M_{\tilde{\gamma}}}) = \frac{1}{T}\left[k_0 + P_c\left[y + \frac{S(\overline{\gamma_M})}{T^{\frac{1}{m}}}\left[t_1^{\frac{1}{m}} + \frac{\alpha t_1^{\frac{(m+1)}{m}}}{(m+1)} \right] + \frac{S(\overline{\gamma_M})\eta}{T^{\frac{1}{m}}}\left(T^{\frac{1}{m}} - t_2^{\frac{1}{m}} \right) \right] + - \right.$$

$$+ \frac{S_c S(\overline{\gamma_M})\eta}{2}(T - t_2)\left(1 - \frac{t_2^{\frac{1}{m}}}{T^{\frac{1}{m}}} \right) + \left(\frac{n_1 + 1}{2n_1} \right) I_p P_c l v q$$

$$\left. + \tau\left[C_T + \left(2sC_f C_V + sC_V C_p w_p q \right) + \left(2se_v + se_t q \right) \times \left(1 - \omega\left(1 - e^{-\chi G_c} \right) \right) \right] + G_c T \right]$$

The rank of $\tilde{\gamma}$ is $R\left(\tilde{T}_{AC}\right)_{(\tilde{\gamma})} = \left[W_{\tilde{\gamma}}\tilde{T}_{AC}S(\overline{\mu}_{\tilde{\gamma}}) + V_{\tilde{\gamma}}\tilde{T}_{AC}S(\overline{\gamma}_{\tilde{\gamma}}) \right] \times \frac{1}{(W_{\tilde{\gamma}} + V_{\tilde{\gamma}})}$

ALGORITHMS

Step 1: Set all the values of the parameters.

Step 2: Set $T=2.4$ and $G_c=9$.

Step 3: Compute the optimal T_{AC} from equation (22) using MATLAB.

Step 4: Increase $T=T+1$, at $G_c=9$ and repeat Step 3 until the minimum value of T_{AC} is reached.

Step 5: Record the new values of T^* and T_{AC} when $G_c=9$ from step 4 and go to Step 6.

Step 6: Increase $G_c=G_c+1$ and taking the new value of T_1^* from step 5 and

And record the values of T_{AC}. Repeat step 6 until the minimum value of T_{AC} is not reached.

Step 7: Find optimum values of T^*, G_c^* and T_{AC}.

Step 8: Stop.

This algorithm is applicable for intuitionistic fuzzy inventory models derived in the present research.

NUMERICAL ILLUSTRATIONS

For the validation of the model, a numerical example is suggested. The optimal values of green technology investment cost, cycle time, and total cost are obtained for the prescribed set of parameters.

For illustration purposes, we consider an inventory system with the following values of the parameters:

$k_0 = 500$, $P_c = 35$, $C_o = 150$, $\gamma = 60$, $m = 4$, $\tau = 3$, $\eta = 5$, $H_r = 2$, $H_o = 1$, $\alpha = 0.05$,

$\beta = 0.01$, $\lambda = 0.1$, $\psi = 2$, $S_c = 24$, $I_p = 0.07$, $l = 0.5$, $v = 0.5$, $d = 30$, $C_T = 0.1$, $C_f = 0.75$,

$C_p = 2.4$, $v_t = 0.1$, $e_v = 0.3$, $e_t = 0.4$, $w_p = 2$, $\omega = 4$, $\chi = 0.7$, $t_1 = 0.4$, $t_2 = 1.5$, $\overline{\gamma}_1 = 60.2$,   .

$\overline{\gamma}_2 = 60.3$, $\overline{\gamma}_3 = 60.4$, $\overline{\gamma}_4 = 60.5$, $\overline{\gamma}_5 = 60.6$, $\overline{\gamma}_1' = 60.1$, $\overline{\gamma}_2' = 60.2$, $\overline{\gamma}_3' = 60.4$, $\overline{\gamma}_4' = 60.6$,

$\overline{\gamma}_5' = 60.7$, $W_{\tilde{\gamma}} = 0.4$, and $V_{\tilde{\gamma}} = 0.5$

Table 2. Optimum results of $T/G_c/T_{AC}$ (crisp model)

T	G_c	$T_{AC}(t_1, T)$
2.8	9	1294.41
3	9	1282.63
3.2	9	1275.69
3.4	9	1272.48
3.6	**9**	**1272.03**
3.8	9	1273.82
4	9	1277.30
3.6	9.2	1271.06
3.6	9.4	1270.24
3.6	9.6	1269.56
3.6	9.8	1268.99
3.6	10	1268.52
3.6	10.2	1268.13
3.6	10.4	1267.83
3.6	10.6	1267.59
3.6	10.8	1267.40
3.6	11	1267.27
3.6	11.2	1268.13
3.6	10.4	1267.83
3.6	10.6	1267.59
3.6	10.8	1267.40
3.6	11	1267.27
3.6	11.2	1267.18
3.6	11.4	1267.13
3.6	**11.6**	**1267.11**
3.6	11.8	1267.12

Table 3. Optimum results of T/G$_c$/T$_{AC}$ (Fuzzy model)

T	G$_c$	T$_{AC}$(t$_1$,T)
3.5	9.2	1191.38
3.5	9.4	1190.83
3.5	9.6	1190.38
3.5	9.8	1190.02
3.5	10	1189.72
3.5	10.2	1189.50
3.5	10.4	1189.33
3.5	**10.6**	**1189.20**
3.5	10.8	1189.26
3.6	10.6	1177.66
3.8	10.6	1176.38
4	10.6	1175.72
4.2	10.6	1174.30
4.4	**10.6**	**1174.10**
4.6	10.6	1174.25

Sensitivity Analysis

Optimum tables for the total cost with discrete values of k_0, P_c, H_r, H_o, e_v, e_t, S_c and C_T, taken one at a time, while other parameters kept unchanged. All the solutions are given in the following tables.

Table 4. Sensitivity analysis for k$_0$ and P$_c$

Effect of change in k$_0$ on T$_{AC}$				Effect of change in P$_c$ on T$_{AC}$			
k$_0$	T	G$_c$	T$_{AC}$(T,G$_c$)	P$_c$	T	G$_c$	T$_{AC}$(T,G$_c$)
450	3.5	11.7	1252.5568	34.5	3.4	11.7	1231.3558
500	3.6	11.6	1267.11	35.0	3.6	11.6	1267.11
600	3.6	11.6	1294.8947	36.0	3.52	11.7	1336.526

Table 5. Sensitivity analysis for H$_r$ and H$_o$

Effect of change in H$_r$ on T$_{AC}$				Effect of change in H$_o$ on T$_{AC}$			
H$_r$	T	G$_c$	T$_{AC}$(T,G$_c$)	H$_o$	T	G$_c$	T$_{AC}$(T,G$_c$)
2.1	3.5	11.7	1266.9226	0.5	3.5	11.7	1258.0579
2	3.6	11.6	1267.11	1	3.6	11.6	1267.11
1.9	3.5	11.7	1266.7623	1.5	3.5	11.7	1275.6271

Table 6. Sensitivity analysis for e_v and e_t

Effect of change in e_v on T_{AC}				Effect of change in e_t on T_{AC}			
e_t	T	G_c	$T_{AC}(T,G_c)$	e_t	T	G_c	$T_{AC}(T,G_c)$
0.09	3.5	11.7	1267.8707	0.295	3.7	10.5	1328.0619
0.1	3.6	11.6	1267.11	0.3	3.6	11.6	1267.11
0.11	3.5	11.7	1265.8143	0.301	3.5	11.7	1254.3863

Table 7. Sensitivity analysis for S_c and e_t

Effect of change in S_c on T_{AC}				Effect of change in C_T on T_{AC}			
S_c	T	G_c	$T_{AC}(T,G_c)$	C_T	T	G_c	$T_{AC}(T,G_c)$
22	3.8	11.6	1219.8905	0.09	1254.9287	11.6	3.5
24	3.6	11.6	1267.11	0.1	3.6	11.6	1267.11
26	3.2	11.8	1284.1793	0.11	3.5	11.7	1254.3980

Figure 4. G_c vs. T_{AC}

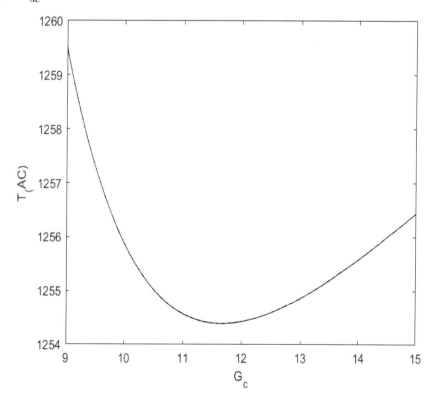

Figure 5. T vs. T_{AC}

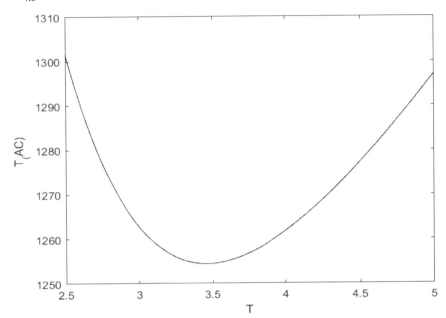

Figure 6. Total cost vs. T and G_c

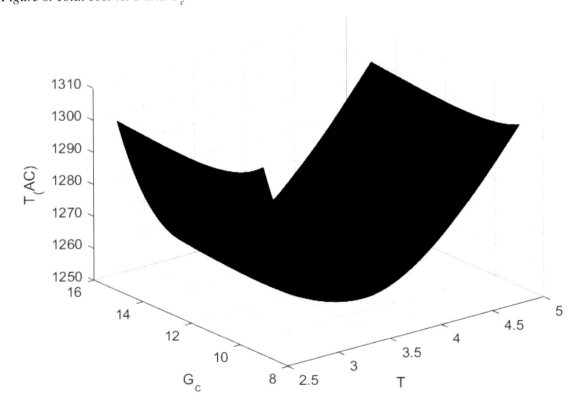

MANAGERIAL INSIGHTS

Formulated on the behavioral changes in Table - 4,5,6 and 7 the following are the managerial insights.

1. When k_0 increases, initially T increases and G_c decreases to two fixed values and throughout the value of T_{AC} increases.
2. When P_c increases, initially T increases and then decreases and the reverse happens for G_c, and T_{AC} increases.
3. When H_r increases, initially both T and T_{AC} increase and then they decrease and the reverse happens for G_c.
4. When H_o increase, initially T increases and then decreases and the reverse happens for G_c but all along T_{AC} increases.
5. When e_v increases, initially T increases and then decreases and the reverse happens for G_c, and T_{AC} decreases.
6. When e_t increases, strictly T decreases and G_c increases, and T_{AC} decreases.
7. When S_c increases, strictly T decreases and initially G_c remains constant and then increases, and T_{AC} increases.
8. When C_T increases, initially T and T_{AC} increases and then decreases and initially G_c remains constant and increases.

CONCLUSION

In this present research, a two ware-house sustainable deteriorating intuitionistic fuzzy and crisp EOQ models under the consideration of power demand, partial back-log and green technology investment are developed. A Weibull distribution with two-parameter is introduced to describe the characteristics of the model. Again, this model opens insights for the vendor that how to transport the products from the OW to the RW and then it goes to the customers efficiently with minimum emissions, which guarantees on the optimum cost and cycle time. Along with these considerations, a pre-payment plan is preferred to fulfil the requirements of the supplier. Primarily, the vendor deposits a part of the cost utilized for purchasing of products as a pre-payment to place the order and the rest of it is done when the product is received. In the present study, we have tried to extend the work of Uthra et al. (2017) and Mashud et al. (2020) with the consideration of power demand. Numerical examples are furnished to establish the optimality conditions meant for costs related to green technology, total time cycle and total cost, and finally it ends at sensitivity analysis.

Additionally, the convexity of the total cost, green technology cost and total time cycle have been ascertained graphically using MATLAB.

Models with numerous kinds of demands like stock dependent, advertisement cost dependent and probabilistic parameters can be proposed. Also, more realistic types of models with two-level trade credit policy, quantity discount, etc., can be included.

REFERENCES

Atanasssov, K. (1989). Intuitionistic fuzzy sets. *Fuzzy Sets and Systems, 20*(1), 87–96. doi:10.1016/S0165-0114(86)80034-3

Bae, S. H., Sarkis, J., & Yoo, C. S. (2011). Greening transportation fleets: Insights from a two-stage game theoretic model. *Transportation Research Part E, Logistics and Transportation Review, 47*(6), 793–807. doi:10.1016/j.tre.2011.05.015

Benjaafar, S., Li, Y., & Daskin, M. (2013). Carbon footprint and the management of supply chains: Insights from simple models. *IEEE Transactions on Automation Science and Engineering, 10*(1), 99–116. doi:10.1109/TASE.2012.2203304

Bonney, M., & Jaber, M. Y. (2011). Environmentally responsible inventory models: Non-classical models for a non-classical era. *International Journal of Production Economics, 133*(1), 43–53. doi:10.1016/j.ijpe.2009.10.033

Bouchery, Y., Ghaffari, A., Jemai, Z., & Dallery, Y. (2012). Including sustainability criteria into inventory models. *European Journal of Operational Research, 222*(2), 229–240. doi:10.1016/j.ejor.2012.05.004

Chakrabarti, T., & Chaudhuri, K. S. (1997). An EOQ model for deteriorating items with a linear trend in demand and shortages in all cycles. *International Journal of Production Economics, 49*(3), 205–213. doi:10.1016/S0925-5273(96)00015-1

Chen, X., Benjaafar, S., & Elomri, A. (2013). The carbon-constrained EOQ. *Operations Research Letters, 41*(2), 172–179. doi:10.1016/j.orl.2012.12.003

Covert, R. P., & Philip, G. C. (1973). An EOQ model for items with Weibull distribution deterioration. *AIIE Transactions, 5*(4), 323–326. doi:10.1080/05695557308974918

Datta, T. K. (2017). Effect of a green technology investment on a production-inventory system with carbon tax. Advances in operations research, 2017. *Article ID, 4834839*, 1–12.

De, S. K., & Mahata, G. (2019). A cloudy fuzzy economic order quantity model for imperfect-quality items with allowable proportionate discounts. *Journal of Industrial Engineering International, 15*(4), 571–583. doi:10.100740092-019-0310-1

Ghare, P., & Schrader, G. (1963). A model for exponentially decaying inventories. *Journal of Industrial Engineering, 14*, 238–243.

Goswami, A., & Chaudhuri, K. (1991). EOQ model for an inventory with a linear trend in demand and finite rate of replenishment considering shortages. *International Journal of Systems Science, 22*(1), 181–187. doi:10.1080/00207729108910598

Hua, G., Cheng, T. C. E., & Wang, W. (2011). Managing carbon footprints in inventory management. *International Journal of Production Economics, 132*(2), 178–185. doi:10.1016/j.ijpe.2011.03.024

Ilic, A., Staake, T., & Fleisch, E. (2009). Using sensor information to reduce the carbon footprint of perishable goods. *IEEE Pervasive Computing, 8*(1), 22–29. doi:10.1109/MPRV.2009.20

Jaggi, C. K., Pareek, S., Khanna, A., & Nidhi, N. (2016). Optimal replenishment policy for fuzzy inventory model with deteriorating items and allowable shortages under inflationary conditions. *Yugoslav Journal of Operations Research*, *26*(4), 1–21. doi:10.2298/YJOR150202002Y

Jaggi, C. K., Tiwari, S., & Shafi, A. A. (2015). Effect of deterioration on two-warehouse inventory model with imperfect quality. *Computers & Industrial Engineering*, *88*(C), 378–385. doi:10.1016/j.cie.2015.07.019

Kacprzyk, J., & Staniewski, P. (1982). Long-term inventory policy- making through fuzzy decision-making models. *Fuzzy Sets and Systems*, *8*(2), 117–132. doi:10.1016/0165-0114(82)90002-1

Kaufmann, A., & Gupta, M. M. (1991). *Introduction to fuzzy arithmetic theory and applications*. International Thomson Computer Press.

Liu, Z. L., Anderson, T. D., & Cruz, J. M. (2012). Consumer environmental awareness and competition in two-stage supply chains. *European Journal of Operational Research*, *218*(3), 602–613. doi:10.1016/j.ejor.2011.11.027

Mahata, G. C., & Goswami, A. (2009a). A fuzzy replenishment policy for deteriorating items with ramp type demand rate under inflation. *International Journal of Operational Research*, *5*(3), 328–348. doi:10.1504/IJOR.2009.025200

Mashud, A. H. M. M., Pervin, M., Mishra, U., & Daryanto, Y. (2021). A sustainable inventory model with controllable carbon emissions in green-warehouse farms. *Journal of Cleaner Production*, *298*(126777), 1–15. doi:10.1016/j.jclepro.2021.126777

Mishra, R. B. (1975). Optimum production lot size model for a system with deteriorating inventory. *International Journal of Production Research*, *13*(5), 495–505. doi:10.1080/00207547508943019

Mishra, U., Wu, J. Z., Tsao, Y. C., & Tsend, M. L. (2020b). Sustainable inventory system with controllable non-instantaneous deterioration and environmental emission rates. *Journal of Cleaner Production*, *244*(118807), 1–29. doi:10.1016/j.jclepro.2019.118807

Patro, R., Acharya, M., Nayak, M. M., & Patnaik, S. (2017). A fuzzy inventory model with time dependent weibull deterioration, quadratic demand and partial backlogging. *International Journal of Management and Decision Making*, *16*(3), 243–279. doi:10.1504/IJMDM.2017.085636

Patro, R., Acharya, M., Nayak, M. M., & Patnaik, S. (2017). A fuzzy imperfect quality inventory model with proportionate discount under learning effect. *International Journal of Intelligent Enterprise*, *4*(4), 303–327. doi:10.1504/IJIE.2017.089211

Ponnivalavan, K., & Pathinathan, T. (2015). Intuitionistic pentagonal fuzzy number. *Journal of Engineering and Applied Sciences (Asian Research Publishing Network)*, *10*(12), 5446–5450.

Sahoo, S., & Acharya, M. (2021). *An inventory model for seasonal deteriorating items with price dependent demand and preservation technology investment in crisp and fuzzy environments. Recent Trends in Applied Mathematics*. Springer Verlag.

Sahoo, S., Acharya, M., & Nayak. M.M. (2019). A three rates of EOQ/EPQ model for instantaneous deteriorating items involving fuzzy parameter under shortages. *International Journal of Innovative Technology and Exploring Engineering, 8*(8S2), 405-418.

Sahoo, S., Acharya, M., & Nayak, M. M. (2020a). Application of Preservation Technology and Disposal Costs for Instantaneous Deteriorating Seasonal Products under Crisp and Fuzzy Environments. *International Journal of Advanced Science and Technology, 29*(8s), 392–405.

Sahoo, S., Acharya, M., & Nayak, M. M. (2020b). A Cloudy Fuzzy Inventory Model for Deteriorating Items with Price Dependent Demand. *TEST Engineering and Management, 83*, 6090–6097.

Shah, N. H., & Cardenas-Barron, L. E. (2015). Retailer's decision for ordering and credit policies for deteriorating items when a supplier offers order-linked credit period or cash discount. *Applied Mathematics and Computation, 259*(15), 569–578. doi:10.1016/j.amc.2015.03.010

Sharmila, D., & Uthayakumar, R. (2016). An Inventory model with three rates of production rate understock and time dependent demand for time varying deterioration rate with shortages. International Journal of Advanced Engineering. *Management Science, 2*(9), 1595–1602.

Skouri, K., Konstantaras, I., Papachristos, S., & Ganas, I. (2009). Inventory models with ramp type demand rate, partial backlogging and Weibull deterioration rate. *European Journal of Operational Research, 192*(1), 79–92. doi:10.1016/j.ejor.2007.09.003

Taleizadeh, A. A., Hazarkhani, B., & Moon, I. (2020). Joint pricing and inventory decisions with carbon emission considerations, partial backordering and planned discounts. *Annals of Operations Research, 290*(3), 95–113. doi:10.100710479-018-2968-y

Tiwari, S., Ahmed, W., & Sarkar, B. (2019). Sustainable ordering policies for non-instantaneous deteriorating items under carbon emission and multi-trade-credit-polices. *Journal of Cleaner Production, 240*(118183), 1–19.

Tiwari, S., Cardenas-Barron, L. E., Khanna, A., & Jaggi, C. K. (2016). Impact of trade credit and inflation on retailer's ordering policies for non-instantaneous deteriorating items in a two-warehouse environment. *International Journal of Production Economics, 176*, 154–169. doi:10.1016/j.ijpe.2016.03.016

Uthra, G., Thangavelu, K., & Shunmugapriya S. (2017). Ranking generalized intuitionistic pentagonal fuzzy number by centroidal approach. *International Journal of Mathematics and Its Applications, 5*(4),589-593.

Vijayan, T., & Kumaran, M. (2008). Inventory model with a mixture of back-orders and lost sales under fuzzy cost. *European Journal of Operational Research, 189*(1), 105–119. doi:10.1016/j.ejor.2007.05.049

Zimmerman, H. J. (1978). Fuzzy programming and linear programming with several objective functions. *Fuzzy Sets and Systems, 1*(1), 45–55. doi:10.1016/0165-0114(78)90031-3

Zimmermann, H. J. (1996). *Fuzzy Set Theory and Its Applications.* Kluwer Academic Publishers. doi:10.1007/978-94-015-8702-0

Chapter 8
AI–Driven COVID–19 Patient Screening With Design Thinking Approach– C3IA Tool:
A Case Study

Sunita Vikrant Dhavale

Defence Institute of Advanced Technology, India

ABSTRACT

In this chapter, the authors discuss a brief literature review on AI-driven COVID-19 patient screening technologies along with their pros and cons. Next, they discuss the need of human-centric design thinking in AI-driven solutions. Next, in this study, a novel C3IA (CNN-based COVID-19 chest image analysis) tool for automatic COVID-19 detection with multi-class classification (COVID/normal/pneumonia) using raw chest x-ray images is proposed. The authors implemented a two-stream CNN architecture with two pre-trained VGG-16 models, which incorporates both segmented and un-segmented image features. The trained model is tested on more than 500 Indian patient x-ray image datasets and confirmed accuracy of 99% in detecting COVID signatures. Further, in this work, the authors discuss how the design thinking approach is followed in various stages while developing the product to provide a user-friendly efficient real-time COVID-19 chest x-ray image analysis for the common citizen.

INTRODUCTION

On December 31, 2019, COVID-19 pandemic eruption in Wuhan, Hubei, China, turned as a rapidly spreader pandemic endangering humankind. Severe acute respiratory syndrome Coronavirus (SARS-CoV) caused severe respiratory disease and death in humans (Khan et. al., 2021). The most common symptoms like dry cough, loss of smell and taste, fever, fatigue, respiratory illness and shortness of breath were experienced by COVID-19 patients. To mitigate the transmission of the novel virus, most of the countries followed lockdowns/curfews with immediate effect along with encouraging various research organizations, higher educational institutes, individuals, scientists, and researchers to work

DOI: 10.4018/978-1-6684-4580-8.ch008

on technological solutions including AI technologies to diminish the COVID-19 pandemic along with discovering effective vaccines (Khan et. al., 2021). Many governments took major steps to accelerate artificial Intelligence (AI) based research in tackling this global health crisis response and healthcare management. In response, AI proved to be crucial technology in building next-generation epidemic preparedness along with a resilient recovery.

Viral nucleic acid detection using the real-time polymerase chain reaction (RT-PCR) and anti-body test are currently the agreed standard method used for COVID-19 diagnosis which are costly, invasive, labor-intensive, time-consuming, diagnostic techniques that require specific instruments. CT Scanning/X-ray imaging modalities has already proven as an adjunctive tool/effective imaging technique for the diagnosis of lung-related diseases like pneumonia and also they does not require any reagents. These technologies can be used for rapid screening of COVID patients as evolution of ground-glass opacification with consolidation in the peripheries and subsequent resolution of the airspaces changes in COVID patients radiological images is seen commonly. Researchers found the symptoms or patterns like right infrahilar airspace opacities, single nodular opacity in the left lower lung region, many irregular opacities in both lungs, ground-glass opacities (GGO), consolidation, and vascular dilation in the lesion, interlobular septal thickening and air bronchogram sign, with or without vascular expansion, Peripheral focal or multifocal GGO affecting both lungs, rounded lung opacities in chest XRay/CT images of various COVID patients (Chakraborty et. al., 2020).

For rapid screening and tracking of unique COVID signatures pertaining to lung irregularities, AI based technological solutions can be employed. With the emergence of machine learning (ML) and deep learning (DL) technologies (subset of AI), the feasibility of AI based data driven solutions is already proven in various domains such as, in product industries, process industries, defence, agriculture, and banking domains. Deep learning (DL) based techniques have proven robust systems for both automated feature engineering and classification of complex imaging data and hence gaining popularity for building automatic diagnosis/assisting tools for clinicians in the medical field.

Recently, many radiology images have been widely used for COVID-19 detection. Chest XRay/CT scan images have been an actively used imaging technique for the diagnosis of lung-related diseases like pneumonia (Tulin et. al., 2020). Tulin et. al., (2020) proposed DarkNet model and reported a classification accuracy of 98.08% for binary classes and 87.02% for multi-class cases. Yicheng et al. (2020) reported the high sensitivity (up to 98%) of chest CT for COVID-19 screening in a series of 51 patients. To speed up the screening, Ophir et al. (2020) employed the DL techniques to detect COVID-19 on CT images. Shi et al. (2021) collected a large-scale COVID-19 CT dataset and developed a ML based method for COVID 19 screening. CT scanning modality suffers from disadvantages like non-portability, high cost, less availability, chance of human to human transmission, and requirement of more technical expertise. Chest Xray is more widely accessible due to its faster imaging time and considerably lower cost than CT, and COVID-19 test kit (Chakraborty et. al., 2020). X-Ray images can be taken at patient place itself/ ICU patients; hence they can be convenient mode for later assessments too. So for real-time low cost massive screening of COVID patients, X-Ray modalities can be used in AI based technological solutions.

Recently, several DL approaches are suggested by researchers to screen and diagnose coronavirus-infected patients using chest X-ray images (Chakraborty et. al., 2020). Apostolopoulos et al. (2020) used transfer learning with pre-trained CNNs for COVID-19 detection and achieved 93.48% and 98.75% classification accuracy in three and two class classifications, respectively. Wang and Lin et al. (2020) proposed and trained COVID-Net DL model with the COVIDx dataset with 92.6% test accuracy in three-class classification. Hemdan et al. (2020) employed transfer learning with ImageNet pre-trained

CNNs for COVID-19 detection and reported good performance of VGG19 and DenseNet121 compared to other pre-trained CNN models. Chakraborty et. al. (2020) Corona-Nidaan, a lightweight DL model, for COVID-19 detection, and the model achieved 95% accuracy for three-class classification with 94% precision and recall for COVID-19 cases.

In this study, a novel real-time user-friendly C3IA (CNN based COVID-19 Chest Image Analysis) tool for automatic COVID-19 patient screening with multi-class classification (COVID/Normal/Pneumonia) is proposed. The remaining paper organized as follows: In Section 2, we will discuss the need of human centric design thinking in AI driven solutions. In Section 3, we introduce the proposed C3IA tool architecture. In Section 4, we present the experimental setup and results. In Section 5, we will discuss how design thinking approach is followed in various stages while developing the product to provide a user friendly efficient real time COVID-19 Chest X-ray Image Analysis for common citizen. Section 6 states the conclusions.

HUMAN CENTRIC DESIGN THINKING IN AI DRIVEN SOLUTIONS

Design Thinking is highly interactive and incremental process and a structured approach to generating and evolving ideas. Design thinking approaches follow user centric product development where user's needs, emotions, feelings, and problems are valued. For successful usage of AI research driven solutions by users, AI research team should focus on AI design thinking to create human-centric AI products and services. Following are some important stages in design thinking approach (Joana et al., 2021),(Dorota et al., 2021), (Robert et al., 2020), (Ala-Kitulaet al., 2017), (Amandaet al., 2019).

1. Empathize- This stage concentrates on feeling empathy with the users of our product. One should understand people, their needs and discover what they feel, think, and expect. One should work with people representing different mindsets, experiences, groups and work to. One should think about how he can improve their lives using AI solutions.
2. Define- In this stage, one can define his target group and target challenge. Explore feasibility of AI application to solve their problems using AI solution. Analyze collected data, build user profiles, ask questions and search for insights to produce actionable problem statements.
3. Ideate- This stage refers about finding innovative solutions for the problems of users. Here, brainstorm all the possible ideas, use team's creativity, and find some new/uncommon way of solving the problem. Diverge on possible solutions. One can formulate which AI algorithms, tools, and techniques will be used in designing this product.
4. Prototype- Once you choose the most interesting ideas convert them into prototypes instead of developing a full-scale AI solution at this stage. Here, one can choose the best trained/fitted AI model to develop a perfect final piece of software.
5. Test- In this last stage, one has to identify and remove the problems with his product by testing the prototype in a close-to-real environment selected in the first stages. One can observe their users – their reactions/ feedbacks/ surveys/usages about developed product. In case of any short comings, go few steps back, may redefine problem and repeat the process.

Design Thinking in human centric AI driven solutions offers increased user satisfaction and greater usage as user is always at the center of product development,

Proposed C3IA Model

In this section, we propose a novel real-time user-friendly C3IA (CNN based COVID-19 Chest Image Analysis) tool for automatic COVID-19 patient screening with multi-class classification (*COVID/Normal/Pneumonia*).

Deep learning relies on large amounts of annotated data. First, we collected the standard dataset provided by MD.ai for chest x-rays images along with annotation masks. For accurate assessment of model performance, the use of 'gold-standard' test data labels is recommended where "gold standard" segmentations for the chest X-ray are generated manually under the supervision of a radiologist. They used the following conventions for outlining the lung boundaries: Both posterior and anterior ribs are readily visible in the CXRs; the part of the lung behind the heart excluded. They followed anatomical landmarks such as the boundary of the hearth, aortic arc/line, and pericardium line and sharp costophrenic angle that follow the diaphragm boundary (Jaeger et al., 2014).

The MD.ai app used to view the DICOM images and get image-level annotation (MD.ai et al., 2021). The MD.ai python client library used to download images and annotations, prepare the datasets, and then train the model for segmentation. The original public dataset available for educational purposes only is downloaded from (MD.ai et al., 2021).

We trained U-Net for Semantic Segmentation of the lung fields for the standard chest X-Rays lung segmentation dataset. Dataset divided in Train dataset and test dataset with 80:20 ratio. We trained U-Net for Semantic Segmentation of the lung fields for these chest x-rays. We created a dataset containing the chest x-rays images of the COVID 19 patients and normal patients.

Unet is implemented using Tensorflow and keras. Using keras U-Net, we received 98%accuracy in lung segmentation. Figure 1 shows the sample output of trained UNET model after segmentation.

Figure 1. a) Original Lung X-Ray Images b) Mask Ground Truth c) Segmentation mask predicted by trained UNet Model, and c) Predicted Lung Segmented Portion

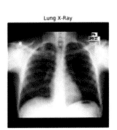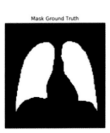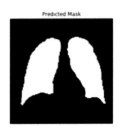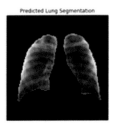

Next, we collected the standard dataset available with 3 different data classification (Normal/COVID/Pneumonia) (Ref: https://github.com/ieee8023/covid-chestxray-dataset, https://github.com/JordanMicahBennett/SMART-CT-SCAN_BASED-COVID19_VIRUS_DETECTOR/). We used trained U-Net model to automatically segment all given lung X-Ray images into segmented lung images using trained UNET model without expert intervention and verify the medical experts' results. We applied a U-Net for Semantic Segmentation of the lung fields on chest x-rays.

Next, we proposed C3IA based on two-stream VGG-16 Model architecture as shown in Figure 2. The VGG-16 models are trained with both segmented and un-segmented images against 3 different data classification (Normal/COVID/Pneumonia). Segmented features will be given more weightage by the model while training without leaving important noisy features from un-segmented parts.

During testing phase any given input chest X-Ray image will be automatically segmented by trained UNet model and both segmented and un-segmented image features will be given as input to the two stream VGG-16 trained model which will predict if there are any COVID signatures present in given input chest X-Ray image. In final stage we started collecting Indian Covid-19 patient dataset from various medical institutes/hospitals in order to test the efficacy of our trained model. We consulted with the medical experts to achieve accuracy in prediction.

Figure 2. Proposed C3IA model

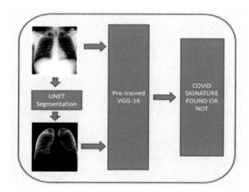

Experimental Results and Analysis

The experiments are carried out on a laptop running Windows 10 with Intel(R) Core(TM) i7-8750H CPU @ 2.20GHz, 16 GB memory, NVIDIA GeForce GTX 1060, Dedicated GPU memory 6.0 GB. C3IA model is trained with 5664 chest X-ray images (1423 Normal, 357 Covid, 3883 Pneumonia). These images are resized to 224x224 and standard data augmentation techniques are applied to tackle data imbalance problems. The model is tested on unseen dataset of more than 600 images (234 Normal, 220 Covid, 390 Pnuemonia) samples. The model achieved 95% accuracy for three-class classification with good precision and recall for COVID-19 cases. Although it is difficult to find symptoms in XRay images during the early stages of COVID-19, well-trained deep learning models can find those hidden signatures well [1] proposed approach is evaluated based on accuracy (Refer Equation 1), precision (Refer Equation 2), recall (Refer Equation 3) and F1-Score (Refer Equation 4).

$$Accuracy = \frac{TruePositive + TrueNegative}{TruePositive + TrueNegative + FalsePositive + FalseNegative} \tag{1}$$

Precision is the fraction of relevant instances that are recovered and is defined as given Equation

$$Precision = \frac{TruePositive}{TruePositive + FalsePositive} \tag{2}$$

Recall is defined as given in Equation 3.

$$\mathrm{Re}\,call = \frac{\mathrm{TruePositive}}{\mathrm{TruePositive} + \mathrm{F}alse\mathrm{N}ega\mathrm{tive}} \qquad (3)$$

To further assess the efficacy of the model, we used 5-fold cross-validation.
Also, we calculated the F-score, which is the harmonic mean of Precision and Recall (as in Equation 4).

$$F - score = \frac{2 \times \mathrm{Pr}\,ecision \times \mathrm{Re}\,call}{\mathrm{Pr}\,ecision + \mathrm{Re}\,call} \qquad (4)$$

Proposed C3IA provides overall accuracy of about 95%. Table 1 shows the C3IA's performance parameter values. Figure 3 shows the training and validation loss as well as training and validation accuracy of model.

Figure 3. Training and validation loss as well as training and validation accuracy of C3IA

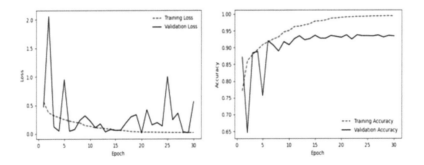

Table 1. Precision, recall, F1-score and accuracy

	Precision	Recall	F1-Score
COVID-19	0.93	0.93	0.93
Normal	0.98	0.93	0.96
Pneumonia	0.97	0.92	0.94
Accuracy			0.95

DESIGN THINKING APPROACH IN C3IA DEVELOPMENT

Practical artificial intelligence has made its way out of the labs and into our daily lives. Apple's Siri, AI powered Google search engines, Microsoft's intelligent personal assistant cortana are some of the AI solutions fielded by the big players in the industry. To make C3IA user-friendly tool, we tried to find answers for following design questions during empathy phase:

1. Do we need to automate COVID patient screening? Ans: Yes, it will help them to analyze their X-Ray reports from anywhere/anytime using their smartphones supporting telemedicine facilities during pandemic;
2. Will the data be private and public data? Ans: Standard dataset is released on many websites for research. However privacy of private patient data needs to be maintained. For testing, use of unseen test data collected from hospitals is required;
3. How one will tune the AI? Ans: Using various performance parameters like precision or recall;
4. Are the end-users technical or non-technical people? Ans: Both;
5. What value are they expecting to derive from the model? Ans: Real-Time Fast Artificial Intelligence based COVID-19 cases detection with great accuracy, Solution should be low-cost, non-invasive, real-time, accurate, Accessible via standard web browser/smartphone, Easy to operate system, Aid medical staff especially situated at rural places, Supports mass level testing,
6. What can be the larger implications of the model? Need large dataset for training, non-availability of standard dataset in given domain, product may not be accepted by user, dedicated cloud resources will be required to purchase in order to make the tool available to users etc.

C3IA was made freely accessible for all Indian citizens on DIAT Website (https://www.diat.ac.in) by developing easy web-based access via smartphones and supporting DIAT's noble humanitarian response in the current global pandemic situation. Figure 4, Figure 5, Figure 6, Figure 7 and Figure 8 shows the User interface design of C3IA product while using it for COVID patient screening. In May 2020, C3IA was made publicly accessible for all users as shown in Figure 4. A simple user interface is created for C3IA tool using FLASK web Server Technology in python to host the web based C3IA tool in public domain as shown in Figure 5, Figure 6 and Figure 7, where any user can upload and view any Chest X-Ray file from their smartphone for COVID analysis.

Figure 4. C3IA access on main institute's webpage

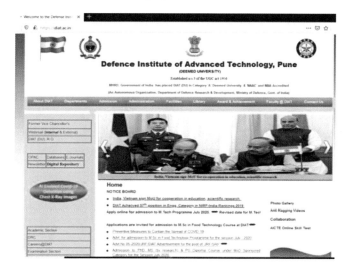

Figure 5. C3IA main user interface

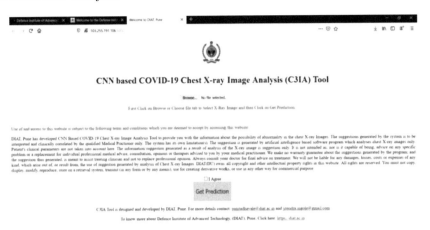

Figure 6. C3IA user interface to select image

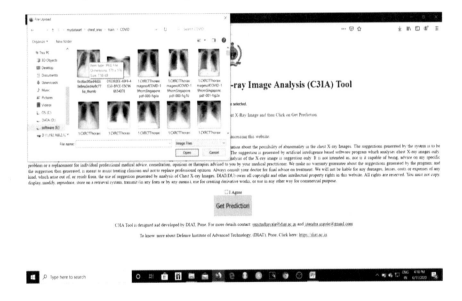

Once they agree to our disclaimer section, they can click on prediction tab. Finally prediction results will be displayed as shown in Figure 8. The output text is displayed in user-friendly as well as clinically verified format. A feedback for was also given so that we can improve the usability of C3IA product to solve the problem. GUI tool interpreted and clinically correlated by the qualified Medical Practitioners only.

C3IA tool received good feedback from many users, various research organizations and doctors.

Figure 7. C3IA user interface after selecting image: view image selected

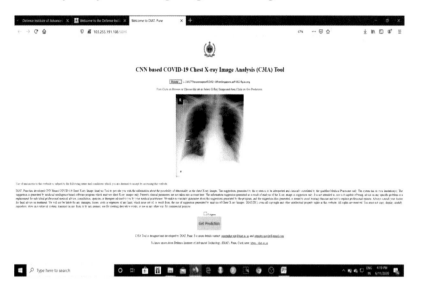

Figure 8. C3IA user interface: display screening output

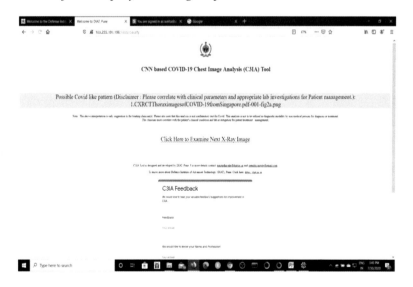

CONCLUSION

This chapter provides insights on how AI driven solutions with Design Thinking Approach are important in today's era. In this study, a novel real-time user-friendly C3IA (CNN based COVID-19 Chest Image Analysis) tool for automatic COVID-19 patient screening with multi-class classification (*COVID/Normal/Pneumonia*) is proposed and presented as a case study of human centric AI driven solution following design thinking approach. We implemented two-stream CNN architecture with two pre-trained VGG-16 net models that incorporate segmented and un-segmented image features. The model achieved 95% accuracy for three-class classification with 94% precision and recall for COVID-19 cases. C3IA

Model is capable of extracting important, relevant features from the chest x-rays images of the COVID 19 patients as well as normal patients. C3IA Model is tested against the COVID infected patient dataset for the performance assessment and is found to have a good accuracy along with good sensitivity and specificity. The COVID infection for these patients is verified by the accepted standard RT-PCR test and results generated by this tool are consistent with the same. C3IA provides user-friendly, real-time, cost-effective, rapid mass COVID patient screening solution as design thinking approaches are followed in all stages. This will not only support remote diagnosis (telemedicine) in case of shortage of domain experts in remote villages. During 2020, C3IA was made freely accessible for all Indian citizens on DIAT Website (https://www.diat.ac.in) supporting noble humanitarian response in current global pandemic situation. However, while designing product, we have not taken into account other clinical parameters of patients. Hence, the information displayed as a result of the X-ray image analysis can be used as a screening test only. In future work, C3IA tool will be enhanced to quantify the disease severity by collecting more of these images from local radiologists and hospitals.

REFERENCES

Ala-Kitula, A., Talvitie-Lamberg, T., Tyrväinen, P., & Silvennoinen, M. (2017). Developing Solutions for Healthcare-Deploying Artificial Intelligence to an Evolving Target. *International Conference on Computational Science and Computational Intelligence (CSCI)*, 1637-1642. 10.1109/CSCI.2017.285

Amanda, J. W. (2019). Design Thinking for a User-Centered Approach to Artificial Intelligence. *She Ji: The Journal of Design, Economics, and Innovation, 5*(4), 394-396. doi:10.1016/j.sheji.2019.11.015

Apostolopoulos, I. D., & Mpesiana, T. A. (2020). *Covid-19: automatic detection from x-ray images utilizing transfer learning with convolutional neural networks.* Physical and Engineering Sciences in Medicine.

Chakraborty, M., Dhavale, S. V., & Ingole, J. (2020). Corona-nidaan: Lightweight deep convolutional neural network for chest x-ray based covid-19 infection detection. *Applied Intelligence.* Advance online publication. doi:10.100710489-020-01978-9 PMID:34764582

Dorota, O. (2021). *Applying Design Thinking to Artificial Intelligence. Why should you use it in your AI-based projects?* https://nexocode.com/blog/posts/applying-design-thinking-to-ai/

Feng, S., Liming, X., Fei, S., Dijia, W., Ying, W., Huan, Y., Huiting, J., Yaozong, G., He, S., & Dinggang, S. (2021). Large-scale screening of covid-19 from community acquired pneumonia using infection size-aware classification. *Physics in Medicine and Biology.* arXiv2003.09860v1

Hemdan, E., Shouman, M. A., & Karar, M. (2020). *Covidx-net: A framework of deep learning classifiers to diagnose covid-19 in x-ray images.* arXiv preprint arXiv:200311055

Jaeger, S., Candemir, S., Antani, S. K., Wang, L. P., & Thoma, G. R. (2014, December 4). Two public chest X-ray datasets for computer-aided screening of pulmonary diseases. *Quantitative Imaging in Medicine and Surgery,* (6), 475–477. doi:10.3978/j.issn.2223-4292.2014.11.20 PMID:25525580

Joana, C. (2021). *The design process of human-centered AI—part 1.* https://bootcamp.uxdesign.cc/human-centered-ai-design-process-part-1-8cf7e3ce00

Joana, C. (2021). *The design process of human-centered AI—part 2.* https://bootcamp.uxdesign.cc/human-centered-ai-design-process-part-2-empathize-hypothesis-6065db967716

Khan, M., Mehran, M. T., Haq, Z. U., Ullah, Z., Naqvi, S. R., Ihsan, M., & Abbass, H. (2021, December). Applications of artificial intelligence in COVID-19 pandemic: A comprehensive review. *Expert Systems with Applications, 185*, 115695. Advance online publication. doi:10.1016/j.eswa.2021.115695 PMID:34400854

MD.ai. (2021). *MD.ai annotator project.* https://public.md.ai/annotator/project/aGq4k6NW

MD.ai. (2021). *Python client library.* https://github.com/mdai/mdai-client-py

Ophir, G., Maayan, F., Hayit, G., Patrick, D. B., Huangqi, Z., Wenbin, J., Adam, B., & Eliot, S. (2020). *Rapid AI development cycle for the coronavirus (COVID-19) pandemic: Initial results for automated detection & patient monitoring using deep learning CT image analysis.* arXiv preprint arXiv:2003.05037

Robert, S., & Tracey, K. (2020). Design Thinking in Software and AI Projects. doi:10.1007/978-1-4842-6153-8

Tulin, O., Muhammed, T., Eylul, A. Y., Ulas, B. B., Ozal, Y., & Acharya, R. (2020). *Automated detection of COVID-19 cases using deep neural networks with X-ray images.* Computers in Biology and Medicine Journal.

Wang, L., & Wong, A. (2020). *Covid-net: A tailored deep convolutional neural network design for detection of covid-19 cases from chest radiography images.* arXiv preprint arXiv:200309871

Yicheng, F., Huangqi, Z., Jicheng, X., Minjie, L., Lingjun, Y., Peipei, P., & Wenbin, J. (2020). Sensitivity of chest CT for COVID-19: Comparison to RT-PCR. *Radiology*, 200–432. PMID:32073353

Chapter 9
Risk–Based Authentication:
A Survey

Vivin Krishnan
CHRIST University (Deemed), India

Sreeja Cherillath Sukumaran
https://orcid.org/0000-0002-6351-2826
CHRIST University (Deemed), India

ABSTRACT

The rapid internet adoption has heralded the era of connected devices and services. Applications and systems are now internet-centric. The bulk of transactions, communications, and even healthcare data are transmitted online. Internet of things (IoT) are being used extensively across domains. With the increasing digital and online traffic, the risk window grows as well. Evolving threat vectors have prompted the need for multi-factor authentication (MFA) systems that utilize multiple modalities to strengthen security. With enterprises opting for bring-your-own-device (BYOD), static MFA proves insufficient. This brought about risk-based authentication (RBA) that follows an adaptive and continuous authentication strategy. With contextual attributes of the user factored in, RBA is more robust and can withstand multiple attacks. NIST, US and NCSC, UK have recommended RBA. This chapter covers authentication methodologies and their evolution. The need for risk-based authentication, with an analysis of current RBA methodologies, their future outlook, and challenges are covered.

INTRODUCTION

Authentication is the process of validating and verifying a user's identity. Authentication is essential to ensure that personal and confidential information is protected and is not open to access by unauthorized entities. With online transactions growing exponentially with the availability of high-speed internet connections, the attack vectors have also grown sophisticated. The rapid adoption of Internet-of-Things (IoT) has accelerated the volume of data being generated and with it, the risk of exposure of this data.

DOI: 10.4018/978-1-6684-4580-8.ch009

Authentication mechanisms are categorized into three types (Gunson et al., 2011):

1.   What You know (Knowledge Factor)

A Knowledge Factor authentication mechanism relies on what the user knows. This knowledge is applied to authenticate with the system. A knowledge-based authentication can utilize a password, a Personal Identification Number (PIN), a pattern drawn on a mobile phone or an answer to a question.

2.   What You Are (Inherence Factor)

Biometric authentication relies on identifying the user based on biometric data captured as the user attempts login. Biometric traits of a user such as a fingerprint, retinal scan, facial traits, etc., are used to identify the user and provide access uniquely. Fingerprint and facial recognition are widely used forms of biometric authentication. Gait pattern detection using sensors is also being adopted as a biometric authentication scheme. This scheme gathers the gait pattern using various sensors and video and uses it to identify unique traits that can then be used to identify the user.

3.   What You Have (Possession Factor)

Possession Factor authentication schemes depend on something the user possesses. This can be a physical object like a smart card or digital entities such as digital certificates or One Time Passwords (OTP). Grid based authentication is a form of possession factor authentication.

This paper covers the existing types of authentications and its evolution. It covers the existing authentication modalities and approaches proposed by various authors. The paper also covers the scenarios that prompted the need for Multi-Factor Authentication and Risk-based Authentication and presents the available works on them. Further, the future of Risk-based authentication in the perspective of Privacy protection legal frameworks is covered.

The sections of this paper are organized as follows. Section 2 covers Knowledge-Factor based authentication. Inheritance-factor based authentication is covered in Section 3. Section 4 covers Possession-factor based authentication. The need for multi-factor authentication and works featuring MFA are covered in Section 5. Section 6 features the significance of Risk-based authentication and evaluation of works covering RBA. The challenges and future ahead of Risk-based authentication in the era of Legal frameworks on protecting end users' privacy is discussed in Section 7.

KNOWLEDGE-FACTOR BASED AUTHENTICATION

Knowledge-factor authentication is the most widely used and most common form of authentication. The most used knowledge factor authentication types are:

1.   Credentials-based validation (Password-based authentication)

a. This authentication type is based on "something you know" or knowledge-factor. This is a widely used authentication scheme and is easy to implement. The user is asked to provide a specific piece of information they know. Users tend to use dictionary words or weak passwords that are easy to remember. It is also typical of users to use the same password across multiple accounts and services (Das et al., 2014). Brute force or dictionary attacks have shown high success rates against weak passwords. Password database leaks are also a major cause of concern (Wiefling et al., 2019) (Thomas et al., 2019).

2. Security Questions based authentication

a. An authentication scheme where the user is expected to provide answers to predefined questions. The questions may be static and system-generated or set by the user.

4. PIN or Patterns

a. With the wide availability of touch screens, mobile phone PINs or patterns that users draw on the mobile screen have become popular as authentication mechanisms.

5. Image-based authentication

a. This authentication scheme involves the end-user choosing an image from a set of images as the authentication key. Upon trying to authenticate, the user is presented with a set of images from which the user chooses the correct image.

Knowledge factor authentication schemes are the simplest to implement. As a result, many works have been developed on Knowledge-factor authentication:

Authors (Gupta et al., 2012) developed a system and application that uses behavioral data obtained from a user's mobile device to create a fingerprint. Attributes such as user's call and messaging details, application usage patterns etc., gathered over time were used to create a digital fingerprint. The users are then asked authentication questions based on the contextual data gathered. While this scheme was among the first to adopt the technique, the approach has the drawback that the invasive data gathering required to obtain the behavioral context may not be agreeable to all users. Also, continuous data collection has a performance cost.

In (Pan &Bangay, 2014), the authors propose using Propp Theory of Narrative to generate security questions. The security questions will serve the purpose of extra authentication in case of account or credentials recovery. In this approach, security questions can be generated without depending on the user's personal information. This prevents this scheme from social engineering attacks. The story is generated when the user registers. The user is supposed to memorize the story, and this becomes a shared secret between the client and the server. When the need for security questions arises, the server frames questions from the generated story. The proposal is further enhanced and implemented by (Anvari et al., 2017).

In (Thorpe et al., 2013), the authors propose an authentication approach where the user chooses a location on the map as their password. The user does not key in string passwords. During registration, they choose a location on the map and are asked to select the location during subsequent logins. If the location is selected correctly on a map within a specified error tolerance factor, the user is authenticated successfully and logs in to the system. The study conducted by the authors showed that the users were able to memorize the location and use it if the logins were within a short span of a few days. However, this system has the chance of the user forgetting the exact location if the logins are not very frequent. Also, the users may not remember the location-password, beyond a few days.

(Shone et al., 2015) proposed an authentication system that uses digital memories of a user to authenticate. In this scheme, the authentication service is configured with a set of users' digital memories in various media forms. The user chooses which digital memories should be stored and used to generate authentication queries. When the user requests for a specific resource, the resource provider contacts the authentication service which then presents the user with a digital memory in any media format and asks the user questions related to the memory. The media on which questions are created is presented to the user without associated metadata. If the user answers correctly, authentication succeeds, and the user is granted access to the resource. This scheme, however, has the drawback that, with the increased online and social media presence of users, an attacker may be able to obtain details that constitute the user's digital memory data set. While the set of security questions that can be generated from a sizable collection of digital memories is large, this system may also have a longer time to authenticate as the user may need to recall data.

(Al-Ameen et al., 2015) showcases an authentication system that helps users with memorable passwords. The system is based on providing the user with cues of their choice. While the system has a higher-order login time, the authors find that the users can recall their passwords with 100% accuracy.

(Hang et al.,2015) proposed the use of location and security questions as the approach for fallback authentication. In this proposal, the system asks security questions derived from the user's personal information but tag the location aspect. The user is expected to answer the question by choosing the location on a map where the event related to the security question happened. If the user can point the location within an accuracy window, the system considers it a successful candidate for login. With this scheme, the authors associate a spatial and temporal context to an event from the user's personal experience. As such, the authors argue the scheme has better resiliency against social engineering attacks. However, the scheme has a high turnaround time as the user is expected to find a precise location on a map.

Authors (Agadakos et al., 2016) propose a system where location is also considered an aspect of authentication. That is, in addition to the user credentials, the user's location is also factored into the authentication flow. Location as a context is considered before granting login or access rights. This prevents cases where an attacker is trying to spoof the way into the system by masquerading as the user. In (Liu et al., 2017), the authors propose a credential-based authentication scheme that uses multiple passwords and a temporal session key. The proposed authentication scheme was tailored to Wireless Sensor networks. The users register multiple passwords during registration. Thereafter, during login, the user uses a combination of a smart card and multiple passwords to authenticate. The scheme also supports mutual authentication. However, the user is required to remember a multitude of passwords and enter them in the right sequence to log in successfully.

(Takada & Hattori, 2020) proposes a novel approach that promotes the use of secure credentials using an incentive system. They achieve this by linking a role-playing game associated with and present in the pattern lock screen of a mobile phone. When the user chooses a strong authentication pattern during registration, the game provides a powerful weapon to the protagonist. The strength of the weapon is proportional to the strength of the credential chosen. When the user logs in with the pattern, fewer attacks are required to win, depending on the strength of the credentials. The authors believe that the incentive in the form of a linked game will encourage the end-users to set stronger credentials.

Image-based or graphical passwords have also been explored in detail in various works. As graphical passwords are easier to recall than memorizing passwords, this authentication scheme provides a better user experience. Some works exploring graphical passwords are shown in Table 1

Table 1. Works on graphical passwords-based authentication

Reference	Approach
(Kikuchi et al., 2002)	Study on the memorability of pictures for authentication.
(Li et al., 2005)	Interactive, image-based authentication scheme.
(Chiasson, 2009)	User authentication using click-based graphical passwords.
(Almulhem, 2011)	Points of interests based graphical passwords system.
(Sun et al., 2012)	Map-based graphical password authentication.
(Umar & Rafiq, 2012)	Recognition-based image authentication system.
(Almuairfi et al., 2013)	Image-based authentication system where keywords are associated with images.
(Wu et al., 2013)	Shoulder-surfing proof graphical password-based authentication system.
(Gurav et al., 2014)	Image-based authentication with images forming characters of the password
(Gokhale & Waghmare, 2016)	Recognition and recall based shoulder-surfing proof Image-based authentication system.
(Shnain& Shaheed, 2019)	Image-based authentication using modified inkblot features with shapes dependent on textual inputs.

Password Less authentication is another paradigm that aims at improving user experience by not having the user memorize and use passwords. Instead, the user enters the unique user name or identifier such as email, and the authentication service sends them an OTP or the user enters a token obtained from a token generator (hardware or software). Password-less authentication offers a higher security level by forgoing the need to remember passwords, which are susceptible to compromise. This approach is also convenient to end-users as it removes the requirement to remember passwords.

In (Shi et al., 2011), authors proposed a system that performs implicit and password-less authentication by capturing a wide array of attributes from the device the user tries to log in from and analyses those via Machine Learning to determine if the user should be allowed access or not. The attributes collected vary from location, user's behavioral patterns on the device - call logs, calendar entries, the pattern of request locations, battery drain analysis and the applications installed on the devices. If the variances are within range, the system allows implicit authentication and rejects if the variance is high.

While Knowledge-Factor authentication is the simplest of the schemes, it is also the weakest . Users tend to use simple passwords that can be broken by brute-force attacks or eavesdropping. Users may also tend to forget the passwords if not used frequently.

INHERENCE-FACTOR AUTHENTICATION

With the wide availability of smartphones equipped with fingerprint sensors and/or facial recognition technology, biometric authentication has become popular. It offers the end-users convenience in that they do not have to memorize passwords. Biometric authentication via fingerprint is quick and convenient. Application vendors have furthered the usage by incorporating biometric authentication (mostly fingerprint) within the application - for login or even as a second-factor authentication.

Authors in (Ali Fahmi et al., 2012) have proposed using ear shape biometrics as a means to identify and authenticate the user uniquely. The authors achieve this by having the front camera of the mobile device capture images without user interaction and use it for implicit authentication. (Gragnaniello et al., 2013) and (Xia et al., 2020) have proposed approaches to detect the liveliness of fingerprint scans so that attackers cannot copy the fingerprints and use them imprinted on silicon or gelatin. Similarly, authors (Henry Zhong et al., 2017) have demonstrated the use of vein patterns captured during fingerprint sensing to identify the user uniquely. While fingerprints may be lifted off surfaces, the attackers cannot copy the vein patterns present under the skin.

A touch and motion sensor-based authentication mechanism is described in (Bo et al., 2013) and (Bo et al., 2014). (Xie, 2014), describes a facial recognition approach where facial muscle movement is factored in to identify an individual uniquely. Facial muscle movement, which is unique to an individual coupled with depth-sensing, is used to prevent attackers from using a replica or video in a login attempt. User authentication based on tapping pattern is an approach proposed in (Zheng et al., 2014). The authors show that every person has a unique tapping behavior, and this can be used to differentiate between the actual owner and an imposter, non-intrusively. A similar authentication mechanism that factors in a user's tapping pattern or sliding pattern representing a song or melody is discussed in (Chen et al., 2015).

A novel biometric scheme for authentication based on chirography is mentioned in (Aronowitz et al., 2014). The approach involves the user writing on a digital screen with their fingers. Subsequently, two more biometric modalities - face and voice are fused with chirography to generate a multimodal biometrics scheme for authentication. (Khan & Hengartner, 2014) proposes an application-centric implicit authentication scheme for mobile phones. The proposal is based on the authors' finding that existing device-centric implicit authentication approaches treat data as a whole and not specific to the user application. The proposal delegates the decision of when to authenticate and how to, to the application. The logic to achieve the proposed model is left to the application provider, giving them the flexibility of implementation. The model intends to offer task-aware authentication. The authors used touch-screen input as the attribute for validation.

(Feng et al., 2015) describes a system that uses multiple modalities from various sensors to determine if the device has been transferred from person to person. The design intends to detect if there has been an identity change by utilizing attributes gathered from touch, audio, and motion sensors. The aggregate of the data collected is used to determine the change of hands. As seen in (Sankaran et al., 2015), there has also been work on taking fingerprint photos on smartphone cameras, extracting fingerprint features by photo enhancement and using it for authentication.

A biometric authentication scheme that combines arm gestures and shape of the user's ear capture via the front camera is specified in (Abate et al., 2016). The ear's unique shape combined with the arm gesture while answering a call provides a unique biometric signature. A similar implicit user authentication employing the user's hand movement pattern has been proposed by (Eremin & Kogos, 2018). The approach aims at implicit authentication merely by identifying the hand movement pattern. The intent is to determine if the device owner is using the phone or not. (Junshuang Yang et al., 2015) covers a similar approach using user motion patterns to authenticate smart devices. A similar approach to authenticate smart wearable devices based on head movements is covered in (Li et al., 2016). Arriving at human identity is detailed in (Neverova et al., 2016) based on data collected from 1500 volunteers over many months. Human kinematics is the basis of the biometric context in this work.

A novel acoustics-based biometric authentication has been proposed by (Chauhan et al., 2017). The technique analyses the breathing patterns of the user when the device is held close to the nose. This approach demonstrated 94% accuracy in tests. Behavioral biometrics gathered via multiple modalities is the basis of the authentication system proposed in (Fridman et al., 2017). The authors consider the text entered, websites visited, applications used, and location gathered via Wi-Fi or GPS to create the user's behavioral profile. The system demonstrates a low Equal Error Rate (ERR) in tests across various subjects. The human body's response to an electric pulse has been used as a biometric signature is proposed in (Martinovic et al., 2017). The system works by applying a small pulse in one palm and measuring the response at the other. The work is based on how each human body has a different reaction to an electrical pulse. The setup, however, needs dedicated gadgets to generate the pulse and obtain a response. Research has been done on more advanced forms of biometrics utilizing Electroencephalography (EEG) for authentication. (Zhang et al., 2018) presents an approach using EEG brainwaves and Neural networks to arrive at a unique biometric signature. While the approach offers uniqueness and accuracy, EEG capturing equipment will be required to obtain the brain waves.

Unlike password-based authentication schemes where the credentials can be reset or changed, biometric traits of an individual cannot be modified. As such, once compromised, an attacker can use duplicated biometric data of a user.

POSSESSION-FACTOR AUTHENTICATION

1. One-time Password (OTP)

a. OTP-based authentication mechanism involves sending an SMS or Push notification-based short-lived one-time password to the user—the user keys in the OTP, are validated by the security service. OTPs are typically used as an additional security layer, but they can also be the primary authentication mode. As the password is generated for that specific transaction (one-time) and is short-lived, OTP is resilient to sniffing attacks. However, if an attacker is in possession of the user's mobile device, this authentication mechanism is compromised.

b. Time-based OTP(TOTP) requires the end user to enter a generated token to be entered to login to the system. The token is generated on-demand and is valid for a short period. Token generation can be performed using hardware in the form of dedicated token generation devices or Authenticator applications installed on mobile devices. TOTP is widely used in two-factor authentication scenarios. The authentication server creates a secret key to the end-user during the configuration phase, who adds it to the Authenticator application. This secret key is typically passed on in the form of Quick Response (QR) codes.

2. Smart Card authentication

a. Smart card authentication uses dedicated hardware that generates strong cryptographic keys. The key generation is usually affected using dedicated hardware chips that are embedded on the smart cards. This helps the users by not requiring them to remember lengthy passwords. Smart cards may need the users to memorize a PIN to use or activate the smart card. As it utilizes dedicated hard chips to generate authentication keys, it is very efficient and can generate strong cryptographic keys. Smart card-based authentication requires dedicated hardware readers. Smart cards may also be lost, misplaced, or stolen and without an authenticating PIN on the smart card, may be targeted by an attacker.

3.   Digital certificate-based authentication

a. Digital certificate-based authentication uses Digital Certificates that identify a specific user or system. Digital certificate-based authentication is typically used in conjunction with another authentication mechanism - such as credentials-based authentication.

b. Digital certificates are generally created with long expiry - ranging from months to years. As such, once configured, it does not need to be changed/re-configured until expiry. This makes it a user-friendly solution.

c. Digital certificate-based authentication is widely used in machine/device authentication. For example, a mobile device or computer may use a digital certificate to authenticate and login into a secure wireless network. In addition, digital certificates are used to authenticate into VPNs or secure gateways in many enterprises.

4.   Grid-based authentication

a. Grid-based authentication involves the authentication service providing the user with a specific Grid that is unique to the user. The Grid has an appearance of an nXn matrix with numbers as each element. During authentication, the user is challenged to enter numbers from random positions. If the grid is relatively large, random positions can be asked without the possibility of an attacker guessing the response. Grids can be conveyed to the user securely during the registration phase. However, if the Grid is compromised, this opens the system to the attacker.

Various works on possession-factor authentication are covered in Table 2:

Table 2. Works on possession-factor based authentication

Reference	Approach
(Syta et al., 2010)	RFID-based authentication with on-demand encryption of files.
(Rahnama et al., 2010)	RFID-based authentication with key changing during every login.
(Song, 2010)	Smart card-based authentication scheme with mutual authentication support.
(Wang & Ma, 2012)	Smart card-based multi-server authentication scheme.
(Li et al., 2013)	Smart card-based remote user password authentication scheme.
(Jiang et al., 2013)	Smart card-based authentication scheme with protection from password guessing attacks.
(Farash, 2014)	Smart card-based authentication for Session Initiation Protocol(SIP).
(Amin et al., 2015)	Anonymity preserving, smart card-based authentication scheme for Telecare Medical System.
(Kumari et al., 2015)	Smart card-based authentication scheme for SIP developed as an improvement over (Farash, 2014).
(Wang et al., 2017)	Smart card-based lightweight authentication scheme with forward secrecy.
(Gope et al., 2018)	Privacy preserving RFID-based authentication for IoT.

While Possession-factor schemes are convenient and have better usability by virtue of the user not having to remember passwords, they are susceptible to loss, physical damage or tampering of the entities.

MULTI-FACTOR AUTHENTICATION

Single-factor authentication schemes are popular on account of their usability and ease of implementation. Credentials-based authentication schemes such as password of PIN are popular, but also happen to be among the weakest (Dasgupta et al., 2016) (Bonneau et al., 2015). There is also the possibility of the user forgetting the passwords. Moreover, as there is a single authentication modality, this is susceptible to various attacks, including shoulder-surfing.

Multi-factor authentication (MFA) utilizes two or more authentication modalities (Abhishek et al., 2013). The combination involves using different authentication schemes that take different channels. Typically, the combination consists of authentication types covering knowledge, inherence, and possession factors. With multiple modalities, it becomes difficult for an attacker to compromise and break all the authentication modalities (Petsas et al., 2015).

Multitude of MFA schemes have been proposed over the years:

(Eldefrawy et al., 2011) proposed a 2FA using passwords and OTP. In their work, the OTP is generated with an initial seed and different nested hash chains. (Ribeiro de Mello et al., 2020) describes an MFA system for Shibboleth Identity providers that provides Time-based OTP, FIDO2 and phone prompt modes of authentication. The authors have developed a solution that is extensible and can be integrated with existing IdPs. (Choi et al., 2017) proposes an MFA algorithm that uses biometric and smart card authentication in addition to the username-password combination. The authors use a bio-hash function to hash the biometric data to obtain a level of error tolerance in case the biometric data is slightly different.

(Dasgupta et al., 2016) proposes a framework for the dynamic selection of authentication schemes by calculating the trustworthiness, performance, and other factors. With the mathematical approach adopted, the framework can prevent repetition in selecting authentication schemes and ensure randomness while still choosing the most optimum authentication factor. A two-factor authentication mechanism that utilizes the user's touch for both knowledge and inherence factors is described (Sun et al., 2014). In this scheme, the user can enter an arbitrary curve anywhere within the screen. The system validates both the curve drawn (knowledge-factor) and the biometrics from the gesture such as pressure applied and geometry of the finger (inherence-factor) to identify the user. This scheme can be helpful for the visually challenged, as the curve can be drawn anywhere on-screen.

(Abdurrahman et al., 2013) proposed an MFA scheme that utilizes a pre-shared number, GPS location and timestamp to generate the OTP for the second authentication factor. A Physical Unclonable Functions (PUF) and voiceprint-based transparent 2FA (T2FA) is proposed in (Zhang et al., 2018). In the first phase, the scheme uses credentials. In the second factor, a PUF based challenge needs to be answered by the user's mobile phone, and thereafter, the ambient noise is captured by both the user's browser and the mobile device. Finally, the second factor passes only if the PUF challenge is answered and both browser and mobile device audio recordings match.

A 2FA based on passwords and the user's behavioral profile is demonstrated by (Acar et al., 2019). The behavioral profile is constructed based on the user's network and host features. As the data gathered for the profile is sensitive, fuzzy hashing and fully homomorphic encryption is used to prevent attackers from gaining the data. Two-factor authentication schemes that utilise sound sensing and ambient sounds are covered in (Zhu et al., 2016) (Zhou et al., 2018)(Choi et al., 2018)(Ren et al., 2021). The proximity of the user device to the system to which he intends to log in is sensed by the ambient sound sensors and used as the second factor in authentication. Password and smart card-based 2FA has been proposed by (Sharma & Kalra, 2018). A password and Elliptic Curve Cryptography with smart card-based 2FA is proposed in (Karthigaiveni&Indrani, 2019). The scheme has been proposed for the IoT-based healthcare domain.

Work done by (Ali & Pal, 2017) showcases a 3FA system that utilizes credentials, biometric and smart card authentication. Similarly, (Liu et al., 2020) and (Taher et al., 2021) present a 3FA authentication scheme for IoT that utilizes password, biometrics and smart devices and performs mutual authentication.

(Shah &Kanhere, 2018) proposes a 2FA system that uses password for the first factor and Wi-Fi channel states for the second factor. In this scheme, the user must place a pre-registered device in close proximity to the primary device. Both devices are expected to record very similar Wi-Fi Channel state information on account of their proximity. If the information matches, the second-factor authentication passes. This scheme requires the user to pre-register a Wi-Fi-enabled second device and always have it along when performing authentication.

(Alsulaiman& El Saddik, 2008) proposed a novel multi-factor authentication based on a virtual three-dimensional (3D) world. The user needs to interact with various 3D objects in the virtual environment. Authentication is performed based on the user's interaction with the objects and the sequence of interactions. Multiple authentication modalities can be incorporated into the scheme.

Multi-Factor Authentication Challenges

(Ometov et al., 2018) analyses the challenges faced by Multi-factor authentication. They note that the operational challenges are mainly usability and integration, followed by security, privacy, robustness, and probabilistic behavior.(Katsini et al., 2016) notes that usability challenges of MFA can be categorized into three:

i)   Task efficiency (e.g., time to register and time to login),
ii)   Task effectiveness (e.g., number of attempts to login) and
iii) User preference (e.g., whether the user prefers a particular authentication scheme over another)

The choice of the authentication modalities should be kept in mind to balance security and usability. For example, if an authentication scheme is found to be hard to use, end users might avoid the MFA approach entirely.

While MFA offers added security over single-factor authentication, it does come with a cost. The choice of modalities is critical in terms of usability and security. Enterprises also have to invest in their infrastructure to provide seamless integration and support for the various authentication schemes (Henricks &Kettani, 2019).

RISK-BASED AUTHENTICATION

MFA improves the security of a system by including multiple authentication modalities, making it difficult for an attacker to break into all the authentication schemes. However, MFA performs a static and sequential authentication of the user. For example, the system may be designed first to challenge the user with a username-password combination and thereupon ask for biometrics. If both the authentication events pass, the system continues through with implicit trust. An attacker may have managed to break the multiple authentication schemes that are applied in sequence. While the authentication challenges may have been answered in a typical MFA system, the system does not factor in other contextual attributes.

Risk-Based Authentication (RBA) is the approach of adaptive authentication, applying varying authentication challenges to an attempt at authentication and resource access. The different authentication challenges are chosen to be commensurate with the level of the access request. The higher the risk from unauthorized access, the stronger and rigorous authentication methods are chosen to challenge the user.

Consider a scenario where a user has requested a resource. He has answered the challenges, but there are contextual attributes that vary from their baseline behavior. For instance, the access appears to have originated in another continent. The time elapsed since the last successful login and the latest does not match the typical geo-velocity a normal user goes through. The user normally accesses the system from a specific mobile device, but currently, the request bears a different device signature. In a typical MFA system, the contextual attributes are not factored into the process of authentication and authorization.

Risk-based authentication involves capturing a plurality of user and auxiliary attributes that include Geo-location, time of login, attempts required to login etc. From these attributes, the system generates a risk score or risk profile for the user request. The risk score represents the level of risk to the system, associated with the user logging and accessing resources. Authentication challenges are chosen corresponding to the risk score. The authentication service typically invokes multi-factor authentication, with the strength of the authentication schemes in-line with the risk factor. The relevance of Risk-based authentication increases as enterprises switch to Bring-Your-Own-Device (BYOD). The rapid expansion of multi-domain Internet-of-Things has also led credence to the adoption of RBA.Risk-based authentication has been recommended by the National Institute of Standards and Technology (NIST, USA) in their Digital Identity Guidelines (Grassi, Fenton, Newton, et al., 2017) and the National Cyber Security Centre (NCSC, UK) (Centre, N. C. S. (2019, April 15) (Wiefling et al., 2021).

Adaptive Authentication

The process of choosing appropriate authentication challenges based on the risk score and profile of the requesting user is called Adaptive Authentication. Adaptive authentication uses contextual information gathered from the user and associated attributes and policies to determine the authentication challenge dynamically.

Machine Learning is being employed widely to determine the risk score based on gathered contextual information and user's behavioral patterns. For example, when a request is made, the user's current contextual information is verified against the behavioral profile gathered over time. This allows calculation of a variance score - a measure of how much the user's current request behavior varies from past behavior - and use that as a basis to arrive at a risk score. The risk score is then used to choose one or more authentication challenges to ensure the authenticity of the user. As the user answers the various authentication challenges, the risk score decreases, and the risk profile is adjusted accordingly.

Evaluation of Risk-Based Authentication Schemes

(Lenzini et al., 2008) presents a system to enhance the trust in location-based adaptive authentication. Information gleaned from various location detectors is used to create a composite trust value, using subjective logic. The proposal depends on the infrastructure to obtain contextual information. A risk-based authentication system that uses Bayesian network models is presented by (Lai et al., 2011). The work proposes using modalities including mouse and keystroke dynamics and user actions to create an identity context to enable risk-based authentication. The system uses a trained Bayesian network model to calculate and arrive at risk scores. (Rocha et al., 2011) presents an adaptive authentication system based on the Spatio-temporal context of the user. Variations and anomalies in authentication are tracked based on the location and time of events. (Traore et al., 2012) (Traore et al., 2013) propose a Risk-based authentication approach that combines mouse dynamics and keystroke dynamics to build a behavioral pattern for the user. Over the study, the authors note that the modalities taken individually give low performance using the Bayesian Network Model. When combined, the performance increases significantly. The study is based on the premise that the other attributes such as IP address, location and historical data may be spoofed or subject to fraud.A risk-based adaptive security for IoT that utilizes Game theory and context-awareness is discussed in (Abie & Balasingham, 2012).

In (Riva et al., 2012), the authors focus on the approach - when to choose which authentication modality for which applications, rather than a new technique. The authors propose that any adaptive authentication system should progressively authenticate based on contextual attributes gathered. It should provide a better user experience by combining multiple modalities such as biometrics, behavioral aspects, continuity of usage and possession. This approach depends on data collection from embedded sensors to determine the threshold and trigger explicit authentication. The authors suggest Machine Learning as the way forward, especially when dealing with contextual data streams gathered from device sensors. To preserve onboard resources, the system may choose to offload processing onto cloud-based services.

A context-aware and scalable authentication framework with a probabilistic selection of authentication modalities is described in (Hayashi et al., 2013). The framework considers passive factors such as location data and active factors that involve user interaction separately. The Bayesian probabilistic framework allows selecting active factors given passive factors. The use of passive factors also contributes to better usability. (Li et al., 2013) discusses a dynamic behavioral profiling-based active authentication methodology. In this approach, behavioral profiling is based on historical application usage. The framework is designed such that it does not reject a user request immediately upon a noted transgression. Instead, a series of consecutive aberrations will trigger the need for further authentication or rejection.

Adaptive authentication based on users' behavior forms the basis of the study in (Abu Bakar &Haron, 2014). The system developed by the authors is called the Unified Authentication Platform (UAP) that factors in contextual attributes such as the location of the login attempts, time of login, types of resource requested and the operating system and browser client attributes. The risk score is calculated based on the weightage assigned to various resources. A dynamic risk-based access control framework for Cloud computing is proposed in (Santos et al., 2014). The framework utilizes a risk engine, risk quantification service and risk policies to act on a request for resources. The framework builds on eXtensible Access Control Markup Language (XACML) architecture.A movement pattern-based RBA system is presented by (Xiong et al., 2014). The risk factor assessment is based on the variance in a user's movement patterns based on spatial entropy from the historical records. The model uses spatial data but does not store it, contributing to better user privacy. A critical analysis of the use of mobile device fingerprinting is presented by (Spooren et al., 2015). The authors analyzed the increasing use of device fingerprinting as a contextual attribute. They observed that mobile devices across brand and model can still generate fingerprints that match or similar. Furthermore, the authors observed that the mobile browser fingerprinting in different mobile devices gave duplicate values in many instances across various vendors. The attributes utilized by fingerprinting algorithms are found to be predictable if the used mobile operating system is known. The study, however, only analyses mobile browsers.A risk-aware, multimodal, cross-device, continuous authentication system is presented by (Hintze et al., 2015). The framework is extensible in that it allows using different biometric modalities for continuous authentication across various trusted devices. Contextual information can be gathered from the other devices a user possesses. Trust between devices is established first and risk assessment is done by fusing the confidence levels obtained from the contexts. A dynamic context fingerprinting for continuous authentication is presented in (Preuveneers&Joosen, 2015). The authors use Hoeffding trees to monitor user identity in minimal-interaction scenarios. The authors used a consent-driven system where every attribute gathered for context has user consent. Further, any sensitive data gathered is hashed to prevent its transmission or availability in plain text. This system operates both at the client-side and server-side gathering attributes for fingerprinting. Finally, the proposal adds extra parameters into the contextual data to resist replay attacks, ensure freshness, integrity etc.

(Ramakrishnan et al., 2015) presents a risk-aware implicit authentication framework that gathers contextual attributes - location, behavioral patterns etc., to lock devices in case of unauthorized access. The system is flexible to allow the lock-out policies based on the obtained contextual data or via manual policies set by the user. The implicit authentication provides usability. (Premarathne et al., 2015) have detailed their work on a location-dependent risk disclosure system that utilizes location as the primary contextual source. The work is aimed mainly at the e-healthcare domain. In their continuous authentication model, the system gathers the location change of the user to calculate the associated risk of data disclosure. Based on the risk from location variance, the user is required to reauthenticate. This system also considers the need for break-glass policies in case of emergencies. (Murmuria et al., 2015) showcases continuous monitoring using machine learning to analyze deviations from behavioral metrics based on power consumption, touch gestures and physical movement within the context of the application. This is based on the observation that behavioral changes are significant when the user switches from one application to another. The model also configures a threshold to account for anomalous behavior, beyond which the user is challenged for authentication. The authors were able to achieve good performance in their experiments.

(Liu et al., 2016) proposes an adaptive single sign-on system that offers a balance between security and ease of use. The system can prevent unauthorized access by using contextual attributes such as location, time, activity, and identity, processed by a machine learning model. (Hintze et al., 2016) describes a location-based risk assessment authentication system that uses location in conjunction with multi-modal biometrics to determine the risk and proportional authentication modalities. The location is tracked based on GSM and Wi-Fi data. The system also follows a Spatio-temporal association, where the user's location is considered at a specific time window. Authors (Misbahuddin et al., 2017) detail the design and work done on a risk-based authentication system that uses machine learning to arrive at the risk score. A contextual behavior profile of the user is constructed by gathering constituent attributes in every request. Once this corpus of data has exceeded a threshold, a machine learning-based risk engine is employed to calculate the risk score of the current request in comparison with the data available. The outcome of the risk engine is used to create the risk profile of the user request and based on that; alternate authentication schemes are triggered. The study employs three machine learning algorithms to compare the operational performance.

(Gebrie& Abie, 2017) proposes a risk-based adaptive authentication for the Internet of Things in the smart health domain. The system analyses variation in channel characteristics to determine risk factors and choose alternative authentication mechanisms. The user and device activities are continuously monitored to ensure variance is captured. The authors employed Naive Bayes Machine Learning algorithm to analyze the data for variations. As the system is specifically designed for IoT, it factors in the resource requirements of the authentication or re-authentication challenges. If the authentication challenge cannot be processed in-device, it is offloaded to an authentication server with more resources. (Atlam et al., 2017) proposes a risk-based access control model for IoT. Every request to IoT is analyzed for the risk posed and its severity, gathered from the context, to choose alternate authentication schemes. The resource's sensitivity, the action requested, and the user's risk history are factored in to arrive at risk score. In (Sepczuk&Kotulski, 2018), the authors study and propose a risk analysis procedure with a novel authentication management model. The contextual data covered attributes such as place, time, type of service and kind of device. The authors use Gaussian approximation of observation probability, to obtain fluctuation in the contextual data. The authors calculate the level of security offered by common authentication mechanisms ranging from PIN to passwords of varying length and biometric authentication. The study involved experiments considering three actors - a normal user, an experienced user, and a hacker. As a result, the authors can infer that the level of risk is commensurate with the contextual data.

(Wiefling et al., 2019) studies Risk-based Authentication approaches of eight internet services. As part of the analysis, the authors gather IP Address, User-Agent, Language, Display Resolution and Login time as the attributes required to build context. The intent was to study how the different service providers reacted to changes in the attributes. The analysis noted if the providers challenged the users with alternate authentication methods and the threshold. The inference from the tests showed that the subject service providers rated IP Addresses as a key marker. Authors (Ashibani& Mahmoud, 2019) developed a behavior-based authentication system that uses application usage patterns from end-user devices' application access logs to determine deviation from normal usage. Machine learning is used to analyze the usage pattern to fix a regular pattern that subsequent requests are validated against. The proposed approach uses application access events and hence small data sets, which achieves faster computation. If an abnormal request pattern is observed, the system challenges the user, reporting the variance to update the model.

(Gupta et al., 2019) covers the application of risk-based authentication schemes in ride-sharing applications. Their DriverAuth system uses multiple biometric modalities to verify the driver before starting a ride. The system, however, considers only Inherence-factor-based modalities to verify the user and in a sequential manner. An adaptive authentication system that utilizes behavioral patterns, device and browser, geolocation and network and risk-based authentication is detailed in (De Silva et al., 2019). Under behavioral data, the system uses keystroke and mouse dynamics and analyzes these using a recurrent neural network and Support Vector Machine (SVM), respectively. In addition, geo-location of the device and geo-velocity between logins are also factored in.

A study on utilizing users' IoT devices to enable continuous authentication is undertaken by (Gonzalez-Manzano et al., 2019). The authors posit that users' increasing reliance on IoT devices and each user being associated with multiple IoTs can be used to enable continuous authentication. (Solano et al., 2019) (Solano et al., 2020)'s work on combining behavioral biometrics and user's device context to identify a user's risk profile via machine learning has shown promising results. While the two contexts have lower accuracy in isolation, the combination has been shown to provide higher accuracy in detection. The device context is obtained using fingerprinting.

In further studies, (Wiefling et al., 2020) analyses the Risk-based Re-authentication methods. In this study, re-authentication based on email as the channel of communication. For re-authentication, the authors studied sending a code within the email body, as part of the subject and via a URL in the email body the user must click. The study also covered user perception and acceptance of the three modes.

As part of the analysis, the authors considered time to answer the challenge and time to complete the re-authentication process in total. In (Rivera et al., 2020), the authors develop a Risk-based authentication system that calculates risk profiles by analyzing the network latency of requests. Machine learning models analyze the latency of the request and decide if the user request originates via a VPN, a possible indicator of unauthorized access. For this, the system runs a script that executes in the end users' browsers when a resource is requested. The script pings an array of resource servers geographically apart. The round trip time from all the pings is gathered and analyzed by a Machine learning algorithm in the authentication server. This serves to build a network latency profile of the user. If an attacker attempts to spoof a normal user's location using VPN or TOR networks, the latency profile will differ. This prompts the system to challenge the user with another authentication challenge. This approach, however, cannot determine if a legitimate user's network latency profile showed variance because of network fluctuations or if the user was on a different data channel.

An implicit authentication scheme based on temporal access patterns is proposed in (Ashibani& Mahmoud, 2020). The authors' working premise on which the study was done is that device-based authentication does not necessarily guarantee strong authentication. This happens as end-users prefer knowledge-factor credentials that are simply easy to remember. In this work, risk-based authentication is based on application usage. Towards this, the applications on the device are categorized based on usage. Since the approach considers application usage patterns, the user intervention required is minimal. It can also adapt to newly introduced applications.

(Buriro et al., 2021) presents a risk-based continuous authentication system that utilizes behavioral biometrics. Towards this, the authors utilize touch timing differences and hand gesture patterns as biometric traits. The primary authentication mode is password-based but allows users to set and use any 8-digit alphanumeric passwords. The behavioral biometrics are gathered as the user enters the credentials. Thereafter, the system continues to monitor a variety of client attributes to check for variations from normal and established behavior. In case of variance beyond a threshold representing a high-risk score, the system terminates the session and prompts the user to re-authenticate.

CHALLENGES AND FUTURE OF RBA

Adaptive and Risk-based Authentication involves gathering and continuously analyzing a slew of information. From the onset, this is computationally more intensive than a regular single or multi-factor authentication. Traditional authentication schemes are generally applied statically and in the case of multi-factor authentication, in sequence. The process login is considered successful if the user can answer challenges successfully. In comparison, an adaptive and risk-aware authentication system obtains a multitude of contextual attributes, processing and classifying them to arrive at a risk score. The alternate authentication modalities need to be chosen and presented to the user without obstructing usability, aiming to minimize unnecessary challenges (Cabarcos et al., 2017). This aspect should be reflected in the choice of the authentication modalities as well. While RBA provides usability and security to end users, it comes at the cost of gathering attributes and data deemed private and confidential. The balance between privacy and security may be tilted towards security, depending on the domain of application. The data captured from the users could include their personal information, including call details, habitual patterns, connections etc.

An extensive array of contextual information needs to be obtained to enable RBA, which consists mostly of attributes deemed private and can be used to trace back to the user. IP Address is an attribute frequently gathered under RBA, which is treated as a private identifier. The risk score calculated as a derivative of the contextual attributes can be treated as an identifier (Wieflinget al., 2021). Regulatory frameworks regarding the data collected from the users and how it is used in place restrictions on RBA vendors and implementations. User consent is key, and the end user is also at will to refuse gratuitous access to data that is deemed private (General Data Protection Regulation (GDPR) – Official Legal Text, 2016) (California Consumer Privacy Act (CCPA), 2018) ISO/IEC 29100:2011. (2016, August 26). With the regulations in place, an RBA system should ensure that the data gathered is minimal and most relevant. The data controller is now also responsible for safekeeping the data collected. This includes data in transit and at rest. The data should be obfuscated or anonymized when with the data controller. The safety of the data from exposure and misuse should also be factored in while implementing RBA. At the same time, reducing the amount of data collected or the number of attributes may compromise the quality or accuracy of the Risk-based service. As such, RBA vendors should consider usability, security, and privacy while designing the system (Wiefling et al., 2020).

CONCLUSION

With rapid digitization and widespread internet adoption, users' private or confidential data needs to be protected more than ever. The risk of unauthorized access or exposure to sensitive information is high. Strong security measures and protocols are the need of the hour, with authentication schemes implemented at every level of access. Through this chapter, the evolution of security and authentication protocols have been covered. The shortcomings of each type of scheme that necessitated the need for newer and stronger authentication schemes were discussed. The current state of the art and the onward outlook along with the challenges that Risk-based authentication schemes face as it looks into the future has been covered.

REFERENCES

Abate, A. F., Nappi, M., & Ricciardi, S. (2016, October). Smartphone enabled person authentication based on ear biometrics and arm gesture. *2016 IEEE International Conference on Systems, Man, and Cybernetics (SMC)*. 10.1109/SMC.2016.7844812

Abdurrahman, U. A., Kaiiali, M., & Muhammad, J. (2013, November). A new mobile-based multi-factor authentication scheme using pre-shared number, GPS location and time stamp. *2013 International Conference on Electronics, Computer and Computation (ICECCO)*. 10.1109/ICECCO.2013.6718286

Abhishek, K., Roshan, S., Kumar, P., & Ranjan, R. (2013). A comprehensive study on multifactor authentication schemes. In *Advances in Computing and Information Technology* (pp. 561–568). Springer Berlin Heidelberg. doi:10.1007/978-3-642-31552-7_57

Abie, H., & Balasingham, I. (2012). Risk-Based Adaptive Security for Smart IoT in eHealth. *Proceedings of the 7th International Conference on Body Area Networks*. 10.4108/icst.bodynets.2012.250235

Abu Bakar, K. A., & Haron, G. R. (2014, August). Adaptive authentication based on analysis of user behavior. *2014 Science and Information Conference.* 10.1109/SAI.2014.6918248

Acar, A., Liu, W., Beyah, R., Akkaya, K., & Uluagac, A. S. (2019). A privacy-preserving multifactor authentication system. *Security and Privacy, 2*(6). Advance online publication. doi:10.1002py2.94

Agadakos, I., Hallgren, P., Damopoulos, D., Sabelfeld, A., & Portokalidis, G. (2016, December 5). Location-enhanced authentication using the IoT. *Proceedings of the 32nd Annual Conference on Computer Security Applications.* 10.1145/2991079.2991090

Al-Ameen, M. N., Wright, M., & Scielzo, S. (2015, April 18). Towards making random passwords memorable. *Proceedings of the 33rd Annual ACM Conference on Human Factors in Computing Systems.* http://dx.doi.org/10.1145/2702123.2702241

Ali, R., & Pal, A. K. (2017). An efficient three factor-based authentication scheme in multiserver environment using ECC. *International Journal of Communication Systems, 31*(4), e3484. doi:10.1002/dac.3484

Ali Fahmi, P. N., Kodirov, E., Choi, D.-J., & Lee, G.-S., MohdFikriAzli, A., & Sayeed, S. (2012, October). Implicit authentication based on ear shape biometrics using smartphone camera during a call. *2012 IEEE International Conference on Systems, Man, and Cybernetics (SMC).* 10.1109/ICSMC.2012.6378079

Almuairfi, S., Veeraraghavan, P., & Chilamkurti, N. (2013). A novel image-based implicit password authentication system (IPAS) for mobile and non-mobile devices. *Mathematical and Computer Modelling, 58*(1–2), 108–116. doi:10.1016/j.mcm.2012.07.005

Almulhem, A. (2011, February). A graphical password authentication system. *2011 World Congress on Internet Security (WorldCIS-2011).* 10.1109/WorldCIS17046.2011.5749855

Alsulaiman, F. A., & El Saddik, A. (2008). Three-Dimensional password for more secure authentication. *IEEE Transactions on Instrumentation and Measurement, 57*(9), 1929–1938. doi:10.1109/TIM.2008.919905

Amin, R., Islam, S. H., Biswas, G. P., Khan, M. K., & Kumar, N. (2015). An Efficient and Practical Smart Card Based Anonymity Preserving User Authentication Scheme for TMIS using Elliptic Curve Cryptography. *Journal of Medical Systems, 39*(11), 180. Advance online publication. doi:10.100710916-015-0351-y PMID:26433889

Aronowitz, H., Li, M., Toledo-Ronen, O., Harary, S., Geva, A., Ben-David, S., Rendel, A., Hoory, R., Ratha, N., Pankanti, S., & Nahamoo, D. (2014, September). Multi-modal biometrics for mobile authentication. *IEEE International Joint Conference on Biometrics.* 10.1109/BTAS.2014.6996269

Ashibani, Y., & Mahmoud, Q. H. (2019). A behavior-based proactive user authentication model utilizing mobile application usage patterns. In *Advances in Artificial Intelligence* (pp. 284–295). Springer International Publishing. doi:10.1007/978-3-030-18305-9_23

Ashibani, Y., & Mahmoud, Q. H. (2020, October 11). An intelligent risk-based authentication approach for smartphone applications. *2020 IEEE International Conference on Systems, Man, and Cybernetics (SMC).* 10.1109/SMC42975.2020.9283267

Atlam, H. F., Alenezi, A., Walters, R. J., Wills, G. B., & Daniel, J. (2017, June). Developing an adaptive risk-based access control model for the internet of things. *2017 IEEE International Conference on Internet of Things (IThings) and IEEE Green Computing and Communications (GreenCom) and IEEE Cyber, Physical and Social Computing (CPSCom) and IEEE Smart Data (SmartData).* http://dx.doi.org/10.1109/ithings-greencom-cpscom-smartdata.2017.103

Bo, C., Zhang, L., Jung, T., Han, J., Li, X.-Y., & Wang, Y. (2014, December). Continuous user identification via touch and movement behavioral biometrics. *2014 IEEE 33rd International Performance Computing and Communications Conference (IPCCC).* http://dx.doi.org/10.1109/pccc.2014.7017067

Bo, C., Zhang, L., Li, X.-Y., Huang, Q., & Wang, Y. (2013). SilentSense. *Proceedings of the 19th Annual International Conference on Mobile Computing & Networking - MobiCom '13.* http://dx.doi.org/10.1145/2500423.2504572

Bonneau, J., Herley, C., van Oorschot, P. C., & Stajano, F. (2015). Passwords and the evolution of imperfect authentication. *Communications of the ACM, 58*(7), 78–87. doi:10.1145/2699390

Buriro, A., Gupta, S., Yautsiukhin, A., & Crispo, B. (2021). Risk-Driven behavioral biometric-based one-shot-cum-continuous user authentication scheme. *Journal of Signal Processing Systems for Signal, Image, and Video Technology, 93*(9), 989–1006. doi:10.100711265-021-01654-2

Cabarcos, P. A., & Krupitzer, C. (2017). On the Design of Distributed Adaptive Authentication Systems. *Thirteenth Symposium on Usable Privacy and Security (SOUPS 2017).* https://www.usenix.org/conference/soups2017/workshop-program/way2017/arias-cabarcos

California Consumer Privacy Act (CCPA). (2018, October 15). State of California - Department of Justice - Office of the Attorney General. https://oag.ca.gov/privacy/ccpa

Centre, N. C. S. (2019, April 15). *Cloud security guidance.* National Cyber Security Centre. https://www.ncsc.gov.uk/collection/cloud-security/implementing-the-cloud-security-principles/identity-and-authentication

Chauhan, J., Hu, Y., Seneviratne, S., Misra, A., Seneviratne, A., & Lee, Y. (2017, June 16). BreathPrint. *Proceedings of the 15th Annual International Conference on Mobile Systems, Applications, and Services.* 10.1145/3081333.3081355

Chen, Y., Sun, J., Zhang, R., & Zhang, Y. (2015, April). Your song your way: Rhythm-based two-factor authentication for multi-touch mobile devices. *2015 IEEE Conference on Computer Communications (INFOCOM).* 10.1109/INFOCOM.2015.7218660

Chiasson, S. (2009). *Usable authentication and click-based graphical passwords.* Carleton University. http://dx.doi.org/ doi:10.22215/etd/2009-06388

Choi, W., Seo, M., & Lee, D. H. (2018). Sound-Proximity: 2-Factor authentication against relay attack on passive keyless entry and start system. *Journal of Advanced Transportation, 2018*, 1–13. doi:10.1155/2018/1935974

Choi, Y., Lee, Y., Moon, J., & Won, D. (2017). Security enhanced multi-factor biometric authentication scheme using bio-hash function. *PLoS One*, *12*(5), e0176250. doi:10.1371/journal.pone.0176250 PMID:28459867

Das, A., Bonneau, J., Caesar, M., Borisov, N., & Wang, X. (2014). The tangled web of password reuse. *Proceedings 2014 Network and Distributed System Security Symposium*. 10.14722/ndss.2014.23357

Dasgupta, D., Roy, A., & Nag, A. (2016). Toward the design of adaptive selection strategies for multi-factor authentication. *Computers & Security*, *63*, 85–116. doi:10.1016/j.cose.2016.09.004

De Silva, H. L. S. R. P., Wittebron, D. C., Lahiru, A. M. R., Madumadhavi, K. L., Rupasinghe, L., & Abeywardena, K. Y. (2019). AuthDNA: An Adaptive Authentication Service for any Identity Server. *2019 International Conference on Advancements in Computing (ICAC)*, 369–375. 10.1109/ICAC49085.2019.9103382

dos Santos, D. R., Westphall, C. M., & Westphall, C. B. (2014, May). A dynamic risk-based access control architecture for cloud computing. *2014 IEEE Network Operations and Management Symposium (NOMS)*, 1-9. 10.1109/NOMS.2014.6838319

Eldefrawy, M. H., Khan, M. K., Alghathbar, K., Kim, T.-H., & Elkamchouchi, H. (2011). Mobile one-time passwords: Two-factor authentication using mobile phones. *Security and Communication Networks*, *5*(5), 508–516. doi:10.1002ec.340

Eremin, A., & Kogos, K. (2018). Incoming call implicit user authentication - User authentication via hand movement pattern. *Proceedings of the 4th International Conference on Information Systems Security and Privacy*. 10.5220/0006555200240029

EU General Data Protection Regulation (GDPR): Regulation (EU) 2016/679 of the European Parliament and of the Council of 27 April 2016 on the protection of natural persons with regard to the processing of personal data and on the free movement of such data, and repealing Directive 95/46/EC (General Data Protection Regulation), OJ 2016 L 119/1

Farash, M. S. (2014). An improved password-based authentication scheme for session initiation protocol using smart cards without verification table. *International Journal of Communication Systems*, *30*(1), e2879. doi:10.1002/dac.2879

Feng, T., Zhao, X., DeSalvo, N., Gao, Z., Wang, X., & Shi, W. (2015, April). Security after login: Identity change detection on smartphones using sensor fusion. *2015 IEEE International Symposium on Technologies for Homeland Security (HST)*. 10.1109/THS.2015.7225268

Fridman, L., Weber, S., Greenstadt, R., & Kam, M. (2017). Active authentication on mobile devices via stylometry, application usage, web browsing, and GPS location. *IEEE Systems Journal*, *11*(2), 513–521. doi:10.1109/JSYST.2015.2472579

Gebrie, M. T., & Abie, H. (2017, September 11). Risk-based adaptive authentication for internet of things in smart home eHealth. *Proceedings of the 11th European Conference on Software Architecture: Companion Proceedings*. 10.1145/3129790.3129801

General Data Protection Regulation (GDPR) – official legal text. (2016, July 13). General Data Protection Regulation (GDPR). https://gdpr-info.eu

Gokhale, A. S., & Waghmare, V. S. (2016). The shoulder surfing resistant graphical password authentication technique. *Procedia Computer Science*, *79*, 875–884. doi:10.1016/j.procs.2016.03.091

Gonzalez-Manzano, L., Fuentes, J. M. D., & Ribagorda, A. (2019). Leveraging user-related internet of things for continuous authentication. *ACM Computing Surveys*, *52*(3), 1–38. doi:10.1145/3314023

Gope, P., Amin, R., Hafizul Islam, S. K., Kumar, N., & Bhalla, V. K. (2018). Lightweight and privacy-preserving RFID authentication scheme for distributed IoT infrastructure with secure localization services for smart city environment. *Future Generation Computer Systems*, *83*, 629–637. doi:10.1016/j.future.2017.06.023

Gragnaniello, D., Poggi, G., Sansone, C., & Verdoliva, L. (2013, September). Fingerprint liveness detection based on Weber Local image Descriptor. *2013 IEEE Workshop on Biometric Measurements and Systems for Security and Medical Applications*. 10.1109/BIOMS.2013.6656148

Grassi, P. A., Fenton, J. L., Newton, E. M., Perlner, R. A., Regenscheid, A. R., Burr, W. E., Richer, J. P., Lefkovitz, N. B., Danker, J. M., Choong, Y.-Y., Greene, K. K., & Theofanos, M. F. (2017). *Digital identity guidelines: Authentication and lifecycle management*. National Institute of Standards and Technology. doi:10.6028/nist.sp.800-63b

Gunson, N., Marshall, D., Morton, H., & Jack, M. (2011). User perceptions of security and usability of single-factor and two-factor authentication in automated telephone banking. *Computers & Security*, *30*(4), 208–220. doi:10.1016/j.cose.2010.12.001

Gupta, P., Wee, T. K., Ramasubbu, N., Lo, D., Gao, D., & Balan, R. K. (2012, March). HuMan: Creating memorable fingerprints of mobile users. *2012 IEEE International Conference on Pervasive Computing and Communications Workshops*. 10.1109/PerComW.2012.6197540

Gupta, S., Buriro, A., & Crispo, B. (2019). DriverAuth: A risk-based multi-modal biometric-based driver authentication scheme for ride-sharing platforms. *Computers & Security*, *83*, 122–139. doi:10.1016/j.cose.2019.01.007

Gurav, S. M., Gawade, L. S., Rane, P. K., & Khochare, N. R. (2014, January). Graphical password authentication: Cloud securing scheme. *2014 International Conference on Electronic Systems, Signal Processing and Computing Technologies*. 10.1109/ICESC.2014.90

Hang, A., De Luca, A., Smith, M., Richter, M., & Hussmann, H. (2015). Where have you been? using location-based security questions for fallback authentication. In *Eleventh Symposium On Usable Privacy and Security (SOUPS 2015)* (pp. 169-183). Academic Press.

Hayashi, E., Das, S., Amini, S., Hong, J., & Oakley, I. (2013). CASA. *Proceedings of the Ninth Symposium on Usable Privacy and Security - SOUPS '13*. http://dx.doi.org/10.1145/2501604.2501607

Henricks, A., & Kettani, H. (2019, October 14). On data protection using multi-factor authentication. *Proceedings of the 2019 International Conference on Information System and System Management*. 10.1145/3394788.3394789

Hintze, D., Findling, R. D., Muaaz, M., Koch, E., & Mayrhofer, R. (2015). Cormorant. *Proceedings of the 2015 ACM International Joint Conference on Pervasive and Ubiquitous Computing and Proceedings of the 2015 ACM International Symposium on Wearable Computers - UbiComp '15.* http://dx.doi.org/10.1145/2800835.2800906

Hintze, D., Koch, E., Scholz, S., & Mayrhofer, R. (2016). Location-Based Risk Assessment for Mobile Authentication. *Proceedings of the 2016 ACM International Joint Conference on Pervasive and Ubiquitous Computing: Adjunct,* 85–88. doi:10.1145/2968219.2971448

Huseynov, E., & Seigneur, J.-M. (2017). Context-Aware multifactor authentication survey. In *Computer and Information Security Handbook* (pp. 715–726). Elsevier. doi:10.1016/B978-0-12-803843-7.00050-8

ISO/IEC 29100:2011. (2011). European Innovation Partnership - European Commission. https://ec.europa.eu/eip/ageing/standards/ict-and-communication/data/isoiec-291002011_en.html

ISO/IEC 29100:2011. (2011). ISO. Retrieved October 9, 2021, from https://www.iso.org/standard/45123.html

Jiang, Q., Ma, J., Li, G., & Li, X. (2013). Improvement of robust smart-card-based password authentication scheme. *International Journal of Communication Systems, 28*(2), 383–393. doi:10.1002/dac.2644

Karthigaiveni, M., & Indrani, B. (2019). An efficient two-factor authentication scheme with key agreement for IoT-based E-health care application using a smart card. *Journal of Ambient Intelligence and Humanized Computing.* Advance online publication. doi:10.100712652-019-01513-w

Katsini, C., Belk, M., Fidas, C., Avouris, N., & Samaras, G. (2016, November 10). Security and usability in knowledge-based user authentication. *Proceedings of the 20th Pan-Hellenic Conference on Informatics.* 10.1145/3003733.3003764

Khan, H., & Hengartner, U. (2014, February 26). Towards application-centric implicit authentication on smartphones. *Proceedings of the 15th Workshop on Mobile Computing Systems and Applications.* 10.1145/2565585.2565590

Kikuchi, H., Hattori, T., & Nakanishi, S. (2002.). User authentication with facial images. Human-friendly identification in the Internet. *Proceedings Joint 9th IFSA World Congress and 20th NAFIPS International Conference* (Cat. No. 01TH8569). http://dx.doi.org/10.1109/nafips.2001.944424

Kumari, S., Chaudhry, S. A., Wu, F., Li, X., Farash, M. S., & Khan, M. K. (2015). An improved smart card based authentication scheme for session initiation protocol. *Peer-to-Peer Networking and Applications, 10*(1), 92–105. doi:10.100712083-015-0409-0

Lai, D. Y. (2011, January 1). *Intelligent online risk-based authentication using Bayesian network model.* http://dspace.library.uvic.ca/handle/1828/3290

Lenzini, G., Bargh, M. S., & Hulsebosch, B. (2008). Trust-enhanced security in location-based adaptive authentication. *Electronic Notes in Theoretical Computer Science, 197*(2), 105–119. doi:10.1016/j.entcs.2007.12.020

Li, F., Clarke, N., Papadaki, M., & Dowland, P. (2013). Active authentication for mobile devices utilising behaviour profiling. *International Journal of Information Security*, *13*(3), 229–244. doi:10.100710207-013-0209-6

Li, S., Ashok, A., Zhang, Y., Xu, C., Lindqvist, J., & Gruteser, M. (2016, March). Whose move is it anyway? Authenticating smart wearable devices using unique head movement patterns. *2016 IEEE International Conference on Pervasive Computing and Communications (PerCom)*. http://dx.doi.org/10.1109/percom.2016.7456514

Li, X., Niu, J., Khurram Khan, M., & Liao, J. (2013). An enhanced smart card based remote user password authentication scheme. *Journal of Network and Computer Applications*, *36*(5), 1365–1371. doi:10.1016/j.jnca.2013.02.034

Li, Z., Sun, Q., Lian, Y., & Giusto, D. D. (2005). A secure image-based authentication scheme for mobile devices. In *Lecture Notes in Computer Science* (pp. 751–760). Springer Berlin Heidelberg. doi:10.1007/11538356_78

Liu, X., Zhang, R., & Liu, Q. (2017). A temporal credential-based mutual authentication with multiple-password scheme for wireless sensor networks. *PLoS One*, *12*(1), e0170657. doi:10.1371/journal.pone.0170657 PMID:28135288

Liu, Z., Bonazzi, R., & Pigneur, Y. (2016). Privacy-based adaptive context-aware authentication system for personal mobile devices. J. *Mobile Multimedia*, *12*(1&2), 159–180.

Liu, Z., Guo, C., & Wang, B. (2020). A physically secure, lightweight three-factor and anonymous user authentication protocol for iot. *IEEE Access: Practical Innovations, Open Solutions*, *8*, 195914–195928. doi:10.1109/ACCESS.2020.3034219

Martinovic, I., Rasmussen, K., Roeschlin, M., & Tsudik, G. (2017). Authentication using pulse-response biometrics. *Communications of the ACM*, *60*(2), 108–115. doi:10.1145/3023359

Misbahuddin, M., Bindhumadhava, B. S., &Dheeptha, B. (2017, August). Design of a risk based authentication system using machine learning techniques. *2017 IEEE SmartWorld, Ubiquitous Intelligence & Computing, Advanced & Trusted Computed, Scalable Computing & Communications, Cloud & Big Data Computing, Internet of People and Smart City Innovation (SmartWorld/SCALCOM/UIC/ATC/CBDCom/IOP/SCI)*. http://dx.doi.org/ doi:10.1109/uic-atc.2017.8397628

Murmuria, R., Stavrou, A., Barbará, D., & Fleck, D. (2015). Continuous authentication on mobile devices using power consumption, touch gestures and physical movement of users. In Research in Attacks, Intrusions, and Defenses (pp. 405–424). Springer International Publishing. doi:10.1007/978-3-319-26362-5_19

Neverova, N., Wolf, C., Lacey, G., Fridman, L., Chandra, D., Barbello, B., & Taylor, G. (2016). Learning human identity from motion patterns. *IEEE Access: Practical Innovations, Open Solutions*, *4*, 1810–1820. doi:10.1109/ACCESS.2016.2557846

Ometov, A., Bezzateev, S., Mäkitalo, N., Andreev, S., Mikkonen, T., & Koucheryavy, Y. (2018). Multi-Factor authentication: A survey. *Cryptography*, *2*(1), 1. doi:10.3390/cryptography2010001

Pan, L., & Bangay, S. (2014, October). Generating repudiable, memorizable, and privacy preserving security questions using the propp theory of narrative. *2014 International Conference on Cyber-Enabled Distributed Computing and Knowledge Discovery*. 10.1109/CyberC.2014.20

Petsas, T., Tsirantonakis, G., Athanasopoulos, E., & Ioannidis, S. (2015, April 21). Two-factor authentication: Is the world ready? *Proceedings of the Eighth European Workshop on System Security*. 10.1145/2751323.2751327

Premarathne, U. S., Khalil, I., & Atiquzzaman, M. (2015). Location-dependent disclosure risk based decision support framework for persistent authentication in pervasive computing applications. *Computer Networks*, *88*, 161–177. doi:10.1016/j.comnet.2015.06.002

Preuveneers, D., & Joosen, W. (2015, April 13). SmartAuth. *Proceedings of the 30th Annual ACM Symposium on Applied Computing*. 10.1145/2695664.2695908

Rahnama, B., Elci, A., & Celik, S. (2010). Securing RFID-based authentication systems using ParseKey+. *Proceedings of the 3rd International Conference on Security of Information and Networks - SIN '10*. 10.1145/1854099.1854142

Ramakrishnan, A., Tombal, J., Preuveneers, D., & Berbers, Y. (2015, December 11). PRISM. *Proceedings of the 13th International Conference on Advances in Mobile Computing and Multimedia*. 10.1145/2837126.2837157

Ren, Y., Wen, P., Liu, H., Zheng, Z., Chen, Y., Huang, P., & Li, H. (2021, May 10). Proximity-Echo: Secure two factor authentication using active sound sensing. *IEEE INFOCOM 2021 - IEEE Conference on Computer Communications*. http://dx.doi.org/10.1109/infocom42981.2021.9488866

Ribeiro de Mello, E., Silva Wangham, M., Bristot Loli, S., da Silva, C. E., Cavalcanti da Silva, G., de Chaves, S. A., & Bristot Loli, B. (2020). Multi-factor authentication for shibboleth identity providers. *Journal of Internet Services and Applications*, *11*(1), 8. Advance online publication. doi:10.118613174-020-00128-1

Riva, O., Qin, C., Strauss, K., & Lymberopoulos, D. (2012). Progressive authentication: deciding when to authenticate on mobile phones. In *21st USENIX Security Symposium (USENIX Security 12)* (pp. 301-316). USENIX.

Rivera, E., Tengana, L., Solano, J., Castelblanco, A., López, C., & Ochoa, M. (2020, November 9). Risk-based authentication based on network latency profiling. *Proceedings of the 13th ACM Workshop on Artificial Intelligence and Security*. 10.1145/3411508.3421377

Rocha, C. C., Lima, J. C. D., Dantas, M. A. R., & Augustin, I. (2011, June). A2BeST: An adaptive authentication service based on mobile user's behavior and spatio-temporal context. *2011 IEEE Symposium on Computers and Communications (ISCC)*. 10.1109/ISCC.2011.5983933

Sankaran, A., Malhotra, A., Mittal, A., Vatsa, M., & Singh, R. (2015, September). On smartphone camera based fingerphoto authentication. *2015 IEEE 7th International Conference on Biometrics Theory, Applications and Systems (BTAS)*. http://dx.doi.org/10.1109/btas.2015.7358782

Sepczuk, M., & Kotulski, Z. (2018). A new risk-based authentication management model oriented on user's experience. *Computers & Security, 73*, 17–33. doi:10.1016/j.cose.2017.10.002

Shah, S. W. A., & Kanhere, S. (2018). Wi-Auth: WiFi based Second Factor User Authentication. *Proceedings of the 14th EAI International Conference on Mobile and Ubiquitous Systems: Computing, Networking and Services.* 10.4108/eai.7-11-2017.2274992

Sharma, G., & Kalra, S. (2018). A lightweight multi-factor secure smart card based remote user authentication scheme for cloud-IoT applications. *Journal of Information Security and Applications, 42*, 95–106. doi:10.1016/j.jisa.2018.08.003

Shi, E., Niu, Y., Jakobsson, M., & Chow, R. (2011). Implicit authentication through learning user behavior. In *Lecture Notes in Computer Science* (pp. 99–113). Springer Berlin Heidelberg. doi:10.1007/978-3-642-18178-8_9

Shnain, A. H., & Shaheed, S. H. (2019). User authentication by secured graphical password implementation in problems e-commerce. *Journal of Computational and Theoretical Nanoscience, 16*(5), 2327–2332. doi:10.1166/jctn.2019.7894

Shone, N., Dobbins, C., Hurst, W., & Shi, Q. (2015, October). Digital memories based mobile user authentication for iot. *2015 IEEE International Conference on Computer and Information Technology; Ubiquitous Computing and Communications; Dependable, Autonomic and Secure Computing; Pervasive Intelligence and Computing.* http://dx.doi.org/10.1109/cit/iucc/dasc/picom.2015.270

Solano, J., Camacho, L., Correa, A., Deiro, C., Vargas, J., & Ochoa, M. (2019). Risk-Based static authentication in web applications with behavioral biometrics and session context analytics. In *Lecture Notes in Computer Science* (pp. 3–23). Springer International Publishing. doi:10.1007/978-3-030-29729-9_1

Solano, J., Camacho, L., Correa, A., Deiro, C., Vargas, J., & Ochoa, M. (2020). Combining behavioral biometrics and session context analytics to enhance risk-based static authentication in web applications. *International Journal of Information Security, 20*(2), 181–197. doi:10.100710207-020-00510-x

Song, R. (2010). Advanced smart card based password authentication protocol. *Computer Standards & Interfaces, 32*(5–6), 321–325. doi:10.1016/j.csi.2010.03.008

Spooren, J., Preuveneers, D., & Joosen, W. (2015, April 21). Mobile device fingerprinting considered harmful for risk-based authentication. *Proceedings of the Eighth European Workshop on System Security.* 10.1145/2751323.2751329

Sun, H.-M., Chen, Y.-H., Fang, C.-C., & Chang, S.-Y. (2012). PassMap. *Proceedings of the 7th ACM Symposium on Information, Computer and Communications Security - ASIACCS '12.* http://dx.doi.org/10.1145/2414456.2414513

Sun, J., Zhang, R., Zhang, J., & Zhang, Y. (2014, October). TouchIn: Sightless two-factor authentication on multi-touch mobile devices. *2014 IEEE Conference on Communications and Network Security.* 10.1109/CNS.2014.6997513

Syta, E., Kurkovsky, S., & Casano, B. (2010). RFID-Based authentication middleware for mobile devices. *2010 43rd Hawaii International Conference on System Sciences.* http://dx.doi.org/10.1109/hicss.2010.320

Taher, B. H., Liu, H., Abedi, F., Lu, H., Yassin, A. A., & Mohammed, A. J. (2021). A secure and lightweight three-factor remote user authentication protocol for future iot applications. *Journal of Sensors*, *2021*, 1–18. doi:10.1155/2021/8871204

Takada, T., & Hattori, Y. (2020, September 28). Giving motivation for using secure credentials through user authentication by game. *Proceedings of the International Conference on Advanced Visual Interfaces*. 10.1145/3399715.3399950

Thomas, K., Pullman, J., Yeo, K., Raghunathan, A., Kelley, P. G., Invernizzi, L., Benko, B., Pietraszek, T., Patel, S., Boneh, D., & Bursztein, E. (2019). Protecting accounts from credential stuffing with password breach alerting. In *28th USENIX Security Symposium (USENIX Security 19)* (pp. 1556–1571). USENIX Association.

Thorpe, J., MacRae, B., & Salehi-Abari, A. (2013). Usability and security evaluation of GeoPass. *Proceedings of the Ninth Symposium on Usable Privacy and Security - SOUPS '13*. 10.1145/2501604.2501618

Traore, I., Woungang, I., Obaidat, M. S., Nakkabi, Y., & Lai, I. (2012, November). Combining mouse and keystroke dynamics biometrics for risk-based authentication in web environments. *2012 Fourth International Conference on Digital Home*. 10.1109/ICDH.2012.59

Traore, I., Woungang, I., Obaidat, M. S., Nakkabi, Y., & Lai, I. (2013). Online risk-based authentication using behavioral biometrics. *Multimedia Tools and Applications*, *71*(2), 575–605. doi:10.100711042-013-1518-5

Umar, M. S., & Rafiq, M. Q. (2012, March). Select-to-Spawn: A novel recognition-based graphical user authentication scheme. *2012 IEEE International Conference on Signal Processing, Computing and Control*. 10.1109/ISPCC.2012.6224382

Wang, B., & Ma, M. (2012). A smart card based efficient and secured multi-server authentication scheme. *Wireless Personal Communications*, *68*(2), 361–378. doi:10.100711277-011-0456-7

Wang, C., Wang, D., Xu, G., & Guo, Y. (2017). A lightweight password-based authentication protocol using smart card. *International Journal of Communication Systems*, *30*(16), e3336. doi:10.1002/dac.3336

Wiefling, S., Dürmuth, M., & Lo Iacono, L. (2020, December 7). More than just good passwords? A study on usability and security perceptions of risk-based authentication. *Annual Computer Security Applications Conference*. 10.1145/3427228.3427243

Wiefling, S., Lo Iacono, L., & Dürmuth, M. (2019). Is this really you? An empirical study on risk-based authentication applied in the wild. In *ICT Systems Security and Privacy Protection* (pp. 134–148). Springer International Publishing. doi:10.1007/978-3-030-22312-0_10

Wiefling, S., Patil, T., Dürmuth, M., & Lo Iacono, L. (2020). Evaluation of risk-based re-authentication methods. In *ICT Systems Security and Privacy Protection* (pp. 280–294). Springer International Publishing. doi:10.1007/978-3-030-58201-2_19

Wiefling, S., Tolsdorf, J., & Lo Iacono, L. (2021). Privacy Considerations for Risk-Based Authentication Systems. In *2021 International Workshop on Privacy Engineering* (pp. 315–322). IEEE.

Wu, T.-S., Lee, M.-L., Lin, H.-Y., & Wang, C.-Y. (2013). Shoulder-surfing-proof graphical password authentication scheme. *International Journal of Information Security, 13*(3), 245–254. doi:10.100710207-013-0216-7

Xia, Z., Yuan, C., Lv, R., Sun, X., Xiong, N. N., & Shi, Y.-Q. (2020). A novel weber local binary descriptor for fingerprint liveness detection. *IEEE Transactions on Systems, Man, and Cybernetics. Systems, 50*(4), 1526–1536. doi:10.1109/TSMC.2018.2874281

Xie, P. (2014). *Facial movement based human user authentication.* Iowa State University. http://dx.doi.org/ doi:10.31274/etd-180810-3817

Xiong, J., Xiong, J., & Claramunt, C. (2014). A spatial entropy-based approach to improve mobile risk-based authentication. *Proceedings of the 1st ACM SIGSPATIAL International Workshop on Privacy in Geographic Information Collection and Analysis - GeoPrivacy '14.* 10.1145/2675682.2676400

Yang, Li, & Xie. (2015, March). MotionAuth: Motion-based authentication for wrist worn smart devices. *2015 IEEE International Conference on Pervasive Computing and Communication Workshops (PerCom Workshops).* http://dx.doi.org/ doi:10.1109/percomw.2015.7134097

Zhang, J., Tan, X., Wang, X., Yan, A., & Qin, Z. (2018). T2FA: Transparent two-factor authentication. *IEEE Access: Practical Innovations, Open Solutions, 6,* 32677–32686. doi:10.1109/ACCESS.2018.2844548

Zhang, X., Yao, L., Kanhere, S. S., Liu, Y., Gu, T., & Chen, K. (2018). MindID. *Proceedings of the ACM on Interactive, Mobile, Wearable and Ubiquitous Technologies, 2*(3), 1–23. doi:10.1145/3264959

Zheng, N., Bai, K., Huang, H., & Wang, H. (2014, October). You are how you touch: User verification on smartphones via tapping behaviors. *2014 IEEE 22nd International Conference on Network Protocols.* http://dx.doi.org/10.1109/icnp.2014.43

Zhong, Kanhere, & Chou. (2017, March). VeinDeep: Smartphone unlock using vein patterns. *2017 IEEE International Conference on Pervasive Computing and Communications (PerCom).* http://dx.doi.org/10.1109/percom.2017.7917845

Zhou, B., Lohokare, J., Gao, R., & Ye, F. (2018, October 15). EchoPrint. *Proceedings of the 24th Annual International Conference on Mobile Computing and Networking.* 10.1145/3241539.3241575

Zhu, X., Yu, S., & Pei, Q. (2016, December). QuickAuth: Two-Factor quick authentication based on ambient sound. *2016 IEEE Global Communications Conference (GLOBECOM).* 10.1109/GLOCOM.2016.7842192

Chapter 10
Prediction of COVID-19 Active, Recovered, and Death Cases Using Artificial Neural Network and Grey Wolf Optimization

Arup Kumar Mohanty

Siksha 'O' Anusandhan (Deemed), India

Sipra Sahoo

Siksha 'O' Anusandhan (Deemed), India

Apurv Taunk

Siksha 'O' Anusandhan (Deemed), India

Mamata Garnayak

Centurion University of Technology and Management, India

Subhashree Choudhury

Siksha 'O' Anusandhan (Deemed), India

ABSTRACT

The 2019 novel corona virus was declared a global pandemic by the World Health Organization (WHO) on March 11th, 2020. The world is stressed out because of this disease's high infectiousness and transmission mode. A predictive model of the COVID-19 outbreak is developed for India using state-of-the-art neural network models. The chapter evaluates the key features to predict the patterns, potential infection rate, and death of the present COVID-19 outbreak in India. In this chapter, machine learning methods such as artificial neural network (ANN) optimized by a bio-inspired optimization algorithm that is grey wolf optimization (GWO) and particle swarm optimization (PSO) have been implemented for the prediction of infection rate and mortality rate for the 5 days, 15 days, and 30 days ahead. The prediction of various parameters obtained by the proposed approach is effective within a certain specific range and would be a useful tool for administration and healthcare providers.

DOI: 10.4018/978-1-6684-4580-8.ch010

INTRODUCTION

The COVID-19 global epidemic, widely identified as a coronavirus outbreak, is a growing global coronavirus disease contagion in 2019 (COVID-19), triggered by extreme acute respiratory coronavirus syndrome 2 (SARS CoV2) (Dey, J. K., et al., 2020, Vaishya, R et al., 2020, Law, P. K. et al., 2020). The outbreak was first reported in Wuhan, China in December 2019. On 30th January the epidemic was declared an international public health emergency by the World Health Organization (Hui, D. S et al., 2020, Atique, S et al., 2020). The World Health Organization announced the disease on 30th January 2020 as a public health emergency of global importance and on 11th March as a pandemic. About 13.8 million cases of COVID-19 as of 17th July 2020 have been reported in more than 188 countries and territories, resulting beyond 589,000 deaths; over and above 7.71 million people have recovered. Globally COVID-19 pandemic is now one of the major concerns around the globe. Due to this pandemic the world is going through a tough situation. The world came to a standstill for this pandemic. Round the globe all are facing a tensed situation. Mortality rate and transmission of the disease is growing rapidly throughout the world though in some countries it has become stable. All countries seek to save their lives by enforcing steps such as travel bans, quarantines, postponements and cancellations of activities, social barriers, examinations, hard and soft lockdowns (Acter, T et al.,2020, Moon, M. J et al.,2020). It has an impact upon the survival of mankind economically and socially. People infected with the virus thus face difficulty in breathing because of fluid and pus in the lung. This happens because of the air sacs swelling in one or both lungs. The most general signs and symptoms of COVID-19 are dry-cough, nausea, fever, and some uncommon symptoms such as body aches, sore throat, diarrhea, the headache of conjunctivitis, skin rash, loss of taste or smell, or discoloration of the finger or toe, difficulty breathing, chest pain etc (Larsen, J. R et al., 2020, Johansson, M. A et al.,2021, da Rosa Mesquita, R et al., 2021). So, if someone has some of those symptoms, COVID-19 test may be referred to. On 7th July 2020, there are 98192 cumulative cases of infection worldwide and 3,045 deaths have been reported.

Artificial Intelligence is an umbrella term where Machine Learning (ML) and deep learning are part of it and play an important role for solving many complex real-world problems. Artificial Intelligence techniques applied in almost all the domains like in business, natural language processing, climate prediction, finance modeling, robotics, gaming, healthcare, genomics and genetics, software engineering, networking, speech, and image processing etc. as every domain need intelligence (Libbrecht, M. W et al.,2015, Ramprasad, R et al., 2017, Carbonell, J. G et al., 1983, Magoulas, G. D et al.,1999, July).The learning of ML techniques is usually based on hit and trial methods very contrary to traditional algorithms, which implement programming instructions such as if-else type of decision statements. Forecasting or prediction is one of the fascinating aspects of ML which have been used to decide the future actions in many application domains such as market condition prediction, climate prediction, disease transmission, and mortality rate prediction, forecasting of economic scenarios etc. (Krollner, B et al., 2010, April, Bontempi, G et al., 2012, July). Artificial Neural Network (ANN) methods and specific regression techniques are widely applicable in foretelling patient problems with a particular disease in the future. There are several studies carried out to predict different diseases using the above-mentioned techniques such as coronary artery disease, cardiovascular disease, and breast cancer forecasting (Chen, M et al., Hao, 2017, Mohan, S et al., 2019, Sriram, T. V et al., 2013). This research primarily focuses on live forecasting of confirmed COVID-19 cases and the research also focuses on COVID-19 pandemic prediction and early intervention. Such prediction systems can be highly useful in taking decisions to control the present scenario in order to direct early responses for very successful management of these diseases.

The subsequent part of the research article has been structured as follows. The related works available in literature has been meticulously surveyed in Section 2. The proposed models, different parameters that are associated with these models and the techniques used for forecasting the cases in this work has been outlined in Section 3. The findings for India are presented in Section 4. Finally, in Section 5 the conclusions are drawn from the entire study.

LITERATURE SURVEY

For COVID-19's current research, development and its impact, many researchers have developed specific forecasting models based on obtained data. Corona virus spread is not a perfect exponential spread, because of which the traditional epidemiological approach used to model the spread of infectious diseases does not explain the COVID-19. Many researchers have applied machine learning algorithms for better prediction. Several reports on predicting infectious diseases are included in the literature. Time-series forecasting approach has been also used with the Auto-Regressive Integrated Moving Average (ARIMA) approach (Fattah, J et al., 2018). The reason this approach being so often used is because statistical features can be beneficial. They are also very versatile since, multiple time series can be represented using different order parameters. The ARIMA method was used in predicting many diseases like Influenza, Brucellosis, Hemorrhagic Fever with Renal Syndrome (HFRS) and COVID-19 He, Z et al.,2018) (Wu, N et al., 2020, Alim, M et al., 2020, Liu, Q et al., 2011, Li, Q et al., 2012,Sharma, R. R et al., 2020). In this study, the Nonlinear Auto regression Neural Network (NARNN) and Auto-Regressive Integrated Moving Average (ARIMA) were designed on instances of COVID-19 in Germany, Denmark, Belgium, France, Finland, Switzerland, the United Kingdom & Turkey. Six model performance metric such as Mean Absolute Percentage Error (MAPE), Normalized Root Mean Square Error (NRMSE), Mean Absolute Error (MSE), Symmetric Mean Absolute Percentage Error (SMAPE), Root Mean Square Error (RMSE) etc. were used to select the most accurate model. The NARNN model is a technique that carries out nonlinear regression. This technique of machine learning was used to forecast different pandemics (Bahri, S et al., 2020, December) (Wu, W et al., 2019)(Soebiyanto, R. P et al., 2010)(Singh, R. K et al., 2020)(Kırbaş, İ et al., 2020). (Jiang, Coffee, Bari et al.2020) have proposed some artificial intelligence methods that forecast patients' risk vulnerability on initial presentation data from two hospitals in Wenzhou, Zhejiang, China (Jiang, X et al., 2020). Yang et al. proposed Susceptible-Exposed-Infectious-Removed (SEIR) model and Artificial Intelligence (AI) approach to forecasting the epidemic curve taking into consideration COVID-19 updated data and 2003 SARS data. Lifting off the Hubei quarantine would steer to another epidemic where the peak period is in the middle of March and extend up to late April (Yang, Z et al., 2020). A dynamic and time series forecasting model based on different mathematical formulas is proposed for COVID-19 for foretelling the short-term transmission of COVID-19 which is very important information for the intervention and prevention of this disease (Keeling, M. J et al., 2021). The result showed that the rate of transmission and regeneration of COVID-19 decreased and increased mortality contributed to additional cases of pneumonia, while the total number of confirmed cases was not susceptible to increased cure rates. Dong et al. built a web-based interactive dashboard which helps in tracking of COVID-19 using the real-time data (Dong, E et al., 2020). Data randomization techniques are being used by a dynamic stochastic general equilibrium (DSGE) model for evaluating the impact of corona virus on the travel & tourism industry and it also achieves trend prediction (Yang, Y et al., 2020). The Long Short Term Memory model is used to predict the end of the Epidemic phase, which uses forward time memory processing with a huge amount of data considering actual factors and characteristic conditions resulting output data that is associated with the factors.

In the paper, epidemiological model basing upon control measures like social distancing and lock down for India is implemented. Time varying effects of these lockdown and social distancing are measured upon COVID-19 transmission rate. ESIR model is implemented for forecasting disease transmission rate taking nine different features and taking the dates of lockdown relaxation dates of different states. After forecasting different prevention measures can be adopted for preventing the disease transmission rate (Tomar, A et al., 2020).

Two models were suggested by Amit et al., such as the Discrete Cosine Transformation (DCT)-based Fourier Decomposition System (FDM)). The DCT acts as an ideal method and model of Susceptible-Infected-Recovered (SIR) to obtain the trend and estimate the number of infected cases for preventive action (Dhanwant, J. N., 2020). Results showed a confidence interval of 95% globally. The proposed study gives positive outcomes with the strength to perform as a strong complement to current predictive monitoring methods for the COVID-19 pandemic. Determination of the total number of positive covid-19 cases and end period of this pandemic across various regions of globe, Gaussian mixture model is used by many researchers (Singhal, A et al., 2020). The Long-Term Short-Term memory model (LSTM) is being used by authors in (Zeroual, A et al., 2020) to calculate the number of COVID-19 cases and to explicate the effectiveness of social isolation and lock-down. In Italy, forecasting of infected cases is carried out using an integrated moving average auto-regressive model (Wangping, J et al., 2020). Fanelli and Piazza presented predictions concerning the proliferation of COVID-19 in France, China & Italy (Wangping, J et al., 2020).

PROPOSED METHODOLOGY

The work described in this paper has been performed upon the data that is publicly available on the website – 'covid19india.org'. The data collection was done in a CSV file and then uploaded to Jupyter Notebook for analysis. The analysis was done using python software version 3.7.1. The input features are daily confirmed cases, daily deceased, daily recovered, tests per million and total samples tested.

Using ANN-GWO and ANN-PSO, the network is then trained. The main difference between ANN-GWO and ANN-PSO is that the GWO technique optimizes the ANN- model better in comparison to the Particle Swarm Optimization. It is evaluated with the test data in the next step, after creating the network. The model is used to forecast the infection rates and death rates for 5 days ahead, 15 days ahead and 30 days ahead. The proposed model has been compared with the projected model of ANN-GWO. The model predicts the infection and death rate for 5 days, 15 days and 30days in advance. The outputs are: Prediction of daily cases 5 days ahead, 15 days ahead and 30 days ahead in advance and the prediction of daily deaths 5 days ahead,15 days ahead and 30 days ahead. Figure.1 illustrates the layout of the proposed model.

Figure 1. Layout of proposed model

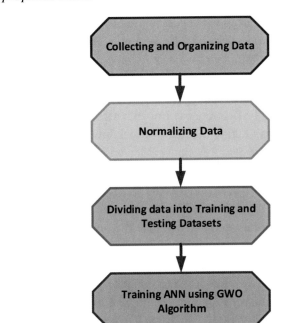

ANN

The word "Artificial Neural Network (ANN)" refers to a subfield of Artificial Intelligence. An ANN is normally a computational network model basing upon the biological neural networks and imitates the structure of human brain. In ANN neurons are interconnected with each other in a different layer like the human brain. These neurons are referred to as nodes. Figure.2 shows the schematic layout of feed forward neural network which is one of the simplest variants of neural networks. They pass information in one direction, through various input nodes named as X1, X2, X3 until it makes it to the output node Y. The network may or may not have hidden node layers, making their functioning more interpretable. It takes multiple inputs and generates an output which is a weighted combination of all the inputs. w1, w2, wn are the weights associated with the input nodes. This output is fed into a transfer function to produce Y (Sairamya, N. J et al., 2019)(Zupan, J et al., 1994)

GWO

Based upon the hunting behavior and leadership nature of the Grey Wolves, the GWO algorithm is developed. Based on the population, it is a more powerful algorithm which has higher convergence quality and gives a near-optimal solution which is compared with the PSO algorithm, Gravitational Search Algorithm (GSA), Genetic Algorithm (GA), ACO algorithm or the Differential Evolutionary (DE) algorithm. A

Figure 2. Layout of neurons in ANN

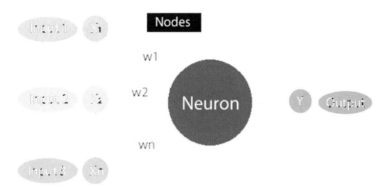

major benefit of this recently proposed algorithm is that it doesn't require the gradient knowledge. It has gained significant popularity (Bontempi, G et al., 2012, July) because it can be quickly applied and has the potential to automate many realistic optimization problems. As it can be easily implemented and has an ability to optimize many practical optimization problems, it has gained considerable attention (Bontempi, G et al., 2012, July)(Panda, N et al., 2019). As inspired by the leadership and hunting behavior of the Grey Wolves, this algorithm contains three phases: 1) Involving wolves' social hierarchy for confronting the prey; 2) Enclosing the prey and 3) Trapping the prey.

The best solution is represented as alpha (α) which is the decision-maker and acts as the leader of wolves which is trailed by the second and third-best solutions defined as beta (β) and delta (δ) and assist the leader wolf in decision making as such in the social hierarchy of the Grey Wolves. Omega (ω) represents the rest of the wolves that follow alpha (α), beta (β), and delta (δ). Mathematically this social ladder of grey wolves is used for modeling the first phase of the algorithm.

In second phase, the mathematical model used for encircling the prey is represented in (1).

$$\vec{w}(t+1) = \vec{w}_P(t) - \vec{A}.\left|\vec{C}.\vec{w}_P(t) - \vec{w}(t)\right|$$ (1)

Where ($\vec{w}$) represents the position vector of a grey wolf, the current iteration is represented by t and $\vec{w}_P$ represents the position vector of the prey. The coefficient vectors $\vec{A}$ & $\vec{C}$ are calculated using (2) and (3).

$$\vec{A} = 2a.\vec{r}_1 - \vec{a}$$ (2)

$$\vec{C} = 2.\vec{r}_2$$ (3)

Where the linear decrement over the iterations is shown by a & $\vec{r}_1, \vec{r}_2$ represent the random vectors as follows:

$$\vec{a}(t) = 2 - 2t / \text{Itr}_{\max} \tag{4}$$

The current iteration is represented by t and Itr_max represents the maximum number of iterations to take place. With respect to the position values of α, β and δ, the position of the remaining wolves is updated. The third phase of the GWO algorithm i.e. 'the hunting of the prey' can be simulated using mathematical formulas as given in (5), (6), (7) and (8).

$$\vec{w}_1 = \vec{w}_\alpha - \vec{A}_1 . \left| \vec{C}_1 . \vec{w}_\alpha - \vec{w} \right| \tag{5}$$

$$\vec{w}_2 = \vec{w}_\beta - \vec{A}_2 . \left| \vec{C}_2 . \vec{w}_\beta - \vec{w} \right| \tag{6}$$

$$\vec{w}_3 = \vec{w}_\delta - \vec{A}_3 . \left| \vec{C}_3 . \vec{w}_\delta - \vec{w} \right| \tag{7}$$

$$\vec{w}_{t+1} = \frac{\vec{w}_1(t) + \vec{w}_2(t) + \vec{w}_3(t)}{3} \tag{8}$$

$\vec{A}_1, \vec{A}_2, \vec{A}_3$ are same as $\vec{A}$ and $\vec{C}_1, \vec{C}_2, \vec{C}_3$ are same as $\vec{C}$.

PSO

Among many Optimization Algorithms, Particle Swarm Optimizations is a computational method which optimizes the problem by iteratively trying to get a candidate solution with respect to a given quality measure. Here the population of solutions called as particles and the particles are moved around the search space according to some basic mathematical formula taking position and velocity of the particle. Each particle's movement is directed by its best-known local location, but it is also pushed towards the best-known search-space positions that are altered as better positions are identified by other particles. This is intended to drive the swarm to the better alternatives (Marini, F et al.,2015) (Eberhart, R et al.,1995).

EXPERIMENTAL SETUP

A description about the datasets used for performing the experimental work is provided in this section along with the description of the different parameters used for implementing the swarm intelligence techniques in the proposed approach. Analysis of the results obtained from the experimental work is done in this section and the different validations such as the accuracy, precision, recall and f-1 score that are used to evaluate the proposed model, the fitness function used for evaluation is also described. This section contains the results that are obtained using the datasets used for the implementation of the above method and the evaluation results obtained are represented in both graphical and tabular format for better visualization and understanding of the system's performance.

The key findings from the proposed approach such as performance comparison between individual trust metrics and the proposed hybrid approach, extent up to which the proposed technique handles the problem of data sparsity is also provided in this section along with the performance description of the model for individual datasets is also provided.

Hardware and Software Specifications

The proposed hybrid system for generating predictions for number of infected patients and number of mortality cases using ANN and ANN GWO was performed in a system having storage of 1Tb, with 8 GB of RAM and no SDD storage used. i5 Processor with 2.7Ghz of processing speed was used along with a Windows-10 operating system.

The task was performed in python (v-3.7.1) along with the libraries- NumPy, this library is for the Python programming language that supports with a large collection of different mathematical functions used upon arrays, also provides support for large multidimensional arrays and matrices, pandas, this library is designed for providing support for data processing and data analytics, provides different data-structures for handling tabular data and time series. Jupyter notebook was used as an editor for this purpose that allows us to code, share, visualize, transform data and statistically model the data and is widely used for different machine learning and data-analytics purposes. The above-mentioned system specifications and software that were used helped to perform the proposed approach and evaluate the same.

Availability of Data and Materials

The work described in this paper has been performed upon the data that is available for the public on the website – 'covid19india.org'. The data collection was done in a CSV file and then uploaded to Jupyter Notebook for analysis. The analysis was done using python software version 3.7.1.

Inputs: Daily confirmed cases, daily deceased, daily recovered, tests per million, total samples tested.

Outputs: Daily cases & deaths 5 days ahead, daily cases & deaths 15 days ahead, daily cases & deaths 30 days ahead.

Results

Figure 3, Figure 4 depict about the predicted infected case and death cases using PSO after 5th day. Figure 5 and Figure 6 describe about the predicted infected cases and death cases using PSO for 15th day. Figure 7 and Figure 8 give description of the predicted infected cases and death cases using PSO for 30 days. Figure 9 and Figure 10 describes about the predicted infected case and death cases using GWO for 5th day. Figure 11 and Figure 12 show the predicted infected case and death cases using GWO for 15th day. Figure 13 and Figure 14 show the predicted infected case and death cases using GWO after 30th day.

These metrics were used to measure the overall performance of the model. The evaluation is done by measuring the mean absolute error of the predictions done by the model and the mean absolute percentage error was calculated to measure the overall accuracy of the model.

1. *MAE:* Mean absolute error can be described as an average of the absolute difference between the actual value and the predicted value obtained from the model. The greater the MAE, the more is

Figure 3. Predicted cases for 5th day using PSO

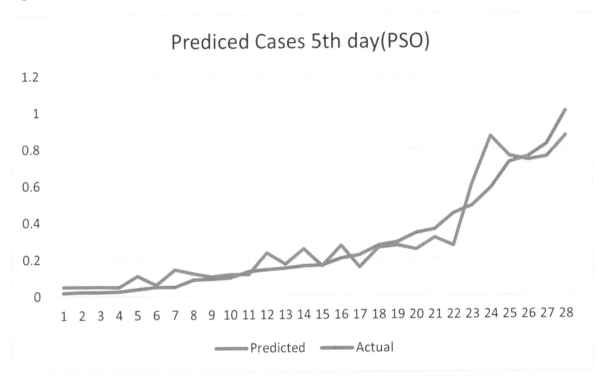

Figure 4. Predicted deaths for 5th day using PSO

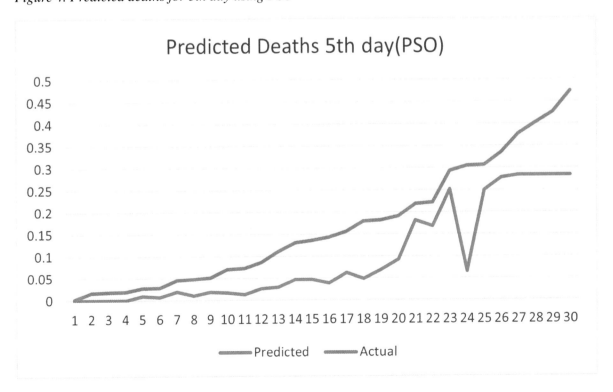

Figure 5. Predicted cases for 15th day using PSO

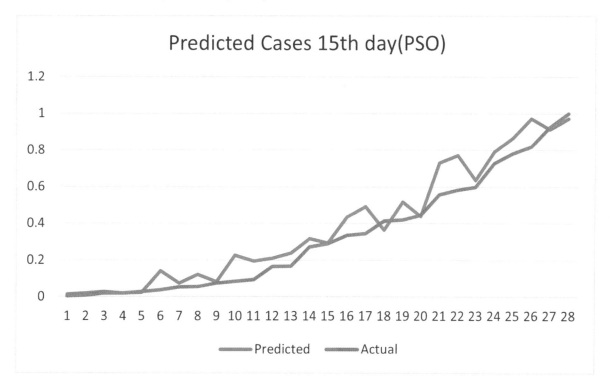

Figure 6. Predicted deaths for 15th day using PSO

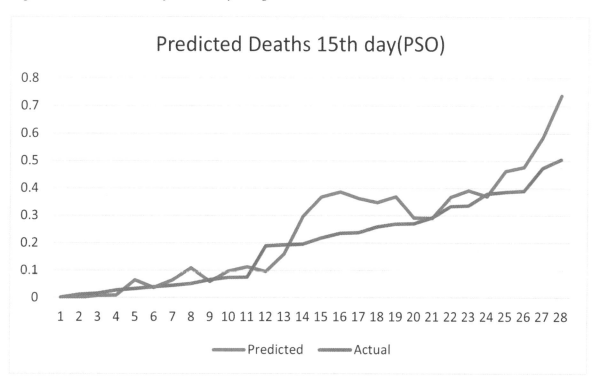

Figure 7. Predicted cases for 30th day using PSO

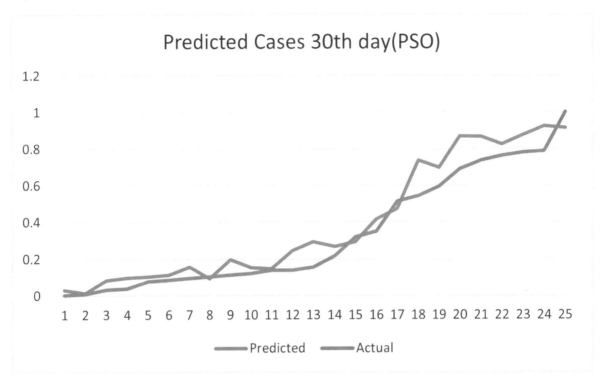

Figure 8. Predicted deaths for 30th day using PSO

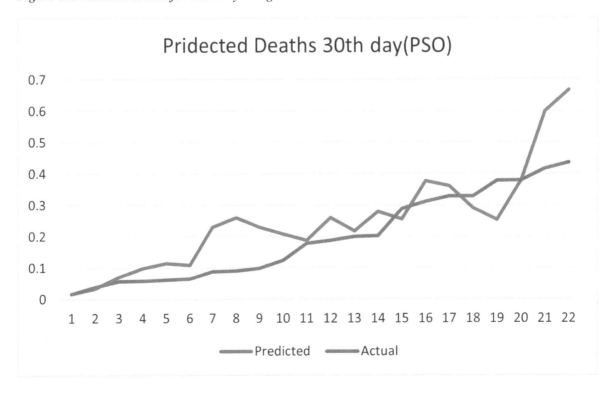

Figure 9. Predicted cases for 5th day using GWO

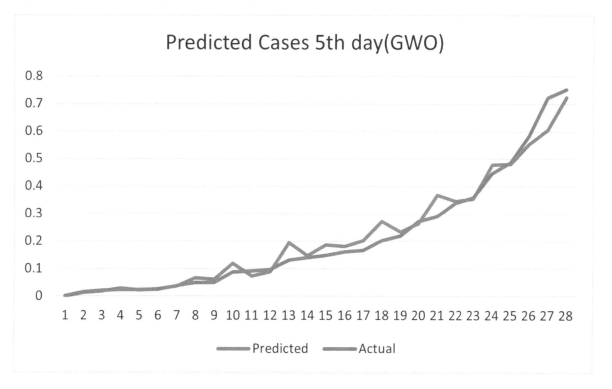

Figure 10. Predicted deaths for 5th day using GWO

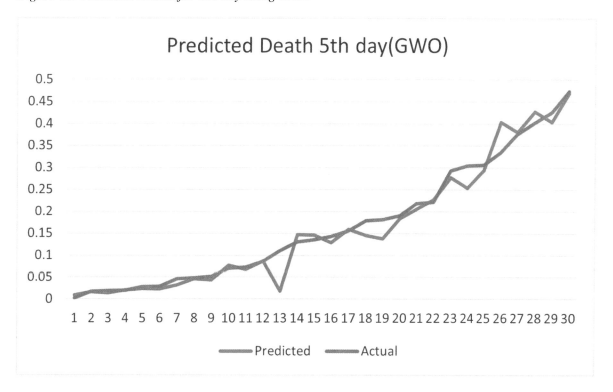

Figure 11. Predicted cases for 15th day using GWO

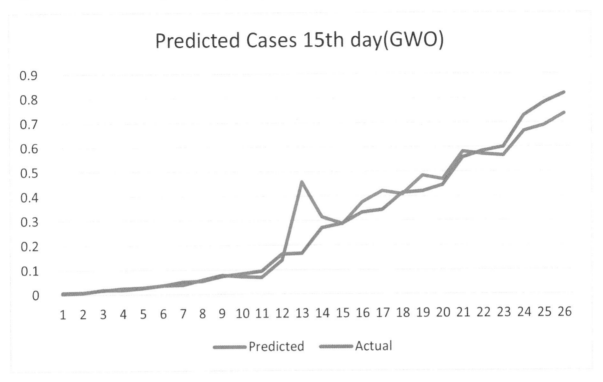

Figure 12. Predicted deaths for 15th day using GWO

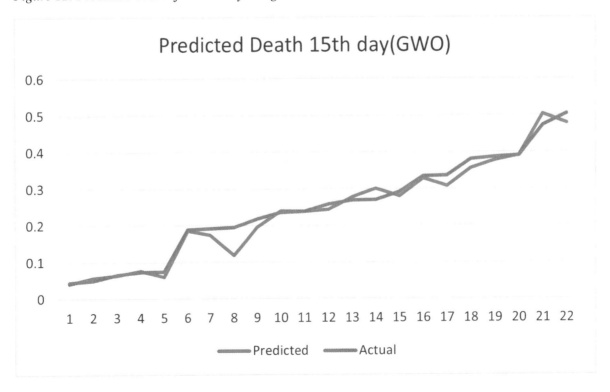

Figure 13. Predicted cases for 30th day using GWO

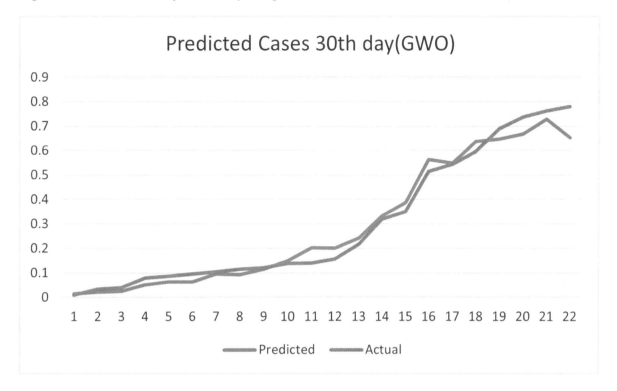

Figure 14. Predicted deaths for 30th day using GWO

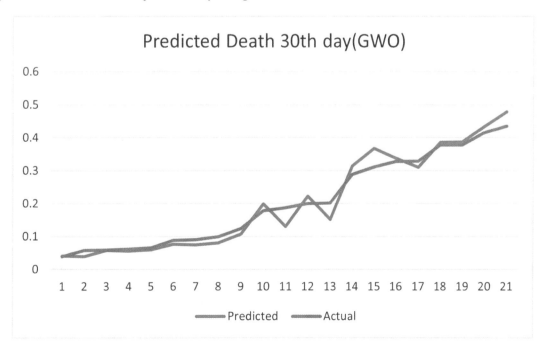

deviation from the actual output. In the following equation p_i is the predicted value and a_i is the actual value.

$$\mathbf{MAE} = \frac{\sum_{i=1}^{n} |\mathbf{p_i} - \mathbf{a_i}|}{\mathbf{n}} \qquad (9)$$

2. **R2 Score:** The R2 Score measures how the model replicates the well-observed results. This is based on the proportion of total variance of results described by the model. The coefficient of determination usually varies from 0 to 1, but it may be negative in some situations.

3. If $\bar{y}$ is the mean of the observed data & y_i be the predicted value:

$$\bar{\mathbf{y}} = \frac{1}{\mathbf{n}} \sum_{i=1}^{n} \mathbf{y_i} \qquad (10)$$

The three sum of squares were then used to measure the variability that is possessed by the data set.

a. The total sum of squares which is proportional with the variance that is possessed by the data is represented by SS_{tot}, described in the below formula:

$$\mathbf{SS_{tot}} = \sum_{i} \left(\mathbf{y_i} - \bar{\mathbf{y}} \right)^2 \qquad (11)$$

b. The regression sum of squares which is also referred as the explained sum of squares is represented by SS_{reg}, described in the below formula:

$$\mathbf{SS_{reg}} = \sum_{i} \left(\mathbf{f_i} - \bar{\mathbf{y}} \right)^2 \qquad (12)$$

c. The sum of squares of residuals which is also referred as residual sum of squares is represented by SS_{res}, described in the below formula:

$$\mathbf{SS_{res}} = \sum_{i} \left(\mathbf{y_i} - \mathbf{f_i} \right)^2 \qquad (13)$$

The definition of the coefficient of determination in the most general form is:

$$\mathbf{R}^2 = 1 - \frac{\mathbf{SS_{res}}}{\mathbf{SS_{tot}}} \qquad (14)$$

As a best case where the modelled values have an exact match with the observed values resulting in the values of R^2 as 1 and SS_{res} equals 0. A base model predicting $\bar{y}$ will have value of R^2 as zero and models predicting even worse will have a negative value for R^2.

3. **MAPE:** To measure the prediction accuracy made by the statistical forecasting method MAPE or The Mean absolute percentage error is used as defined by in the below given formula, however the MAPE is usually expressed in ratio.

$$\mathbf{M} = \frac{1}{\mathbf{n}} \sum_{i=1}^{n} \left| \frac{\mathbf{A_t} - \mathbf{F_t}}{\mathbf{A_t}} \right| \tag{15}$$

A_t here represents actual value while the forecasted value is represented by F_t.

4. **Accuracy:** Accuracy is the measure of how accurate predictions are made by the model. It can be calculated as:

$$\text{Accuracy} = 1 - M \tag{16}$$

Where M is the MAPE of the model.

The following tables contain the evaluation scores for both the algorithms used for each of the predictions done. Table 1 shows the evaluation of performance for number of cases prediction. Table 2 depicts the evaluation of performance for number of deaths prediction

Figure 15. MAE of both models for number of cases

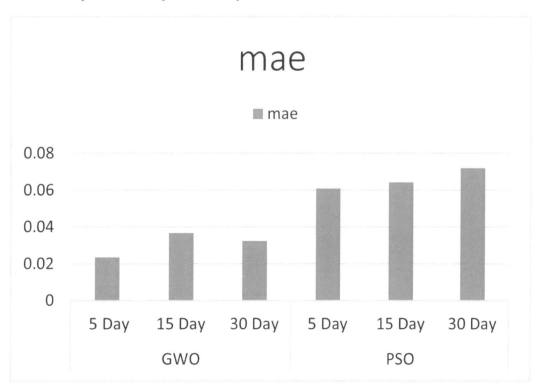

Figure 16. R2 Score of both models for number of cases

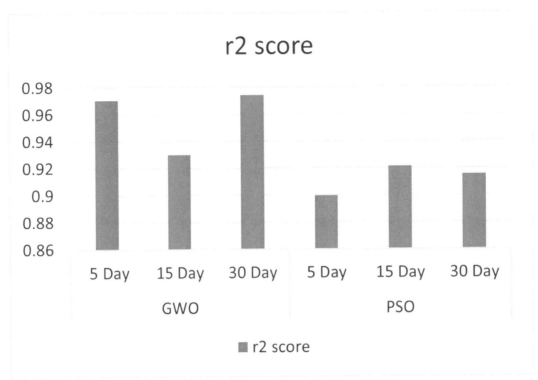

Figure 17. Accuracy of both models for number of cases

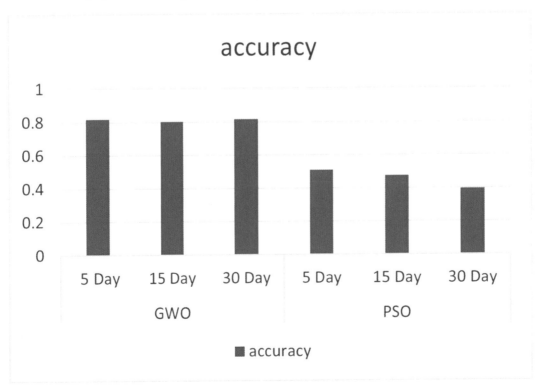

Figure 18. MAE of both models for number of deaths

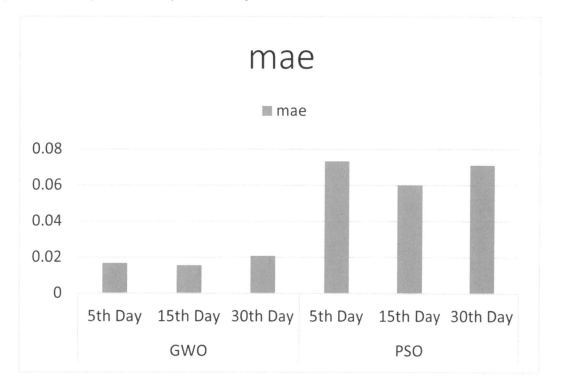

Figure 19. R2 Score of both models for number of deaths

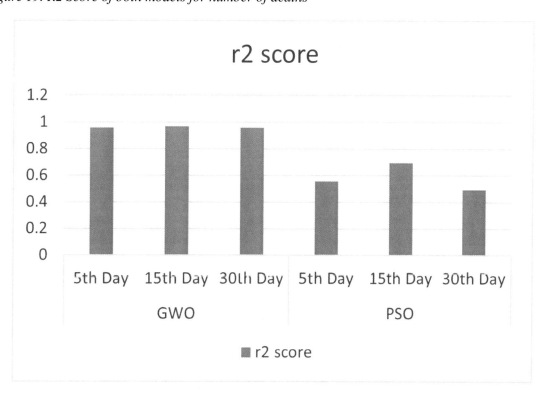

Figure 20. Accuracy of both models for the number of deaths

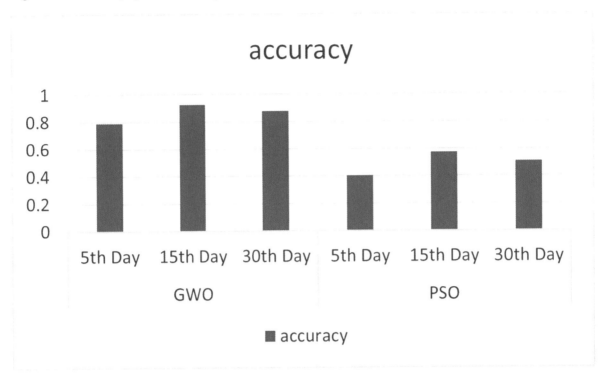

Table 1. Evaluation of performance for number of cases prediction

Optimizer	Days	MAE	R2 Score	MSE	RMSE	MAPE	Accuracy
GWO	5	0.02344	0.970601	0.001302	0.036089	0.181082	0.8189184
	15	0.036738	0.9299699	0.004688	0.068469	0.195918	0.8040816
	30	0.032285	0.9742608	0.001783	0.042231	0.184005	0.8159954
PSO	5	0.061034	0.8996117	0.00729	0.085381	0.491297	0.5087029
	15	0.064176	0.9212076	0.007314	0.085525	0.525755	0.4742451
	30	0.071932	0.9153618	0.007807	0.088359	0.604427	0.395573

Table 2. Evaluation of performance for number of deaths prediction

Optimizer	Days	MAE	R2 Score	MSE	RMSE	MAPE	Accuracy
GWO	5	0.01679	0.9605021	0.000729	0.027005	0.206947	0.7930533
	15	0.015611	0.9695407	0.000521	0.022822	0.074029	0.9259714
	30	0.020799	0.9587383	0.000712	0.026684	0.120573	0.8794267
PSO	5	0.07332	0.5554446	0.008208	0.090597	0.596202	0.403798
	15	0.060214	0.6942447	0.006771	0.082284	0.42622	0.5737802
	30	0.0712	0.4925808	0.009144	0.095623	0.491747	0.5082532

Figure 15, 16 and 17 represents the MAE, R2 and accuracy performance of both the models for predicting number of cases respectively. Figure 18, 19 and 20 illustrates the MAE, R2 and accuracy performance of both the models for predicting number of deaths respectively.

CONCLUSION

A data-driven estimation/forecasting approach was used in this paper for estimating the potential number of positive COVID-19 cases in India for 5 days ahead, 15 days ahead & a month ahead. Optimizing the ANN using the GWO & PSO algorithms, a forecast prediction was made for the number of positive, recovered & deceased cases across India. It has been observed that the spread of the virus can be substantially reduced by using preventive measures like social distancing & lockdown.

The predictions would certainly be affected due to any changes made in the policy regarding the reopening of society, social distancing norms or if there is any new research method that can alter the spread of virus. The predicted results from the models may vary dramatically from the actual ones. Clearly, more research is needed in the wider validation of this conclusion by updating the actual current COVID-19 data into the model.

REFERENCES

Acter, T., Uddin, N., Das, J., Akhter, A., Choudhury, T. R., & Kim, S. (2020). Evolution of severe acute respiratory syndrome coronavirus 2 (SARS-CoV-2) as coronavirus disease 2019 (COVID-19) pandemic: A global health emergency. *The Science of the Total Environment*, *730*, 138996. doi:10.1016/j.scitotenv.2020.138996 PMID:32371230

Alim, M., Ye, G. H., Guan, P., Huang, D. S., Zhou, B. S., & Wu, W. (2020). Comparison of ARIMA model and XGBoost model for prediction of human brucellosis in mainland China: A time-series study. *BMJ Open*, *10*(12), e039676.

Atique, S., Bautista, J. R., Block, L. J., Lee, J. J., Lozada-Perezmitre, E., Nibber, R., O'Connor, S., Peltonen, L.-M., Ronquillo, C., Tayaben, J., Thilo, F. J. S., & Topaz, M. (2020). A nursing informatics response to COVID-19: Perspectives from five regions of the world. *Journal of Advanced Nursing*, *76*(10), 2462–2468. doi:10.1111/jan.14417 PMID:32420652

Bahri, S., Kdayem, M., & Zoghlami, N. (2020, December). Deep Learning for COVID-19 prediction. In *2020 4th International Conference on Advanced Systems and Emergent Technologies (IC_ASET)* (pp. 406-411). IEEE.

Bontempi, G., Taieb, S. B., & Le Borgne, Y. A. (2012, July). Machine learning strategies for time series forecasting. In *European business intelligence summer school* (pp. 62–77). Springer.

Carbonell, J. G., Michalski, R. S., & Mitchell, T. M. (1983). An overview of machine learning. *Machine Learning*, 3–23.

Chen, M., Hao, Y., Hwang, K., Wang, L., & Wang, L. (2017). Disease prediction by machine learning over big data from healthcare communities. *IEEE Access: Practical Innovations, Open Solutions, 5,* 8869–8879.

da Rosa Mesquita, R., Francelino Silva, L. C. Jr, Santos Santana, F. M., Farias de Oliveira, T., Campos Alcântara, R., Monteiro Arnozo, G., ... Freire de Souza, C. D. (2021). Clinical manifestations of CO-VID-19 in the general population: Systematic review. *Wiener Klinische Wochenschrift, 133*(7), 377–382. doi:10.100700508-020-01760-4 PMID:33242148

Dey, J. K., Mukherjee, A., Dey, S. K., Udayat, M. P., Pramanik, A., & Giri, S. (2020). *An assessment of the efficacies and therapeutic interventions of homoeopathic medicines in combating viral disorders with implications in the treatment of SARS-CoV-2 (Covid-19), a global pandemic.* Academic Press.

Dhanwant, J. N., & Ramanathan, V. (2020). *Forecasting covid 19 growth in india using susceptible-infected-recovered (sir) model.* arXiv preprint arXiv:2004.00696.

Dong, E., Du, H., & Gardner, L. (2020). An interactive web-based dashboard to track COVID-19 in real time. *The Lancet. Infectious Diseases, 20*(5), 533–534.

Eberhart, R., & Kennedy, J. (1995, November). Particle swarm optimization. In *Proceedings of the IEEE international conference on neural networks* (Vol. 4, pp. 1942-1948). IEEE.

Fanelli, D., & Piazza, F. (2020). Analysis and forecast of COVID-19 spreading in China, Italy and France. *Chaos, Solitons, and Fractals, 134,* 109761.

Fattah, J., Ezzine, L., Aman, Z., El Moussami, H., & Lachhab, A. (2018). Forecasting of demand using ARIMA model. *International Journal of Engineering Business Management, 10,* 1847979018808673.

He, Z., & Tao, H. (2018). Epidemiology and ARIMA model of positive-rate of influenza viruses among children in Wuhan, China: A nine-year retrospective study. *International Journal of Infectious Diseases, 74,* 61–70.

Hui, D. S., Azhar, E. I., Madani, T. A., Ntoumi, F., Kock, R., Dar, O., ... Petersen, E. (2020). The continuing 2019-nCoV epidemic threat of novel coronaviruses to global health—The latest 2019 novel coronavirus outbreak in Wuhan, China. *International Journal of Infectious Diseases, 91,* 264–266. doi:10.1016/j.ijid.2020.01.009 PMID:31953166

Jiang, X., Coffee, M., Bari, A., Wang, J., Jiang, X., Huang, J., ... Huang, Y. (2020). Towards an artificial intelligence framework for data-driven prediction of coronavirus clinical severity. Computers. *Materials & Continua, 63*(1), 537–551.

Johansson, M. A., Quandelacy, T. M., Kada, S., Prasad, P. V., Steele, M., Brooks, J. T., ... Butler, J. C. (2021). SARS-CoV-2 transmission from people without COVID-19 symptoms. *JAMA Network Open, 4*(1), e2035057–e2035057.

Keeling, M. J., Hill, E. M., Gorsich, E. E., Penman, B., Guyver-Fletcher, G., Holmes, A., ... Tildesley, M. J. (2021). Predictions of COVID-19 dynamics in the UK: Short-term forecasting and analysis of potential exit strategies. *PLoS Computational Biology, 17*(1), e1008619.

Kırbaş, İ., Sözen, A., Tuncer, A. D., & Kazancıoğlu, F. Ş. (2020). Comparative analysis and forecasting of COVID-19 cases in various European countries with ARIMA, NARNN and LSTM approaches. *Chaos, Solitons, and Fractals*, *138*, 110015.

Krollner, B., Vanstone, B. J., & Finnie, G. R. (2010, April). Financial time series forecasting with machine learning techniques: A survey. ESANN.

Larsen, J. R., Martin, M. R., Martin, J. D., Kuhn, P., & Hicks, J. B. (2020). Modeling the Onset of Symptoms of COVID-19. *Frontiers in Public Health*, *8*, 473.

Law, P. K. (2020). COVID-19 pandemic: Its origin, implications and treatments. *Open Journal of Regenerative Medicine*, *9*(02), 43–64. doi:10.4236/ojrm.2020.92006

Li, Q., Guo, N. N., Han, Z. Y., Zhang, Y. B., Qi, S. X., Xu, Y. G., ... Liu, Y. Y. (2012). Application of an autoregressive integrated moving average model for predicting the incidence of hemorrhagic fever with renal syndrome. *The American Journal of Tropical Medicine and Hygiene*, *87*(2), 364.

Libbrecht, M. W., & Noble, W. S. (2015). Machine learning applications in genetics and genomics. *Nature Reviews. Genetics*, *16*(6), 321–332. doi:10.1038/nrg3920 PMID:25948244

Liu, Q., Liu, X., Jiang, B., & Yang, W. (2011). Forecasting incidence of hemorrhagic fever with renal syndrome in China using ARIMA model. *BMC Infectious Diseases*, *11*(1), 1–7.

Magoulas, G. D., & Prentza, A. (1999, July). Machine learning in medical applications. In *Advanced course on artificial intelligence* (pp. 300–307). Springer.

Marini, F., & Walczak, B. (2015). Particle swarm optimization (PSO). A tutorial. *Chemometrics and Intelligent Laboratory Systems*, *149*, 153–165.

Mohan, S., Thirumalai, C., & Srivastava, G. (2019). Effective heart disease prediction using hybrid machine learning techniques. *IEEE Access: Practical Innovations, Open Solutions*, *7*, 81542–81554.

Moon, M. J. (2020). Fighting COVID-19 with agility, transparency, and participation: Wicked policy problems and new governance challenges. *Public Administration Review*, *80*(4), 651–656. doi:10.1111/puar.13214 PMID:32836434

Panda, N., & Majhi, S. K. (2019). How effective is spotted hyena optimizer for training multilayer perceptrons. *Int J Recent Technol Eng*, 4915-4927.

Ramprasad, R., Batra, R., Pilania, G., Mannodi-Kanakkithodi, A., & Kim, C. (2017). Machine learning in materials informatics: recent applications and prospects. *NPJ Computational Materials, 3*(1), 1-13.

Sairamya, N. J., Susmitha, L., George, S. T., & Subathra, M. S. P. (2019). Hybrid Approach for Classification of Electroencephalographic Signals Using Time–Frequency Images With Wavelets and Texture Features. In Intelligent Data Analysis for Biomedical Applications (pp. 253-273). Academic Press.

Sharma, R. R., Kumar, M., Maheshwari, S., & Ray, K. P. (2020). EVDHM-ARIMA-based time series forecasting model and its application for COVID-19 cases. *IEEE Transactions on Instrumentation and Measurement*, *70*, 1–10.

Singh, R. K., Rani, M., Bhagavathula, A. S., Sah, R., Rodriguez-Morales, A. J., Kalita, H., ... Kumar, P. (2020). Prediction of the COVID-19 pandemic for the top 15 affected countries: Advanced autoregressive integrated moving average (ARIMA) model. *JMIR Public Health and Surveillance, 6*(2), e19115.

Singhal, A., Singh, P., Lall, B., & Joshi, S. D. (2020). Modeling and prediction of COVID-19 pandemic using Gaussian mixture model. *Chaos, Solitons, and Fractals, 138*, 110023.

Soebiyanto, R. P., Adimi, F., & Kiang, R. K. (2010). Modeling and predicting seasonal influenza transmission in warm regions using climatological parameters. *PLoS One, 5*(3), e9450.

Sriram, T. V., Rao, M. V., Narayana, G. S., Kaladhar, D. S. V. G. K., & Vital, T. P. R. (2013). Intelligent Parkinson disease prediction using machine learning algorithms. *International Journal of Engineering and Innovative Technology, 3*(3), 1568–1572.

Tomar, A., & Gupta, N. (2020). Prediction for the spread of COVID-19 in India and effectiveness of preventive measures. *The Science of the Total Environment, 728*, 138762.

Vaishya, R., Javaid, M., Khan, I. H., & Haleem, A. (2020). Artificial Intelligence (AI) applications for COVID-19 pandemic. *Diabetes & Metabolic Syndrome, 14*(4), 337–339. doi:10.1016/j.dsx.2020.04.012 PMID:32305024

Wangping, J., Ke, H., Yang, S., Wenzhe, C., Shengshu, W., Shanshan, Y., ... Yao, H. (2020). Extended SIR prediction of the epidemics trend of COVID-19 in Italy and compared with Hunan, China. *Frontiers in medicine, 7*, 169.

Wu, N., Green, B., Ben, X., & O'Banion, S. (2020). *Deep transformer models for time series forecasting: The influenza prevalence case.* arXiv preprint arXiv:2001.08317.

Wu, W., An, S. Y., Guan, P., Huang, D. S., & Zhou, B. S. (2019). Time series analysis of human brucellosis in mainland China by using Elman and Jordan recurrent neural networks. *BMC Infectious Diseases, 19*(1), 1–11.

Yang, Y., Zhang, H., & Chen, X. (2020). Coronavirus pandemic and tourism: Dynamic stochastic general equilibrium modeling of infectious disease outbreak. *Annals of Tourism Research, 83*, 102913.

Yang, Z., Zeng, Z., Wang, K., Wong, S. S., Liang, W., Zanin, M., ... He, J. (2020). Modified SEIR and AI prediction of the epidemics trend of COVID-19 in China under public health interventions. *Journal of Thoracic Disease, 12*(3), 165.

Zeroual, A., Harrou, F., Dairi, A., & Sun, Y. (2020). Deep learning methods for forecasting COVID-19 time-Series data: A Comparative study. *Chaos, Solitons, and Fractals, 140*, 110121.

Zupan, J. (1994). Introduction to artificial neural network (ANN) methods: What they are and how to use them. *Acta Chimica Slovenica, 41*, 327–327.

Chapter 11
Serverless Architecture for Healthcare Management Systems

Anisha Kumari

Department of Computer Science and Engineering, National Institute of Technology, Rourkela, India

Bibhudatta Sahoo

Department of Computer Science and Engineering, National Institute of Technology, Rourkela, India

ABSTRACT

Serverless computing is an emerging cloud service architecture for executing distributed applications, where services are provided based on a pay-as-you-go basis. It allows the developers to deploy and run their applications without worrying about the underlying architecture. Serverless architecture has been popular due to its cost-effective policies, auto-scaling, independent, and simplified code deployment. The healthcare service can be made available as a serverless application that consists of distributed cloud services achieving the various requirements in the healthcare industry. The services offered may be made available on premise on a cloud infrastructure to users and health service providers. This chapter presents a novel model for serverless architecture for healthcare systems, where the services are provided as functional units to various stakeholders of the healthcare system. Two case studies related to healthcare systems that have adopted serverless frameworks are discussed.

INTRODUCTION

Serverless computing is a comparatively current computation model or paradigm which emerges from the rapid and continuous advancement of the Cloud. Such a type of service is provided by serverless computing with which users or developers can write and deploy application logic without the provision or management of containers or servers (Baldini, et al., 2017)(Bienko, Greenstein, Holt, Phillips, & others, 2015). Adopting the serverless model holds a significant effect on various aspects of software engineering in particular the pricing model, the development process, and QoS (Quality of Service) assurance

DOI: 10.4018/978-1-6684-4580-8.ch011

(Gadepalli, Peach, Cherkasova, Aitken, & Parmer, 2019)(Ivan, Vasile, & Dadarlat, 2019). Even though serverless computing has various advantages and benefits, such as no up-front provisioning, zero server management, high availability, pay only for the resources used, and auto scalability, it has also certain shortcomings which should also be taken into consideration: As currently offered by providers, it is inappropriate for long term tasks through the limited-time service can run; furthermore, there is increasing complexity of the underlying architecture, which is strengthened by the lack of suitable operational tools (Jangda, Pinckney, Brun, & Guha, 2019)(Brenner & Kapitza, 2019)(Hall & Ramachandran, 2019).

Serverless computing is one of the most useful buzzword in the era of cloud computing which present an architecture and deployment model to run the code by abstracting underlying infrastructure and the resources. In this platform developer does not concern about operational environment which includes resource configuration, environmental setup, security, reliability, encrypted messaging etc(Carreira, Fonseca, Tumanov, Zhang, & Katz, 2018)(Manvi & Shyam, 2014). It has been widely adapted by number of MNCs for their project to have more economical outputs. It poses a lot of challenges as well as opportunities to develop scalable application where user can focus only on writing business logic without worrying about the infrastructure. Serverless computing model can be thought of as the intermediary between PaaS and SaaS (Kim & Lee, 2019)(Gadepalli, Peach, Cherkasova, Aitken, & Parmer, 2019). It is based on function as a service model where an application can be developed by composing number of discrete functions which can be executed independently at a separate container at the server side. Sometimes, it makes it difficult for developer to understand the execution environment of their application as most of the control are abstracted from the user. Data and application security is another concern in case of serverless platform as users are totally unaware of the location of the servers where the data and applications are residing(Jain & Menache, 2016)(Van Eyk, et al., 2018). In serverless framework, functions are treated as the unit of execution, which can run in separate container to provide an isolation environment (McGrath & Brenner, 2017)(Mistry, Stelea, Kumar, & Pasquier). Developers are facing challenging in writing serverless application as the framework is very limited to pre-packaged library(Christoforou & Andreou, 2018)(Ivan, Vasile, & Dadarlat, 2019).

Serverless architecture is observed to be more flexible as compared to platform as a service and less stringent to the software as a service (Cusumano, 2010). In software as a service, applications are executed as a unit of execution where all the processing rely on API calls through which certain software are provided as a service (Hall & Ramachandran, 2019). All the code integration are not fixed with any hosted server. In fact, they are executed through AP calls. This approach has been used by many giant firms like Google, Yahoo etc. In comparison to SaaS, serverless provides an flexible environment which allow the developers to write and execute code in less expensive and auto-scalable manner. Serverless computing model has been widely accepted at many companies like Google, Yahoo, IBM, Microsoft etc. With the advancement of information and communication technology, health care systems has grown significantly over the past decade by capturing the huge amount of digital data (Lakhan, Khoso, Arain, & Kanwar, 2021)(Shafiei, Khonsari, & Mousavi, 2019). The healthcare business is transitioning to value-based care, which necessitates the collection of new data. Costs must be minimized for healthcare services to be accessible to a growing number of people (Thirunavukkarasu, Champion, Horan, Seyedmahmoudian, & Stojcevski, 2018), (Golec, Ozturac, Pooranian, Gill, & Buyya, 2021). All of this is feasible thanks to cutting-edge technologies like AI, machine learning, and serverless computing. The healthcare IT business can profit from serverless technology in a variety of ways. Serverless computing has the potential to drastically alter the healthcare industry. In healthcare tech start-ups, here are some of the primary advantages of employing serverless technology (Sewak & Singh, 2018)(Crespo-Cepeda, Agapito, Vazquez-Poletti, & Cannataro, 2019).

1. **Improves the Interoperability:** The amount of data in the healthcare industry is enormous and growing all the time. The use of serverless technologies has made storing massive volumes of data simple. Outside of the hospital, the data can be accessed, cleansed, and modified for use in other investigations.
2. **Quick Growth or Rapid Changes:** If you launch a medical app, it's hard to predict all the features users will need. You can try to implement them all at once, but it will require a lot of time and cost a fortune well before the app is launched and you receive any income. With serverless technologies, a development team can quickly alter, update, or fix the app without affecting its performance. In other words, instead of guessing, you can match the app with real user expectations.
3. **High-Latency Background Tasks:** Using serverless architecture for healthcare applications that process loads of data or multimedia may be a natural choice. Thanks to scalable storage and asynchronous data processing, your users will continue enjoying premium app performance, regardless of how much data is being uploaded at the moment.
4. **Client-Heavy Applications**: The shift toward value-based care has made patient engagement and experience a top priority for many healthcare organizations, resulting in more patient-centred applications. With serverless architecture, the app's functionality can berun on local servers closer to users, reducing latency and improving performance.
5. **Better security:** There is a risk of a data breach or other security incidents while using servers in the traditional way. Because the servers are protected by large IT companies like Amazon, serverless computing has far fewer security risks.

The chapter is organized in the following structure. Section 2 presents various aspects of serverless computing and its characteristics. Section 3 articulates the serverless architecture. The role of Function as a Service (FaaS) in serverless architecture is discussed in section 4. Section 5 gives the idea about basic healthcare management system in cloud. The role of serverless architecture for healthcare system is discussed in Section 6. In Section 7, the mapping of function as a service to healthcare system is discussed. Section 8 formalize Serverless architecture for web-based application for healthcare management. Section 9 discusses various case studies of serverless application for healthcare system.Section 10 summarizes the conclusion and future work of the study.

SERVERLESS COMPUTING AND ITS CHARACTERISTICS

A Serverless computing differs from the traditional cloud computing concept (we call it as a serverful in this chapter) in the sense that the infrastructure and platforms in which resources operate, are transparent to customers. In this way, customers are only concerned about the desired performance of their application and the rest is referred to the service provider. Engineers have to be conscious of these structures while selecting a platform. Some of the characteristics of serverless computing are discussed below (Gadepalli, Peach, Cherkasova, Aitken, & Parmer, 2019)(Hong, Srivastava, Shambrook, & Dumitraş, 2018)(Bila, Dettori, Kanso, Watanabe, & Youssef, 2017):

1. **Cost**:In the serverless pricing model, the cost is usually calculated for the resources consumption only when the applications are executed through serverless functions. So when the applications is idle, the cost may be measured as zero which is the most attractive features in serverless platform. Metal-based services or resources, such as memory or CPU, as well as price models, such as less expensive discounts, vary from provider to provider.

2. **Performance and Limits**: The serverless architecture is found to be more scalable as compared to other deployment models. However, it also limits the resource requirements by the business logic to control the incoming traffic which can able to provide better service. The limitation may be increased in future based on the user demands.

3. **Programming Languages**: Another attractive feature of serverless framework is that it allows the users to write the code diverse number of programming language which includes Java, Python, Go, Ruby, Java Script, C#, Swift etc. It has large number of APIs written in different number of languages. Some serverless frameworks allow to write programs in any language which can be integrated to Docket image that supports diverse sets of APIs (Kumari, Behera, Sahoo, & Sahoo, 2022).

4. **Composability**: Building application is quite efficient as compared to other models in cloud as it allows the users to write code in modular manner without worrying about the composability. User can write the function independently for different types of business logic. Serverless framework provides an different ways of composability where a function execution may be requested from another function. All these things will be taken care by the serverless framework. In this way, it allows the developers to build complex application in a simpler way.

5. **Deployment**: Ease of deployment is another attractive feature of serverless framework where usersneeds to packages all the source file in the form of Docker image in the form of binary file. The AWS CloudFormation is used to deployment of source code (Dalbhanjan, 2015). It also allows the users to automate the deployment process by continuous integration and continuous deployment (CI/CD) system (Singh, Gaba, Kaur, & Kaur, 2019).

6. **Security and Accounting**: Security is one of the major concerns when user deploy their code for execution in cloud. Serverless framework has elegant mechanism for separate the performance of tasks of different users. Based on the actual resource consumption, the accounting information is communicated in a separate channel (Hong, Srivastava, Shambrook, & Dumitraş, 2018).

7. **Monitoring and Debugging:** Every architecture supports the correction of basic errors by using print statements recorded in the log file. Additional skills may be provided to help users identify issues, track errors, and better understand the work environment (Hendrickson, et al., 2016).

8. **Auto-scaling:** It is expected from a cloud platform to be capable of scaling resources instantly, automatically, and available on demand. Serverless models are come complete containerization with minimal initial delay, allowing for the provision of thousands of events within a few seconds. Likewise, in the absence of application requests traffic, operating conditions reach zero to keep inactive application execution.

Compared with IaaS frameworks, serverless environments offer different tradeoffs in terms of flexibility, control, and cost. Specifically, it compels clients or developers to consider carefully the cost of business logic when modifying their applications, rather than delays, flexibility, and scalability that is where a considerable development attempt has conventionally been utilized (Shahrad, Balkind, & Wentzlaff, 2019).

A serverless platform benefits both clients as well as providers. From a client's point of view, it is found to be more cost effective as compared to other deployment models due to its flexible pricing model. According to the pricing model of serverless, billing is setup only for the actual resource consume. It does not account for the idle times. Another major advantage is that client is not responsible for configuring and management of container or the server at the backend (Hong, Srivastava, Shambrook, & Dumitraş, 2018)(Rajan, 2018). The responsibility is usually migrated from client to the server side. Developers can focus only on the business logic without worrying about any kind of infrastructure. As the functions at the server side are executed in stateless manner, the service providers have more control over the application stack which allow them to configure security in transparent manner.

Despite of serveral advantages, some limitation related to transparency are there in serverless platform. It is quite challenging to measure the actual performance of serverless application as a very limited performance and cost models have been emerged recent years. This leads to confusion in deciding in adaption of serverless in business solutions (Brenner & Kapitza, 2019)(Malawski, Gajek, Zima, Balis, & Figiela, 2020). Based on the performance analysis of standalone application developers can make the choices for solutions to the business problems. Another limitation lies in compatibility of complex and large application in serverless framework. As it is based on function as a service model where an application to be developed in a modular fashion, some complex applications may not be supported in the framework. It might not support the latest version of python or few libraries may not be available in the framework which makes challenging for developing an complex application.

SERVERLESS ARCHITECTURE

Serverless architecture is a new paradigm for software design where the client or the developers are allowed to upload and execute their code without worrying about the servers and the infrastructure (Gadepalli, Peach, Cherkasova, Aitken, & Parmer, 2019) . It can also be called as function as a service deployment model in the era of cloud service provider. Developers are offloading the responsibility of managing the server, configuring infrastructure, security patches to the service providers. They can only focus on writing the business logic. The architecture is also found to be cost efficient as compared to other deployment models as it is based on pay-as-you-go basis(Al-Roomi, Al-Ebrahim, Buqrais, & Ahmad, 2013). User doesn't have to pay for the idle time. They only have the pay for the exact amount of resources consume while the application is running at the server side. The backbone of serverless architecture is the function-as-a-service model, where users can focus on writing the application in the form of set of discrete functions, where each function may be corresponding to a specific task in the application.

Each of these functions are required to upload to the cloud along with set of events through which functions can start executing. The events may be in the form of http request or any king of updates in the database or any king of notification from any IoT device etc(Khandelwal, Kejariwal, & Ramasamy, 2020)(Behera & Rath, 2016). Upon triggering, the serverless vendors execute the function on a running server or the container (Kaewkasi, 2018). If no server is running, a new server may be provisioned for execution. All the triggers are to be paas through the API gateway on which the specific features of the application as defined earlier are processed. It may be related to resource scheduling, the auto-scaling or the logging the events. Based on the request received from the API gateway the appropriate action will be taken care by the cloud vendor. The scheduler will decide which execution node or the container are to be provided to serve the request. The auto-scaling module is executed when the application demands for the additional resources. Once the execution environment is configured, the corresponding function is start running. The execution environment is usually abstracted from the client side. Once the execution of the application is completed, all the resources that have been allocated are deprovisioned and the created environment is destroyed. The state between the function calls are destroyed. Hence, it is also known as stateless execution framework. The execution process in serverless architecture is presented in Figure. 1.

Figure 1. Serverless architecture

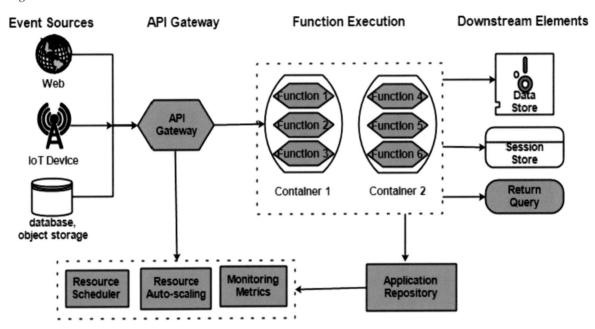

FUNCTION AS A SERVICE (FAAS) COMPUTING MODEL

A serverless computing paradigm is a rising approach for growing cloud-primarily based applications. IBM defines it as "a method to computing which offloads responsibility for commonplace infrastructure management tasks (scheduling, provisioning, patching, scaling, and many others.) to cloud vendors and gear, allowing developers to focus their effort as well time on the enterprise logic particular to their programs or procedure"(Rimal, Choi, & Lumb, 2009)(Ristov, Pedratscher, & Fahringer, 2021). Server-less computing calls for much less proficiency than other self-controlled tactics. Users do no longer control without delay the runtime and infrastructure of the system, however, as a substitute, delegate its operations to the cloud vendor. Moreover, cloud companies can install finer-grain pricing regulations (e.g., based on service requests) for any of the presented services, which usually leads to decreasing costs for developers.

One can make a distinction between several serverless computing paradigms: (1) Function as a Service (FaaS) implemented as an example by means of AWS Lambda (Hendrickson, et al., 2016), (2) Software as a Service (SaaS), through Google Cloud and (3)Database as A Service (DBaaS), as to be had through Microsoft Azure for PostgreSQL. FaaS can be taken into consideration as a hybrid among

Platform as a Service (PaaS) and the Software as a Service (SaaS) provider version: infrastructure, as well as information, is fully controlled via the cloud vendor, even as the software is handled through the clients or developers(Korhonen, 2017)(Kumari, Sahoo, Behera, Misra, & Sharma, 2021). FaaS systems or Function-as-a-Service permit developers to create and host an application (consisting of a single function or set of functions) that scales dynamically. These applications are meant to carry out a single function on demand and then forestall running till needed once more. Such systems provide enormous cost financial savings to application developers, permitting them to pay for only the instances all through which their serverless applications are executing. Moreover, web hosting companies can also recognize widespread savings in resource intake, for the reason that serverless functions do no longer require continuously running dedicated containerized or virtualized hardware resources(Kumanov, Hung, Lloyd, & Yeung, 2018). Even though at the start designed for the cloud, these frameworks are properly suited for fog/edge computing environments, in which assets are necessarily constrained. Figure 2 illustrates a standard FaaS framework. In the standard FaaS model, developers pass the setup, maintenance, along with the control of a compute node (like containers, virtual machines, or even bare metal). Instead, clients offer business logic for specific functions to be deployed and developed to the cloud. Specific activities such as storage, database situations, or HTTP requests cause function execution. Then, the cloud vendor handles the requests, scaling as well as the availability of resource requirements. Though the benefit of the serverless model, it is currently tough to determine a selected FaaS provider based on standards along with pricing scheme, performance, or workload adaptability.

Figure 2. Traditional FaaS architecture. The key points to benchmark are: performance of a worker (i.e., execution speed of a function) and quality of the auto-scaling mechanism.

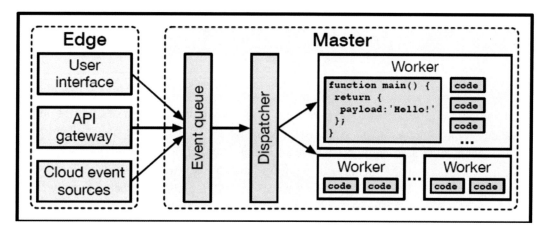

HEALTHCARE MANAGEMENT SYSTEM IN CLOUD

Cloud computing refers to Internet infrastructure and on-demand availability of services, which allows the clients to utilize accessible cloud computing services and resources anytime from anywhere (Behera, Jena, Rath, & Misra, 2021). It is a new paradigm of offering cloud computing resources, now not a brand-new technology. Examples of typically utilized non-healthcare services or applications like Google Docs, Microsoft Hotmail, etc. even as some better-recognized applications in health-care consist of Google Health platform, Microsoft HealthVault, etc(Fox, et al., 2009). Despite that, in comparison to traditional cloud computing, the serverless paradigm offers new benefits such as computing resources to be had on-call for, removal of an up-the-front commitment utilizing clients, and price for a short duration to execute the client's business logic. Various blogs, articles, forums, research works have pronounced serverless application in an enterprise, commercial enterprise, national protection, transportation, education, security, etc. Health care, as with every other service operation, requires systematic as well as continuous innovation to remain efficient, cost-powerful, and convenient, and to offer outstanding services.

Figure 3. The health system architecture in cloud environment

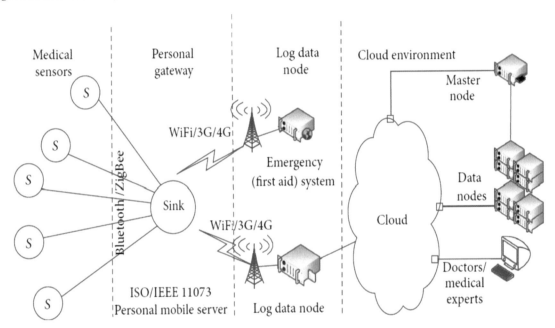

A wide number of research have been carried out in solving the problem of digitization in the era of healthcare sector (Behera, Sahoo, Naik, Rath, & Sahoo, 2021). Cloud service has been emerged as a promising technology in providing various healthcare related services over the Internet. It can reduce electronic healthcare cost which includes, networking, hardware, software, proprietary licenses etc. It has been observed from many literatures that bioinformatics sector is getting number of benefits in adopting serverless computing model (Regan, 2019)(Rausch, Rashed, & Dustdar, 2021). Biomedical industries are facing difficulties in meeting the deadline to fulfill the research objectives especially when analyzing vast amount of genome data and with computational resource which are expensive in nature. Serverless platform is emerged to right solution for solving many such problems in the era of healthcare sectors (Gupta, Phade, Courtade, & Ramchandran, 2020). Despite of number of benefits, it is associated with lots of challenges and issues in implementation which should be pointed out.

It can be observed from the literature that a number of framework for healthcare sectors have been emerged by the cloud vendors to provide better service in healthcare sector (Gan, et al., 2019)(Gunasekaran, Mishra, Thinakaran, Kandemir, & Das, 2020). Different deployment models like PaaS. IaaS and SaaS are proving different kinds of services to healthcare sector. Each of them are applied at diverse number of domains. One of the popular application in healthcare system is related to automate the process of patient data collection where IoT is integrated with cloud deployment models (Cheng, Fuerst, Solmaz, & Sanada, 2019)(Huang, Mi, & Hua, 2020). It has number of advantages such as, it reduces the overhead for manual collection of samples, eradicate the mistakes due to typing error and the ease of deployment. A separate set of cloud protocols have been developed to provide security for mobile and other multimedia devices (Kaffes, Yadwadkar, & Kozyrakis, 2019). A number of sensors can be planted on the mobile devices which will able to send the health-related information at the cloud. The cloud server can be used to store and process the data to extract the health behavior of user which can be send back to the client side to the healthcare personals for taking appropriate actions. The cloud framework has been used to provide immediate attention of doctor in a fraction of second which consequently improve the healthcare system. The layered architecture for integration of IoT based cloud architecture with the healthcare system is shown in Figure 3.

The layered architecture as shown in Figure 3 consist of numerous sensors to collect patient information using wireless protocols. The sensors can be used to measure the pulse rate, oxygen level, sugar level heart rate etc. Each of sensor collect various information and propagated toward the local area gateway using Bluetooth or the wireless protocols. Sometime the user's telephone can be used as the personal gateway which can be used to send the personal health related information to the cloud. The sensor resides on the mobile device periodically collect and send the data to the cloud which can be accessed by any legitimate users. The data collected through sensor can be put into the message queue which may have various health related parameters. Apart from the actual data, the message queue is required to have metadata which includes mobile IP address, location, destination logical address etc. It can be collected through cloud specific optimized algorithms. After processing the messages, the actual instruction or the recommendation can be generated for the patient or the other stake holders. The information from the cloud service may be compressed and secured to provide end to end encryption delivery, which can be displayed on the mobile devices of the user. A specific set of cloud services may be provided to the patient for intensive care. In addition to that, the doctors and care givers can have direct communication with the patient when required.

SERVERLESS COMPUTING FOR HEALTHCARE MANAGEMENT SYSTEM

The healthcare business is transitioning to value-based care, which necessitates the collection of new data. Costs must be minimized for healthcare services to be accessible to a growing number of people. All of this is feasible thanks to cutting-edge technologies like AI, machine learning, and serverless computing (Jonas, et al., 2019). The healthcare IT business can profit from serverless technology in a variety of ways. The pandemic-related events of 2020-21 have certainly changed how various industry sectors are thinking about digital transformation. A recent survey by McKinsey said that COVID-19's impact had accelerated digitalization to such an extent that some companies were reporting that their integration schedule had been brought forward by three to four years. According to McKinsey, this demonstrated an aggressive attitude to a required digital transformation, with healthcare proving to be one of the most eager industries for change. As a result of the pandemic, the survey noted, companies had seen demonstrated value in digital investments, citing smooth operations, faster service and better customer experience as reasons why digital was the way forward. If we take healthcare as the example, hospitals are introducing online appointment booking, tele-consultations (AKA tele-health), remote diagnosis, remote monitoring and the full-scale digitization of patient records, to name but a few. Insurance companies have also shifted to the digital world, with policy purchase, claim initiation, claim verification and approval – all available digitally. Both sides of the healthcare coin – providers and insurance – need an effective digital strategy, especially when you factor in time-to-market, lowering costs and ROI.

MAJOR CONCERNIN HEALTHCARE SYSTEM

In speaking to migrant health care corporations or deploying their solutions to the cloud, we learn that they are usually not sure about how to start a difficult transition journey. First, corporations measure the capabilities as well as the resources required for extending the cloud model solution. The conception of converting and dismantling the common answer into a fast-paced environment matters of concern. Second, corporations may be interested in maintaining and acquiring cloud compliance - particularly with regard to FDA CFR Part 11 and HIPAA - meanwhile not under the direct control of local virtual servers. Cost savings is the third one but not the last. Healthcare management systems rely upon the following three aspects which are used to address the above concerns:

Enhancing Speed of Delivery and Scalability

Serverless architecture possibly leading several advantages if you configure it properly. Serverless applications on the scale of the server that does not automatically supply with growing usage and demand. Additionally, in the case of a few two-week sprints, functionality and infrastructure can be provided in a cloud-based environment - usually through infrastructures such as a business logic, which represents providing and managing infrastructure with descriptive code that facilitates translation control, testing, and rollbacks. Such frameworks are AWS CloudFormation, Terraform, Pulumi, Azure Resource Manager, etc. Scalable serverless solutions might be utilized throughout the digital healthcare environment. For example, Medicare & Medicaid Services uses AWS Cloud services to host infrastructure that can handle hundreds of thousands of users at once. The corporations which are dealing with large data sets, the same powerful AWS features may be employed to build data repositories for better data collection, secure storage, and processing in an inexpensive way and analyzing large amounts of data.

Ensuring Compliance

Healthcare enters the digital train through programs such as collaborating with the goal of well-designed serverless cloud architectures. For proceedings as AWS, as an illustration, the main objective is having as many services as possible and no longer work while maintaining HIPAA along with other compliance. The AWS HIPAA program allows covered organizations — as well as business partners under the U.S. Health Insurance Portability and Accountability Act of 1996 (HIPAA) —to utilize the AWS secure environment to process, manage, and store protected health information (PHI). According to customer feedback, AWS is making attempt to add more services to the HIPAA system, which includes serverless techniques.

Cost Optimization

Because there is no requirement to configure and manage the infrastructure, clients may easily download and upgrade products, reduce costs and increase speed to live. Infrastructure is often extremely complex, and the monthly cost of repairing and repairing it is stagnant - and unacceptably high. While DevOps Vicert works to transform one of our clients' digital health solutions, they move to the cloud, resulting in significant improvements in time and durability as well as a significant reduction in care costs. The clients increased their monthly service time to 99.9% with experiencing a strong downtime in the application. By deployment on the cloud and using special serverless solutions (like AWS Lambda, Azure functions, open whisk, etc.), improved security and faster upgrades for both - results in savings, easier and faster deployment, higher reliability, as well as service expiration.

SERVERLESS ARCHITECTUREFOR HEALTHCARE MANAGEMENT SYSTEM

Figure 4. Serverless architecture for healthcare management system

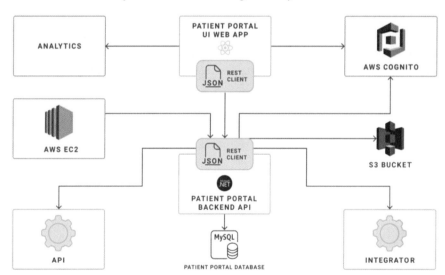

The serverless technologies rely on the most advanced services to provide the automatization, flexibility, and personalization most needed in the medical field. It can be adopted successfully in several different organizations - for product companies, from startups to businesses, and from payers to suppliers. Beneath the lid, serverless technology relies on portable servers but is managed by cloud vendors like IBM, Amazon, Google, Microsoft, etc., and not the company itself. It means that the procedure for the provision and storage of infrastructure remains separate from internal procedures. This separated concern is one of the principal reasons many fast-developing health tech solutions use serverless technologies. If they rely on the serverless model, the corporation can build and deploy applications without having to manage downtime and compromised infrastructure and related security. It is particularly significant as health care organizations expand applications to wider areas as well as most difficult correlations.

Therefore, speed, cost savings, repetition, and scaling are unfavorable to success. By taking an example of a patient portfolio application. In contrast to the traditional cloud framework, where serverless technology is used, the site might be managed by several services that are based on usage as well as demand. In addition, authentication can be used using managed authentication services, such as Cognito, while on the AWS Aurora Serverless, it can be used. The results are lower cost of easier maintenance, increased expansion, and building a portfolio. Various components of serverless healthcare management system is shown in Figure 4.

VARIOUS COMPONENTS FOR SERVERLESS FRAMEWORK FOR HEALTHCARE SYSTEM

Cloud platforms enable modern businesses to embrace agility and innovate. They allow businesses to experiment; quickly try out new ideas; and scale rapidly when an idea takes off. Just as importantly, their usage-based payment model makes it easy to decommission the ones that don't work. Try new things, see what works, and fail fast: the mantra of agile businesses. In the past, compliance and privacy issues slowed innovation in the healthcare industry. That is changing. Offerings from all of the large cloud vendors now support HIPAA (Health Insurance Portability and Accountability Act) and even HITRUST (Health Information Trust Alliance Common Security Framework), thus allowing companies to quickly assemble secure solutions from off-the-shelf components. It is easier than ever to build secure, compliant cloud applications that protect sensitive personal health information. Security and compliance are built into all of the major cloud platforms, allowing secure, scalable, and manageable products to be built on Microsoft's Azure, Google Cloud Platform (GCP), Amazon Web Services (AWS), and many of the other cloud platforms. Additionally, with interoperability between the platforms increasing, a best-of-breed approach leveraging components from two or more platforms is possible. However, for this article we are focused on our recent experience using AWS for a healthcare startup.

Data Storage

Data storage is at the core of most products and AWS offers quite a few ways of persisting data needed by an application (Amazon, 2015). We've found these solutions work well and are HIPAA compliant:

1. **DynamoDB** is a fully managed NoSQL database, with the ability to use key-value stores, document stores like JSON, and graph databases. While it is not HITRUST-certifiable, it is HIPAA-eligible. DynamoDB requires very little overhead and is extremely easy to use, especially with other AWS services (Sivasubramanian, 2012).
2. **Relational Database Services** (RDS) is a fully managed service that provides on-demand scalable, highly available relational database engines. RDS makes it easy to provision data stores to provide multi-tenant databases and master data. In addition, RDS has several database engines options, including Aurora DB, MySQL, PostgreSQL, Oracle, and MS SQL Server.
3. **Elasticache** for Redis is in-memory data storage for scaling web applications. It offers two flavors of in-memory data storage. In just one example, we have used Redis to store notifications while the user is off-line, so they are not lost. When the user returns to the system, the missed notifications are presented from Redis.

ServerlessIntegration

Serverless solutions free organizations and engineers from managing servers and frameworks and simplify compliance.

1. **API Gateway** is used to publish, maintain, and monitor API written on AWS Lambda. With API Gateway, transmitting PHI (Protected Health Information) to and from web servers is secure and encrypted.
2. **Lambda** is a serverless architecture used to run code without provisioning or managing servers. It allows digital solution engineers to quickly ship applications in a variety of languages including Node, .Net, Java, Python and more, without provisioning virtual machines and installing runtimes. Lambda also ensures PHI remains secure by using encrypted protocols such as HTTPS and by providing authentication and authorization support to the API Gateway itself.
3. **Amazon MQ** is a managed message queue broker for Apache ActiveMQ. Message queues enable applications to communicate asynchronously. Each system, regardless of platform or programing language, can integrate via a message queue in a broker. Amazon MQ allows easy configuration to provision Apache ActiveMQ on AWS.

Infrastructure Deployment and Monitoring

Managing solutions and data is every bit as critical to compliance as having secure technology building blocks. AWS offers a suite of solutions manage the deployment of components and monitor data access and usage.

1. **CloudWatch** is a monitoring and observability service used to set alarms, trigger action, discover insight, troubleshoot issues. CloudWatch is primarily used to monitor operational logs from various services running within this architecture (Schad, Dittrich, & Quiané-Ruiz, 2010).
2. **Terraform** is an open-source infrastructure as a code (IaC) tool used to deploy the solution infrastructure safely and repetitively across multiple environments (Brikman, 2019).
3. **Elastic Kubernetes Service** (EKS) is a fully managed Kubernetes service available on AWS that allows users to deploy, manage, and scale containerized **applications (Mulligan, 2020).**

HEALTHCARESERVICES WITH FUNCTION AS A SERVICE

Health care system need efficient distribution of services in fast and efficient manner. Health services include emergency service, diagnosis, analysis, preventive, home care etc. Each of these services should be patient centered and high quality. All the stakeholders include healthcare workers, hospitals, medical professional requires several serverless services at many scales based on their needs. Each serverless service may be provided as function as a service framework. Some of them are described as below:

Appointment Booking Service

Serverless framework can be used to develop web application through which services can be provided for booking the appointment. Healthcare service providers requires to have hipaa-compliant application which can be deployed and executed in scalable and cost-effective manner. AWS APIs gateway can be used to create and publish the services for any point of scale which should able to handle hundreds to thousands of API calls. It also provides another service like traffic management, access control, authorization to provide security to healthcare data. The core business logic for booking service application can be deployed in AWS Lambda which can be processed through either container or the Virtual machine.

Remote Monitoring Service

One way that COVID-19 has impacted the healthcare sector was through an increased requirement for remote patient monitoring. In this use case, smart health monitoring devices became a necessary part of patient care, albeit that these devices had to deal with the challenge of ingesting data at scale and processing that information in real-time to deliver urgent care to those infected. In the visual below, you can see the reference architecture for a remote patient monitoring system on AWS, which (again) provides serverless services and HIPPA Compliance.

Security Services

Privacy is one of the major concerns in healthcare sector especially when the data is exchanged between the stakeholders. Security services may be provided by the container in serverless environment which allows the software to be patched. The server without patch at the backend may leads to high security risk especially in healthcare services (Behera, Sahoo, Mahapatra, Rath, & Sahoo, 2018).

Ease of Access and Availability

Serverless is observed to be most promising solution in term of ease of access and availability of healthcare information. The Availability issues at any point of time may be challenging when the information is located at single server. This can be overcome by replicating multiple instances at several server. However, itmightleads to cost inefficient. In order to provide the cost effective, reliability and fault tolerant access, serverless architecture provide GB-Second pricing model. Serverless storage service keep the copy of instances at multiple data centers, which solve the problem of common source failure. DynamoDB database automatically backup and restore the data which makes available at any point of time (Sivasubramanian, 2012). Serverless framework also provide auto-scaling techniques which allow the clients to keep any amount of data at an ease.

Virtual Reality

VR has become a billion-dollar business. It is time that the healthcare industry jumps in on that too. Virtual reality helps patients deal with pain and suffering. VR can also be used to give a tour of the medical facilities. VR is a highly engaging technology and healthcare can benefit from it. So many people get anxious and worried about visiting a hospital, so giving them a tour of the procedure through VR can be really helpful.

Wearable

Wearable technology has come a long way. From wearing for fun to wearing for health tracking. People have started to take care of themselves seriously. Almost everyone has smart watches to track their physical activity. It also keeps a track of heart rate. Apple released 'Movement Disorder API' which can be helpful in getting insights into Parkinson's disease.

Voice Search

Voice Search has been helping patients with booking appointments and get rides for the hospital. Voice search works as a personal assistant for the patients. Young patients might not require this technology but it works like a miracle for the elderly. They can rely on it entirely. Nuance Communications is a US-based company that provides automated telephone directory services,speech recognition, and telephone call steering systems. So these are some of the technologies that are taking over the healthcare industry and helping out people. With the use of technology, every patient can get personalized attention. Technology has improved healthcare so far; in the future we will see more innovations in healthcare.

HEALTHCARE SYSTEM

Traditionally web applications were deployed on dedicated. For executing a standard web application users' request, it could be forwarded to the backend (server) wherein the application is deployed, after processing the request, the server might return a response to the users or clients. Moreover, it could be a database system executing upon either one or many data centers, servers, containers, etc. with handling the requirement of storage of utility. For enhancing traffic load and redundancy, load balancing can be utilized as a component of the framework. The role of a load balancer would be discovering those servers, in which the application is deployed, dropped, and redirected the service requests a long way off from it; along with it is also able to allocate service requests easily among numerous servers also.

Serverless Architecture for Web-Based Application for What is the Need of Serverless in Web-Based Application?

The Serverless paradigm eliminates the requirements for deploying applications on particular servers, also removes computer resource managers away from the engineers, and delegates the responsibility of external computer service vendors. Despite the term "serverless", the whole concept is still used in a group of servers, which is excluded. Since the functions are assigned to cloud vendors, it is not required to configure and manage servers. The serverless paradigm can be considered as the combination of BaaS (Backend as a service) and FaaS (Function as a service) (Jonas, et al., 2019). Backend as a service describes the applications which integrate services along with cloud-based applications, controlling the backend context (Mustafa, Nazir, Hayat, Madani, & others, 2015)(Popović & Hocenski, 2010). With Function as a service, well known as serverless functions, it is the responsibility of the developers to focus only on their business code.Serverless computing saves a lot because the vendors only charge for the duration it takes to complete each request. It can be concluded if a serverless application receive any requests, it will not cost for ideal capacity - a primary advantage to the standard cloud. In a serverless environment cloud vendors may take full advantage of their server configuration to have minimal downtime, they can transfer those cost savings to their users. In serverless computing, developers are permitted to develop, deploy and also execute the business logic without worrying about complicated infrastructure management procedures. It simplifies those developers are only responsible for developing business code that will be used in areas of health care at a faster rate, bringing technical advancement quickly.

ARCHITECTURE FOR SERVERLESS WEB BASED APPLICATION

The features of AWS Cognito can be leveraged to protect the web application. It provides authentication and security services to new as well as existing clients. It can be customized to scaling up the number of concurrent users. The customized interface at the edge of web application can be provided by Cloud-Front. CloudFront component of AWS service can be used as content delivery networks which process and deliver the content at various access points across the globe (Shackelford, 2015)(Tanna & Singh, 2018). It allows the user to access the content in less response time by storing the content near to the vicinity of the user even if the application hosted somewhere far away. Amazon storage service S3 can be used at the back end to store unstructured file such as image analysis, patient information in every interval etc(Mohan, et al., 2019). Serverless framework can also be used to perform all kinds of linear and non-linear data analysis which is crucial for healthcare sector. The architecture for web-based healthcare application which leveraged the feature of serverless framework is presented in Figure. 5.

The frontend part of the web application is managed by a Javascript tool known as VueJs(Younge, Von Laszewski, Wang, Lopez-Alarcon, & Carithers, 2010). It is found to be more efficient as compared to other tools as it allows the application to be processed in modular fashion. It breaks the functionality into simple and reusable modules. The web application allows to have static as well as dynamic domain. The construction of static domain is taken care by NuxtJs which perform over VueJs tools. It is integrated with Amazon S3 where static web application be hosted at a very low cost. However, It may depends on the size of the application. The beauty of AWS S3 is that it allows the application to be dynamic where various updates can be carried out over the time. Serverless architecture provide various APIs which can be used to download healthcare information and process them using Lambda function. The serverless function are usually called through REST API (Zhang, Zhu, Zhang, & Liu, 2019). Apart from the AWS S3, Dynamo DB is also integrated at the backend to handle large amount of structured data which may be obtained in the form of Relational table or the XML format. It is same as the serverless NOSQL database.

The overall processing of the web application is carried out by the Lambda operations which are the major part of Function as a service or the serverless functions. Any request from the client needs to pass through API gateways which is used to trigger the event. Whenever an event is triggered, the corresponding function is activated and executed to perform the action. The updates in static file is sent to DynamoDB where the updated reated to graph analysis is sent to AWS S3 storage. The Lambda function in this architecture may related to perform sorting, searching, analyzing the healthcare information stored in either DynamoDB or AWS S3. It also allows the health workers to upload the patient data and stored them at the backend and after performing the analysis the resultant graphs can be shown to authentic people using AWS Cognito. It can be shown on application analysis page for better interaction. The processing steps in healthcare web application are shown in Figure 6.

Figure 5. Serverless framework for web-based application

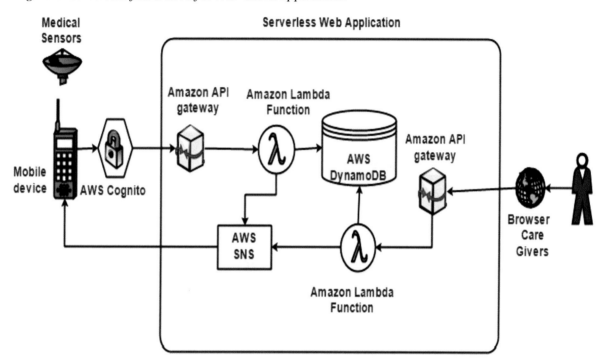

CASE STUDIES OF SERVERLESS APPLICATION FOR HEALTHCARE SYSTEM

Case Study I: Fast Healthcare Interoperability Resources (FHIR)

Fast Healthcare interoperability resources (FHIR) is one of the elegant digitized solutions for managing and exchanging healthcare related information between various parties in secure manner. It ensures the privacy and ease of accessibility to the legitimate stake holders of healthcare systems. One of the serverless vendor i.e., AWS provides serverless platform for integrating API for FHIR interfaces. It allows the developers to access number of resource types and operations. It also provides various architecture pattern to develop integration of other solution to the existing healthcare solution. Serverless framework for FHIR allow the users (healthcare providers, vendors, developers etc.) to access patient and healthcare data from any kind of interfaces such as various browser, mobile device, laptop from any corner of the world. This solution also provides customized AWS APIS to tune the parameters based on the requirements of the organization. The prototypes of the solution need to be deployed in the serverless environment to access the storage services like S3, Dynamo DM etc. through FHIR API. The healthcare services can be obtained through several Lambda functions which can be invoked through AWS APIs. The processing steps along with various components for FHIT is presented in Figure 6.

Figure 6. Serverless configuration for FHIR messaging interface

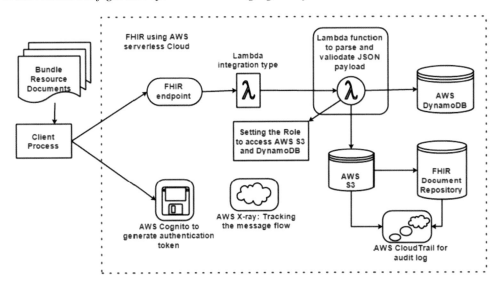

The serverless pattern deployed by Amazon's CloudFormation tools can be used to provide services for FHIR request through APIS. The following components are provided to serve different kind of services as follows:

1. Amazon Cognito pools are used to provide authentication by verifying the user's identity and the group it belongs to.
2. Amazon APIs are provided to routing the request towards the Lambda function which can be invoked by the event a trigger.
3. Two very specified AWS Lambda functions are used in the serverless solution for FHIR. One of them is used to process the FHIR request by routing the path towards the storage services like Amazon S3 to store unstructured data, DynamoDB services to create, delete, update operation on healthcare data or to OpenSearch Service to indexing the search process for faster access by the stack holders. The other Lambda function is used to read the updates and make changes in the indexing component.
4. The DynamoDB storage unit is used to store all the unstructured healthcare data. Whenever any updates are carried out the DynamoDB, the same is reflected back to the OpenSearch service. Sometimes Amazon's S3 is used to store binary data from healthcare resource such as X-ray or any ECG graphs etc (Sivasubramanian, 2012).
5. The indexing and the search process for the incoming request from FHIR APIs are provided by Amazon OpenSearch service.
6. Various Key management services are used to encrypt all the storage components like S3, DynamoDB or the OpenSearch service.
7. The CloudWatch service from the Amazon is used to log all API requests from the stakeholders of healthcare system.

Case Study II: IoT Based Remote Monitoring System Using Serverless Architecture

A number of healthcare applications has been integrated with IoT which leveraged the features of serverless frameworks (Al-Masri, Diabate, Jain, Lam, & Nathala, 2018) (Adzic & Chatley, 2017). In traditional hospitals (and hospice situations), patients come into the hospital or doctor's office when they are not feeling well or, in a worst-case scenario, they need urgent care and are brought directly into Emergency. Digital wearable devices such as smartwatches, digital blood pressure and weight scales have made it possible for patients to self-diagnose problems long before they become urgent cases that require emergency care. However, self-diagnosis can be dangerous, and it is always preferable to have doctors view remote sensor data and perform diagnosis prior to clinic or hospital admittance. The challenge is to make such data available to doctors in real-time. The patients will typically be engaged in their daily tasks in a non-hospital environment (either at home/work or in a senior facility, for example). The future of cardiovascular care is envisioned in the following way by experts in the delivery of such care:

1. Incorporating remote monitoring for cardiovascular patients, using devices that record vital signs, heart rhythms like atrial fibrillation, coronary artery disease detecting heart blockages, and congestive heart failure symptoms, without being in the office or hospital.
2. Enabled by IoT and Cloud Technology, these remote physiologic monitors in conjunction with best practices at the clinic, have the potential to reduce patient hospitalizations and improve care.

This case study consists of number of cloud-based IoT device which has been integrated on AWS, which includes device transmitter code that simulates heart rates at the patient location, and sends the data to the AWS Cloud, where the data is stored in a NoSQL database, anomalies are detected in real-time via Streams processing, and results can be displayed in a dashboard at the doctor's office. Archival for offline analytics is also made available. The integration of IoT and serverless framework for Remote health monitoring system is presented in Figure 7.

Components for Remote Monitoring System

The solution comprises the following:

- A front-end simulator program creates data by emulating a 'sensor'
- The sensor information will comprise the device details (unique identifier for the patient and device) and heart rate readings
- This data will feed into the AWS IoT Core at predefined intervals
- Based on the rules defined, data will be sent downstream to trigger various real-time events such as email notifications where applicable
- Downstream data will be partitioned and sorted into a NoSQL database table, which will be used to enable rapid storage and retrieval of time-series information, and to allow for critical decision-making in near-real time. Goal is to pay attention to scalability, availability, and reliability
- Based on the defined rules, real-time data will be routed to Kinesis Streams, where Kinesis Stream Application will sort data streams based on high and low heart rate and route to a separate Lambda

function for real-time SNS and email notifications. Routed real-time sorted streams will be stored in a separate table in the NoSQL database.

- Dashboards will display the patient wise readings and will be designed to be made available to administrators with authorized access, for insights and action.
- Downstream data will also be sent via an alternative path for archival and offline analytics with secure access as needed by medical personnel for research and regulatory purposes.

Figure 7. Integration of IoT and serverless in remote health monitoring system

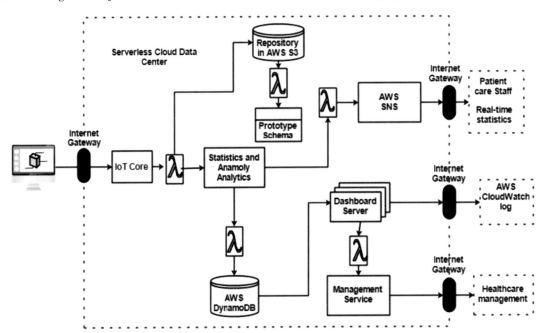

CONCLUSION

Serverless is has been emerging as a promising solution for maintaining digitized environment in healthcare sector where several healthcare services can be provided in low cost and faster response time. Serverless provider may have various types of services based on the client requirement such as on-demand, on-reserve or the instance services. Healthcare sector popularly use on-demand service model of serverless which can handle the peak load at any point of time. It may be noted that different application in healthcare system like ECG, EEG, E-blood analysis etc. requires different pricing model. In this chapter, the serverless architecture for healthcare system is presented. Two case studies related to healthcare system such as Remote monitoring system and Fast Healthcare Interoperability Resources (FHIR) interface are presented which abundantly use the services from various serverless vendors like Amazon, IBM, Microsoft etc. In the present day, serverless architecture is found to be an efficient framework to provide various healthcare services. However, it poses a number of challenges in integrating IoT with serverless in healthcare system. As the serverless framework rely on number of independent stateless functions, they failed to communicate each other by exchanging data which is one of the major concern in healthcare management system. Another challenge in serverless healthcare management system lies in maintaining the tradeoff between cost and deadline of various healthcare applications. Although it poses various challenges, it has been emerging as potential tool for handling various services in healthcare system, the identified research challenges may be considered as one of the research directions in the era of serverless framework in healthcare system.

REFERENCES

Adzic, G., & Chatley, R. (2017). Serverless computing: economic and architectural impact. *Proceedings of the 2017 11th joint meeting on foundations of software engineering*, 884–889. 10.1145/3106237.3117767

Al-Masri, E., Diabate, I., Jain, R., Lam, M. H., & Nathala, S. R. (2018). A serverless IoT architecture for smart waste management systems. *2018 IEEE International Conference on Industrial Internet (ICII)*, 179–180. 10.1109/ICII.2018.00034

Al-Roomi, M., Al-Ebrahim, S., Buqrais, S., & Ahmad, I. (2013). Cloud computing pricing models: A survey. *International Journal of Grid and Distributed Computing*, 6(5), 93–106. doi:10.14257/ijgdc.2013.6.5.09

Amazon, E. C. (2015). *Amazon web services*. Available in: Error! Hyperlink reference not valid.

Baldini, I., Castro, P., Chang, K., Cheng, P., Fink, S., & Ishakian, V. (2017). Serverless computing: Current trends and open problems. In Research Advances in Cloud Computing (pp. 1–20). Springer.

Behera, R. K., Jena, M., Rath, S. K., & Misra, S. (2021). Co-LSTM: Convolutional LSTM model for sentiment analysis in social big data. *Information Processing & Management*, 58(1), 102435. doi:10.1016/j.ipm.2020.102435

Behera, R. K., & Rath, S. K. (2016). An efficient modularity-based algorithm for community detection in social network. *Internet of Things and Applications (IOTA), International Conference on*, 162–167. 10.1109/IOTA.2016.7562715

Behera, R. K., Sahoo, K. S., Mahapatra, S., Rath, S. K., & Sahoo, B. (2018). Security issues in distributed computation for big data analytics. In *Handbook of e-Business Security* (pp. 167–190). Auerbach Publications. doi:10.1201/9780429468254-7

Behera, R. K., Sahoo, K. S., Naik, D., Rath, S. K., & Sahoo, B. (2021). Structural Mining for Link Prediction Using Various Machine Learning Algorithms. *International Journal of Social Ecology and Sustainable Development*, 12(3), 66–78. doi:10.4018/IJSESD.2021070105

Bienko, C. D., Greenstein, M., Holt, S. E., Phillips, R. T., & ... (2015). *IBM Cloudant: Database as a Service Advanced Topics*. IBM Redbooks.

Bila, N., Dettori, P., Kanso, A., Watanabe, Y., & Youssef, A. (2017). Leveraging the serverless architecture for securing linux containers. *2017 IEEE 37th International Conference on Distributed Computing Systems Workshops (ICDCSW)*, 401–404. 10.1109/ICDCSW.2017.66

Brenner, S., & Kapitza, R. (2019). Trust more, serverless. *Proceedings of the 12th ACM International Conference on Systems and Storage*, 33–43. 10.1145/3319647.3325825

Brikman, Y. (2019). *Terraform: Up & Running: Writing Infrastructure as Code*. O'Reilly Media.

Carreira, J., Fonseca, P., Tumanov, A., Zhang, A., & Katz, R. (2018). A case for serverless machine learning. *Workshop on Systems for ML and Open-Source Software at NeurIPS*.

Cheng, B., Fuerst, J., Solmaz, G., & Sanada, T. (2019). Fog function: Serverless fog computing for data intensive iot services. *2019 IEEE International Conference on Services Computing (SCC)*, 28–35. 10.1109/SCC.2019.00018

Christoforou, A., & Andreou, A. S. (2018). An effective resource management approach in a FaaS environment. ESSCA@ UCC, 2–8.

Crespo-Cepeda, R., Agapito, G., Vazquez-Poletti, J. L., & Cannataro, M. (2019). Challenges and opportunies of amazon serverless lambda services in bioinformatics. *Proceedings of the 10th ACM International Conference on Bioinformatics, Computational Biology and Health Informatics*, 663–668. 10.1145/3307339.3343462

Cusumano, M. (2010). Cloud computing and SaaS as new computing platforms. *Communications of the ACM*, *53*(4), 27–29. doi:10.1145/1721654.1721667

Dalbhanjan, P. (2015). *Overview of deployment options on aws*. Amazon Whitepapers.

Fox, A., Griffith, R., Joseph, A., Katz, R., Konwinski, A., & Lee, G. (2009). *Above the clouds: A Berkeley view of cloud computing*. Dept. Electrical Eng. and Comput. Sciences, University of California, Berkeley, Rep. UCB/EECS, 28, 2009.

Gadepalli, P. K., Peach, G., Cherkasova, L., Aitken, R., & Parmer, G. (2019). Challenges and opportunities for efficient serverless computing at the edge. *2019 38th Symposium on Reliable Distributed Systems (SRDS)*, 261–2615. 10.1109/SRDS47363.2019.00036

Gan, Y., Zhang, Y., Cheng, D., Shetty, A., Rathi, P., & Katarki, N. (2019). An open-source benchmark suite for microservices and their hardware-software implications for cloud & edge systems. *Proceedings of the Twenty-Fourth International Conference on Architectural Support for Programming Languages and Operating Systems*, 3–18. 10.1145/3297858.3304013

Golec, M., Ozturac, R., Pooranian, Z., Gill, S. S., & Buyya, R. (2021). iFaaSBus: A security and privacy based lightweight framework for serverless computing using IoT and machine learning. *IEEE Transactions on Industrial Informatics*.

Gunasekaran, J. R., Mishra, C. S., Thinakaran, P., Kandemir, M. T., & Das, C. R. (2020). Implications of Public Cloud Resource Heterogeneity for Inference Serving. *Proceedings of the 2020 Sixth International Workshop on Serverless Computing*, 7–12. 10.1145/3429880.3430093

Gupta, V., Phade, S., Courtade, T., & Ramchandran, K. (2020). *Utility-based Resource Allocation and Pricing for Serverless Computing*. arXiv preprint arXiv:2008.07793.

Hall, A., & Ramachandran, U. (2019). An execution model for serverless functions at the edge. *Proceedings of the International Conference on Internet of Things Design and Implementation*, 225–236. 10.1145/3302505.3310084

Hendrickson, S., Sturdevant, S., Harter, T., Venkataramani, V., Arpaci-Dusseau, A. C., & Arpaci-Dusseau, R. H. (2016). Serverless computation with openlambda. *8th USENIX Workshop on Hot Topics in Cloud Computing (HotCloud 16)*.

Hong, S., Srivastava, A., Shambrook, W., & Dumitraș, T. (2018). Go serverless: Securing cloud via serverless design patterns. *10th USENIX Workshop on Hot Topics in Cloud Computing (HotCloud 18)*.

Huang, Z., Mi, Z., & Hua, Z. (2020). HCloud: A trusted JointCloud serverless platform for IoT systems with blockchain. *China Communications*, *17*(9), 1–10. doi:10.23919/JCC.2020.09.001

Ivan, C., Vasile, R., & Dadarlat, V. (2019). Serverless computing: An investigation of deployment environments for web apis. *Computers*, *8*(2), 50. doi:10.3390/computers8020050

Jain, N., & Menache, I. (2016, September). *Resource management for cloud computing platforms*. Google Patents.

Jangda, A., Pinckney, D., Brun, Y., & Guha, A. (2019). Formal foundations of serverless computing. *Proceedings of the ACM on Programming Languages*, *3*, 1–26.

Jonas, E., Schleier-Smith, J., Sreekanti, V., Tsai, C.-C., Khandelwal, A., & Pu, Q. (2019). *Cloud programming simplified: A berkeley view on serverless computing*. arXiv preprint arXiv:1902.03383.

Kaewkasi, C. (2018). *Docker for Serverless Applications. In Containerize and orchestrate functions using OpenFaas, OpenWhisk, and Fn.* Packt Publishing Ltd.

Kaffes, K., Yadwadkar, N. J., & Kozyrakis, C. (2019). Centralized core-granular scheduling for serverless functions. *Proceedings of the ACM Symposium on Cloud Computing*, 158–164. 10.1145/3357223.3362709

Khandelwal, A., Kejariwal, A., & Ramasamy, K. (2020). Le Taureau: Deconstructing the Serverless Landscape & A Look Forward. *Proceedings of the 2020 ACM SIGMOD International Conference on Management of Data*, 2641–2650. 10.1145/3318464.3383130

Kim, J., & Lee, K. (2019). Functionbench: A suite of workloads for serverless cloud function service. *2019 IEEE 12th International Conference on Cloud Computing (CLOUD)*, 502–504) 10.1109/CLOUD.2019.00091

Korhonen, M. (2017). *Analyzing Resource Usage on Multitenant Cloud Cluster for Invoicing*. University Of Oulu, Faculty Of Information Technology And Electrical Engineering.

Kumanov, D., Hung, L.-H., Lloyd, W., & Yeung, K. Y. (2018). *Serverless computing provides on-demand high performance computing for biomedical research*. arXiv preprint arXiv:1807.11659.

Kumari, A., Behera, R. K., Sahoo, B., & Sahoo, S. P. (2022). Prediction of link evolution using community detection in social network. *Computing*, *104*(5), 1–22. doi:10.100700607-021-01035-4

Kumari, A., Sahoo, B., Behera, R. K., Misra, S., & Sharma, M. M. (2021). Evaluation of Integrated Frameworks for Optimizing QoS in Serverless Computing. *International Conference on Computational Science and Its Applications*, 277–288. 10.1007/978-3-030-87007-2_20

Lakhan, A., Khoso, F. H., Arain, A. A., & Kanwar, K. (2021). Serverless based functions aware framework for healthcare application. *International Journal (Toronto, Ont.)*, 9.

Malawski, M., Gajek, A., Zima, A., Balis, B., & Figiela, K. (2020). Serverless execution of scientific workflows: Experiments with hyperflow, aws lambda and google cloud functions. *Future Generation Computer Systems*, *110*, 502–514. doi:10.1016/j.future.2017.10.029

Manvi, S. S., & Shyam, G. K. (2014). Resource management for Infrastructure as a Service (IaaS) in cloud computing: A survey. *Journal of Network and Computer Applications*, *41*, 424–440. doi:10.1016/j.jnca.2013.10.004

McGrath, G., & Brenner, P. R. (2017). Serverless computing: Design, implementation, and performance. *2017 IEEE 37th International Conference on Distributed Computing Systems Workshops (ICDCSW)*, 405–410. 10.1109/ICDCSW.2017.36

Mistry, C., Stelea, B., Kumar, V., & Pasquier, T. (n.d.). *Demonstrating the Practicality of Unikernels to Build a Serverless Platform at the Edge*. Academic Press.

Mohan, A., Sane, H., Doshi, K., Edupuganti, S., Nayak, N., & Sukhomlinov, V. (2019). Agile cold starts for scalable serverless. *11th USENIX Workshop on Hot Topics in Cloud Computing (HotCloud 19)*.

Mulligan, D. (2020). *Results tracker app and deployment on EKS*. Elastic Kubernetes Service.

Mustafa, S., Nazir, B., Hayat, A., Madani, S. A., & ... (2015). Resource management in cloud computing: Taxonomy, prospects, and challenges. *Computers & Electrical Engineering*, *47*, 186–203. doi:10.1016/j.compeleceng.2015.07.021

Popović, K., & Hocenski, Ž. (2010). Cloud computing security issues and challenges. *The 33rd international convention mipro*, 344–349.

Rajan, R. A. (2018). Serverless architecture-a revolution in cloud computing. *2018 Tenth International Conference on Advanced Computing (ICoAC)*, 88–93. 10.1109/ICoAC44903.2018.8939081

Rausch, T., Rashed, A., & Dustdar, S. (2021). Optimized container scheduling for data-intensive serverless edge computing. *Future Generation Computer Systems*, *114*, 259–271. doi:10.1016/j.future.2020.07.017

Regan, G. (2019). A serverless architecture for wireless body area network applications. *Model-Based Safety and Assessment: 6th International Symposium, IMBSA 2019, Thessaloniki, Greece, October 16–18, 2019 Proceedings*, *11842*, 239.

Rimal, B. P., Choi, E., & Lumb, I. (2009). A taxonomy and survey of cloud computing systems. *2009 Fifth International Joint Conference on INC, IMS and IDC*, 44–51. 10.1109/NCM.2009.218

Ristov, S., Pedratscher, S., & Fahringer, T. (2021). AFCL: An Abstract Function Choreography Language for serverless workflow specification. *Future Generation Computer Systems*, *114*, 368–382. doi:10.1016/j.future.2020.08.012

Schad, J., Dittrich, J., & Quiané-Ruiz, J.-A. (2010). Runtime measurements in the cloud: Observing, analyzing, and reducing variance. *Proceedings of the VLDB Endowment International Conference on Very Large Data Bases, 3*(1-2), 460–471. doi:10.14778/1920841.1920902

Sewak, M., & Singh, S. (2018). Winning in the era of serverless computing and function as a service. *2018 3rd International Conference for Convergence in Technology (I2CT)*, 1–5. 10.1109/I2CT.2018.8529465

Shackelford, A. (2015). CloudFront and DNS Management. In Beginning Amazon Web Services with Node. In JS (pp. 93–120). Springer.

Shafiei, H., Khonsari, A., & Mousavi, P. (2019). *Serverless computing: A survey of opportunities, challenges and applications.* arXiv preprint arXiv:1911.01296.

Shahrad, M., Balkind, J., & Wentzlaff, D. (2019). Architectural implications of function-as-a-service computing. *Proceedings of the 52nd Annual IEEE/ACM International Symposium on Microarchitecture*, 1063–1075. 10.1145/3352460.3358296

Singh, C., Gaba, N. S., Kaur, M., & Kaur, B. (2019). Comparison of different CI/CD tools integrated with cloud platform. *2019 9th International Conference on Cloud Computing, Data Science & Engineering (Confluence)*, 7–12. 10.1109/CONFLUENCE.2019.8776985

Sivasubramanian, S. (2012). Amazon dynamoDB: a seamlessly scalable non-relational database service. *Proceedings of the 2012 ACM SIGMOD International Conference on Management of Data*, 729–730. 10.1145/2213836.2213945

Tanna, M., & Singh, H. (2018). *Serverless Web Applications with React and Firebase: Develop real-time applications for web and mobile platforms.* Packt Publishing Ltd.

Thirunavukkarasu, G. S., Champion, B., Horan, B., Seyedmahmoudian, M., & Stojcevski, A. (2018). Iot-based system health management infrastructure as a service. *Proceedings of the 2018 International Conference on Cloud Computing and Internet of Things*, 55–61. 10.1145/3291064.3291070

Van Eyk, E., Toader, L., Talluri, S., Versluis, L., Uţă, A., & Iosup, A. (2018). Serverless is more: From paas to present cloud computing. *IEEE Internet Computing, 22*(5), 8–17. doi:10.1109/MIC.2018.053681358

Younge, A. J., Von Laszewski, G., Wang, L., Lopez-Alarcon, S., & Carithers, W. (2010). Efficient resource management for cloud computing environments. *International conference on green computing*, 357–364. 10.1109/GREENCOMP.2010.5598294

Zhang, M., Zhu, Y., Zhang, C., & Liu, J. (2019). Video processing with serverless computing: a measurement study. *Proceedings of the 29th ACM Workshop on Network and Operating Systems Support for Digital Audio and Video*, 61–66. 10.1145/3304112.3325608

Chapter 12
An Approach on Image Steganography Based on the Least Significant Bit Algorithm

Karthik Chelakkara Murugan
CHRIST University (Deemed), India

Debabrata Samanta
ⓘ https://orcid.org/0000-0003-4118-2480
CHRIST University (Deemed), India

Mausumi Goswami
CHRIST University (Deemed), India

ABSTRACT

Steganography is the practice of communication by covering information within other information mediums. The goal of steganography is to hide information in such a way that it remains hidden so that it looks normal from a commoner's perspective. It has been prevalent since ancient times, with the first use dating back to 440 BC in Greece. The etymology of steganography is a combination of the Greek words: steganos, "covered," and graphia, "writing." The modern usage of steganography, termed digital steganography, hides information in files stored on a computer. A standard steganography algorithm has three essential components: carrier, message, and key. Carrier is the file that carries the message and an optional key to add a layer of authentication. Researchers have implemented steganography utilizing different carriers, for example, image, audio, and text. The carrier may or may not have any relation with the confidential information. Image steganography is a type of steganography that deals with hiding a message in an image file. The image, as a result, ends up with noise.

DOI: 10.4018/978-1-6684-4580-8.ch012

INTRODUCTION

In this research paper, an automated steganography detection system is proposed that can collect and detect steganography images shared in Social Networking Service Instant Messengers (SNS IMs).In the "Background and Related Works" section, the paper describes the traditional botnets and the difference between traditional botnets and stego-botnets (steganography-based botnets).There are 3 different types of Traditional Botnets described in the paper(A. A. Lopez-Hernandez et al. 2020), (A. H. S. Saad et al. 2021).IRC Botnets: Early botnets, based on the Internet Relay Chat model. HTTP Botnets: Botnets based on the HTTP architecture(Y. Zhang et al. 2020), (Yildirim, Melih et al. 2021), (Z. Zhang et al. 2020). More difficult to detect the communication due to large amount of HTTP traffic.P2P Botnets: Botnets based on P2P architecture. Communication in this type can take place between 2 bots, and the communication can also take place between the individual bots and the Bot Master(A. S. Ansari et al. 2020), (Abd El-Latif, Ahmed A., et al. 2020). In all the Traditional Botnets, there exists a Bot Master, and the commands are sent by the Bot Master and executed by bots in the individual devices. Steganography-Based Botnets is a novel Botnet system where the control and communication take place with commands hidden in multimedia(Abdulkudhur Mohammed et al. 2021), (AlKhodaidi et al. 2021). Since the communication is hidden, the confidentiality of the botnet is improved. In this model, the Bot Master sends commands through a steganography file in an SNS IM environment, and the message is received to the bot in the device, and the communication also takes place vice versa(Ashraf, Zubair, et al. 2020), (Dalal et al. 2021), (Elshoush, Huwaida T., et al. 2022).

DESIGN OF THE PROPOSED SYSTEM

The proposed system is designed in two phases:

1. Automated Collection System
2. Automated Detection System

Automated Collection System: In this phase, a stego-bot master sends the image files in an SNS IM, and is received by the end-user. This then is stored in the internal storage, and collected in an "Inspection Server", after which we move onto the next phase. An SNS IM chatroom is set up in KakaoTalk Instant Messenger application. The smartphone, also termed "Defender" joins the chatroom(Eyssa, Asmaa Abdelmonem, et al. 2020), (Fu, Zhangjie, et al. 2020). Then, the images are sent randomly to the chatroom at some set intervals of time (120 min) to the KakaoTalk chatroom. These images then are stored in the internal storage of the Defender device(G. F. Siddiqui et al. 2020), (Gutub et al. 2020), (Gutub et al. 2020). The storage location is found, and the images are stored in hex format, which is then converted to .png or .jpg after the extension of the file is determined using the Hex Editor. After converting the images to .jpg and .png format, the images are sent to the "Inspection Server". This is done by using a synchronisation application known as FolderSync. This application synchronises the internal storage and moves the files to PC(Hsieh et al. 2022), (J. Cui et al. 2021), (J. Liu et al. 2020). Therefore, Automated Collection Component is completed.

Automated Detection System: The images that have been moved to the Inspection Server are checked individually for steganographic messages hidden in them, and the output is given based on whether the messages exist or not. Once the image files are moved to the Inspection Server, the ADC examines whether the collected image files contain hidden steganography messages(J. R. Jayapandiyan et al. 2020), (J. Zhang et al. 2022), (Karthikeyan, N., et al. 2021). The ADC is implemented using the Python programming language, and the libraries utilised for steganography detection are Stegano, and Crypto steganography(Ke et al. 2021), (L. Zhou et al. 2020), (Li, Fengyong, et al. 2022). The detection is found to be easily scalable, as more libraries can be added with the addition to the ADC(L. Zhou et al. 2020), (Li, Fengyong, et al. 2022). The ADC finds steganography image files from the collected files. For each image file, the ADC checks whether a hidden message can be extracted from the image file. After inspection, the ADC displays the results periodically. The results show whether there are any hidden messages with a "Y" or "N" for yes/no, and if "yes", the hidden message is displayed if it can be extracted by the ADC.

FLOW OF EXECUTION

Flowchart for Automated Collection Component and Automated Detection Component. Figure 1 shows the flow of the Automated Collection Component.

Figure 1. Automated collection component

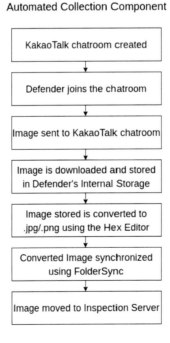

Automated Collection Component

Below Figure 2 shows Automated Detection Component

Figure 2. Automated detection component

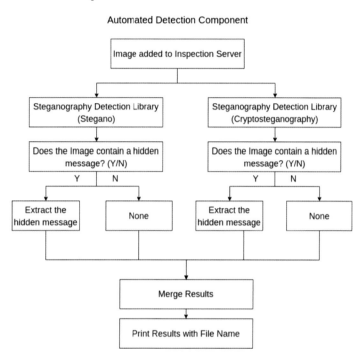

This part of the implementation phase checks each image sent to the Inspection Server and checks for any hidden messages in the image, using Python Programming language and two steganography libraries, Stegano and Cryptosteganography (Qi, Baojun, et al. 2020), (Reshma, V. K., et al. 2020), (Rustad, Supriadi, et al. 2021). The detection is shown to be easily scalable, and more libraries can be implemented in the ADC.

Implementation of the Proposed System

Here are the system details:

- SNS IM: KakaoTalk Instant Messenger
- Device: Samsung Galaxy S10
- Inspection Server: Lenovo Ideapad
- Synchronisation application: FolderSync
- Steganography detection libraries: Stegano, Cryptosteganography
- Stegano-Images: 4 PNG by Stegano, 4 BMP by Cryptosteganography
- Programming Language: Python3

Experimental Results and Analysis

Among the images that were added, the libraries detected that the images contained hidden messages.

Result: For all steganography image files, both libraries displayed "Y". For messages hidden by Stegano, Cryptosteganography failed to extract the message. For messages hidden by Cryptosteganography, Stegano failed to extract the message. Therefore, their model was successful, since the displayed output was the same as what was embedded onto the image file(Li, Li, et al. 2021), (Li, Qi, et al. 2021). This part of the implementation phase involves with collection of steganography images and transfer of the images from a defender to the Inspection Server(M. Sharifzadeh et al. 2020), (Mukherjee, Subhadip, et al.2021).

1. **Chatroom Creation:** A chatroom is created on the SNS. The SNS used in this implementation is KakaoTalk. This is the start of the implementation phase, and the stego-images will be sent to it.
2. **Defender Joins:** The Defender joins the chatroom via their preferred device (smartphone or PC). The device used for the implementation in the paper is Samsung Galaxy S10 5G. This is where the images will be downloaded and stored.
3. **Image Sending Process:** An image is sent to the chatroom. The Defender views the images. These images will be detected for steganography messages hidden.
4. **Image Download and Location Detection:** The image sent to the chatroom is downloaded and stored in the Defender's Internal Storage. The location is found to be at "Internal storage/Android/data/com.kakao.talk/contents/Mg==" (N. Subramanian et al. 2021), (N. Subramanian et al. 2021), (Pattanaik, Balachandra, et al. 2021). This location will be synced with a PC to send it to the Inspection Server.
5. **Conversion to .PNG/.JPG Image:** The image stored is initially in a hex format with no extension. The image is converted to a .jpg/.png file by locating the extension in the Hex Editor(Pramanik, Sabyasachi, et al. 2020), (Pustokhina, Irina V., et al.2022), (Q. Li et al., 2020). (Ex: JFIF implies that the extension is .jpg)
6. **Image Synchronization:** The converted image (.png/.jpg) is synchronized using FolderSync, which sends the images to the Inspection Server.
7. **Image Moved to Inspection Server:** The image is finally moved to the Inspection Server using the synchronization application (FolderSync), periodically, whenever a connection is available.
8. **Image Added to Inspection Server:** Image is added to the Inspection Server. The Automated Detection Component finds the image and checks for steganography. The implementation is based on 2 Steganography libraries in Python, Stegano and Cryptosteganography.

Detection Process

1. **Stegano:**
   a. **Steganography Detection Library (Stegano):** The image is checked by the library Stegano. This library checks for images with plain-text messages and decrypts the plain-text message if it finds a hidden message(S. Dhawan et al. 2021), (S. E. El-Khamy et al. 2020).
   b. **Message Detection:** If the image contains a hidden message, the ADC outputs the character "Y", which denotes a hidden message.
   c. **Message Extraction:** If a message exists, the program extracts the message. If the message is encrypted using steganography, the encrypted message is extracted without decrypting it.

2. Cryptosteganography
   a. **Steganography Detection Library (Cryptosteganography):** The library Cryptosteganography checks the image. This library checks for images with hidden messages. This library can only extract cryptographic messages and decrypt them.
   b. **Message Detection:** If the image contains a hidden message, the ADC outputs the character "Y", which denotes a hidden message.
   c. **Message Extraction:** If a message exists, the ADC extracts it. If the message is in plain-text, Cryptosteganography fails to extract it, and the output is set to "Unknown".
3. OUTPUT PROCESS:
   a. **Merge Results:** The libraries' results of the steganography check are merged.
   b. **Print Results:** The merged results are printed with the file name that the ADC has checked.

HOW STEGANOGRPAHY IS BETTER

In terms of confidentiality, Steganography is better than cryptography since an intruder would not know that communication is occurring, and it is harder to detect. Cryptography techniques, no matter how robust, can be intercepted, and using steganography, the communication can be made harder to detect(Sabeti, Vajiheh, et al. 2022), (Sahu, Aditya Kumar, et al. 2021). In addition to this, Steganography can be employed on other file types as well, such as audio, video, text and image files. This technology is best used in the field of digital watermarking, where the ownership of a file can be confirmed by embedding a message onto the file(Sharma, Himani, et al. 2021), (Sharma et al. 2021), (Sharma, Vijay Kumar, et al. 2022).Whenever required, one can check if the message is embedded onto the file by decoding it.If this technology is coupled with cryptography, the confidentiality of the data would potentially be drastically increased(Shashikiran, B. S., et al. 2021), (Sukumar, Arunkumar, et al. 2021), (Tan, Lei, et al. 2020). This can be achieved by encrypting the message using cryptography, then embedding the encrypted message onto a multimedia file.In the above case, a steganography file would be an attacker would not only have to realise that communication is occurring but also extract the encrypted message from the file, and then decrypt it as well(W. Lu et al. 2021), (W. Su et al. 2021), (X. Ding et al. 2020). The security of the message increases manifolds this way.

MATHEMATICAL FORMULAE RELATED TO STEGANOGRAPHY

Standard Steganography Embedding Process

$C * K * M \rightarrow S, S = Embed(C, K, M)$

Where:
C – Cover
M – Message
K – Key (optional, can be set to null if not required)
S – Stego-file

Standard Steganography Extraction Scheme

Extract(S, K) = M

Where:
    C – Cover
    M – Message
    K – Key (optional, can be set to null if not required)
    S – Stego-file

LSB Steganography

$$r_{ij} = \frac{r_{ij}}{2} + m_k, \mathrm{k} = \mathrm{k}+1$$

$$g_{ij} = \frac{g_{ij}}{2} + m_k, \mathrm{k} = \mathrm{k}+1$$

$$b_{ij} = \frac{b_{ij}}{2} + m_k, \mathrm{k} = \mathrm{k}+1$$

Where:
    i – Row in image
    j – Column in image
    r_{ij}, g_{ij}, b_{ij} – the bit in the i-th row and j-th column of the R, G, and B channel respectively (in 8-bit binary) m_k is the k-th bit in the message (Note that k should be lesser than the number of bytes in the image)

Mean-Squared Error (MSE)

$$MSE = \frac{1}{(M * N)} \sum_{i=1}^{M} \sum_{j=1}^{N} \left(p_{ij} - q_{ij}\right)^2$$

Where:
    MSE – Mean-Squared Error
    M – Number of rows in the image
    N – Number of columns in the image
    i – Current row in image
    j – Current column in image
    p – Normal image
    q – Stego-image

Peak Signal-to-Noise Ratio (PSNR)

$$PSNR = 10 * log_{10}\left(\frac{Max^2}{MSE}\right)$$

Where:

Max - Maximum pixel intensity value, which is 255

MSE - Mean-Squared Error

SAMPLE WORKING OF LSB STEGANOGRPAHY

Algorithm

- **Conversion to Binary:**

```
messageToBinary(message)
        IF type of message is a string
                CONVERT message to 8-bit binary
        ELSE IF type of message is a byte
                CONVERT message to 8-bit binary
        ELSE IF type of message is an integer
                CONVERT message to 8-bit binary
        ELSE
                RETURN error
        ENDIF
```

- **Encoding:**

```
hide(image, secret_message)
        READ image as file;
        SET number of bytes = rows in image * columns in image * 3 // 8
        IF length of secret_message is greater than the number of bytes
                Raise ValueError("Insufficient bytes in image, need a bigger
image or lesser data")
        ENDIF
        APPEND secret_message by "####" (Any special characters would work as
delimiter)
        SET data_index = 0
        SET binary_secret_message = messageToBinary(secret_message) (Converts
the secret message to binary)
        SET data_len = length of binary_secret_message
FOR row in image:
```

```
            FOR pixel in row:
            //Converts each pixel data to 8-bit binary and assigns to r,g,b,a
                    r, g, b, a = messageToBinary(pixel)
            //Appending binary_secret_message bit value to r-pixel
                    IF data_index IS LESSER THAN data_len:
                            SET pixel[0] = int(r[:-1] + binary_secret_
message[data_index],2)
                                INCREMENT data_index by 1
                    ENDIF
            //Appending binary_secret_message bit value to g-pixel
                    IF data_index IS LESSER THAN data_len:
                            SET pixel[1] = int(g[:-2] + binary_secret_
message[data_index],2)
                            INCREMENT data_index by 1
                    ENDIF
            //Appending binary_secret_message bit value to g-pixel
                    IF data_index IS LESSER THAN data_len
                            SET pixel[2] = int(b[:-2] + binary_secret_
message[data_index],2)
                                INCREMENT data_index by 1
                    ENDIF
                    IF data_index IS GREATER THAN OR EQUAL TO data_len
                            BREAK
                    ENDIF
        ENDFOR
        RETURN image
ENDFOR
```

- **Decoding:**

```
Reveal(image)
        READ image as file;
        SET binary_data = ""
        FOR row in image:
                FOR pixel in row:
                //Converts each pixel to 8-bit binary and assigns to r,g,b,a
                        SET r,g,b,a = messageToBinary(pixel)
                        APPEND binary_data with the last r-bit
                        APPEND binary_data with the last g-bit
                        APPEND binary_data with the last b-bit
                ENDFOR
        ENDFOR
        SET all_bytes to the number of bytes decoded
        SET decoded_data = ""
```

```
FOR byte in all_bytes:
        SET decoded_data += chr(int(byte, 2)
        IF decoded_data[-4:] == "####" (Delimiter)
                BREAK
        ENDIF
ENDFOR
RETURN decoded_data[:-4]
```

- **Flowchart:**
  Figure 3 shows flow of the sample code.

Figure 3. Sample code flow

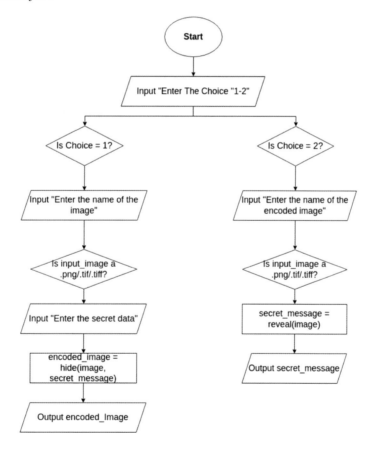

Figure 4 and 5 show the output of the code for a PNG file.

Figure 6 is the sample PNG file that was used to embed the message upon.

Figure 7 is the output image after embedding the message.

Figure 8 and 9 show the output of the code for a TIFF file.

Figure 10 is the sample TIFF file that was used to embed the message upon, sourced from www. filesamples.com.

Figure 4. Code output for PNG file

```
-------------- Steganography Implementation --------------
1. Encode Data
2. Decode Data

Enter the choice:1



Enter the name of the image: samplepng.png


  Enter the secret data to embed into the image: This is a sample image with the extension .PNG.


Maximum bytes to encode: 180000
-------------------- Encoding data --------------------
The encoded image is:  encoded_samplepng.png
```

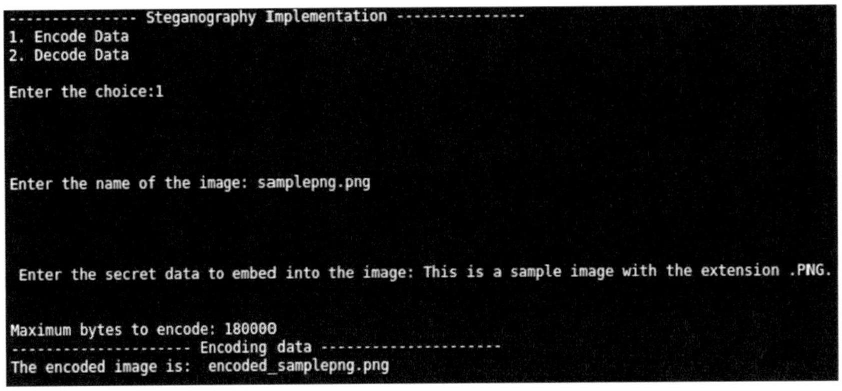

Figure 5. Code output for PNG file

```
-------------- Steganography Implementation --------------
1. Encode Data
2. Decode Data

Enter the choice:2



  Enter the name of the encoded image: encoded_samplepng.png

-------------------- Decoding data --------------------
Decoded data:  This is a sample image with the extension .PNG.
```

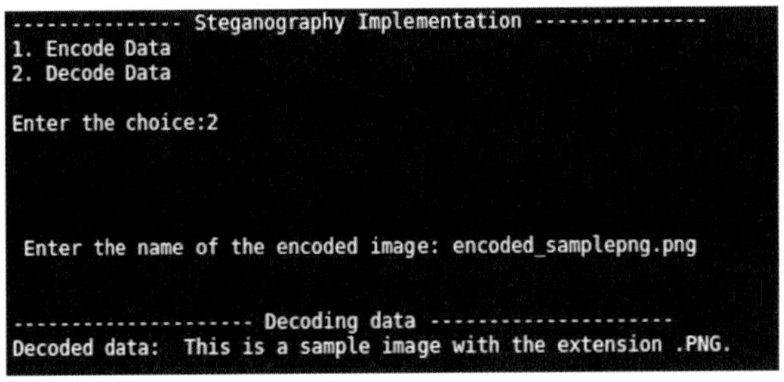

Figure 6. Sample PNG Image; **Source***: www.wikipedia.com*

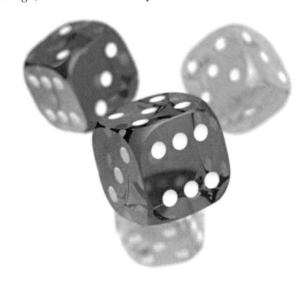

Figure 7. Sample PNG output

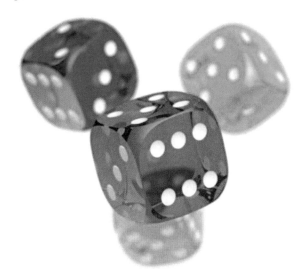

Figure 8. Code output for TIFF file

```
-------------- Steganography Implementation --------------
1. Encode Data
2. Decode Data

Enter the choice:1



Enter the name of the image: sampletiff.tiff



 Enter the secret data to embed into the image: This is a sample image with the extension .TIFF.

Maximum bytes to encode: 8820000
-------------------- Encoding data --------------------
The encoded image is:  encoded_sampletiff.tiff
```

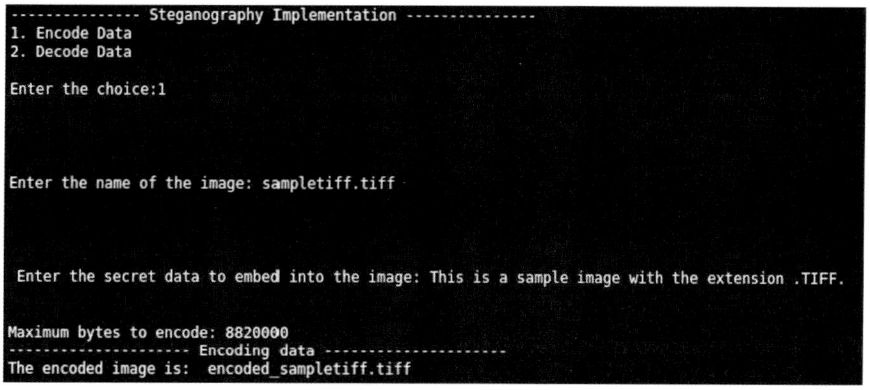

Figure 9. Code output for TIFF file

```
-------------- Steganography Implementation --------------
1. Encode Data
2. Decode Data

Enter the choice:2



 Enter the name of the encoded image: encoded_sampletiff.tiff


-------------------- Decoding data --------------------
Decoded data:  This is a sample image with the extension .TIFF.
```

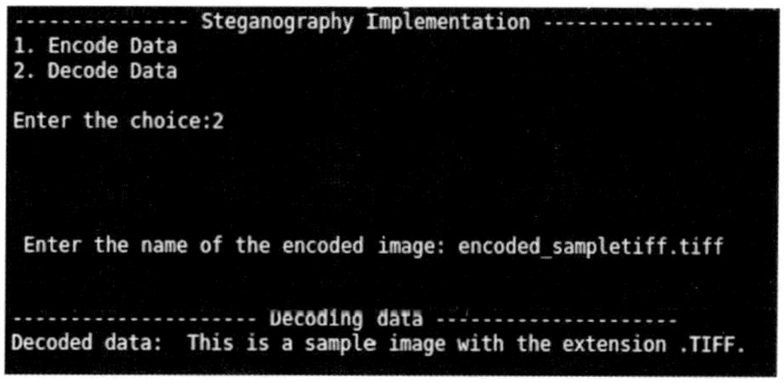

Figure 10. Sample TIFF Image; **Source:** *www.filesamples.com*

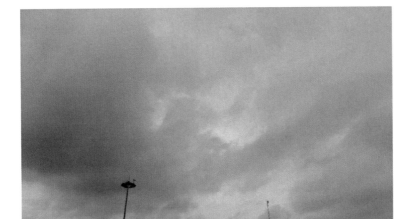

Figure 11 is the output TIFF image after embedding the message.

Figure 12and 13show the output of the code for a BMP file.

Figure 14 is the sample BMP image that was used to embed the message upon, sourced from www. filesamples.com.

Figure 15 is the output BMP image after embedding the message.

Figure 11. Sample TIFF output

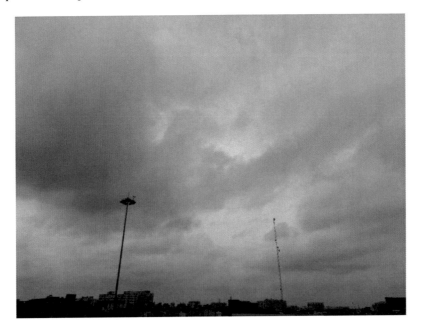

Figure 12. Code output for BMP file

```
-------------- Steganography Implementation --------------
1. Encode Data
2. Decode Data

Enter the choice:1



Enter the name of the image: samplebmp.bmp



 Enter the secret data to embed into the image: This is a sample image with the extension .BMP.

Maximum bytes to encode: 921600
--------------------- Encoding data ---------------------
The encoded image is:   encoded_samplebmp.bmp
```

Figure 13. Code output for BMP file

```
-------------- Steganography Implementation --------------
1. Encode Data
2. Decode Data

Enter the choice:2



 Enter the name of the encoded image: encoded_samplebmp.bmp

--------------------- Decoding data ---------------------
Decoded data:  This is a sample image with the extension .BMP.
```

Figure14. Sample BMP Image **Source:***www.filesamples.com*

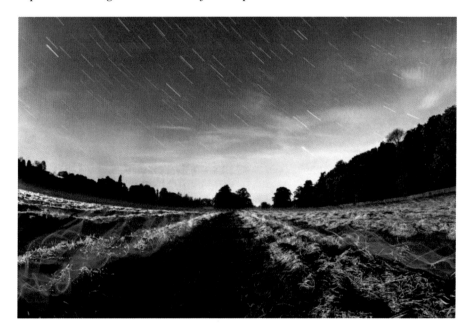

Figure 15. Sample BMP output

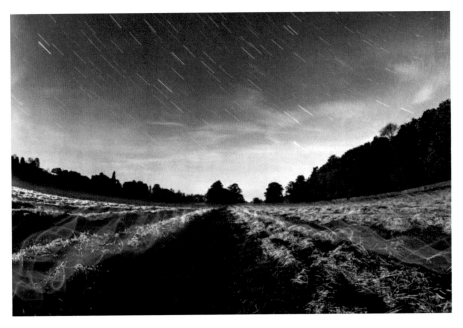

CONCLUSION

Steganography is the process of hiding information within other information mediums in order to communicate with others. Steganography's purpose is to conceal information in such a way that it appears natural to the average person. It's been around since the beginning of time, with the earliest recorded use in Greece in 440 BC. Steganography derives from the Greek words steganos, which means "covered," and graphia, which means "writing." Digital Steganography is a modern use of Steganography that hides data in computer files. The Carrier, Message, and Key components of a conventional steganography algorithm are all necessary. Carrier refers to the file that contains the message as well as an optional key for adding an extra degree of security.

REFERENCES

Abd El-Latif, A. A. (2020). Secret Images Transfer in Cloud System Based on Investigating Quantum Walks in Steganography Approaches. *Physica A: Statistical Mechanics and Its Applications, 541.* . doi:10.1016/j.physa.2019.123687

Abdulkudhur & Al Saffar. (2021). LSB Based Image Steganography Using McEliece Cryptosystem. *Materials Today: Proceedings.* . doi:10.1016/j.matpr.2021.07.182

AlKhodaidi & Gutub. (2021). Refining Image Steganography Distribution for Higher Security Multimedia Counting-Based Secret-Sharing. *Multimedia Tools and Applications, 80*(1), 1143–73. . doi:10.1007/s11042-020-09720-w

Ansari, A. S., Mohammadi, M. S., & Parvez, M. T. (2020). A Multiple-Format Steganography Algorithm for Color Images. *IEEE Access: Practical Innovations, Open Solutions, 8*, 83926–83939. doi:10.1109/ACCESS.2020.2991130

Ashraf, Z. (2020). Interval Type-2 Fuzzy Logic System Based Similarity Evaluation for Image Steganography. *Heliyon, 6*(5). . doi:10.1016/j.heliyon.2020.e03771

Cui, J., Zhang, P., Li, S., Zheng, L., Bao, C., Xia, J., & Li, X. (2021). Multitask Identity-Aware Image Steganography via Minimax Optimization. *IEEE Transactions on Image Processing, 30*, 8567–8579. doi:10.1109/TIP.2021.3107999 PMID:34469298

Dalal & Juneja. (2021). Steganography and Steganalysis (in Digital Forensics): A Cybersecurity Guide. *Multimedia Tools and Applications, 80*(4), 5723–71. . doi:10.1007/s11042-020-09929-9

Dhawan, S., Chakraborty, C., Frnda, J., Gupta, R., Rana, A. K., & Pani, S. K. (2021). SSII: Secured and High-Quality Steganography Using Intelligent Hybrid Optimization Algorithms for IoT. *IEEE Access: Practical Innovations, Open Solutions, 9*, 87563–87578. doi:10.1109/ACCESS.2021.3089357

Ding, X., Xie, Y., Li, P., Cui, M., & Chen, J. (2020). Image Steganography Based on Artificial Immune in Mobile Edge Computing With Internet of Things. *IEEE Access: Practical Innovations, Open Solutions, 8*, 136186–136197. doi:10.1109/ACCESS.2020.3010513

El-Khamy, S. E., Korany, N. O., & Mohamed, A. G. (2020). A New Fuzzy-DNA Image Encryption and Steganography Technique. *IEEE Access: Practical Innovations, Open Solutions, 8*, 148935–148951. doi:10.1109/ACCESS.2020.3015687

Elshoush, H. T. (2022). A New High Capacity and Secure Image Realization Steganography Based on ASCII Code Matching. *Multimedia Tools and Applications, 81*(4), 5191–237. . doi:10.1007/s11042-021-11741-y

Eyssa, A. A. (2020). An Efficient Image Steganography Approach over Wireless Communication System. *Wireless Personal Communications, 110*(1), 321–37. . doi:10.1007/s11277-019-06730-2

Fu, Z. (2020). The Secure Steganography for Hiding Images via GAN. EURASIP Journal on Image and Video Processing. doi:10.118613640-020-00534-2

Gutub & Al-Ghamdi. (2020). Hiding Shares by Multimedia Image Steganography for Optimized Counting-Based Secret Sharing. *Multimedia Tools and Applications, 79*(11), 7951–85. . doi:10.1007/s11042-019-08427-x

Gutub & Al-Shaarani. (2020). Efficient Implementation of Multi-Image Secret Hiding Based on LSB and DWT Steganography Comparisons. *Arabian Journal for Science and Engineering, 45*(4), 2631–44. . doi:10.1007/s13369-020-04413-w

Hsieh & Wang. (2022). Constructive Image Steganography Using Example-Based Weighted Color Transfer. *Journal of Information Security and Applications, 65*. . doi:10.1016/j.jisa.2022.103126

Jayapandiyan, J. R., Kavitha, C., & Sakthivel, K. (2020). Enhanced Least Significant Bit Replacement Algorithm in Spatial Domain of Steganography Using Character Sequence Optimization. *IEEE Access: Practical Innovations, Open Solutions, 8*, 136537–136545. doi:10.1109/ACCESS.2020.3009234

Karthikeyan, N. (2021). Assessment of Composite Materials on Encrypted Secret Message in Image Steganography Using RSA Algorithm. *Materials Today: Proceedings.* . doi:10.1016/j.matpr.2021.04.260

Ke & Yin. (2021). On the Security and Robustness of 'Keyless Dynamic Optimal Multi-Bit Image Steganography Using Energetic Pixels.' *Multimedia Tools and Applications, 80*(3), 3997–4005. . doi:10.1007/s11042-020-09807-4

Li, F. (2022). GAN-Based Spatial Image Steganography with Cross Feedback Mechanism. *Signal Processing, 190.* doi:10.1016/j.sigpro.2021.108341

Li, L. (2021). Adversarial Batch Image Steganography against CNN-Based Pooled Steganalysis. *Signal Processing, 181.* . doi:10.1016/j.sigpro.2020.107920

Li, Q. (2021). Image Steganography Based on Style Transfer and Quaternion Exponent Moments. *Applied Soft Computing, 110.* . doi:10.1016/j.asoc.2021.107618

Li, Q., Wang, X., Wang, X., Ma, B., Wang, C., Xian, Y., & Shi, Y. (2020). A Novel Grayscale Image Steganography Scheme Based on Chaos Encryption and Generative Adversarial Networks. *IEEE Access: Practical Innovations, Open Solutions, 8*, 168166–168176. doi:10.1109/ACCESS.2020.3021103

Liu, J., Ke, Y., Zhang, Z., Lei, Y., Li, J., Zhang, M., & Yang, X. (2020). Recent Advances of Image Steganography With Generative Adversarial Networks. *IEEE Access: Practical Innovations, Open Solutions, 8*, 60575–60597. doi:10.1109/ACCESS.2020.2983175

Lopez-Hernandez, Martinez-Gonzalez, Hernandez-Reyes, Palacios-Luengas, & Vazquez-Medina. (2020). A Steganography Method Using Neural Networks. *IEEE Latin America Transactions, 18*(3), 495-506. doi:10.1109/TLA.2020.9082720

Lu, Xue, Yeung, Liu, Huang, & Shi. (2021). Secure Halftone Image Steganography Based on Pixel Density Transition. *IEEE Transactions on Dependable and Secure Computing, 18*(3), 1137-1149. doi:10.1109/TDSC.2019.2933621

Mukherjee, S. (2021). Pencil Shell Matrix Based Image Steganography with Elevated Embedding Capacity. *Journal of Information Security and Applications, 62.* . doi:10.1016/j.jisa.2021.102955

Pattanaik, B. (2021). Contrasting the Performance Metrics of Discrete Transformations on Digital Image Steganography Using Artificial Intelligence. *Materials Today: Proceedings.* . doi:10.1016/j.matpr.2020.12.076

Pramanik, S. (2020). Application of Bi-Orthogonal Wavelet Transform and Genetic Algorithm in Image Steganography. *Multimedia Tools and Applications, 79*(25), 17463–82. . doi:10.1007/s11042-020-08676-1

Pustokhina, I. V. (2022). Blockchain-Based Secure Data Sharing Scheme Using Image Steganography and Encryption Techniques for Telemedicine Applications. In Wearable Telemedicine Technology for the Healthcare Industry. Academic Press. doi:10.1016/B978-0-323-85854-0.00009-5

Qi, B. (2020). A Novel Haze Image Steganography Method via Cover-Source Switching. *Journal of Visual Communication and Image Representation, 70.* . doi:10.1016/j.jvcir.2020.102814

Reshma, V. K. (2020). Optimized Support Vector Neural Network and Contourlet Transform for Image Steganography. *Evolutionary Intelligence*. . doi:10.1007/s12065-020-00387-8

Rustad, S. (2021). Inverted LSB Image Steganography Using Adaptive Pattern to Improve Imperceptibility. *Journal of King Saud University - Computer and Information Sciences*. . doi:10.1016/j.jksuci.2020.12.017

Saad, A. H. S., Mohamed, M. S., & Hafez, E. H. (2021). Coverless Image Steganography Based on Optical Mark Recognition and Machine Learning. *IEEE Access: Practical Innovations, Open Solutions*, *9*, 16522–16531. doi:10.1109/ACCESS.2021.3050737

Sabeti, V. (2022). An Adaptive Image Steganography Method Based on Integer Wavelet Transform Using Genetic Algorithm. *Computers & Electrical Engineering, 99*. . doi:10.1016/j.compeleceng.2022.107809

Sahu, A. K. (2021). Multi-Directional Block Based PVD and Modulus Function Image Steganography to Avoid FOBP and IEP. *Journal of Information Security and Applications, 58*. . doi:10.1016/j.jisa.2021.102808

Sharifzadeh, M., Aloraini, M., & Schonfeld, D. (2020). Adaptive Batch Size Image Merging Steganography and Quantized Gaussian Image Steganography. *IEEE Transactions on Information Forensics and Security*, *15*, 867–879. doi:10.1109/TIFS.2019.2929441

Sharma, H. (2021). Multi-Image Steganography and Authentication Using Crypto-Stego Techniques. *Multimedia Tools and Applications, 80*(19), 29067–93. doi:10.1007/s11042-021-11068-8

Sharma, V. K. (2022). Hilbert Quantum Image Scrambling and Graph Signal Processing-Based Image Steganography. *Multimedia Tools and Applications*. . doi:10.1007/s11042-022-12426-w

Sharma & Batra. (2021). An Enhanced Huffman-PSO Based Image Optimization Algorithm for Image Steganography. *Genetic Programming and Evolvable Machines, 22*(2), 189–205. . doi:10.1007/s10710-020-09396-z

Shashikiran, B. S. (2021). Minimal Block Knight's Tour and Edge with LSB Pixel Replacement Based Encrypted Image Steganography. *SN Computer Science, 2*(3), 139. . doi:10.1007/s42979-021-00542-7

Siddiqui, G. F., Iqbal, M. Z., Saleem, K., Saeed, Z., Ahmed, A., Hameed, I. A., & Khan, M. F. (2020). A Dynamic Three-Bit Image Steganography Algorithm for Medical and e-Healthcare Systems. *IEEE Access: Practical Innovations, Open Solutions, 8*, 181893–181903. doi:10.1109/ACCESS.2020.3028315

Su, W., Ni, J., Hu, X., & Fridrich, J. (2021, March). Image Steganography With Symmetric Embedding Using Gaussian Markov Random Field Model. *IEEE Transactions on Circuits and Systems for Video Technology*, *31*(3), 1001–1015. doi:10.1109/TCSVT.2020.3001122

Subramanian, N., Cheheb, I., Elharrouss, O., Al-Maadeed, S., & Bouridane, A. (2021). End-to-End Image Steganography Using Deep Convolutional Autoencoders. *IEEE Access: Practical Innovations, Open Solutions*, *9*, 135585–135593. doi:10.1109/ACCESS.2021.3113953

Subramanian, N., Elharrouss, O., Al-Maadeed, S., & Bouridane, A. (2021). Image Steganography: A Review of the Recent Advances. *IEEE Access: Practical Innovations, Open Solutions*, *9*, 23409–23423. doi:10.1109/ACCESS.2021.3053998

Sukumar, A. (2021). Robust Image Steganography Approach Based on RIWT-Laplacian Pyramid and Histogram Shifting Using Deep Learning. *Multimedia Systems, 27*(4), 651–66. . doi:10.1007/s00530-020-00665-6

Tan, L. (2020). Steganalysis of Homogeneous-Representation Based Steganography for High Dynamic Range Images. *Multimedia Tools and Applications, 79*(27), 20079–105. . doi:10.1007/s11042-019-08257-x

Yildirim, M. (2021). Steganography-Based Voice Hiding in Medical Images of COVID-19 Patients. *Nonlinear Dynamics, 105*(3), 2677–2692. doi:10.1007/s11071-021-06700-z

Zhang, Fu, & Ni, Liu, & Yang. (2020). A generative method for steganography by cover synthesis with auxiliary semantics. *Tsinghua Science and Technology, 25*(4), 516–527. doi:10.26599/TST.2019.9010027

Zhang, J., Zhao, X., He, X., & Zhang, H. (2022). Improving the Robustness of JPEG Steganography With Robustness Cost. *IEEE Signal Processing Letters, 29*, 164–168. doi:10.1109/LSP.2021.3129419

Zhang, Y., Luo, X., Guo, Y., Qin, C., & Liu, F. (2020, August). Multiple Robustness Enhancements for Image Adaptive Steganography in Lossy Channels. *IEEE Transactions on Circuits and Systems for Video Technology, 30*(8), 2750–2764. doi:10.1109/TCSVT.2019.2923980

Zhou, L., Feng, G., Shen, L., & Zhang, X. (2020). On Security Enhancement of Steganography via Generative Adversarial Image. *IEEE Signal Processing Letters, 27*, 166–170. doi:10.1109/LSP.2019.2963180

Chapter 13
A Novel Approach for an IoT-Based U-Healthcare System

Rasmita Jena
Udayanath College of Science and Technology (Autonomous), India

Anil Kumar Biswal
https://orcid.org/0000-0001-7341-216X
School of Computer Science, National Institute of Science and Technology (Autonomous), Berhampur, India

Debabrata Singh
Institute of Technical Education and Research (ITER), Siksha 'O' Anusandhan (Deemed), India

ABSTRACT

Among the living organisms, the most important metabolic process is health, or what we can say as the power of living and the basic right to get quality healthcare. In the coming era, the internet will play an important role in monitoring and executing the issues related to the health system of humans through automated sensor response using IoT. IoT connects device to device, things to things, as well as the human body to the network system through the sensors. It can be used to monitor human health-related issues like sugar level, blood pressure level, fever and keep track of a patient's pulse rate and any disease that may be harmful to human life. Today, due to a lack of resources in the world, people are facing many problems related to health.

INTRODUCTION

The good Health quality is the primary requirement of human being. In the principle of the World Health Organization (WHO), health is expressed as a better bonding between the various beings like physical, mental and social-well-being, rather than only the absence of physical inabilities."(Kalarthi, Z. M. 2016) (Salahuddin, M. A. et al. 2018). This paper presents the traditional u-healthcare system in Internet of Things (IoT) environment using the mobile gateway. The Internet of Things connects different devices such as mechanical and digital, objects to object, animals or people to communicate and transfer data

DOI: 10.4018/978-1-6684-4580-8.ch013

without intervention of human to human and human to computer. The health condition of human is most important segment during human lifetime. But current generation people can suffer in many diseases such as heart related problem, COVID-19, blood pressure and any chronic disease in any time but it is not possible by all for immediate consult to the doctor at any time due to unavailability of doctor for the increasing population (Singh, D. et al. 2020). At the critical conditions when doctors and treatment both are unavailable for all the patients, those who are living in remote locations leads to many problems (Gelogo, Y. E. et al. 2015) (Dewangan, K. et al. 2018).

Remote health monitoring and emergency notification can be enabled through the IoT system. Blood pressure, any chronic disease, and heart rate can all be monitored remotely using specialised sensors in a remote health monitoring system (Khamparia, A. et al. 2021). for senior citizens, a specialized sensor needs to be fitted in the body of the human to monitor the health care system, which will assure and secure proper treatment to regain the loss of mobility.

Wearable gadgets have piqued the interest of both the academic and industrial communities. Because of the high degree of curiosity, these devices have become highly common in everyday life. This developed smart wearable health equipment can be linked to the body to observe a person's actions without interfering with or restricting the user's movement (Singla, K. et al. 2021). Wearable devices are small computers that people wear on their bodies, such as clothing, smartwatches, bracelets, wrist bands, or eyewear. Nowadays, there is a smartly equipped fitness device available that can be used to track daily activities. These devices are mostly made up of pedometer sensors, which count the number of steps taken by a person based on hand or hip motion.

The basic goal is to collect sensory data from the body's living organs for local analysis, and then transport the analysed data to a distant medical server (Yeole, A. S. et al. 2016). This can be done by using IoT devices, body sensors such as a smart watch, a smart phone or any Personal Monitoring Device (PMD), a cloud storage platform and encryption algorithm. Through the IOT device, body sensors collect health-related information from the patient's body and transport it to an authentic mobile application, where an encrypting algorithm encrypts the information before it is delivered and stored on the cloud over the internet or through the Wi-Fi module. When data is received by an authentic person's mobile application, it is decrypted using a decryption algorithm (Gelogo, Y. E. et al. 2015) (Kirupa Shankar et al. 2021).

BACKGROUND STUDY

U-Health Care System

The preliminary study suggests that a health management system should provide a health system through which users can get health services anytime and anywhere for better health management (Samanta, D. et al. 2021). The technology used to provide convenient health services to both remote and urban areas in a very efficient and accurate way is the U-healthcare system. People can avail of any medical services and monitor their health condition without going to a hospital or clinic, which is depicted in figure 1.

Ubiquitous healthcare is a new branch of technology that monitors and improves patients' physical and mental health through the use of a huge variety of environmental and body sensors and actuators (Tripathi, V. et al. 2017). The importance of ubiquitous healthcare is that it provides an environment for healthcare for everyone, everywhere, anytime, and in which technology enables ubiquitous healthcare to be not only omnipresent but also smoothly incorporated into daily life.

In order to achieve this goal of omnipresent healthcare, tiny sensors are being developed to capture data on physical parameters such as heart rate, blood pressure, and even blood and urine chemical levels (Subramaniam, S. et al. 2022). These sensors can be worn (by incorporating them into the patient's clothing), implanted, or installed in the patient's home and workplace (such as in furniture, electrical pieces of equipment, and production). The actuators go a step further by inducing behaviours such as the use of small amounts of medicine into the circulation or electrical stimulation of brain regions (Vijayalakshmi, A. et al. 2021). This is a smart conversation-based mobile health monitoring system that very skilfully monitors the health condition on a regular basis, without any caretakers. Patient information is acquired through a mobile or wearable device and is then used by healthcare practitioners to deliver care to their patients.

Devices like mobile phones, laptops, and PDAs are implemented in medical centres, healthcare centres, and emergency or unavoidable situations at anytime and anywhere to get the required data in a secure and transparent manner in ubiquitous computing. The U-health care system is architected by the following technology:

1. Body Area network(BAN)

Body Sensor Networks (BSN) are another name for Body Area Networks (BAN). The sensors in this system are embedded inside the body as a chip or can be worn to sense the patient's body in order to gather biosignals or physiological circumstances such as pulse rate, blood pressure, sugar level, and body temperature (Gelogo, Y. E. et al. 2015).

It is categorized into two parts such as;

a. **Wireless Body Area Network:**WBAN employs two types of devices: specifically, sensors and actuators. Sensors are utilized without any connection between the central node and the body sensor. So the biosensor information acquired from the patient's body is translated into low-frequency electromagnetic waves and sent to the central node or external processing unit (Soni, A. N. 2018).

All of the data collected will be instantly forwarded to the doctors for further analysis. If an emergency situation arises, the doctor will promptly notify the patient via computer system, laptop, PDA, or mobile by sending suitable messages or alarms.

b. **Personal Monitoring Devices (PMD):** A computer, a cell phone, or a PDA can be used as a patient's personal monitoring device (PMD). The information acquired from WBSN via Bluetooth or ZigBee will be processed by PDM logic to determine whether or not it should be sent to IMS. Nowadays, personal computers and smart mobile phones are embedded through the GPRS/Edge/SMS technology. The Internet is used by PMD to communicate with the Intelligent Medical Server (IMS). Whereas the patients are requested for service through PMD and services are provided by IMS (Gelogo, Y. E. et al. 2015) (Mishra, A. et al. 2021).

Figure 1. U-health care service model

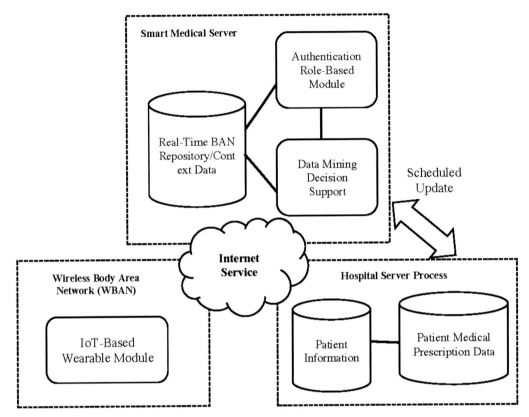

2. Intelligent Medical Server(IMS)

It is recognized as the Intelligent Mobile Health Monitoring System's backbone (IMHMS). It will receive data from the patient's personal monitoring devices as well as past treatment records (PMD). Then, a doctor or a specialist examines the patient and stores the results of the examination and therapy in the database's central node (Mitra, R. et al. 2019) (Baker, S. B. et al. 2017). The examination data will be processed, which is dependent on the features or distribution of the data and also using various data mining techniques such as neural networks, association principals, and decision trees, and feedback will be sent to Personal Monitoring Devices (PMD) and the medical authority if there is any critical situation and for any necessary action. Basically, specializedphysicians control and monitor IMS, and in some cases, patients can assist trained IMS as well as authorities by supplying information particular to him/her and making health policy decisions (Gardaevi, G. et al. 2020) (Samantaray, M. et al. 2021).

By utilising the Radio Frequency Identification (RFID) automation approach, IMS will provide assurance to the patient regarding the confidentiality of the patient's health-related data. RFID tags, or transponders, rely on radio waves to store and remotely retrieve data. It can be traced from a long distance (meters) that is not nearer to the readers. Thus, RFID can provide security features to each patient by using RFID tags (Gelogo, Y. E. et al. 2015).

3. Hospital System

In the U-healthcare system, the third technology is the hospital system, where a number of agents and supportive staff are working to register, retrieve, change, and update the data. The hospital personnel will provide preventive actions to take for the corresponding patient based on the IMS output or report.

RELATED STUDY

In the field of U-health care system significantly monitors patients' health conditions. This system can be used to observe a patient's heart rate, respiration level in percentage, sinus, and body temperature by utilizing a processing device such as an Arduino Uno and various sensors such as heartbeat, sPO2, temperature, and eye blink sensors. The system's disadvantage is that no specific information is explained for individual patients.

(Jeong, J. S. et al. 2016) (Islam, M. M. et al. 2020) In the IoT setting, a healthcare monitoring system was built. The system may be applied to gather data on human health such as pulse rate, ECG, body temperature, and respiration by utilizing various sensors such as a pulse sensor, temperature sensor, blood pressure sensor, ECG sensor, and Raspberry Pi. The acquired data will be forwarded to a Raspberry Pi for processing and the patient's personal monitoring device for action. This system has a demerit in that there is no platform for displaying data.

(Mishra, K. N. et al. 2020) developed a non-invasive technology, a pulse rate detection system. The plethysmography procedure is used in this system, and the results are shown digitally, just like with real monitoring equipment. When compared to other non-invasive techniques, this procedure is more trustworthy for the patient.

(Wu, F. et al. 2019) developed an android-based approach for monitoring pulse rate. An android phone's light and camera were employed in this technology to track and calculate the flow of blood based on cardiac output, and the wireless integrated device converted a human pulse rate to a computer by allowing the human to verify their pulse rate. The design technique is without a doubt excellent, but it is unreliable when continuous heart ratemonitoring is required.

(Kang, S. H. et al. 2021) proposed a smartphone-based sensing system for cardiovascular illness. The prototype produced could only track coronary rhythm in real time, not heart rate over time, and could not detect any cardiovascular disease.

(Bhardwaj, H. et al. 2021) described a smartphone-based health constraint observation framework that can be accessed via a mobile device. In this framework, the sensor detects analogue data and transmits it towards the Arduino Uno board. The captured analogue data value was transformed to digital data using a convertor. The physical properties were then transferred to the built-in device through Bluetooth. The system's disadvantage is that the module used in Bluetooth devices does not cover a vast range.

An IoT safety monitoring gadget was introduced (Mishra, A. et al. 2018). The Arduino board was utilized in this way to collect data from a patient utilizing a DS18B20 sensor and a pulse sensor. The DS18B20 sensor observes the patient's body temperature, while the heart rate sensor measures the patient's pulse level. The Wi-Fi module was then utilized to upload data from the Arduino to the cloud. The sensors cannot be executed properly due to the presence of an Arduino Uno in the system, which is a disadvantage of this technique.

PROPOSED SYSTEM

In general, light-emitting diodes (LEDs) and photodiodes are used in pulse oximeters to find the patient's pulse rate and amount of oxygen through sensing the patient's finger with a spring-loaded clip or an adhesive band, as shown in figure 2. Wearable technology such as smart phones and smart watches now incorporate several inbuilt sensors such as accelerometers, gyroscopes, step counters, and heart rate monitors, which are used to assess the patient's heart rate (Shah, S. A. et al. 2018) (Jeong, J. S. et al. 2016). Internal sensors in the Moto 36012 smart watch sense the patient's health-related data, which is then transferred to the internal memory of the smartphone in a CSV (comma-separated values) arrangement with a preferred label name.

Figure 2. **P***roposed wearable u-health care system*

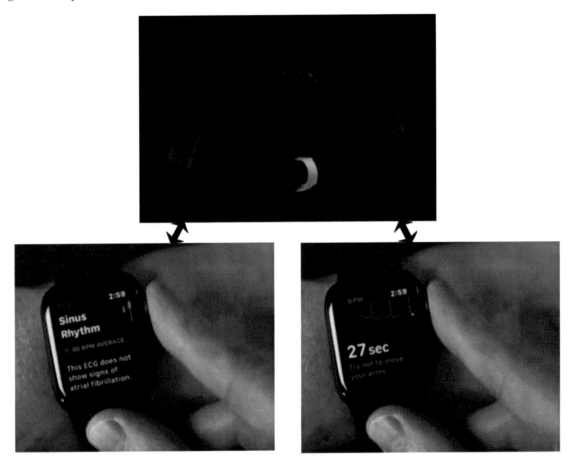

A total of 9000 seconds (1000 seconds for each activity) of sensor data is collected and tagged when each of the eight activities is carried out with the smart watch set to capture 50 samples of sensor data per second. The photo plethysmography (PPG) light is used in many smart watches to assess the flow of blood rate into the heart by pumping beneath the skin's surface. PPG is a technical term that refers to the quantity of light scattered by blood flow when illuminated by the skin.

From the moment the device is turned on, the step counter sensor collects vital information on the number of steps taken in stationary acts (such as writing, keyboard usage, etc.) and non-stationary actions (such as walking, jogging, vacuuming, etc.). Step counter applications make use of the internal accelerometer sensor of the smart device. The application stores the data in memory and investigates the patterns that emerge as a result. The heart rate sensor is designed to help distinguish between running and other activities.

Nowadays, there is a huge range of health equipment accessible that can be used to track daily activities. These devices are mostly made up of pedometer sensors, which count the number of steps taken by a person based on hand or hip motion. These pedometer-equipped devices have proven to be superior activity trackers. This increases the precision of the device and allows it to calculate more than just the walking distance.

The field of designing health-observing equipment and architecture is progressing toward the miniaturization of gadgets that measure vital signs and securely interact with a server. With the implementation of IoT-based smart wearable fitness bands, they are used to gather and track human health data like walking and running distance, calories consumed and expended, pulse rate, sleeping time, and so on, which is directly linked and updated on the computer or smart phone. Figure 3 shows how some cell phones can track health-related activities.

Figure 3. Smart wearable device for tracking body fitness features

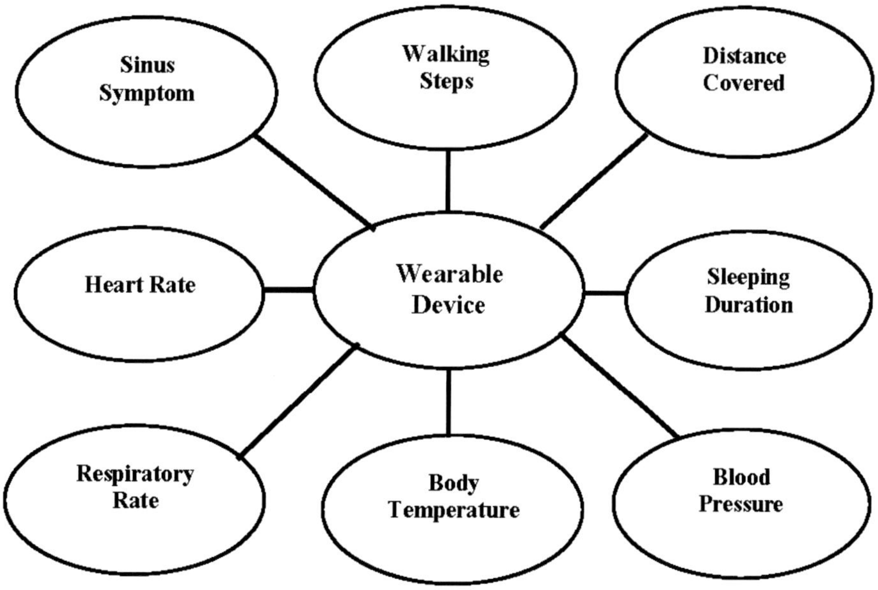

Components

The different component or sensors use to collect information from patient's Body are as follows:

1. **Arduino UNO:** It is a microcontroller board that can be activated through USB or an outer power supply. It functions as a web server by uploading the server code and is powered by a 5-volt battery

(Biswal, A. K. et al. (2021a)). Jumper wires can be used to make physical connections between Arduino GPIO pins, electric devices, and other modules that operate between 1.8 and 5.5 volts. The microcontroller device can read and write data from 32KB of flash memory, 1KB of EEPROM, 23 general I/O lines, and 32 general purpose working registers (Kirupa Shankar et al. 2021) (Biswal, A. K. et al. (2021b)).

2. **ESP8266W:** A jumper-connected 32-bit microcontroller working at 80160MHz from a 3.3v power source is wired, and serial commands are given to it via the Arduino Uno. The AT commands are explored more below.
    ◦ AT+RST: Configuration reset
    ◦ ATCIPSEND: Sends data to the server.
    ◦ AT+CWMODE: Enables AP mode.
    ◦ AT+CIPSERVER: Configures it as an IFI webserver module.

3. **Pulse Sensor:** A pulse sensor is generally implemented to find medical emergencies such as heart attacks, pulmonary embolisms, and vasovagal syncope. The pulse sensor may read data from several parts of the body, including the chest, wrist, earlobe, and fingertip. In general, a wrist sensor in the form of a wrist watch is a more pleasant and long-term wearable system than a chest-worn system wearable (Singh, D. et al. 2022). The most accurate pulse rate can be generated from the earlobe and fingertip. Based on the plethysmography theory, the heartbeat sensor was developed and operates on 3.3v. It can connect to the Arduino Uno breadboard and the couple of LEDs, LDR, and microcontroller, which are used to estimate the pulse rate on the basis of optoelectronics. The heartbeat sensor will be touched to human skin or the tip of the index finger will be placed on the sensor to detect the changes in blood volume. The infrared radiation will discharge as a result of the IR drive, and the surface will reflect the infrared light. The circuit then detects and transmits the beat rate. A healthy human heart beat rate ranges between 60 and 100 beats per minute.

4. **Body Temperature:** A wearable sensor, such as a body temperature sensor, can detect hypothermia, heat stroke, and fever-like diseases. In the previous study, it was discovered that body temperature may be monitored using thermistor-type sensors, negative-temperature-coefficient (NTC) type temperature sensors, and positive temperature coefficient (PTC) sensors. It is clear that thermistors are suitable sensors to measure body temperature for monitoring the human body in all instances (Biswal, A. K. et al. (2021c)). Several studies have concluded that body temperature sensors should be developed by combining a temperature sensor in textiles with sensors printed onto thin, flexible polymers with an adhesive backing that can attach directly to human skin. The LM35 is a body temperature analogue sensor with an output voltage, and the right pin is linked to the body temperature, which is connected directly to the ground. The center pin will provide us with an analogue microcontroller that corresponds to the temperature in Celsius, which is superior to Kelvin's linear temperature sensors in centigrade. Because it is not possible for a beneficiary to remove a huge steady voltage from display (Singh, D. et al. 2021) (Bhanipati, J. et al. 2021).

5. **Blood pressure sensor:** Blood pressure (BP) is an important vital sign that frequently measures human health status in both hypotension and hypertension. A Sphygmomanometer is a manual circulatory strain screen for measuring blood pressure at a very low cost. Sphygmomanometer cuffs can be attached and removed(Huang, B. et al. 2022). The pack comprises an arm sleeve, a crushed bulb to swell the sleeve, and a stethoscope for the patient. The reading electrical signs are changed over to an advanced structure to be perused by the Raspberry Pi (Khan Mamun et al. 2022).

6. **MPU-6050 GY-521 Accelerometer + Gyroscope:** It is a 3-axis accelerometer that does not have cross-axis alignment issues and is embedded with a Digital Motion Processor (DMP) board. This DMP board is capable of executing and solving sophisticated algorithms. In addition, it includes a 3-axis gyroscope that is connected to it(Lucangeli, L. et al. 2021). The sensor has three 16-bit ADCs (Analog to Digital Converters) built in to convert the gyroscope and accelerometer readings to digital. This sensor connects with the Raspberry Pi at 400kHz through the I2C (Inter-integrated Circuit) protocol(Ribeiro, O. et al. 2021). It also included a temperature sensor and an on-chip oscillator with a 1% variance across the working temperature range.

ENERGY CONSUMPTION FOR WEARABLE DEVICE

Batteries are chosen from one of three battery physical structures categories: (i) cylindrical cell (CYC), (ii) button cell (BC), and (iii) coin cell (CC). So the power of wearable fitness bands could be maintained by these three structure of battery. Nominal voltage (V), maximum current (mA), minimal current (mA), minimal capacity (mAh), and dimension (diameter and height (mm x mm)) are the primary parameters for low-power wireless design. The external structure of the battery, liable on its power storage ability, dominates the device volume (mAh). Because the battery cannot be discharged due to any potential loads that has own internal resistance capacity.

Figure 4 depicts the many components of a fitness band that necessitate a voltage supply to function properly.

Figure 4. Smart wearable band consists of source of battery operation

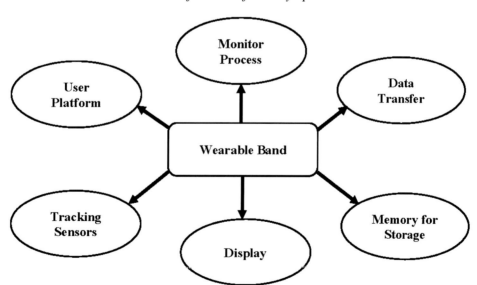

Input Voltage and Maximum Current

Initially, a wearable device is an electronic device that is operated at an optimal battery voltage. The optimum battery voltage is not equivalent to the minimal voltage of the battery that is caused due to the internal voltage drop in the fitness band. So, the purposed microcontroller and wearable device are operated within a voltage range of 1.9 to 3.7 V. By using a voltage converter (DC to DC) to provide external voltage with the help of a battery or organized in such a way that the transferred voltage is built (Yempally, S. et al. 2021).

Furthermore, CR_{avg}(max) is denoted as the maximum current source that a battery needs to confine the usage of its default current. In theory, a 400 mAh battery-powered wearable device can provide around 2 mA for 400 hours or approximately 400 mA for 120 minutes. In practice, all batteries have a smart method for current utilization and if extra current is required, then it is specified but not exactly 400 mAh. The framework's usual voltage requirement must be smaller than the comparative CR_{avg}(max) for the specific battery. Furthermore, if it is required to connect a number of batteries in parallel, maybe with diodes to prevent any non-battery devices from charging at the same time.

A battery can provide more than CR_{avg}(max) for small periods of time, up to an extreme pulse value of CR_{pulse}(max). CR_{pulse}(max) should be large enough to ensure that variations in source voltage, which will diminish as current usage rises, do not exceed the functioning range of the circuit in the wearable device.

Lifetime and Effectiveness of Device

By combining the aforementioned effects, the feasible battery limit (BL_{eff}) can be determined. The framework's normal current utilization (CR_{sys}) matches the maker's prescribed rate (also referred to as the minimal current or the normal release current). BL_{eff} estimation is then an element of CR_{sys}, and it will be lesser than its nominal rate when CR_{sys} exceeds the minimal current. When the critical conditions are met, the battery's lifespan, BLS (CR_{sys}), which can be derives as;

$$BLS\left(CR_{sys}\right) = \frac{BL_{eff}\left(CR_{sys}\right)}{CR_{sys}}$$

DISCUSSION

In terms of India, the country is only now starting to utilize wearable device technology. The wearable device market in India accounts for 90% of the total wearable market. GOQii, Xiaomi, and Fitbit are the leading participants in the Indian market. Fitness bands, on the whole, are durable and require little upkeep. The existing players' most intuitive gadgets will be used.

The market strategy of wearable technology is in a race when it comes to giving value to their goods, whether it's capabilities like pulse rate monitoring, water resistance, or respiration tracking. Beyond that, developers like GOQii are offering free expert guidance, like nutrition guidance, and other facilities in that band. But in this development, sectors are also working under the pressure of Chinese merchants, which puts pressure on enterprises to cut their pricing. As a result, technologists are designing and introducing innovative features and experiences to the sector, which will eventually become commoditized. To deliver a seamless device, wearable devices should be creative and smartly work through the internet.

They should have enough self-esteem capacity to provide information to consumers in an intelligent manner. The primary goal of wearable devices is to generate results via daily use without interfering with the user's ability to do his or her own duties. The wearable devices also have the added facility of measuring the user's psychological state, whether cool or tense, and providing appropriate replies. Whereas the existing wearable devices are needed for improvising through methods such as gamification, social incentives, enhancing services, and so on.

CONCLUSION

In this paper, we have mentioned and proposed a model for monitoring patients' heart rates and discussed some sensors for the setup of emergency clinics. It has been concluded that the use of photo plethysmography (PPG) in many smart watches to measure the heart rate of patients may not be as accurate as compared to medical grade electrocardiogram (ECG). This wearable technology is designed with the following attributes: very silky and lightweight, water resistant, multiple charging facilities, accuracy (moving up and down stairs), and also to monitor main parameters (pulse rate, body temperature, sinus and so on).

Nonetheless, with the advent of new gadgets and next-generation technologies, the present pace of wearable fitness device improvement is increasing swiftly. In this system, future work can be done to make the overall device more reliable for users and will enable much more work to be done automatically rather than manually. This will enhance system performance.

REFERENCES

Baker, S. B., Xiang, W., & Atkinson, I. (2017). Internet of things for smart healthcare: Technologies, challenges, and opportunities. *IEEE Access: Practical Innovations, Open Solutions*, 5, 26521–26544. doi:10.1109/ACCESS.2017.2775180

Bhanipati, J., Singh, D., Biswal, A. K., & Rout, S. K. (2021). Minimization of Collision Through Retransmission and Optimal Power Allocation in Wireless Sensor Networks (WSNs). In *Advances in Intelligent Computing and Communication* (pp. 653–665). Springer.

Bhardwaj, H., Bhatia, K., Jain, A., & Verma, N. (2021, July). IOT Based Health Monitoring System. In *2021 6th International Conference on Communication and Electronics Systems (ICCES)* (pp. 1-6). IEEE.

Biswal, A. K., Singh, D., & Pattanayak, B. K. (2021). IoT-Based Voice-Controlled Energy-Efficient Intelligent Traffic and Street Light Monitoring System. In *Green Technology for Smart City and Society* (pp. 43–54). Springer.

Biswal, A. K., Singh, D., Pattanayak, B. K., Samanta, D., Chaudhry, S. A., & Irshad, A. (2021). Adaptive fault-tolerant system and optimal power allocation for smart vehicles in smart cities using controller area network. *Security and Communication Networks*.

Biswal, A. K., Singh, D., Pattanayak, B. K., Samanta, D., & Yang, M. H. (2021). IoT-Based Smart Alert System for Drowsy Driver Detection. *Wireless Communications and Mobile Computing*, 2021.

Dewangan, K., & Mishra, M. (2018). Internet of things for healthcare: A review. *International Journal of Advanced in Management. Technology and Engineering Sciences*, 8(3), 526–534.

Gardašević, G., Katzis, K., Bajić, D., & Berbakov, L. (2020). Emerging wireless sensor networks and Internet of Things technologies—Foundations of smart healthcare. *Sensors (Basel)*, 20(13), 3619. doi:10.339020133619 PMID:32605071

Gelogo, Y. E., Hwang, H. J., & Kim, H. K. (2015). Internet of things (IoT) framework for u-ealthcare system. *International Journal of Smart Home*, 9(11), 323–330. doi:10.14257/ijsh.2015.9.11.31

Huang, B., Chen, W., Lin, C. L., Juang, C. F., & Wang, J. (2022). MLP-BP: A novel framework for cuffless blood pressure measurement with PPG and ECG signals based on MLP-Mixer neural networks. *Biomedical Signal Processing and Control*, 73, 103404.

Islam, M. M., Rahaman, A., & Islam, M. R. (2020). Development of smart healthcare monitoring system in IoT environment. *SN Computer Science, 1*, 1-11.

Jeong, J. S., Han, O., & You, Y. Y. (2016). A design characteristics of smart healthcare system as the IoT application. *Indian Journal of Science and Technology*, 9(37), 52. doi:10.17485/ijst/2016/v9i37/102547

Kalarthi, Z. M. (2016). A review paper on smart health care system using internet of things. *International Journal of Research in Engineering and Technology*, 5(03), 8084.

Kang, S. H., Baek, H., Cho, J., Kim, S., Hwang, H., Lee, W., ... Suh, J. W. (2021). Management of cardiovascular disease using an mHealth tool: A randomized clinical trial. *NPJ Digital Medicine*, 4(1), 1–7.

Khamparia, A., Singh, P. K., Rani, P., Samanta, D., Khanna, A., & Bhushan, B. (2021). An internet of health things-driven deep learning framework for detection and classification of skin cancer using transfer learning. *Transactions on Emerging Telecommunications Technologies*, 32(7), e3963.

Khan Mamun, M. M. R., & Alouani, A. T. (2022). Cuffless Blood Pressure Measurement Using Linear and Nonlinear Optimized Feature Selection. *Diagnostics (Basel)*, 12(2), 408.

Kirupa Shankar, K. M. (2021). A Novel Approach For Secure & Smart Healthcare Using Internet Of Things Infrastructure. *Turkish Journal of Computer and Mathematics Education*, 12(11), 5992–5997.

Lucangeli, L., D'Angelantonio, E., Camomilla, V., & Pallotti, A. (2021, June). SISTINE: Sensorized Socks for Telemonitoring of Vascular Disease Patients. In *2021 IEEE International Workshop on Metrology for Industry 4.0 & IoT (MetroInd4. 0&IoT)* (pp. 192-197). IEEE.

Mishra, A., & Chakraborty, B. (2018). AD8232 based smart healthcare system using internet of things (IoT). *International Journal of Engineering Research & Technology (Ahmedabad)*, 7(4), 13–16.

Mishra, A., Singh, C., Dwivedi, A., Singh, D., & Biswal, A. K. (2021, October). Network Forensics: An approach towards detecting Cyber Crime. In *2021 International Conference in Advances in Power, Signal, and Information Technology (APSIT)* (pp. 1-6). IEEE.

Mishra, K. N., & Chakraborty, C. (2020). A novel approach towards using big data and IoT for improving the efficiency of m-health systems. In *Advanced computational intelligence techniques for virtual reality in healthcare* (pp. 123–139). Springer. doi:10.1007/978-3-030-35252-3_7

Mitra, R., & Ganiga, R. (2019). A novel approach to sensor implementation for healthcare systems using internet of things. *International Journal of Electrical & Computer Engineering, 9*(6).

Ribeiro, O., Gomes, L., & Vale, Z. (2021, April). IoT-Based Human Fall Detection Solution Using Morlet Wavelet. In *Sustainable Smart Cities and Territories International Conference* (pp. 14-25). Springer.

Salahuddin, M. A., Al-Fuqaha, A., Guizani, M., Shuaib, K., & Sallabi, F. (2018). *Softwarization of internet of things infrastructure for secure and smart healthcare.* arXiv preprint arXiv:1805.11011.

Samanta, D., Karthikeyan, M. P., Banerjee, A., & Inokawa, H. (2021). Tunable graphene nanopatch antenna design for on-chip integrated terahertz detector arrays with potential application in cancer imaging. *Nanomedicine (London), 16*(12), 1035–1047.

Samantaray, M., Biswal, A. K., Singh, D., Samanta, D., Karuppiah, M., & Joseph, N. P. (2021, December). Optical Character Recognition (OCR) based Vehicle's License Plate Recognition System Using Python and OpenCV. In *2021 5th International Conference on Electronics, Communication and Aerospace Technology (ICECA)* (pp. 849-853). IEEE.

Shah, S. A., Ren, A., Fan, D., Zhang, Z., Zhao, N., Yang, X., Luo, M., Wang, W., Hu, F., Rehman, M., Badarneh, O., & Abbasi, Q. H. (2018). Internet of things for sensing: A case study in the healthcare system. *Applied Sciences (Basel, Switzerland), 8*(4), 508. doi:10.3390/app8040508

Singh, D., Bhanipati, J., Biswal, A. K., Samanta, D., Joshi, S., Shukla, P. K., & Nuagah, S. J. (2021). Approach for Collision Minimization and Enhancement of Power Allocation in WSNs. *Journal of Sensors.*

Singh, D., Biswal, A. K., Samanta, D., Singh, D., & Lee, H. N. (2022). Juice Jacking: Security Issues and Improvements in USB Technology. *Sustainability, 14*(2), 939.

Singh, D., Prusty, S. K., Sarangi, S. S., Sahoo, S., & Biswal, A. K. (2020). *Anxiety, Psychological Effects and Prevention during COVID-19 in India.* Academic Press.

Singla, K., Arora, R., & Kaushal, S. (2021). An approach towards IoT-based healthcare management system. In *Proceedings of the sixth international conference on mathematics and computing* (pp. 345-356). Springer.

Soni, A. N. (2018). Smart Devices Using Internet of Things for Health Monitoring. *International Journal of Innovative Research in Science, Engineering and Technology, 7*(5), 6355–6361.

Subramaniam, S., Majumder, S., Faisal, A. I., & Deen, M. J. (2022). Insole-Based Systems for Health Monitoring: Current Solutions and Research Challenges. *Sensors (Basel), 22*(2), 438.

Tripathi, V., & Shakeel, F. (2017, December). Monitoring health care system using internet of things-an immaculate pairing. In *2017 International Conference on Next Generation Computing and Information Systems (ICNGCIS)* (pp. 153-158). IEEE.

Vijayalakshmi, A., Jose, D. V., & Unnisa, S. (2021). Wearable Sensors for Pervasive and Personalized Health Care. In *IoT in Healthcare and Ambient Assisted Living* (pp. 123–143). Springer.

Wu, F., Wu, T., & Yuce, M. R. (2019). An internet-of-things (IoT) network system for connected safety and health monitoring applications. *Sensors (Basel)*, *19*(1), 21. doi:10.339019010021 PMID:30577646

Yempally, S., Singh, S. K., & Velliangiri, S. (2021, October). Review of an IoT-based Remote Patient Health Monitoring System. In *2021 Smart Technologies, Communication and Robotics (STCR)* (pp. 1-5). IEEE.

Yeole, A. S., & Kalbande, D. R. (2016, March). Use of Internet of Things (IoT) in healthcare: A survey. In *Proceedings of the ACM Symposium on Women in Research 2016* (pp. 71-76). 10.1145/2909067.2909079

Chapter 14
Smart Healthcare System Using Containerized Internet of Medical Things

Manoj Kumar Patra

https://orcid.org/0000-0002-7435-2282

National Institute of Technology, Rourkela, India

Bibhudatta Sahoo

https://orcid.org/0000-0001-8273-9850

National Institute of Technology, Rourkela, India

Ashok Kumar Turuk

National Institute of Technology, Rourkela, India

ABSTRACT

There has been a rapid development of healthcare systems in recent times. The main objective of the intelligent healthcare system is to manage, monitor intelligently, and respond to the requirement of the medical ecosystem. In a smart healthcare system, access to different healthcare services and delivery of those services are done by adopting various technologies. Information and communication technology (ICT) has greatly influenced today's healthcare system. The term smart healthcare system comes to the fore because of the integration and application of technologies such as the internet of medical things (IoMT), cloud computing, edge computing, containerization, big data, artificial intelligence, etc. In a smart healthcare system, several medical devices are equipped for collection and management of medical data, remote patient monitoring, tracking health status and location of patients, and monitoring and controlling medical devices to act according to the patients' suitability.

DOI: 10.4018/978-1-6684-4580-8.ch014

INTRODUCTION

The traditional healthcare system cannot meet people's expectations in the modern technology era. This may be because of the rapid increase of populations all over the world or lesser use of technology. Even though we have good doctors, technology, and good infrastructure, everyone can't avail the medical facilities. Providing healthcare services at a reasonable cost and enhancing the ease of access to the healthcare system is a challenging task. Some people can't afford it, and some can't approach it. So, the term smart healthcare comes into the picture to make the healthcare system available and approachable to everyone at any point. A smart healthcare system provides healthcare services to the people and educates people to self-manage some minor health issues in emergency and make them aware of their health. The intelligent management of the medical ecosystem using technology such as the Internet of Medical Things(IoMT), cloud computing, edge computing, containerization, Big Data, Artificial Intelligence, Machine Learning, and different wearable medical devices is termed as a smart healthcare system. The smart healthcare system allows the facility to interconnect medical devices and access medical information, patient data, hospital details, etc., online. A smart healthcare system provides communication between patients and doctors to exchange information remotely. Smart healthcare system reduces the cost of treatment irrespective of geographical location by allowing report monitoring of patients and remotely controlling the medical ecosystems.

In the last few decades, there has been an increasing adaption of information and communication technology (ICT) in the healthcare domain to make the healthcare system readily available to everyone and every time. The use of ICT in healthcare improves service quality, maintains the e-healthcare record, and makes it cost-effective. The e-healthcare record stores details about patients, including their medication history such as prescriptions, last diagnoses report, previous and latest lab test reports, last recommended medicines, and any adverse effect caused in the recent past due to medication, etc. The patient need not carry the previous prescription while visiting a doctor. The doctor can access all details of a patient online from the medical database using a computer or any other electronic device. The term smart healthcare system comes to the fore because of the integration and application of technologies such as the Internet of Medical Things(IoMT), Cloud computing, Edge Computing, Containerization, Big Data, Artificial Intelligence, etc. In a smart healthcare system, several medical devices are equipped to collect and manage medical data, remote patient monitoring, track health status and location of patients, and monitor and control medical devices to act according to the patients' suitability. On the Internet of Medical Things, several medical devices and applications are connected using networking technology and continuously produce a massive amount of data. The IoMT allows analyzing, managing, storing, and transmitting those data, making IoMT a connected healthcare infrastructure.

The main contribution of this chapter is the following.

- A novel architecture for the smart healthcare system is presented that aims to integrate four technologies; cloud computing, edge computing, containerization, i.e., OS-level virtualization, and Internet of Medical Things.
- We introduced the concept of containerization at the edge of the smart healthcare system. We described how the container at the edge would improve the latency requirement and improve response time.
- A brief description of containerization is presented and how it is better than traditional hardware virtualization.

- We found some key technologies that can be used in the smart healthcare system and their impact on it. The technologies include the Internet of Medical Things, Machine Learning, Big Data, Cloud Computing, Artificial Intelligence, Embedded Systems, and 5G communication technology.
- We discuss different challenges involved in a smart healthcare system that need to be taken care of and considered while designing a healthcare system.

CHALLENGES IN DIGITAL SMART HEALTHCARE SYSTEMS

There are several challenges involved in the smart healthcare system that need to be taken care of and considered while designing the healthcare system. These are discussed below.

Societal Factors

In a smart healthcare system, technology will play a vital role, no doubt, but we cannot depend on technology for everything. Everything can't be seen from the technology point of view. Some people do not understand technology and can't afford the cost of technology. So, the digital healthcare system should be delivered with minimal cost, and it should be easy to use (Aickelin et al., 2019). Apart from that, health literacy and digital literacy among people are also very important factors. Especially in uneducated and elderly people, digital literacy is very low. So, to use the digital healthcare system at the social level, a substantial effort is required to educate and make people understand the digital healthcare system. Different initiatives need to be taken (Lennon et al., 2017) to upskill the healthcare professional by educating them. The general public, healthcare professionals, and stakeholders should realize the suitability of a smart healthcare system. For broad adoption, the smart healthcare system systems should be inclusive and engage many users to improve smart healthcare solutions for all.

Security and Privacy of Data

In IoMT, thousands of devices are connected over the internet and communicate with each other. The smart devices in IoMT communicate with each other and generate and share a tremendous amount of data over the internet. Unauthorized access to medical data can cause a severe threat to patients and is very risky for patients' medication (Zeadally et al., 2016). Any change in medical data will lead to wrong decisions, severely harming the patient. The medical devices in IoMT continuously send patients' data and information about the surrounding of a patient to the cloud. There is a chance of a third-party attack during data transmission, and this issue needs to be taken care of very seriously. In the recent past, various wireless networking technologies (Zeadally and Bello, 2019), such as Zigbee, Wi-Fi, BLE, etc., have been used to interconnect different sensors and medical devices in the smart healthcare system. Different security mechanisms must be enforced to prevent any third-party attack. Patients may not like to share their personal information such as family details, medical history, genomic data, etc. To ensure security and privacy, the personal information of patients should be protected (Nambiar et al., 2017).

The security and privacy of medical data is an important concern for patients and healthcare professionals. The healthcare professional or the physician can't make the right decision about the disease if the patient data is compromised or modified. Medical test results such as cancer or HIV are considered to be very personal, and the patient may not like to share this information. The use of connected technology in smart healthcare creates a concern of compromising the confidentiality of patients' data (Sonune et al., 2017). In a smart healthcare system, patient data will be shared between doctors located in different geographical locations and between different applications. Improper network settings and misconfiguration of medical devices can cause concern and affect the patients' data. The medical data of a patient might need to be shared with different agencies and pharmacies for buying medicines or medical devices for treatment. If the agencies and pharmacies do not enforce the security and privacy of data, there is a chance of compromise. This will affect the adoption of a smart healthcare system when medical data privacy is a concern for the patient. A third party manages the network through which medical data is transmitted, and the network is often highly heterogeneous. This makes the protection and privacy of patients' data even more challenging (Williams and McCauley, 2016).

Health Information Exchange Barriers

To enhance the healthcare service delivery in a smart healthcare system, we need to exchange health information among different hospitals and health organizations. The health information can be exchanged using either of the following method (Williams et al., 2012); direct exchange, query-based exchange, and consumer mediated exchange. Important health information such as test results is transferred through direct exchange. When doctors need the previous health record of a patient or to conduct any unplanned treatment, doctors need to ask for the previous health information or access health record, and query-based information exchange occurs. The consumer-mediated health information exchange occurs when the patient accesses their own health information, updates their profile, sees the billing information, tracks the health condition, and takes action accordingly.

The main obstacle in deploying Health Information Exchange is the security and privacy of patient data and maintaining the confidentiality of health information. Some of the major concerns with health information exchange are, firstly, abuse of access rights by an authorized insider. For example, the medical details of important celebrities and renounced politicians often go into the media's hands. This happens because the hospital people share health information with unauthorized people to gain something in exchange for personal benefits or irresponsibility. Secondly, access to information by unauthorized insiders (Strauss et al., 2015). For example, the former employee of a health organization has been resigned but has not yet restricted his access to health information. They may retrieve the health information and share it with a third party for money or to gain something else.

Communication of Medical Devices

Inter medical device communication is one of the significant challenges in the smart healthcare system. Many medical devices are equipped with sensors and actuators to collect data. They are connected to the internet to send those data for further processing. The medical devices often communicate with each other and server to share data. Different manufacturers use different protocols for their medical devices for communication. So, devices from different manufacturers may not necessarily be able to communicate with each other. To overcome these issues, the Internet of Medical Things(IoMT) comes into the picture. The inclusion of heterogeneous devices in smart healthcare systems opens up challenges related to connectivity. IoMT used several wireless technologies to inter-connect medical devices. There may a chance of collision when a medical device in a WLAN comes across another WLAN with the same frequency. The collision can cause many severe effects, such as a reduction in network performance, and may lead to a hazardous situation related to healthcare. Therefore, it should be ensured that all medical devices in IoMT are working properly using different wireless and wired communication technology (Gawanmeh, 2016). In an IoMT domain, communication is required between users, service providers, and themselves. In an interconnected smart healthcare system, data flows with both one-to-one and one-to-many connections. This creates a complex system that requires exchanging information between several interfaces. All systems should cooperate with each other for better information exchange. The medical device in IoMT should be compatible with many protocols and different transmission formats to share data with one other, authentication, and encryption purpose. Efficient management of medical devices is very essential to support plug and play use in IoMT (Williams and McCauley, 2016).

Collection and Management of Data

In the smart healthcare system, thousands of medical devices will be used. This medical device, including sensors, will be implemented inside the patient body as well as in the surrounding of the patient. These medical devices will generate and collect a massive amount of medical data, and this leads to several data management challenges. The health data generated from medical sensors planted inside a patient body are constantly changing because the state of the human body is changing. The collected data are in a different format; for example, Electro Cardio Graph data are encoded in XML format, but the data received from different cameras are stored in different image formats. A connected smart healthcare system consists of heterogeneous medical devices that produce data in a large volume, different variety, different sources, and uncertain data. So, the smart healthcare system needs to be designed in such a way that it will be able to handle these continuously varying data. If the medical data are not analyzed properly, the correct information cannot be extracted from it, and we do not realize its usefulness. The effort of collecting and storing a tremendous amount of data and computing resources is a total waste. A good analysis of those medical data can give valuable information about the patient, and that information can be used further for their treatment. There are different data analytics tools developed by researchers and health service providers (Nambiar et al., 2017) to extract useful information from a huge amount of patient data. Since data collected are in a different format and in large volume and velocity, analyzing them is challenging. Data integrity is also important because if the data is inaccurate, it will lead to wrong decision making and planning. Some information, such as patient health variables, needs to be updated frequently (Hipaa, 2019). Other information, such as contact information and geographical location, is passive and needs not to be updated frequently. So, the integrity of data should be maintained during this frequent update. We have to make sure that data has come from authenticated sources during data collection (Tse et al., 2018).

Design and Implementation

The design and implementation smart healthcare system includes information and communication technology, design of network, embedded systems design, bioengineering and different technique for large data analytics. The implementation of such a huge heterogeneous system requires multi-disciplinary knowledge and skilled people in different fields. The smart healthcare system also needs to be updated time to time to address the dynamic requirement of patient.

TECHNOLOGY FOR SMART HEALTHCARE SYSTEMS

Technology plays an essential role in implementing a smart healthcare system. Several technologies are taking healthcare to the next level. A few of them are discussed below;

Internet of Medical Things

The Internet of Medical Things(IoMT) connects medical devices through the internet and shares data among them. It interconnects medical devices, healthcare applications, and different health services to create a smart healthcare infrastructure. All devices in IoMT are connected to the cloud, where collected data are stored and analyzed. The IoMT has received tremendous attention from scientists and researchers. This is due to the exponential increase in the number of connected medical devices and their ability to generate, collect, and send those data to the cloud for further processing (Patra, Sahoo, Sahoo, & Turuk, 2021). The main advantage of IoMT is accurate diagnoses, low cost for treatment, and fewer mistakes. The health devices are paired with health applications and allow sharing health data with doctors to regularly track their health. Patients can communicate and share their health data with doctors remotely. This improves the patient experience, reduces the cost, and eliminates the in-person visit of the doctor again and again. An overview of IoMT is shown in Figure 1.

Figure 1. Internet of medical things(IoMT)

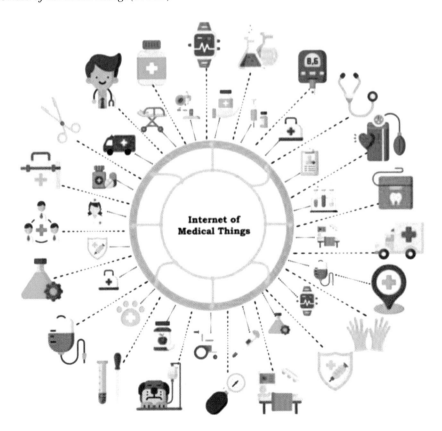

Machine Learning

Machine learning has gained significant importance in smart healthcare systems in the recent past. A lot of medical data is generated daily for a single patient. Using the machine learning technique, the management, analysis, and organizing of data will be easy. Since data analysis will be faster, the treatment will also be provided to the patient earlier. Machine learning will reduce human involvement to some extent, reducing human error. There are different important tasks in the healthcare system that machine learning can handle very easily are; prediction, classification, anomaly detection, recommendation, etc.

In prediction, ML uses current data of the patient to predict the future possibilities of health status. The classification using machine learning in the healthcare system can help to label and determine the type of medication someone is dealing with. Anomaly in healthcare can be wrong physiological reading, leading to some emergency conditions. The detection of anomalous data in healthcare data is crucial and can be done using machine learning. The recommendation engine in healthcare will offer required medical treatment, relevant hospitals for a particular disease, medical instruments, medical shops, etc. There are several opportunities for machine learning in healthcare systems. ML reduces a lot of work of healthcare professionals. This allows them to focus on patient care instead of spending time searching for information or any kind of medical record. The use of machine learning increases the accuracy of medical diagnosis. This has been proved during COVID-19 by predicting the mortality of patients with 92% accuracy. ML can also provide a more precise medication plan for the patient. Different medical cases require different types of treatment for effective and side-effect free treatment. Robotic treatment is another important use of machine learning in the healthcare system. Surgery such as heart operation needs great precision, and a robot can fulfill such requirements. Using ML, robotic surgery can be performed effectively and reduce surgical risk. Machine learning algorithms are widely used in clinical research to determine the best sample for test data collection, analyze real-time test data, and minimize patient data errors.

There are several challenges of ML in healthcare systems, as shown in Figure 2. Firstly, the most important inputs to develop a precise machine learning algorithm are good quality data. The precision of machine algorithms depends on the data used as input for the algorithm. The medical data are not always correct and standardized. So, lack of quality data leads to inaccurate algorithm design. So, the input data needs to be cleaned, structured, and validated for machine algorithm design before applying. Secondly, building machine learning tools that as medical workflow friendly. It is censorious to develop ML tools that would be user-friendly and suitable for medical workflow. To make the healthcare ML tool trustworthy and effective, the necessary feedback should be taken from people who will work with the tool. Thirdly, to make ML successful in healthcare, a big team of skilled people should be built with good skill sets. The skillset includes data science, data analytics, machine learning expert, etc. Apart from all these, good cooperation among the team members is required to deliver valuable products. Figure 2 shows Challenges of ML in Healthcare

Big Data

Big data is one of the disruptive technologies that has revolutionized smart healthcare systems in the recent past. There are several benefits and key applications of using big data in a smart healthcare system. Big data and data analytics can solve many known as well as emerging problems in smart healthcare. It is predicted that the worth of big data analytics will be more than $68B by 2024, driven by tremendous health data and management tools. Big data in the healthcare industry is generated from different sources such as electronic health records, wearable medical devices, patient portals, generic databases, smartphones, etc. The different source of big data in healthcare is shown in Figure 3. This is an ocean of data, and the objective is how to use this data for the treatment of patients. Structured storage with an efficient analytics tool will benefit in many ways. The patients will be healthier, make decisions by doctors, produce medicines and medical devices, perform more efficient operations, and do many more things with proper big data analytics. Some of the key benefits of using big data analytics in healthcare are; reducing medical error, reducing medical cost, real-time monitoring of patients, more authentic treatment, early-stage detection of disease, treatment cost prediction, treatment risk prediction, better staff management services, etc.

The knowledge extracted from healthcare big data provides detailed insights into a patient that was not known earlier. There are different use cases of big data in healthcare systems which are described one by one.

Figure 2. Challenges of ML in healthcare

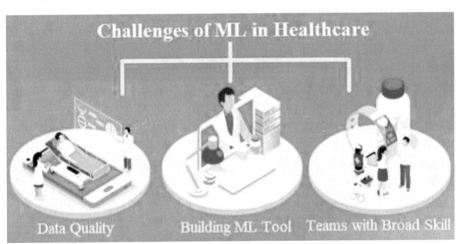

Hospital Management

Hospital management becomes easy with the use of big data analytics in healthcare. It will significantly reduce the cost of operation and improve the quality of services. The data analytics can predict the requirement of medical staff in a particular department at a particular time. So that more staff can be deployed if the requirement is high and distribute the staff during the normal time period. Data analytics can be used to keep track of the performance of the employee, and you can use data analytics to find out who needs more training or any kind of support in their work.

Real-Time Monitoring

In IoMT, several wearable devices collect health data such as body temperature, heart rate, sugar level, blood pressure, pulse, etc. By analyzing these collected data, one can get the real-time health status of a patient. So even doctors can monitor a patient's health status remotely using the data collected by wearable medical devices. The patient need not visit the doctor physically to give health information.

Diagnostics

A disease diagnosis can be made more precisely and quickly using big data analytics. In the usual treatment process, the doctors ask the patients about their illness and examine their symptoms, but they may consult with their colleagues if the case is complex. The doctor just needs to collect the patient data and feed it into an algorithm using big data. That algorithm will analyze the patient data and suggest relevant diagnoses eliminating unnecessary tests.

Modeling and Forecasting

Medical decision-making is a crucial task in healthcare. Big data and different predictive models such as the prognostic model can help make clinical decisions better. Some predictive models are used to determine a treatment's future outcome, and few models are used to predict the future risk.

Telemedicine

The term telemedicine is also referred to as telehealth. It is the idea of delivering healthcare services such as medical tests, medical consultation, medicine, etc., to patients remotely. Big data and data analytics has huge importance in telemedicine. A doctor can perform a critical surgery using a robot being physically present far away from the patient. There are several benefits of telemedicine. Doctors can avoid unnecessary paperwork and consultation to save time. A patient can be monitored and contacted anytime from anywhere. Patients need not be admitted in the hospital they stay in their homes, and telemedicine also reduces costs.

Electronic Health Record

One of the largest sources of big data in the smart healthcare industry is Electronic Health Records (EHR). Big data can analyze the EHR and extract crucial information. The doctors can use big data to instruct the patient for the next lab test and keep track of the patient's health.

Strategic Planning and Decision Making

Better strategic planning and decision in the healthcare field play a vital role. The goal of strategic planning is to find out the current status of a health organization, decide where it will be after a certain period, and create a roadmap to achieve it. By using big data, patients' past and current data can be analyzed to find the possible difficulties in the future and make a strategic plan for that.

Below figure 3 shows Source of Healthcare BigData.

Figure 3. Source of healthcare bigdata

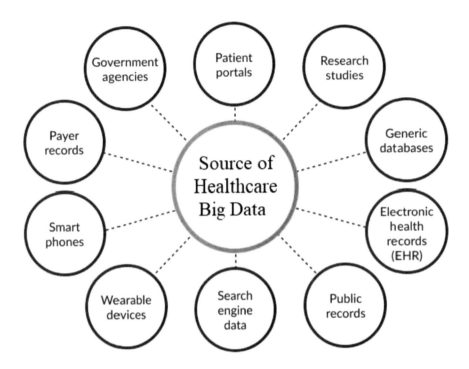

Cloud Computing

As per Global Markets Insights Inc., the healthcare cloud computing market will be worth $55 billion by 2025. Health cloud computing refers to the provisioning of health services through the internet by a remote server. The server will facilitate different services to patients and physicians, such as storing health data in the server process and managing health data remotely. The healthcare organization need not install an onsite data center. Health cloud computing provides storage to keep medical data and HER safely and efficiently. Using cloud computing, doctors can share the medical data of a patient and view the same data simultaneously. Medical data and patient's medical report stored in cloud storage so the patient can access it anytime from anywhere. Cloud can store a huge amount of data with minimum cost saving a significant data storage cost. The users only need to pay the amount for the resources they use. Cloud computing provides faster access, modification, and update health data in cloud storage. Patient can update their medical data as well as personal data easily. The requirement of health organizations changes dynamically. Cloud computing provides storage, computing, and software services to the users. It offers hassle-free scalability and flexibility; users can dynamically increase or reduce the cloud resources based on their requirements.

Artificial Intelligence

The use of Artificial Intelligence(AI) in the healthcare domain has been increased in the recent past. There is a discussion among scientists and researchers about whether the AI Doctor will replace the actual human doctor in the future. Many people believe that AI doctors may not replace human doctors, but AI will definitely help doctors make medical decisions and make the health care system smatter.

Embedded Systems

The combination of software and hardware designs the embedded system to perform a particular task. An embedded system can be attached to a very large system to work together. Different types of embedded systems can be used in the healthcare domain, such as real-time embedded systems, stand-alone embedded systems, mobile embedded systems, and networked embedded systems. These classifications are based on functional and performance requirements. The real-time embedded system provides results in time, i.e., it has a hard deadline. If it can't produce results before the deadline, the system will fail. One example of a real-time embedded system is radiotherapy. The stand-alone embedded system does not require a host system to hold it. It takes input data in the form of a digital or analog signal, processes the data, and produces the output. One example of a stand-alone embedded system is a thermometer for measuring temperature. The networked embedded systems are connected with the resources through the internet. For portable medical devices, mobile embedded systems are used. In the healthcare domain mobile embedded systems are used in different wearable medical devices (Upadhyay et al., 2015).

5G Technology

The role of 5G technology in smart healthcare is huge. Many technologies, such as WiFi, Bluetooth, Wireless Sensor Networks, ZigBee, etc., support communication with different ranges in the Internet of Medical Things. There are many important factors that need to be considered while selecting a particular technology for IoMT (Akpakwa et al., 2017). A few essential factors that need to be considered with higher priority are data rate, communication range, latency, throughput, etc. The authors in (H. Ullah et al., 2019) presented three different case studies; 5G in V2X communication, 5G in healthcare, and 5G in drones. An investigation of the effect of 5G in healthcare is carried out by considering remote surgery, remote health monitoring, remote diagnoses, and remote prescription by using 5G communication technology. The impact of 5G in smart healthcare is far more than other technology such as WiFi or Bluetooth.

EDGE COMPUTING OVER CLOUD COMPUTING FOR HEALTHCARE

With adequate storage and computing capability, cloud computing has empowered the healthcare system to a great extent. In spite of several advantages, the use of cloud computing in many healthcare applications is limited, particularly when the application is latency-sensitive, hard real-time, and data-driven. Even a small period of cloud unavailability in some healthcare systems, which could be caused by a malfunction in cloud servers or a lack of Internet connectivity, could be life-threatening. Some healthcare applications, such as seizure detection, may require a large volume of data on a daily basis. Sending such a large volume of data to the cloud is neither secure nor cost-effective when the communication media is the internet. Furthermore, in applications that require a quick response, the round-trip time created by sending raw data to the cloud, forming inferences, and returning the inferences to the user is unacceptable (Hongxu Yin et al., 2018).

New computing paradigms, namely Edge computing, have recently emerged to solve the drawbacks mentioned above of cloud computing. Edge computing, a horizontally distributed architecture, is presented to bring scalable processing and storage power nearer to the users. Edge computing makes use of computing, networking, and storage resources across the edge-to-cloud continuum. It makes use of both edge-side and Cloud resources and additional resources available in Fog nodes, which are computing nodes positioned between the edge and the cloud. Fog-based applications in healthcare have four major advantages over typical Cloud-based services:

- **Low Latency:** Fog-based applications make use of a number of resources that are close to the user. This reduces the round-trip time imposed by delivering data to remote resources, allowing a variety of low-latency services to be implemented with minimal dependency on remote on-Cloud resources.
- **Resilience to failures:** Availability is a significant concern in designing and implementing real-time applications in smart healthcare systems. In the event of a failure, relying on distributed resources throughout the edge-to-cloud continuum allows for quick service recovery. Important work can be transferred to local resources when a fault is detected in the Fog computing paradigm.
- **Privacy:** Close-to-the-user resources allow sensitive raw data to be processed before being shared with third-party servers, considerably improving patient privacy. For example, noise can be introduced to raw data to disguise private information, or privacy-sensitive data can be filtered.
- **Cost Efficiency:** By utilizing close-to-the-user resources, fog computing eliminates the demand for cloud services while also dramatically lowering the edge-to-cloud data transfer overhead.

As noted above, some of the recent research projects have focused on the benefits of edge computing in real-life smart healthcare systems. The authors in (P. Dong et al., 2020) researches a healthcare system based on edge computing in IoMTs with the goal of lowering system-wide costs. Authors in (J. Li et al., 2020) presented a safe architecture for SDN-based edge computing in IoMT enabled smart healthcare systems. A lightweight authentication system is used to authenticate IoMT devices. After authentication, patients' data is transferred to the edge server for further processing. The Edge servers work together to balance the load and have an SDN controller designed to make intelligent decisions. SDN-based Edge computing allows for greater Edge collaboration and resource usage through appropriate network architecture. It improves system performance by lowering average response time, latency, packet delivery ratio, better throughput, and low network overhead.

PROPOSED CONTAINERIZED EDGE-CLOUD ARCHITECTURE

This section presents the proposed containerized edge-cloud architecture with the Internet of Medical Things for smart healthcare systems. The proposed architecture is presented in Figure 4.

The proposed architecture is mainly divided into three layers; The IoMT layer is the bottom-most layer and is responsible for collecting medical data using different types of medical devices. On top of it, a smart healthcare system is present. The smart healthcare system act as an intermediary between the IoMT layer and the cloud layer. The topmost layer is the cloud layer that supports containerized edge layer.

Figure 4. Proposed containerized edge-cloud architecture

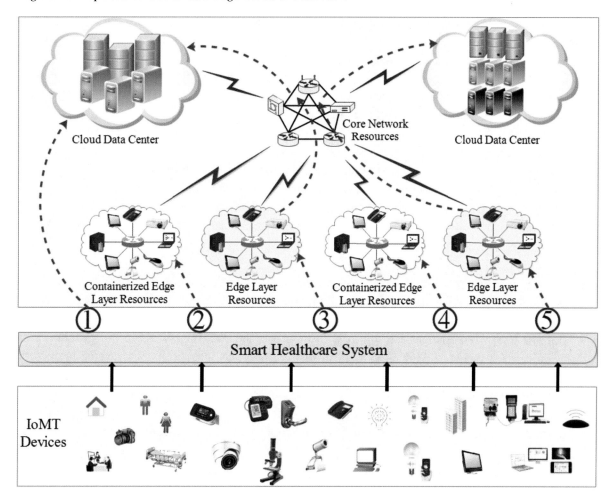

The IoMT layer is a collection of different medical devices connected over the internet. It collects all the medical data and sends those data to the cloud for storing, processing, and analysis purposes. The medical devices in IoMT are connected to the internet and communicate with the cloud layer vis smart healthcare system. In the proposed architecture, devices are interconnected, and communication among medical devices is possible. They can also communicate with the healthcare system, as described in Figure 4. The smart medical device in the IoMT layer could be a temperature sensor that continuously monitors a patient's room temperature. The room temperature data can be used to make a decision, such as whether to switch ON the AC or remain OFF. The AC will automatically switch ON when the room temperature goes above a certain predefined temperature. A surveillance camera monitors a patient's sleeping position and continuously sends images of the patient's sleeping position. If there found any difficulty in sleeping, the bed may adjust automatically to provide better comfort to the patient. A patient may wear some smart medical devices, and those devices will send the data related to patient's body. An ambulance in a city running from one hospital to another will be connected smart healthcare system. They will continuously send data such as current location, speed of moving, next destination, how much time it will take to reach the destination, etc., to the cloud. Those data will further be analyzed for decision making. There will be several other smart devices that will send medical data cloud for further processing through the smart healthcare system. So, the main function of IoMT is to inter-connect all medical devices, collect medical data from the surroundings and send it to the cloud for further processing.

The second layer represents the smart healthcare system. A generalized system structure is shown in Figure 5. Different people interact with the system to avail different healthcare services and to get any health-related information. In the proposed system, four different types of people can interact with the system; Admin, Doctor, Patient, and other public users.

- **Admin Portal:**The admin in a smart healthcare system holds the whole system's total control. The role of an admin is to filter the data coming from the IoMT layer and forward them to the cloud layer. Few data which are irrelevant and not valid for medical decision making are deleted here. The admin sends the only data which are useful for further research or contains some vital information. The admin can add, edit, and delete an individual record from the database. Admin can create a new account for doctors, patients, and normal users, keeping their credentials, including login details.
- **Doctor Portal:**In the doctor portal, doctors can log in with their credentials. They can edit their personal details such as name, specialization, consultation time, etc. The doctor can also see the list of people taking appointments.
- **Patient Portal:**The patient can log in with their username and password in the patient portal. They can see their profile details, medical history, previous test results, and available doctors' profiles. The patient can choose a doctor and make an appointment for a consultation. The patient can edit their personal information.
- **User Portal:**In the user portal, the ordinary public can see the general information about the hospitals, public notice, working hours, available doctors, available vacant beds in hospitals, etc..

Then we have a medical cloud computing layer that provides storage, infrastructure, analytical tools, and container service at the edge level. Some applications require a small number of resources and immediate response in the smart healthcare system. To address such type of request containerized edge layer is present nearer to the users. There are two types of computing resources available; containerized and non-containerized. The execution of any request in a container provides security by isolating it from others. Containers are fast and lightweight applications. In the next section, a brief introduction of the container is presented.

As described in Figure 5, the smart healthcare system can interact with cloud systems in three different ways. The number '1' represents the communication of the smart healthcare system with the cloud. Generally, the cloud is far away from the healthcare system. All servers present in the cloud provide large storage and computing power. So, the application or task that requires large storage and more computing power is directed to the cloud. Their results are stored in the cloud for a longer period of time. They can't be executed in the edge layer. The number '2' and '4' represents the communication with the edge layer. The application or task which requires moderate computing power and storage is executed in the edge layer computing devices. The edge layer is comparatively nearer to the healthcare system than the cloud layer and provides a faster response than the cloud layer. The numbers '3' and '5' represent the containerized edge layer communication. There will be some applications or tasks that quickly respond and require less memory and computing power. Such type of task can be executed in the containerized application at the edge layer. Containers are application-specific provide better security and immediate response. So the smart healthcare system interacts with the cloud system based on the resource requirement and response time.

The main idea of the proposed architecture is to integrate three technologies, cloud computing, edge computing, and the Internet of Medical Things, all together along with containerization. Implementing containers at the edge will reduce the response time, reduce the wastage of memory, and improve the overall performance of the healthcare system. The containerization at the edge will be very much convenient for small size tasks and those task that require quick response.

Figure 5. Smart healthcare system

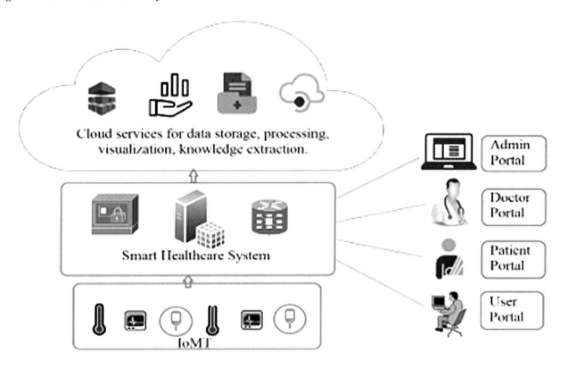

CONTAINERIZATION FOR HEALTHCARE IN CLOUD COMPUTING

Virtualization in cloud computing can be done either using hardware virtualization or software virtualization. Containerization in cloud computing is software virtualization that virtualizes the operating system. So, it is also called OS-level virtualization.

In hardware virtualization, the hypervisor is used to create multiple virtual machines from a single physical machine. The hypervisor is placed on top of hardware, and it acts as an intermediary between virtual machines and hardware. Each virtual machine in hardware virtualization has its own operating system making a virtual machine heavily weighted. Since each virtual machine has its own operating system, it takes more time to startup. From the security point of view, it is completely isolated from other virtual machines, and hence there is no chance of interference with other virtual machines. All communication between the virtual machine and the physical machine takes place through the hypervisor.

On the other hand, in software virtualization, a container engine is used to create multiple containers from a single physical machine. The container engine is placed on top of the host operating system, and it acts as an intermediary between containers and the host operating system. All containers in software virtualization share the same host operating system and do not have their own operating system. This makes a container lightweight and takes very less time to start than a virtual machine. From the security point of view, containers are less isolated than virtual machines because they share the same operating system. All communication between containers and the physical machine takes place through the container engine (Patel, Patra, & Sahoo, 2020). The architecture of a virtual machine and a container is presented in Figure 6.

Figure 6. Hardware vs. software virtualization

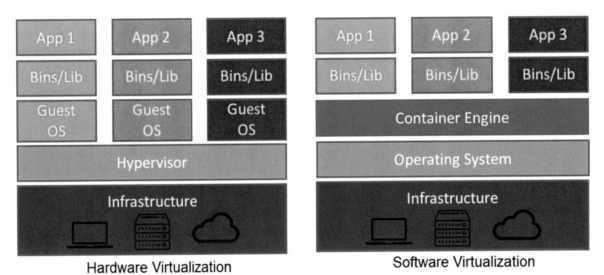

Hardware Virtualization

Software Virtualization

CONCLUSION AND FUTURE POSSIBILITIES

It is a well-known fact that the introduction and deployment of these technologies in the health-care sector provides major benefits to all health-care stakeholders, including inexpensive health care, cost-effective health services, and many others. While the health-care industry is becoming more interested in harnessing IoMT and big data technology to improve efficiency, there are a number of obstacles to overcome before digital health care becomes a widespread reality. In a smart healthcare system, latency and dependability are the two most important elements to consider. In this chapter we found some key technologies that can be used in the smart healthcare system and their impact on it. The technologies include the Internet of Medical Things, Machine Learning, Big Data, Cloud Computing, Artificial Intelligence, Embedded Systems, and 5G communication technology. We discuss different challenges involved in a smart healthcare system that need to be taken care of and considered while designing a healthcare system. Then we emphasize why edge computing over cloud computing is preferable in a smart health-care system. A novel architecture for the smart healthcare system is presented that aims to integrate four technologies; cloud computing, edge computing, containerization with Internet of Medical Things. We introduced the concept of containerization at the edge of the smart healthcare system and described how the container at the edge would improve the latency requirement and improve response time. In conclusion, smart healthcare has a bright future. Individual users may benefit from smart healthcare since it allows them to better control their own health. Medical services will be available when they are needed, and the cost of those treatments will be very less. Smart healthcare can cut expenses, relieve personnel pressure, accomplish unified material and information management, and improve the patient's medical experience for medical institutions.

REFERENCES

Aickelin, U., Chapman, W. W., & Hart, G. K. (2019). *Health Informatics—ambitions and purpose.* Frontiers in Digital Health.

Akpakwu, G. A., Silva, B. J., Hancke, G. P., & Abu-Mahfouz, A. M. (2017). A survey on 5G networks for the Internet of Things: Communication technologies and challenges. *IEEE Access: Practical Innovations, Open Solutions, 6,* 3619–3647. doi:10.1109/ACCESS.2017.2779844

Dong, P., Ning, Z., Obaidat, M. S., Jiang, X., Guo, Y., Hu, X., Hu, B., & Sadoun, B. (2020, September/October). Edge Computing Based Healthcare Systems: Enabling Decentralized Health Monitoring in Internet of Medical Things. *IEEE Network, 34*(5), 254–261. doi:10.1109/MNET.011.1900636

Gawanmeh, A. (2016). Open issues in reliability, safety, and efficiency of connected health. *First IEEE Conference on Connected Health: Applications, Systems and Engineering Technologies,* Washington, DC. 10.1109/CHASE.2016.60

Hipaa. (2019). *Health information privacy.* Available at: www.hhs.gov/hipaa/index.html

Lennon, M. R., Bouamrane, M. M., Devlin, A. M., O'connor, S., O'donnell, C., Chetty, U., Agbakoba, R., Bikker, A., Grieve, E., Finch, T., Watson, N., Wyke, S., & Mair, F. S. (2017). Readiness for delivering digital health at scale: Lessons from a longitudinal qualitative evaluation of a national digital health innovation program in the United Kingdom. *Journal of Medical Internet Research, 19*(2), e6900. doi:10.2196/jmir.6900 PMID:28209558

Li, J., Cai, J., Khan, F., Rehman, A. U., Balasubramaniam, V., Sun, J., & Venu, P. (2020). A Secured Framework for SDN-Based Edge Computing in IoT-Enabled Healthcare System. *IEEE Access: Practical Innovations, Open Solutions, 8,* 135479–135490. doi:10.1109/ACCESS.2020.3011503

Nambiar, A. R., Reddy, N., & Dutta, D. (2017). Connected health: opportunities and challenges. *IEEE International Conference on Big Data,* 1658-1662.

Patel, D., Patra, M. K., & Sahoo, B. (2020). GWO Based task allocation for load balancing in containerized cloud. In 2020 International Conference on Inventive Computation Technologies (ICICT), pp. 655-659. IEEE.

Patra, M. K., Sahoo, S., Sahoo, B., & Turuk, A. K. (2021). Cloud-Edge Centric Service Provisioning in Smart City Using Internet of Things. In *Advances in Parallel & Distributed Processing, and Applications* (pp. 619–631). Springer.

Sonune, S., Kalbande, D., Yeole, A., & Oak, S. (2017). Issues in IoT healthcare platforms: a critical study and review. *IEEE International Conference on Intelligent Computing and Control (I2C2)*. 10.1109/I2C2.2017.8321898

Strauss, A. T., Martinez, D. A., Garcia-Arce, A., Taylor, S., Mateja, C., Fabri, P. J., & Zayas-Castro, J. L. (2015). A user needs assessment to inform health information exchange design and implementation. *BMC Medical Informatics and Decision Making*, *15*(1), 1–11. doi:10.118612911-015-0207-x PMID:26459258

Tse, D., Chow, C. K., Ly, T. P., Tong, C. Y., & Tam, K. W. (2018). The challenges of big data governance in healthcare. *17th IEEE International Conference on Trust, Security and Privacy in Computing and Communications*, New York, NY. 10.1109/TrustCom/BigDataSE.2018.00240

Ullah, H., Gopalakrishnan Nair, N., Moore, A., Nugent, C., Muschamp, P., & Cuevas, M. (2019). 5G Communication: An Overview of Vehicle-to-Everything, Drones, and Healthcare Use-Cases. *IEEE Access: Practical Innovations, Open Solutions*, *7*, 37251–37268. doi:10.1109/ACCESS.2019.2905347

Upadhyay & Dhapola. (2015). Embedded Systems And its Application in Medical Field. *Emerging Trends in Computer Science and Information*, *3*.

Williams, C., Mostashari, F., Mertz, K., Hogin, E., & Atwal, P. (2012). From the office of the national coordinator: The strategy for advancing the exchange of health information. *Health Affairs*, *31*(3), 527–536.

Williams, P. A., & McCauley, V. (2016). *Always connected: the security challenges of the healthcare internet of things*. 3rd IEEE World Forum on the Internet of Things, Reston, VA.

Yin, Akmandor, Mosenia, & Jha. (2018). *Smart Healthcare, now*. Academic Press.

Zeadally, S., & Bello, O. (2019). Harnessing the power of internet of things based connectivity to improve healthcare. Internet of Things. doi:10.1016/j.iot.2019.100074

Zeadally, S., Isaac, J. T., & Baig, Z. (2016). Security attacks and solutions in electronic health (e-health) systems. *Journal of Medical Systems*, *40*(12), 1–12. doi:10.100710916-016-0597-z PMID:27730389

Chapter 15
Medical Information Modeling for Diabetes Based on Logistic Regression

Karthika Natarajan
Vellore Institute of Technology, India

Anjali Gautam
Vellore Institute of Technology, India

Pravalika Somisetty
Vellore Institute of Technology, India

Ramya Venigalla
Vellore Institute of Technology, India

Veeramachaneni Jhansi Lekha
Vellore Institute of Technology, India

ABSTRACT

In this digital health technology world, many health applications are being developed. Artificial intelligence (AI) plays an important role for such important. Popular AI techniques include ML for handling structured and unstructured data. Machine learning detects health issues by studying many health records and data of the patients, hence increasing the efficiency of detection of chronic diseases in the medical field. Medical information modeling is to predict the medical needs in future and is a representation of a complex system into a simplified representation. Diabetes is one of the major diseases in the world population. It is a chronic disease associated with abnormally high levels of glucose in the blood. Gestational diabetes is a temporary condition associated with pregnancy. Several parameters are considered for the study (i.e., age, BMI, insulin levels, BP, number of pregnancies, glucose levels, etc.). Results can be obtained by using machine learning approaches like logistic regression and naive bayes.

DOI: 10.4018/978-1-6684-4580-8.ch015

INTRODUCTION

Artificial intelligence methods in combination with the latest technologies, including medical devices, mobile computing, and sensor technologies, have the potential to enable the creation and delivery of better management services to deal with chronic diseases. One of the most lethal and prevalent chronic diseases is diabetes mellitus, which is characterized by dysfunction of glucose homeostasis. Since the advent of ML, applications of AI have expanded, creating opportunities for personalized medicine rather than algorithm-only based medicine (Ernest, Y.B. et al. 2019) (Gertrud, S. B. et al. 1992). Predictive models can be used for diagnosis of diseases, prediction of therapeutic response and potentially preventative medicine in the future. AI may improve diagnostic accuracy, improve efficiency in provider workflow and clinical operations, facilitate better disease and therapeutic monitoring, improve procedure accuracy and overall patient outcomes (Huma, N . et al. 2020)(Jensen, D.M. et al. 2008)(Davis, EA. et al. 1997).

SETTING THE STAGE

In the Digital health technology, mainly the health applications or apps are being evolved. These are used by people to manage their health conditions (Quan, Z. et al. 2018) (A.H. Mokdad. et al. 2000)(Chakir, F. et al. 2020). Many devices are coming to light for the people having diabetes or who's main motive is to monitor their diet, safety and clinical validity. But we haven't been able to figure out the point how they are doing the tasks because the majority of mobile health apps are not subject to regulation, data for assessment of accuracy, defined as the ability to correctly differentiate patient and healthy cases (Dorothee, D. et al. 2004)(José, G. B. D. et al. 2014)(Ghazal, T.M. et al. 2021).

AI methods in combination with latest technologies like sensor technologies, medical devices can detect and help to treat chronic diseases (Fefie. D. et al. 2009). Research in the past few years led to development in the medical field using different medical information modeling techniques.

CASE DESCRIPTION

The prevalence of gestational diabetes mellitus (GDM) is rising in lockstep with the rise in overweight and obesity among women of childbearing age. GDM develops when a pregnant woman's insulin response is insufficient to compensate for her normal insulin resistance (Merav, C. et al. 2012). Treatment and prevention of GDM, as well as the long and short-term effects of gestational diabetes on both the mother and the baby (Feig, D.S. et al. 2008)(Ioannis, K. et al. 2017). Gestational diabetes mellitus (GDM) affects roughly 5% of pregnancies, however the percentage varies greatly depending on the criteria utilized and the demographic parameters of the population (Kavishwar, B. W.et al. 2012)(Gorgal, R. et al. 2012). The importance of paying close attention to GDM cannot be overstated, and the goal of this review is to cover a wide variety of clinical concerns connected to GDM (Mitushi S. et al. 2020) (Ferrara, A. et al. 2007).

More Concerns

Determining the true prevalence of GDM is difficult. As a result, the prevalence is higher in the United States than in other countries. GDM screening and diagnostic tests, on the other hand, are critical in identifying women who are at risk of acquiring the disease and, as a result, reducing or preventing the risk of adverse events for both mother and child associated with GDM. Past GDM, previous large for gestational age babies, diabetes (of any sort) in first degree relatives, pre-pregnancy adipositas, belonging to a particular ethnic group associated with a high prevalence of GDM, glucosuria, and high maternal age are all the characteristics that are used in most of the countries. There are a number of known risk factors for GDM, including a higher pre-pregnancy BMI and a higher BMI at 28 weeks, both of which are strongly linked to greater insulin resistance at 28 weeks (Kampmann, U. et al. 2015) (Griffin, M.E. et al. 2000).

Even More Concerns

GDM is linked to not just poor pregnancy outcomes, but also to a higher risk of long-term complications for both women and their children (Fei, J. et al. 2017)(Sweety, B. E. et al. 2019). Women who are overweight or obese have a higher risk of developing GDM, which can lead to difficulties during pregnancy; also, it is becoming increasingly obvious that maternal metabolic features are important predictors of insulin resistance during pregnancy (Ornoy, A. et al.2011)(Ivan, C . et al. 2018).

CURRENT CHALLENGES FACING THE ORGANIZATION

In detail, describe some of the challenges and problems that the organization faced at the completion of the project/experience. Furthermore, it would be helpful to the reader if you describe the current status of the aforementioned challenges and problems. Table 1 shows Algorithm Performance Metrics (IGI, 2021)

Table 1. Algorithm performance metrics (IGI, 2021)

S.No	Algorithm	Remarks	Title, Year, Author	Area of Improvement
1.	SVM	Outperforms rule-centred classifiers in prediction of accuracy SVM's are such one of best classifiers when it comes to an increased accuracy of prediction. (Lauenborg, J., et al. 2009)	Modelling Medical Decision making by SVM, Explaining by Rules of Evolutionary Algorithms with Feature Selection. Oct 2012 Ruxandra Stoeana and Catalin Stoeana	As sometimes diseases are temporary but the models perform for the permanent ones, accuracy is not completely accurate
2.	Bayes	Focuses on comprehensive quantitative analysis of many types of problems in medical research and decision making At each stage of model, medical concepts are modelled algebraically, complete with prior distribution (Moshe, P. et al.).	Modeling in Medical Decision Making -A Bayesian approach 2003 Giovanni Parmigiani	It is without attention to what outcome is, as it is difficult to evaluate the model concerning the treatment of problem Bayesian analysis is not only way to interweave information from many sources Less comprehensive models linked by expert judgement are also effective

continues on following page

Table 1. Continued

S.No	Algorithm	Remarks	Title, Year, Author	Area of Improvement
3.	KNN	Multi Label learning model is believed to be more suitable classification model It is to search for k training instance nearest to testing instance and then predict label of test instance according to the nearest instance labels. (Mustafa, A. et al.2021)	Applying k-Nearest Neighbour in Diagnosing Heart Disease Patients June 2012 Mai Shouman, Tim Turner, and Rob Stocker	It quickly judges labels directly by nearest instances without any principle to determine label set based on statistical information from label sets of neighbouring instances. (Reddi, R.et al. 2016)
4.	Logistic Regression	It is widely regarded as the statistic of choice for situations in which the occurrence of a binary outcome is to be predicted from one or more independent variables It is much appropriate for models involving disease state and decision making and hence it is widely used in studies in the medical field. (Vuong, Q.H. et al. 2019)(Wenchao, X. et al. 2017)	A Review of the Logistic Regression Model with Emphasis on Medical Research Ernest Yeboah Boateng and Daniel A. Abaye	If moderate or small samples are taken then they overestimate the effect they measure so in most cases large samples are taken as more independent variables need to be added

COMPUTER CODE

```python
### Importing Libraries and Utilities
import numpy as np
import pandas as pd
import seaborn as sns
from matplotlib import pyplot as plt
from sklearn.metrics import accuracy_score
from sklearn.preprocessing import MinMaxScaler, LabelEncoder, StandardScaler,
RobustScaler
from sklearn.linear_model import LogisticRegression
from sklearn.metrics import accuracy_score, roc_auc_score, confusion_matrix,
classification_report, plot_roc_curve
from sklearn.model_selection import train_test_split, cross_validate
pd.set_option('display.max_columns', None)
pd.set_option('display.float_format', lambda x: '%.3f' % x)
pd.set_option('display.width', 500)
### Load data
df = pd.read_csv("diabetes.csv")
### Check data
def check_df(dataframe: object, head: object = 5) -> object:
print("#### Shape ####")
    print(dataframe.shape)
print("#### Types ####")
    print(dataframe.dtypes)
print("#### Head ####")
    print(dataframe.head(head))
print("#### Tail ####")
    print(dataframe.tail(head))
print("#### NA ####")
```

```
    print(dataframe.isnull().sum())
print("#### Quantiles ####")
print(dataframe.quantile([0, 0.05,0.1, 0.25, 0.50,0.75, 0.90, 0.95, 0.99,
1]).T)
check_df(df)
```

Below figure 1(a) and figure(b) shows Load and Check data

Figure 1a. Load and check data

```
#### Shape ####
(768, 9)
#### Types ####
Pregnancies                int64
Glucose                    int64
BloodPressure              int64
SkinThickness              int64
Insulin                    int64
BMI                        float64
DiabetesPedigreeFunction   float64
Age                        int64
Outcome                    int64
dtype: object
#### Head ####
   Pregnancies  Glucose  BloodPressure  SkinThickness  Insulin   BMI  DiabetesPedigreeFunction  Age  Outcome
0            6      148             72             35        0  33.600                     0.627   50        1
1            1       85             66             29        0  26.600                     0.351   31        0
2            8      183             64              0        0  23.300                     0.672   32        1
3            1       89             66             23       94  28.100                     0.167   21        0
4            0      137             40             35      168  43.100                     2.288   33        1
#### Tail ####
     Pregnancies  Glucose  BloodPressure  SkinThickness  Insulin   BMI  DiabetesPedigreeFunction  Age  Outcome
763           10      101             76             48      180  32.900                     0.171   63        0
764            2      122             70             27        0  36.800                     0.340   27        0
765            5      121             72             23      112  26.200                     0.245   30        0
766            1      126             60              0        0  30.100                     0.349   47        1
767            1       93             70             31        0  30.400                     0.315   23        0
```

Figure 1b. Load and check data

```
#### NA ####
Pregnancies                0
Glucose                    0
BloodPressure              0
SkinThickness              0
Insulin                    0
BMI                        0
DiabetesPedigreeFunction   0
Age                        0
Outcome                    0
dtype: int64
#### Quantiles ####
                          0.000   0.050   0.100   0.250   0.500    0.750    0.900    0.950    0.990    1.000
Pregnancies               0.000   0.000   0.000   1.000   3.000    6.000    9.000   10.000   13.000   17.000
Glucose                   0.000  79.000  85.000  99.000 117.000  140.250  167.000  181.000  196.000  199.000
BloodPressure             0.000  38.700  54.000  62.000  72.000   80.000   88.000   90.000  106.000  122.000
SkinThickness             0.000   0.000   0.000   0.000  23.000   32.000   40.000   44.000   51.330   99.000
Insulin                   0.000   0.000   0.000   0.000  30.500  127.250  210.000  293.000  519.900  846.000
BMI                       0.000  21.800  23.600  27.300  32.000   36.600   41.500   44.395   50.759   67.100
DiabetesPedigreeFunction  0.078   0.140   0.165   0.244   0.372    0.626    0.879    1.133    1.698    2.420
Age                      21.000  21.000  22.000  24.000  29.000   41.000   51.000   58.000   67.000   81.000
Outcome                   0.000   0.000   0.000   0.000   0.000    1.000    1.000    1.000    1.000    1.000
```

```
df.groupby(['Outcome']).agg({"Age":["mean","median"],
                             "Glucose":["mean","median"],
                             "Pregnancies":["mean","median"],
                             "BMI":["mean","median"],
                             "SkinThickness":["mean","median"]})
```

Figure 2. Grouping data

	Age		Glucose		Pregnancies		BMI		SkinThickness	
	mean	median	mean	median	mean	median	mean	median	mean	median
Outcome										
0	31.190	27	109.980	107	3.298	2	30.304	30.050	19.664	21
1	37.067	36	141.257	140	4.866	4	35.143	34.250	22.164	27

```
### Exploratory Data Analysis
def grab_col_names(dataframe, cat_th=10, car_th=20):
cat_cols = [col for col in dataframe.columns if dataframe[col].dtypes == "O"]
num_but_cat = [col for col in dataframe.columns if dataframe[col].nunique()
<cat_th and
dataframe[col].dtypes != "O"]
cat_but_car = [col for col in dataframe.columns if dataframe[col].nunique()
>car_th and
dataframe[col].dtypes == "O"]
cat_cols = cat_cols + num_but_cat
cat_cols = [col for col in cat_cols if col not in cat_but_car]
num_cols = [col for col in dataframe.columns if dataframe[col].dtypes != "O"]
num_cols = [col for col in num_cols if col not in num_but_cat]
print(f"Observations: {dataframe.shape[0]}")
print(f"Variables: {dataframe.shape[1]}")
print(f'cat_cols: {len(cat_cols)}')
print(f'num_cols: {len(num_cols)}')
print(f'cat_but_car: {len(cat_but_car)}')
print(f'num_but_cat: {len(num_but_cat)}')
    return cat_cols, num_cols, cat_but_car
cat_cols, num_cols, cat_but_car = grab_col_names(df)
```

Figure 3. Exploratory data analysis

```
Observations: 768
Variables: 9
cat_cols: 1
num_cols: 8
cat_but_car: 0
num_but_cat: 1
```

```
# Analysis of Categorical Variables
def cat_summary(dataframe, col_name, plot=False):
print(pd.DataFrame({col_name: dataframe[col_name].value_counts(),
                    "Ratio": 100*dataframe[col_name].value_counts()/
len(dataframe)}))
    if plot:
plt.style.use('seaborn-darkgrid')
        fig, ax = plt.subplots(1,2)
        ax = np.reshape(ax,(1,2))
ax[0,0] = sns.countplot(x=dataframe[col_name],color="yellow",ax=ax[0,0])
        ax[0,0].set_ylabel('Count')
        ax[0,0].set_xticklabels(ax[0,0].get_xticklabels(), rotation=-45)
ax[0,1] = plt.pie(dataframe[col_name].value_counts().values,
labels=dataframe[col_name].value_counts().keys(),
                        colors=sns.color_palette('bright'), shadow=True,
autopct='%.0f%%')
plt.title("Percent")
fig.set_size_inches(10,6)
fig.suptitle('Analysis of Categorical Variables',fontsize=13)
plt.show()
for col in cat_cols:
cat_summary(df,col,plot=True)
```

Figure 4. Analysis of categorical variables

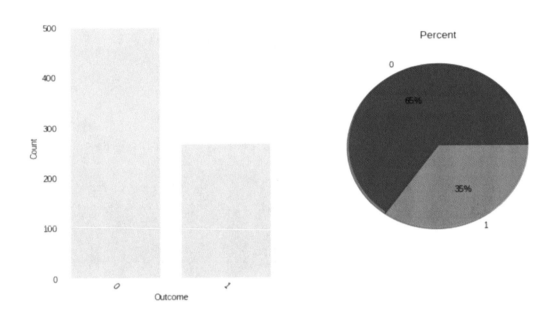

```
# Analysis of Numerical Variables
def num_summary(dataframe, numerical_col):
plt.style.use('seaborn-darkgrid')
    fig, ax = plt.subplots(1,2)
    ax = np.reshape(ax,(1,2))
ax[0,0] = sns.histplot(x=dataframe[numerical_col],color="red",bins=20,ax=
ax[0,0])
    ax[0,0].set_ylabel('Count')
    ax[0,0].set_title('Distribution')
ax[0,1] = sns.boxplot(y=dataframe[numerical_col],color="purple",ax=ax[0,1])
    ax[0,1].set_title('Quantiles')
fig.set_size_inches(12,6)
fig.suptitle('Analysis of Numerical Variables',fontsize=14)
plt.show()
for col in df[num_cols]:
num_summary(df,col)
```

Figure 5. Analysis of numerical variables for pregnancies

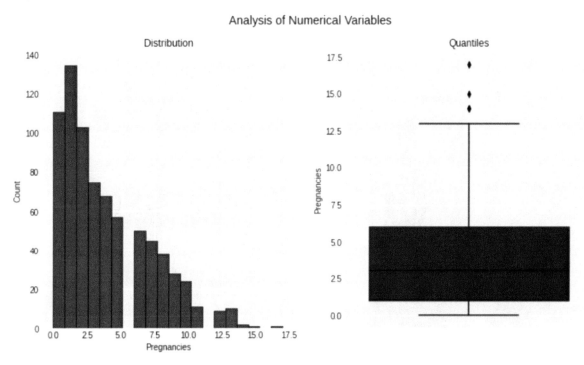

Below figure 6 shows Analysis of Numerical Variables for Glucose

Figure 6. Analysis of numerical variables for glucose

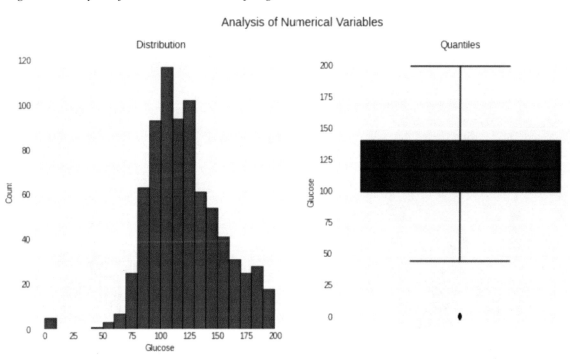

Below figure 7 shows Analysis of Numerical Variables for Blood Pressure

Figure 7. Analysis of numerical variables for blood pressure

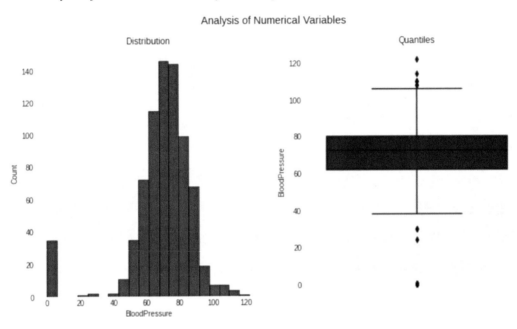

Below figure 8 shows Analysis of Numerical Variables for Skin Thickness

Figure 8. Analysis of numerical variables for skin thickness

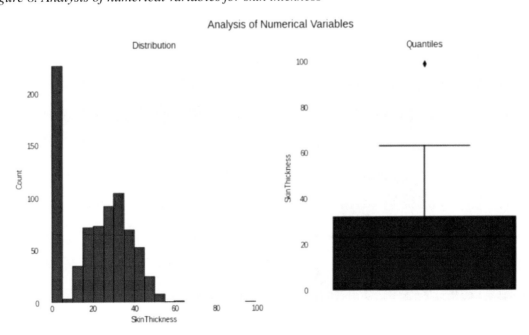

Below figure 9 shows Analysis of Numerical Variables for Insulin

Figure 9. Analysis of numerical variables for insulin

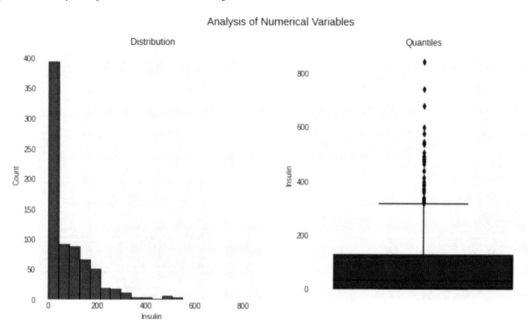

Below figure 10 shows Analysis of Numerical Variables for BMI

Figure 10. Analysis of numerical variables for BMI

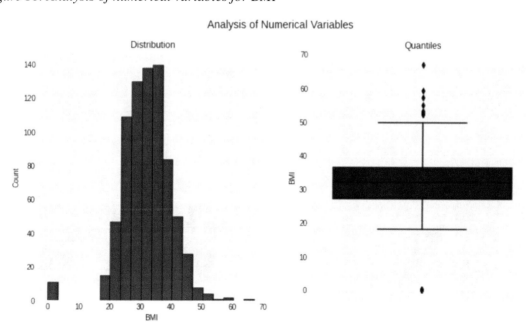

Below figure 11 shows Analysis of Numerical Variables for Diabetes Pedigree Function

Figure 11. Analysis of numerical variables for diabetes pedigree function

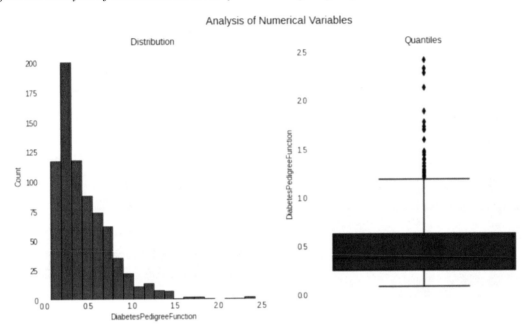

Below figure 12 shows Analysis of Numerical Variables for Age

Figure 12. Analysis of numerical variables for age

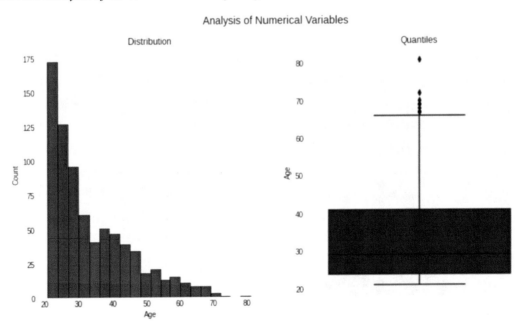

```
# Analysis of Correlation
def correlated_map(dataframe,plot=False):
corr = dataframe.corr()
    if plot:
sns.set(rc={'figure.figsize':(8,8)})
sns.heatmap(corr,cmap="YlGnBu",annot=True,linewidths=.7)
plt.xticks(rotation=60,size=10)
plt.yticks(size=10)
plt.title('Correlation Map',size=18)
plt.show()
correlated_map(df,plot=True)
```

Figure 13. Analysis of correlation

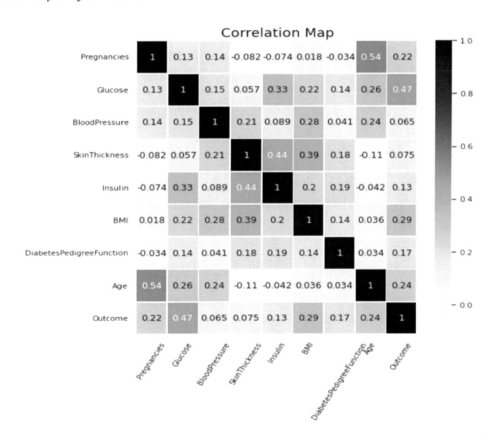

```
### Data Preprocessing
# Missing Values
def missing_values_table(dataframe, na_name=False):
na_columns = [col for col in dataframe.columns if dataframe[col].isnull().
sum() > 0]
```

```
n_miss = dataframe[na_columns].isnull().sum().sort_values(ascending=False)
    ratio = (dataframe[na_columns].isnull().sum()/dataframe.shape[0]*100).
sort_values(ascending=False)
missing_df = pd.concat([n_miss,np.round(ratio,2)],axis=1,keys=['n_
miss','ratio'])
print(missing_df, end="\n")
    if na_name:
        return na_columns
missing_values_table(df, na_name=True)
```

Figure 14. Missing values

```
                          Empty DataFrame
                          Columns: [n_miss, ratio]
                          Index: []
                          []
```

```
# Outliers
def outlier_thresholds(dataframe, col_name, q1=0.05, q3=0.95):
    quartile1 = dataframe[col_name].quantile(q1)
    quartile3 = dataframe[col_name].quantile(q3)
interquantile_range = quartile3 - quartile1
up_limit = quartile3+1.5*interquantile_range
low_limit = quartile1-1.5*interquantile_range
    return low_limit, up_limit
for col in num_cols:
    print(outlier_thresholds(df,col))
```

Figure 15. Outliers

```
                    (-15.0, 25.0)
                    (-74.0, 334.0)
                    (-38.249999999999986, 166.95)
                    (-66.0, 110.0)
                    (-439.5, 732.5)
                    (-12.09249999999999, 78.2875)
                    (-1.3483999999999996, 2.621599999999999)
                    (-34.5, 113.5)
```

```
def replace_with_thresholds(dataframe, variable):
low_limit, up_limit = outlier_thresholds(dataframe, variable)
dataframe.loc[(dataframe[variable] <low_limit), variable] = low_limit
dataframe.loc[(dataframe[variable] >up_limit), variable] = up_limit
for col in num_cols:
replace_with_thresholds(df,col)
df.describe().T
```

Figure 16. Description of data

	count	mean	std	min	25%	50%	75%	max
Pregnancies	768.000	3.845	3.370	0.000	1.000	3.000	6.000	17.000
Glucose	768.000	120.895	31.973	0.000	99.000	117.000	140.250	199.000
BloodPressure	768.000	69.105	19.356	0.000	62.000	72.000	80.000	122.000
SkinThickness	768.000	20.536	15.952	0.000	0.000	23.000	32.000	99.000
Insulin	768.000	79.637	114.243	0.000	0.000	30.500	127.250	732.500
BMI	768.000	31.993	7.884	0.000	27.300	32.000	36.600	67.100
DiabetesPedigreeFunction	768.000	0.472	0.331	0.078	0.244	0.372	0.626	2.420
Age	768.000	33.241	11.760	21.000	24.000	29.000	41.000	81.000
Outcome	768.000	0.349	0.477	0.000	0.000	0.000	1.000	1.000

```
### Feature Extraction
# BMI
bmi_labels = ["Under_weight","Normal_weight","OverWeight","Obesity_
class_1","Obesity_class_2","Obesity_class_3"]
df['BMI_Cat'] = pd.cut(df['BMI'],[-1,18.5,25,30,35,40,df['BMI'].
max()],labels=bmi_labels)
cat_summary(df,"BMI_Cat",plot=True)



# Age
df["New_Age_Cat"] = df["Age"].apply(lambda x: "young_Male" if x < 30 else
("mature_Male" if 30 <= x <= 50 else "senior_Male"))
cat_summary(df,"New_Age_Cat",plot=True)



# Glucose
df["Glucose_Cat"] = df["Glucose"].apply(lambda x: "Normal" if x < 140 else
("IGT" if 140 <= x <= 200 else "DM"))
cat_summary(df,"Glucose_Cat",plot=True)
```

Figure 17. Analysis of categorical variables for BMI

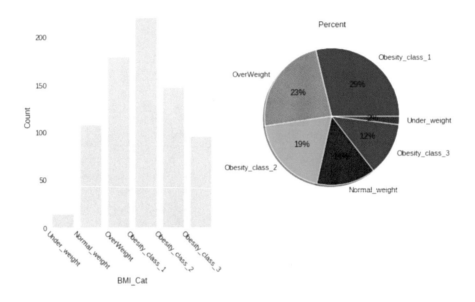

```
                BMI_Cat  Ratio
Obesity_class_1     221  28.776
OverWeight          180  23.438
Obesity_class_2     148  19.271
Normal_weight       108  14.062
Obesity_class_3      96  12.500
Under_weight         15   1.953
```

```
# Blood Pressure
bp_labels = ["Optimal","Normal","High_normal","Grade_1_hypertension","Grade_2_
hypertension","Grade_3_hypertension"]
df['Blood_Pressure_Cat'] = pd.cut(df['BloodPressure'],[-1,80, 85,90,100,110,df
['BloodPressure'].max()],labels=bp_labels)
cat_summary(df,"Blood_Pressure_Cat",plot=True)



### Encoding
# Label Encoding
def label_encoder(dataframe,binary_col):
labelencoder = LabelEncoder()
dataframe[binary_col] = labelencoder.fit_transform(dataframe[binary_col])
    return dataframe
binary_cols = [col for col in df.columns if df[col].dtype not in [int, float]
and df[col].nunique() == 2]
len(binary_cols)
```

Figure 18. Analysis of categorical variables for age

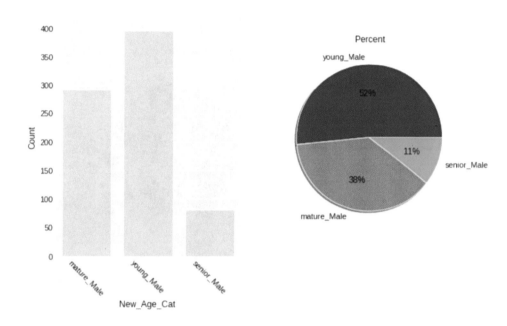

```
            New_Age_Cat  Ratio
young_Male          396  51.562
mature_Male         291  37.891
senior_Male          81  10.547
```

Figure 19. Analysis of categorical variables for glucose

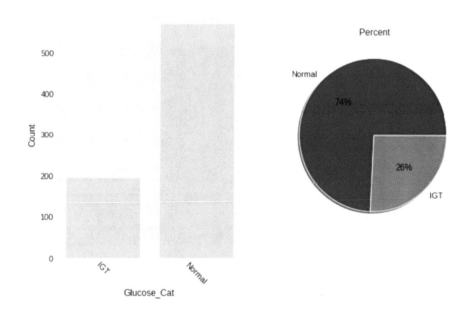

```
          Glucose_Cat  Ratio
Normal            571  74.349
IGT               197  25.651
```

Figure 20. Analysis of categorical variables for blood pressure

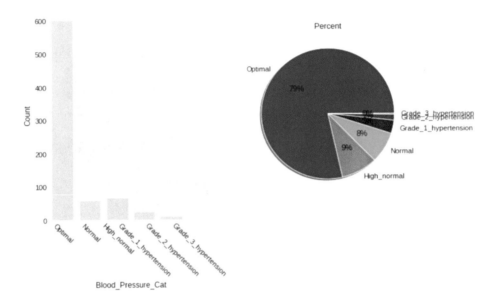

```
                    Blood_Pressure_Cat  Ratio
Optimal                          603  78.516
High_normal                       68   8.854
Normal                            59   7.682
Grade_1_hypertension              25   3.255
Grade_2_hypertension              11   1.432
Grade_3_hypertension               2   0.260
```

Figure 21. Length of binary column

1

```
for col in binary_cols:
label_encoder(df, col)
df.head()
```

Figure 22. Label encoding

	Pregnancies	Glucose	BloodPressure	SkinThickness	Insulin	BMI	DiabetesPedigreeFunction	Age	Outcome	BMI_Cat	New_Age_Cat	Glucose_Cat	Blood_Pressure_Cat
0	6.000	148.000	72.000	35.000	0.000	33.600	0.627	50.000	1	Obesity_class_1	mature_Male	0	Optimal
1	1.000	85.000	66.000	29.000	0.000	26.600	0.351	31.000	0	OverWeight	mature_Male	1	Optimal
2	8.000	183.000	64.000	0.000	0.000	23.300	0.672	32.000	1	Normal_weight	mature_Male	0	Optimal
3	1.000	89.000	66.000	23.000	94.000	28.100	0.167	21.000	0	OverWeight	young_Male	1	Optimal
4	0.000	137.000	40.000	35.000	168.000	43.100	2.288	33.000	1	Obesity_class_3	mature_Male	1	Optimal

```
# One-Hot Encoding
def one_hot_encoder(dataframe, categorical_cols, drop_first=False):
dataframe = pd.get_dummies(dataframe, columns=categorical_cols, drop_
first=drop_first)
    return dataframe
ohe_cols = [col for col in df.columns if 10 >= df[col].nunique() > 2]
df = one_hot_encoder(df,ohe_cols,drop_first=True)
df.head()
```

Figure 23. One-hot encoding

	Pregnancies	Glucose	BloodPressure	SkinThickness	Insulin	BMI	DiabetesPedigreeFunction	Age	Outcome	Glucose_Cat	BMI_Cat_Normal_weight	BMI_Cat_Overweight
0	6.000	148.000	72.000	35.000	0.000	33.600	0.627	50.000	1	0	0	0
1	1.000	85.000	66.000	29.000	0.000	26.600	0.351	31.000	0	1	0	1
2	8.000	183.000	64.000	0.000	0.000	23.300	0.672	32.000	1	0	1	0
3	1.000	89.000	66.000	23.000	94.000	28.100	0.167	21.000	0	1	0	1
4	0.000	137.000	40.000	35.000	168.000	43.100	2.288	33.000	1	1	0	0

BMI_Cat_Overweight	BMI_Cat_Obesity_class_1	BMI_Cat_Obesity_class_2	BMI_Cat_Obesity_class_3	New_Age_Cat_senior_Male	New_Age_Cat_young_Male	Blood_Pressure_Cat_Normal
0	1	0	0	0	0	0
1	0	0	0	0	0	0
0	0	0	0	0	0	0
1	0	0	0	0	1	0
0	0	0	1	0	0	0

Blood_Pressure_Cat_High_normal	Blood_Pressure_Cat_Grade_1_hypertension	Blood_Pressure_Cat_Grade_2_hypertension	Blood_Pressure_Cat_Grade_3_hypertension
0	0	0	0
0	0	0	0
0	0	0	0
0	0	0	0
0	0	0	0

```
cat_cols, num_cols, cat_but_car = grab_col_names(df)
```

Figure 24. Exploratory data analysis

```
Observations: 768
Variables: 22
cat_cols: 14
num_cols: 8
cat_but_car: 0
num_but_cat: 14
```

```
# Standard Scaler
scaler = StandardScaler()
df[num_cols] = scaler.fit_transform(df[num_cols])
check_df(df)
```

Figure 25a. Standard scalar description

```
#### Shape ####
(768, 22)
#### Types ####
Pregnancies                                    float64
Glucose                                        float64
BloodPressure                                  float64
SkinThickness                                  float64
Insulin                                        float64
BMI                                            float64
DiabetesPedigreeFunction                       float64
Age                                            float64
Outcome                                          int64
Glucose_Cat                                      int64
BMI_Cat_Normal_weight                            uint8
BMI_Cat_OverWeight                               uint8
BMI_Cat_Obesity_class_1                          uint8
BMI_Cat_Obesity_class_2                          uint8
BMI_Cat_Obesity_class_3                          uint8
New_Age_Cat_senior_Male                          uint8
New_Age_Cat_young_Male                           uint8
Blood_Pressure_Cat_Normal                        uint8
Blood_Pressure_Cat_High_normal                   uint8
Blood_Pressure_Cat_Grade_1_hypertension          uint8
Blood_Pressure_Cat_Grade_2_hypertension          uint8
Blood_Pressure_Cat_Grade_3_hypertension          uint8
dtype: object
```

Figure 25b. Standard scalar description

```
#### Head ####
    Pregnancies  Glucose  BloodPressure  SkinThickness  Insulin    BMI  DiabetesPedigreeFunction    Age  Outcome  Glucose_Cat  BMI_Cat_Normal_weight  BMI_Cat_OverWeight  BMI_Cat_Obes
0        0.640     0.848         0.150          0.907   -0.698  0.204                     0.468  1.426        1            0                      0                   0
1       -0.845    -1.123        -0.161          0.531   -0.698 -0.684                    -0.365 -0.191        0            1                      0                   1
2        1.234     1.944        -0.264         -1.288   -0.698 -1.103                     0.604 -0.106        1            0                      1                   0
3       -0.845    -0.998        -0.161          0.155    0.126 -0.494                    -0.921 -1.042        0            1                      0                   1
4       -1.142     0.504        -1.505          0.907    0.774  1.410                     5.485 -0.020        1            1                      0                   0
#### Tail ####
    Pregnancies  Glucose  BloodPressure  SkinThickness  Insulin    BMI  DiabetesPedigreeFunction    Age  Outcome  Glucose_Cat  BMI_Cat_Normal_weight  BMI_Cat_OverWeight  BMI_Cat_Ob
763      1.828    -0.623         0.356          1.723    0.879  0.115                    -0.909  2.532        0            1                      0                   0
764     -0.548     0.035         0.046          0.405   -0.698  0.610                     0.398 -0.531        0            1                      0                   0
765      0.343     0.003         0.150          0.155    0.283 -0.735                     0.685 -0.276        0            1                      0                   1
766     -0.845     0.160         0.471         -1.288   -0.698 -0.240                     0.371  1.171        1            1                      0                   0
767     -0.845    -0.873         0.046          0.656   -0.698 -0.202                     0.474 -0.871        0            1                      0                   0
#### NA ####
Pregnancies                 0
Glucose                     0
BloodPressure               0
SkinThickness               0
Insulin                     0
BMI                         0
DiabetesPedigreeFunction    0
Age                         0
Outcome                     0
Glucose_Cat                 0
BMI_Cat_Normal_weight       0
BMI_Cat_OverWeight          0
BMI_Cat_Obesity_class_1     0
BMI_Cat_Obesity_class_2     0
```

Figure 25c. Standard scalar description

```
BMI_Cat_Obesity_class_3                      0
New_Age_Cat_senior_Male                      0
New_Age_Cat_young_Male                       0
Blood_Pressure_Cat_Normal                    0
Blood_Pressure_Cat_High_normal               0
Blood_Pressure_Cat_Grade_1_hypertension      0
Blood_Pressure_Cat_Grade_2_hypertension      0
Blood_Pressure_Cat_Grade_3_hypertension      0
dtype: int64
#### Quantiles ####
```

	0.000	0.050	0.100	0.250	0.500	0.750	0.900	0.950	0.990	1.000
Pregnancies	-1.142	-1.142	-1.142	-0.845	-0.251	0.640	1.531	1.828	2.719	3.907
Glucose	-3.784	-1.311	-1.123	-0.685	-0.122	0.606	1.443	1.881	2.351	2.444
BloodPressure	-3.573	-1.572	-0.781	-0.367	0.150	0.563	0.977	1.080	1.907	2.735
SkinThickness	-1.288	-1.288	-1.288	-1.288	0.155	0.719	1.221	1.472	1.932	4.922
Insulin	-0.698	-0.698	-0.698	-0.698	-0.430	0.417	1.142	1.869	3.856	5.718
BMI	-4.060	-1.294	-1.065	-0.596	0.001	0.585	1.207	1.574	2.382	4.456
DiabetesPedigreeFunction	-1.190	-1.001	-0.927	-0.689	-0.300	0.466	1.228	1.996	3.704	5.884
Age	-1.042	-1.042	-0.956	-0.786	-0.361	0.660	1.511	2.107	2.872	4.064
Outcome	0.000	0.000	0.000	0.000	0.000	1.000	1.000	1.000	1.000	1.000
Glucose_Cat	0.000	0.000	0.000	0.000	1.000	1.000	1.000	1.000	1.000	1.000
BMI_Cat_Normal_weight	0.000	0.000	0.000	0.000	0.000	0.000	1.000	1.000	1.000	1.000
BMI_Cat_OverWeight	0.000	0.000	0.000	0.000	0.000	0.000	1.000	1.000	1.000	1.000
BMI_Cat_Obesity_class_1	0.000	0.000	0.000	0.000	0.000	0.000	1.000	1.000	1.000	1.000
BMI_Cat_Obesity_class_2	0.000	0.000	0.000	0.000	0.000	0.000	1.000	1.000	1.000	1.000
BMI_Cat_Obesity_class_3	0.000	0.000	0.000	0.000	0.000	0.000	1.000	1.000	1.000	1.000
New_Age_Cat_senior_Male	0.000	0.000	0.000	0.000	0.000	0.000	1.000	1.000	1.000	1.000
New_Age_Cat_young_Male	0.000	0.000	0.000	0.000	1.000	1.000	1.000	1.000	1.000	1.000
Blood_Pressure_Cat_Normal	0.000	0.000	0.000	0.000	0.000	0.000	0.000	1.000	1.000	1.000
Blood_Pressure_Cat_High_normal	0.000	0.000	0.000	0.000	0.000	0.000	0.000	1.000	1.000	1.000
Blood_Pressure_Cat_Grade_1_hypertension	0.000	0.000	0.000	0.000	0.000	0.000	0.000	0.000	1.000	1.000
Blood_Pressure_Cat_Grade_2_hypertension	0.000	0.000	0.000	0.000	0.000	0.000	0.000	0.000	1.000	1.000
Blood_Pressure_Cat_Grade_3_hypertension	0.000	0.000	0.000	0.000	0.000	0.000	0.000	0.000	0.000	1.000

```
### Model
y = df["Outcome"]
X = df.drop(["Outcome"],axis=1)
log_model = LogisticRegression().fit(X,y)
# Model Validation: 10-Fold Cross Validation
cv_results = cross_validate(log_model,X,y,cv=10,
                            scoring=["accuracy","precision","recall","f1","r
oc_auc"])
# Predict
y_pred = log_model.predict(X)
# Model Evaluation
# Confusion Matrix
def plot_confusion_matrix(y, y_pred):
    acc = round(accuracy_score(y, y_pred),2)
    cm = confusion_matrix(y, y_pred)
sns.heatmap(cm,annot=True,fmt=".0f")
plt.xlabel('y_pred')
plt.ylabel('y')
plt.title('Accuracy Score: {0}'.format(acc),size=13)
plt.show()
plot_confusion_matrix(y, y_pred)
```

```
print(classification_report(y, y_pred))
```

Figure 26. Confusion matrix

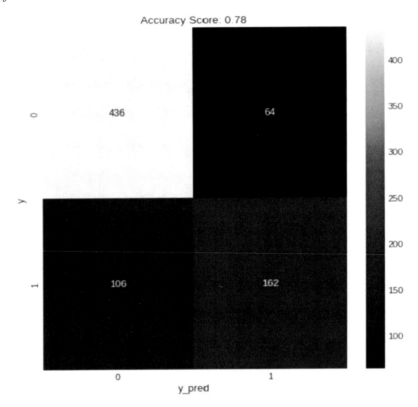

```
y_prob = log_model.predict_proba(X)[:,1]
roc_auc_score(y, y_prob)
```

Figure 27. Classification report

	precision	recall	f1-score	support
0	0.80	0.87	0.84	500
1	0.72	0.60	0.66	268
accuracy			0.78	768
macro avg	0.76	0.74	0.75	768
weighted avg	0.77	0.78	0.77	768

```
X.columns
random_user = X.sample(1,random_state=42)
log_model.predict(random_user)
```

Figure 28. Probability of outcome

```
0.8544626865671641
```

```
feature_imp = pd.DataFrame({'Value': log_model.coef_[0], 'Feature': X.columns})
plt.figure(figsize=(10,6))
sns.set(font_scale=1)
sns.barplot(x="Value", y="Feature", data=feature_imp.sort_values(by="Value",
          ascending=False)[0:8])
plt.title('Features')
plt.tight_layout()
plt.show()
```

Figure 29. Random user prediction

```
array([0])
```

CONCLUSION

The frequency of overweight and obesity in women of reproductive age basically has risen dramatically over the world. Women who particularly are pretty overweight or obese literally are fairly more sort of likely to for the most part acquire Gestational diabetes mellitus, which can cause difficulties during pregnancy, birth, and neonatal care in a very major way. Obese pregnant women and women with Gestational diabetes mellitus mostly are difficult to mostly manage clinically, putting additional strain on the healthcare system in an actually big way. Furthermore, it is becoming increasingly very clear that maternal metabolic characteristics particularly are important determinants of insulin resistance during pregnancy and in offspring, and that interventions, particularly exercise, weight loss, and a healthy diet before, during, and after pregnancy, may be a definitely key to breaking the vicious cycle that contributes to the obesity, insulin resistance, and type 2 diabetes epidemics in a subtle way. In this paper we generally get to definitely know about the prediction of gestational diabetes using logistic regression so that we could essentially get to for the most part know the accuracy of the gestational diabetes and its permanent ness or temporarily in a big way.

Figure 30. Bar plot of features and its value

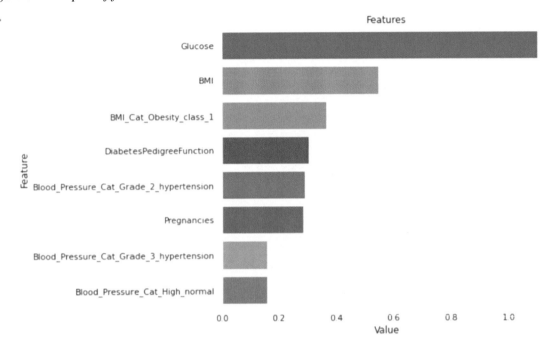

REFERENCES

Chakir, F., & Rachid, E. (2020). Machine Learning and Deep Learning applications in E-learning Systems: A Literature Survey using Topic Modeling Approach. *2020 6th IEEE Congress on Information Science and Technology (CiSt)*, 267-273. https://ieeexplore.ieee.org/xpl/conhome/9357063/proceeding

Davis, E. A., Keating, B., Byrne, G. C., Russell, M., & Jones, T. W. (1997). Hypoglycemia: Incidence and clinical predictors in a large population-based sample of children and adolescents with IDDM. *Diabetes Care*, 20(1), 22–25. doi:10.2337/diacare.20.1.22 PMID:9028688

Dorothee, D., Reinhard, H., Julia, H., & Olga, K. (2004). Assessment of glycemic control by continuous glucose monitoring system in 50 children with type 1 diabetes starting on insulin pump therapy. *Pediatric Diabetes*, 5(3), 117–121. doi:10.1111/j.1399-543X.2004.00053.x PMID:15450005

Ernest, Y.B., & Daniel, A. (2019). A Review of the Logistic Regression Model with Emphasis on Medical Research. *Journal of Data Analysis and Information Processing*, 190-207.

Fefie, D. (2009). From data to knowledge in e-health applications: An integrated system for medical information modelling and retrieval. *Medical Informatics and the Internet in Medicine*, 231–251. PMID:14668128

Fei, J., Yong, J., Hui, Z., Yi, D., Hao, L., Sufeng, M., Yilong, W., Qiang, D., Haipeng, S., & Yongjun, W. (2017). Artificial intelligence in healthcare: Past, present and future. *SVN Stroke and Vascular Neurology, BMJ Journals*. https://svn.bmj.com/content/2/4/230

Feig, D. S., Zinman, B., Wang, X., & Hux, J. E. (2008). Risk of development of diabetes mellitus after diagnosis of gestational diabetes. *Canadian Medical Association Journal, 179*(3), 229–234. doi:10.1503/cmaj.080012 PMID:18663202

Ferrara, A. (2007). Increasing prevalence of gestational diabetes mellitus: A public health perspective. *Diabetes Care, 30*(2), S141–S146. doi:10.2337/dc07-s206 PMID:17596462

Gertrud, S. B., Robert, H.L., Rosemary, W., & Deborah, L. (1992). Race/Ethnicity and Other Risk Factors for Gestational Diabetes. *American Journal of Epidemiology, 135*(9), 965–973. doi:10.1093/oxfordjournals.aje.a116408

Ghazal, T. M., Hasan, M. K., Alshurideh, M. T., Alzoubi, H. M., Ahmad, M., Akbar, S. S., Al, K. B., & Akour, I. A. (2021). IoT for Smart Cities: Machine Learning Approaches in Smart Healthcare—A Review. *Future Internet, 13*(8), 218. doi:10.3390/fi13080218

Gorgal, R., Gonçalves, E., Barros, M., Namora, G., Magalhães, A., Rodrigues, T., & Montenegro, N. (2012). Gestational diabetes mellitus: A risk factor for non-elective cesarean section. *Journal of Obstetrics and Gynaecology Research, 38*(1), 154–159.

Griffin, M. E., Coffey, M., Johnson, H., Scanlon, P., Foley, M., Stronge, J., O'Meara, N. M., & Firth, R. G. (2000). Universal vs. risk factor-based screening for gestational diabetes mellitus: Detection rates, gestation at diagnosis and outcome. *Diabetic Medicine, 17*(1), 26–32.

Huma, N., & Sachin, A. (2020). Deep learning approach for diabetes prediction using PIMA Indian dataset. *J Diabetes Metab Disord*, 391-403. https://pubmed.ncbi.nlm.nih.gov/32550190/

Ioannis, K., Olga, T., Athanasios, S., Nicos, M., Ioannis, V., & Ioanna, C. (2017). Machine Learning and Data Mining Methods in Diabetes Research. *Computational and Structural Biotechnology Journal, 15*, 104–116.

Ivan, C., & Josep, V. (2018). Artificial Intelligence for Diabetes Management and Decision Support: Literature Review. *Journal of Medical Internet Research, 20*(5).

Jensen, D. M., Korsholm, L., Ovesen, P., Beck, N. H., Mølsted, P. L., & Damm, P. (2008). Adverse pregnancy outcome in women with mild glucose intolerance: Is there a clinically meaningful threshold value for glucose? *Acta Obstetricia et Gynecologica Scandinavica, 87*(1), 59–62. doi:10.1080/00016340701823975 PMID:18158628

José, G. B. D., Marius, R., Wayne, S. C., Teresa, E. P., Sheryl, T., Ann, F., Jane, M. P., Paul, L. D., & Paul, L. H. (2014). Effects of Age, Gender, BMI, and Anatomical Site on Skin Thickness in Children and Adults with Diabetes. *PLoS One, 9*(1), e86637. Advance online publication. doi:10.1371/journal.pone.0086637 PMID:24466182

Kampmann, U., Madsen, L. R., Skajaa, G. O., Iversen, D. S., Moeller, N., & Ovesen, P. (2015). Gestational diabetes: A clinical update. *World Journal of Diabetes, 6*(8), 1065–1072. doi:10.4239/wjd.v6.i8.1065 PMID:26240703

Kavishwar, B. W., Vijayraghavan, S., & Ashok, W. D. (2012). Modeling Paradigms for Medical Diagnostic Decision Support: A Survey and Future Directions. *Journal of Medical Systems, 36*, 3029–3049. https://link.springer.com/article/10.1007/s10916-011-9780-4

Lauenborg, J., Grarup, N., Damm, P., Borch, J. K., Jørgensen, T., Pedersen, O., & Hansen, T. (2009). Common type 2 diabetes risk gene variants associate with gestational diabetes. *J Clin Endocrinol Metab, 94*(1), 145-50.

Merav, C., Eyal, C., Sigal, F., Zamir, H., Uri, N., & Eshel, B.J. (2012). Artificial Neural Networks Based Controller for Glucose Monitoring during Clamp Test. *PLOS ONE*. https://journals.plos.org/plosone/article?id=10.1371/journal.pone.0044587

Mitushi, S., & Sunita, V. (2020). Diabetes Prediction using Machine Learning Techniques. *International Journal of Engineering Research & Technology*. https://www.ijert.org/diabetes-prediction-using-machine-learning-techniques

Mokdad, Ford, Bowman, Nelson, Engelgau, & Vinicor. (2000). Diabetes trends in the U.S.: 1990-1998. *Diabetes Care 1, 23*(9), 1278–1283. doi:10.2337/diacare.23.9.1278

Moshe, P., Tadej, B., Eran, A., Olga, K., Natasa, B., Shahar, M., Torben, B., Magdalena, A.S., Ido, M., Revital, N., & Thomas, D. (n.d.). Nocturnal Glucose Control with an Artificial Pancreas at a Diabetes Camp. *The New England Journal of Medicine*. https://www.nejm.org/doi/10.1056/NEJMoa1206881#article_citing_articles

Mustafa, A., & Rahimi, A. M. (2021). Automated Machine Learning for Healthcare and Clinical Notes Analysis. *Computers, 2021*(10), 24. doi:10.3390/computers10020024

Ornoy, A. (2011). Prenatal origin of obesity and their complications: Gestational diabetes, maternal overweight and the paradoxical effects of fetal growth restriction and macrosomia. *Reproductive Toxicology (Elmsford, N.Y.), 32*(2), 205–212.

Quan, Z., Kaiyang, Q., Yamei, L., Dehui, Y., Ying, J., & Hua, T. (2018). Predicting Diabetes Mellitus With Machine Learning Techniques. *Frontiers in Genetics, 9*, 515. https://www.ncbi.nlm.nih.gov/pmc/articles/PMC6232260/

Reddi, R., & Jasmina, B. (2016). Screening and Diagnosis of Gestational Diabetes Mellitus, Where Do We Stand. *Journal of Clinical and Diagnostic Research : JCDR, 10*(4), QE01–QE04.

Sarker, I. H., Hoque, M. M., Uddin, M. K., & Tawfeeq, A. (2021). Mobile Data Science and Intelligent Apps: Concepts, AI-Based Modeling and Research Directions. *Mobile Networks and Applications, 26*(1), 285–303. doi:10.100711036-020-01650-z

Sweety, B. E., Srimathi, H., & Bagavandas, M. (2019). A Survey Of Machine Learning Algorithms In Health Care. *International Journal of Scientific & Technology Research, 8*(11).

Vuong, Q. H., Ho, M. T., Vuong, T. T., La, V. P., Ho, M. T., Nghiem, K. C., Tran, B. X., Giang, H. H., Giang, T. V., Latkin, C., Nguyen, H. K. T., Ho, C. S. H., & Ho, R. C. M. (2019). Artificial Intelligence vs. Natural Stupidity: Evaluating AI Readiness for the Vietnamese Medical Information System. *Journal of Clinical Medicine, 8*(2), 168. doi:10.3390/jcm8020168 PMID:30717268

Wenchao, X., & Yilin, B. (2017). Medical Health Big Data Classification Based on KNN Classification Algorithm. *IEEE Access: Practical Innovations, Open Solutions.* Advance online publication. doi:10.1109/ACCESS.2019.2955754

Chapter 16

Understanding of the Exploratory Graph Theoretical Approach for Data Analysis With Supervised and Unsupervised Learning

Kiran Hemanthraj Muloor
LTI, India

Somesh Kumar Sahu
https://orcid.org/0000-0003-2171-0338
LTI, India

Rajshree Dahal
CHRIST University (Deemed), India

ABSTRACT

Information is a vital part of optimizing the effectiveness, profitability, and dynamic abilities of organizations of all sizes, which leads to expanded deals, profits, and benefits. Currently, organizations deal with immense datasets, but owning a lot of data doesn't boost the business unless ventures investigate the available data and drive authoritative development. It is possible to automate exploratory data analysis to save a lot of time and effort, since we no longer need to write code for each visualization and statistical analysis. Automation of the process generates a report that includes all the visualization and data analysis as well.

DOI: 10.4018/978-1-6684-4580-8.ch016

INTRODUCTION

The exploratory data analysis [EDA] process was first developed in 1970 by Tukey and John Wilder. It is a method used prior to analyzing and creating a model to gain a complete understanding of the data. Simple quantitative and graphical techniques can be used to identify and explore the gaps in the data. According to Tukey, too much emphasis in statistics is placed on statistical hypothesis testing (confirmatory data analyses); instead, the data should be used to suggest hypotheses for further testing. Using EDA, the characteristics, behaviors, features, and features of the data are identified, reviewed, modified, and corrected before putting the data into any statistical model or analysis. EDA techniques have been incorporated into data mining (Tukey, 1977b).

To demonstrate how simple graphics and quantitative methods can be used to openly explore data, John W. Tukey brought the term "Exploratory Data Analysis" into existence.

Typical graphical techniques include

- Data visualization (e.g., stem-and-leaf diagrams, histograms, scatter plots)
- Statistical plotting (such as mean, box and residual plots)
- The positioning of multiple plots in order to enhance cognition

Data analysis is a life cycle that includes numerous stages. Exploratory data analysis is one of the stages that help the analyst understand the domain and data better so that he or she can derive insights and provide solutions based on the information provided by the data. Figure 1 shows details about 7 stages of Data analytics process.

Figure 1. 7 stage data analytics process

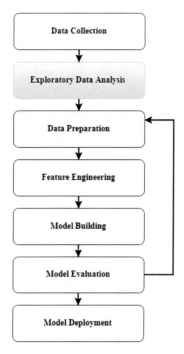

Although there is no unified structure for analyzing data, multiple steps are involved in achieving a problem-solving process based on data analysis. Data Analytics primarily consists of 6 stages excluding Model Deployment. Each stagehas their own significance in the world of analysis. Let's have a detailed look into these stages.

1. **Data Collection**: At this phase of the data analytics life cycle, the objective of the data will be defined, as will the means and means by which it will be achieved. By analyzing the data, one can identify the core objectives of a firm, what it is looking to accomplish, and what it needs to achieve to accomplish those objectives. The team gains an understanding of the business domain during this phase, as well as checking whether the business unit or institution has undertaken similar projects in the past to apply learned lessons.

In order to be an effective data manager, you must identify potential uses and demands for your company's information, such as where the data comes from, what the data can tell you, and what the business benefits will be by using it. Rather than focusing on data as it stands, as a data analyst you need to focus on enterprise data requirements. Additionally, it is your responsibility to assess the tools and systems you will need to read, organize, and analyze the data you receive.

This phase will involve a number of activities including framing the business problem as an analytics challenge and formulating initial hypotheses (IHs) that will be tested and learned from the data that can be collected. It is therefore essential to ensure that the drawn-in objective is achieved during the subsequent phases.

2. **Exploratory Data Analysis:** Any Data Analysis or Data Science project begins with an exploratory data analysis, or EDA, as an initial step. The objective of EDA is to investigate a dataset, identify patterns and anomalies (outliers), and finally formulate hypotheses based on the knowledge we have about the dataset.

In the case of EDA, statistics are generated for numerical data in the dataset and various chart representations are created so that a better understanding of the data can be achieved. Data professionals commonly use exploratory data analysis (EDA), also known as exploratory data mining (EDM)(Matchev et al., 2022), to prepare themselves before attempting to model a dataset. Alternatively, the term is sometimes used to refer to data exploration. EDA is the process of examining a dataset to find out more about its characteristics. When an EDA is conducted, data analysts are able to make assumptions and predictions about the dataset. In many cases, enterprise data analysis (EDA) includes data visualization, such as creating histograms, scatter plots and box plots (Rao et al., 2021).

3. **Data Preparation:** At this stage, all of the data-related issues will be taken into consideration. Experts are primarily focused on the requirements of information at this stage rather than business requirements, which are more common at this stage. Data preparation and processing is the process that involves gathering, processing, and purifying the gathered data so that it can be used. In this phase, you'll have to verify that you have the needed data readily available so that you can begin the process of processing it. This is one of the most crucial parts of the process. The first stage in data preparation is collecting relevant data, which is the first step in the analytics life cycle. This is

followed by the next stage of the analytics lifecycle called analytics analysis. (Becher et al., 2000). The following approaches are used to acquire data:

Data acquisition: It is a process of collecting data from external sources such as the internet in order to gather data.

Data Entry: In order to prepare any data points that have been recently collected, this process involves preparing the preliminary data using digital systems or manual entry tools.

Data Reception: It does so by gathering and capturing data from digital devices that are attached to the Internet such as control systems and Internet of Things.

4. **Feature Engineering**: In machine learning, feature engineering is a method that allows users to simplify the task of analyzing data. The process of feature engineering refers to the selection, manipulation, and transformation of raw data into features that can be used to perform supervised learning applications. It might be necessary to train and design more effective features in order for machine learning to work well in new tasks (Al-Kandari & Jolliffe, 2005).

For this particular problem, we are mainly interested in making it more transparent so that it can be digestible for people with no background in data or analytics. Nevertheless, more features could be developed for the data visualization prepared for people without such knowledge to be more digestible. Nevertheless, the concept of transparency is a much more complex one when it comes to machine learning models since the models often require different approaches for handling the various types of data. In machine learning, feature engineering is a procedure that is used to transform the data into a form that is easier to understand(Bezerra et al., 2019).

5. **Model Building**: Data sets are developed for testing, training, and production purposes in this step of the data analytics architecture. In the following step, the data analytics experts meticulously build and operate the model they created previously. Models are built and executed using various tools and techniques, such as decision trees, regression techniques, and neural networks. To verify that the model matches the datasets, experts also run a trial run of the model.
6. **Model Evaluation**: In this phase, you should verify that the tests you have run in phase one satisfy those criteria. In the communication step, major stakeholders work together to determine whether the project was a success or a failure. Identifying and evaluating key findings from the analysis, measuring the associated business value, and producing a narrative to summarize and communicate the results is required of the project team.

In order to help businesses, achieve their goals, the data analytics lifecycle is composed of six phases, each of which is designed to explain how information is collected, processed, utilized, and analyzed. Data analysts, however, do face difficulties in their attempts to work with the information when there is no standard set of phases for the architecture of data analytics (Rao et al., 2021).

The process of data analysis begins with the exploratory analysis of the information obtained from the survey. During the analysis process, one of our primary objectives is to understand the data we have - things such as formulating the right questions to ask, understanding how to manipulate the data sources in order to figure out the right answer, etc. In order to get a better understanding of our research, a visual approach is key, since trends, patterns, and outliers come to light more easily. Data explorers can assist in the identification of mistakes, the difference between exceptions within data sets, the discovery of connections within the data sets, the discovery of important elements, the discovery of patterns, and the ability to uncover new insights hidden within the data set.

UNDERSTANDING OF EXPLORATORY DATA ANALYSIS

Visualizing and analysing data can be done in many different ways by data professionals. Data scientists and other data professionals use exploratory data analysis to understand datasets before modelling. Exploratory Data Analysis (EDA)(Wasay et al., 2015) is an approach to data analysis that employs a number of different techniques to:

- Consider what the data seems to be saying and make an informed decision based on it,
- Recognize the underlying structures and their relationships
- Determine the most important variables,
- Identify outliers, anomalies, and anomalous behavior by analyzing the data,
- Suggest appropriate models that could be used with conventional statistics.

The exploratory data analysis method consists of analyzing data sets to summarize their main features, often using statistical graphics and other methods of visualizing data. EDA is a technique of data analysis, which consists of several different techniques, in order to:

- Analyze the data to find out what it seems to indicate,
- Investigate the underlying structures
- Determine the most relevant variables,
- Analyze anomalies and outliers,
- Make recommendations for suitable conventional statistics models.

It is imperative to know three rules when it comes to analysing data. In order to avoid making incorrect claims about your data, you should follow the following three guidelines:

Take a look at the data that you have and decide what you want to learn by looking at it. Let's say you want to know for certain that the world is round. Would you like to prove the circumference of the planet or at least how it would appear to be round? The formal way of stating a hypothesis is to formulate this question. The next thing is to analyse your data to determine whether the central tendency is obvious. In most cases, the mean and median are used to quantify both the central tendency and the central tendency. Your hypothesis in Step 1 will determine which one you should use. When trying to prove that the planet is round, you can look at either the average volume or the average circumference.

Not all cases are governed by the central tendency. When you have taken the average, you will need to analyse the data that differ from it. Check the numbers that did not meet the median expectation if you measured a median. Check for anomalies to see if your conclusions are incorrect. You might be able to identify a problem if your child gets a 70 on a test in school. It seems reasonable, right? Furthermore, if we look at the exceptions, you will be able to see that they are getting 100 points in three classes (this is awesome!), and 40 points in three others (also great!). Therefore, the average must be interpreted with caution.Figure 2 shows about Process involved to perform Exploratory Data Analysis

Figure 2. Process involved to perform exploratory data analysis

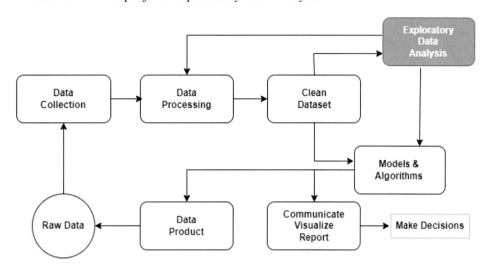

Raw Data is collected for any data analysis, there are several ways for data collection. Collecting data is a key step in exploratory data analysis. It involves finding and loading data into the platform. Data can be found on various public websites or purchased from private organizations. Data collection can be done in a number of ways. Other methods involve directly asking customers for information, while others involve monitoring your interactions with customers and observing their behavior. Depending on the data you collect, you will decide which to use.

Cleansing your dataset means getting rid of unwanted variables and values and removing irregularities. Anomalies such as these skew the data disproportionately and thus adversely impact the results. Here are some steps you can take to clean the data:

- Eliminating missing values, outliers, and unnecessary rows/columns.
- Our data will be reindexed and reformatted.

A variety of methods can be used to analyse and manipulate data in order to draw relevant conclusions using various techniques, such as statistical analysis, regression analysis, neural networks, text analysis, etc. Following the completion of this stage, you will begin to observe trends, correlations, variances, and patterns that will provide answers to the questions you had when you began the project. Researchers, as well as average business users, can both benefit from the use of the numerous technologies available for managing their data. Many types of software are available for business intelligence and visualization, data mining, and predictive analytics.

Finally, the most important step is to interpret your results. A researcher develops action plans based on findings during this stage. You would understand if your clients prefer boxes that are red or green, plastic or paper, for example. Moreover, you can also discover some limitations at this stage and work on them. This stage involves the dissemination of the key findings to all or part of the stakeholders. Using this information, you can determine if the results of the project support the inputs of the model or if it is a failure.

EDA has the following objectives:

1. Describe the causes of observed phenomena and suggest hypotheses
2. Inferential statistics are based on assumptions
3. Provide support in selecting appropriate statistical tools and techniques
4. The data collected in this survey or experiment will be used to collect more information

As a matter of fact, all three approaches begin with a science/engineering problem and conclude with a conclusion based on science/engineering. Although there are differences in the intermediate steps and the order in which the steps are completed, there is a general pattern.

According to classical analysis,

1. the sequence is for Classic Analysis
    Problem > Data > Model > Analysis > Conclusions,
2. the sequence is for EDA
    Problem > Data > Analysis > Model > Conclusions
3. the sequence is for Bayesian
    Problem > Data > Model > Prior Distribution > Analysis > Conclusions

The collection of data is generally followed by the application of a model (normality, linearity, etc.) based on the data, and then any subsequent analyses, estimations, or tests are based upon the parameters of the model. The approach to data collection is not governed by a particular model; rather, it is determined by a subsequent analysis of which model will be appropriate. It is also important to note that Bayesian analysis entails the integration of scientific and engineering expertise into the analysis by imposing a probability distribution on the parameters of the model that is applied at every iteration of the model. As a result of integrating the prior distribution and the collected data, this analysis then can be used to infer or test assumptions regarding the parameters of the model. Ultimately, the goal of every data analyst is to be able to combine elements of all of these approaches (along with other approaches) in a way that achieves maximum benefit. In order to highlight the key differences between these two approaches, we have positioned them differently, both to highlight their similarities, and also to highlight the differences between them.

GRAPH THEORETICAL APPROACH TO DATA ANALYSIS:

The branch of the graph deals with vertices and edges. A graph G is considered to be an ordered set of vertices set V and edge set E and given by, G= (V, E). The analysis of data through graphical means of nodes and links has gained lots of interest in the last few years. The representation of raw data into graph connections or networks helps in better visualization of the aspects that it consists of irrespective of the size of the data. Further, this helps us in advance actionable perceptions and makes us take better figuresmotivatedconclusionsbuilt on them. Moreover, various programming software like R-programming and Python has already built up the various network packages for using graph theory for data analysis because of the positive traits of the graphical approach for a particular data. In data analysis, we are to provide the best possible solution that is efficient in every way cost-wise or time-wise. The analysis of the problem by graph theory helps in arranging the data in a systematic and ordered manner thus help-ing in achieving the efficiency factor. Table 1 has some real-time problems that may be presented as bulk data considering the huge number of factors they take into account. The graph-based approach is also given for the same:

The concepts like betweenness, centrality, parallel connections, shortest path, least cost path, and average path length help in a deeper analysis of a given data. These conditions are helpful in better understanding and using the data to derive multiple solutions for a given problem.

Table 1. Real-time problems

Field of Data/ Network	Vertex Features	Edge Features
Stock Chain Network	Storehouses are the vertices - conditions: locations, capacity, connectivity, manual, automatic.	Vehicles are the edges -conditions: permit, year of manufacture, the total cost on the driver, maintenance, miles travelled.
Airlines	Airportsare the vertices- conditions: Total number of passengers on an everyday basis, Staff Population, Number of Terminals, Seating capacity, Store networks, Total number of flights hold capacity.	Routes/ Links are the edges – conditions: type of plane, frequency, routes, fuel usage, distance travelled, empty seats.
Social Network	Users are the network conditions: connections, likes, dislikes, followed, unfollowed, circles.	Interactions are the edges – conditions: Time, duration, medium of connection.

EDA FOR DIFFERENT DATA TYPES

Exploratory data analysis refers to a process in which all preliminary investigations are performed, such as recognizing patterns, detecting outliers, testing hypotheses, and evaluating assumptions, using summary statistics and graphical representations as a basis for evaluation. In order to gain as many insights from the data as possible, it is important to understand the data first. Before getting dirty with the data, EDA is about making sense of the data at hand.We have access to a large data source. From different data sources, we can find different types of data. However, we should know more about the data's characteristics. These characteristics are determined by variables. We can easily categorize or divide variables based on a few parameters. Basically, variables fall into two categories: categorical and numerical

Types of Variables in the Data

A data type is an important statistician's concept that needs to be understood in order to correctly apply statistical measurements to your data and, as a result, to make correct conclusions regarding it. Data consists of two types of variables - numerical and categorical. In numerical data, there are continuous and discrete values. For categorical data, there are nominal and ordinal values. Figure 3 shows about types of variables.

Numerical

Data that can be quantified and expresses itself numerically, but not in words or as text, is numerical data. Numbers that do not have a logical end are called continuous numbers. These include variables like monetary amounts or heights.

Figure 3. Types of variables

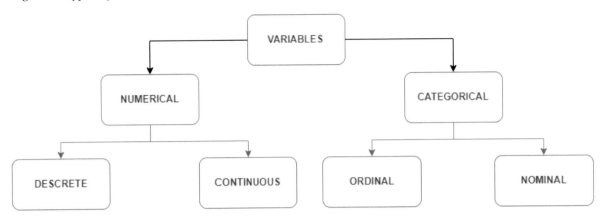

Discrete numbers have no logical end and are the opposite. Variables such as the number of days in the month or the number of bugs logged are examples. It's important to note that correlation is not the same as causation - you probably heard that before. Thus, a correlation between two variables does not mean that one variable will cause the other to react. A relationship may exist between them, but there may also be other factors to consider.

Categorical

Data that is not a number, such as a string of text or date, is categorical data. Nominal and ordinal values for these variables can be derived, although this isn't done often. The order of a value is referred to as an ordinal value. An example of an ordinal value is a priority assigned to a bug such as "Critical" or "Low" or the ranking of a race such as "First" or "Third". Values with no set order are called nominal values, and they are the opposite of ordinal values. There are a number of variables that represent nominal values, including "State" and "Occupation".

There is also a category of categorical data that is called binary in addition to ordinal and nominal values. This category of data only has two possible values - true or false. Different ways of expressing this can be used, such as "True" and "False" or 1 and 0 respectively. The classification machine learning models heavily use binary data. Some binary variables include whether a person is currently subscribing to a service or not and whether they have purchased a car (Eda, 2006; Rao et al., 2021).

Types of EDA

An exploration of data analysis techniques has been devised to assist in this situation. A majority of these techniques work by masking certain aspects of the data and revealing others. Exploratory data analysis can generally be divided into two categories. Methods can either be non-graphical or graphical. Secondly, the methods are either univariate or multivariate (usually just bivariate) (Cleff, 2014; Ëáë& Ý, 2001; Tukey, 1977a).

A non-graphic approach usually involves the computation of the summary statistics, but a graphical approach can include the visualization of the data through diagrams or pictures along with the summary statistics. By using more than one variable in tandem, this method can be used to analyse two or more variables at once. Most of the time, multivariate methods are used when multiple variables (types of data) are subjected to the same analysis at the same time. It is generally accepted that a multivariate EDA is composed of two variables, but there are instances when three or more variables are included in an EDA. In order to reduce the risk of interpretation error, it is always a good practice to perform univariate EDAs on each component before performing the multivariate EDA. After the cross-classification described above, the following four categories could be created as a result of the above cross-classification. Furthermore, each category of variables was further segmented as to the function (outcome or explanation) and type (categorical or quantitative) of the variable(s) being analysed. In EDA, both numerical and graphic methods are employed. Graphs require the representation of the data visually or diagrammatically, whereas statistics require the presentation of summary statistics. Also, these two methods can also be classified as single-variate and multiple-variate approaches.

The multivariate methods are methods that take into account more than one variable (data column) at the same time, whereas the univariate methods only take into account one variable (data column). It is pertinent to note that there are four types of EDAs, namely the graphical univariate, the graphical multivariate, the non-graphic univariate, and the non-graphic multivariate. Using quantitative analysis is more objective while using visual analysis is more subjective. Figure 4 shows types of EDA.

Figure 4. Types of exploratory data analysis

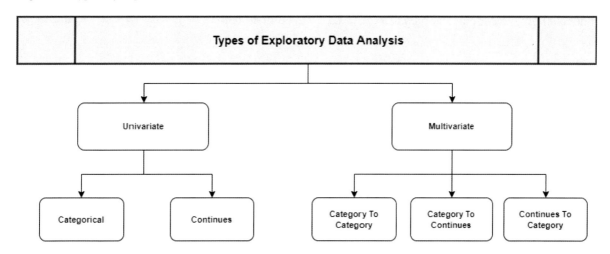

1. **Univariate non-graphical:** This is the easiest of the four options. The data examined in this type of analysis consists of just one variable. Analyzing data is primarily focused on finding patterns and describing the data.
2. **Univariate graphical:** Comparatively, this method provides a comprehensive picture of data whereas other methods do not utilize a graphical representation. An important characteristic of this type of analysis is that it relies primarily on histograms, stem and leaf plots, and box plots, to illustrate its results. A histogram shows the range of values and the number of cases for each range of values, as well as the range of values. The stem and leaf plot of the data can provide a visual representation of the shape of the distribution as well as the data values. Within each quarter of the age group,

the box plot shows the minimum, first quartile median, third quartile median, and maximum for each one of those values (Dibia&Demiralp, 2019).

3. **MultivariateNon-graphical:** By utilizing cross-tabulation and statistics, the multivariate non-graphic type of EDA visualizes the relationship between multiple variables of data.

4. **Multivariate graphical**: An EDA that illustrates the relationships between two or more datasets is called a Correlation Diagram. Accordingly, the bar chart was constructed so that each group represented the level of one variable, and each bar within the group represented the level of another variable within that group.

Stages in EDA

Exploratory Data Analysis, or EDA, is a fundamental step to becoming proficient in Data Analysis and Data Science. Using EDA, we investigate the dataset to find patterns, anomalies (outliers), and hypotheses based on our understanding of the dataset. To help understand the data better, EDA involves summarizing numerical data and creating various graphics. First, EDA is used after the data has been collected, before any models have been chosen for the structural elements or stochastic components. Second, it can also be used to check for deviations from common assumptions(El et al., 2020).

There are multiple stages in Exploratory Data Analysis, this includes missing value imputation, outlier detection, variable transformation, etc(Verbeeck et al., 2020). Figure 5 shows the procedures for understanding, cleaning, and preparing your data are outlined below.

Figure 5. Procedures for understanding, cleaning, and preparing your data

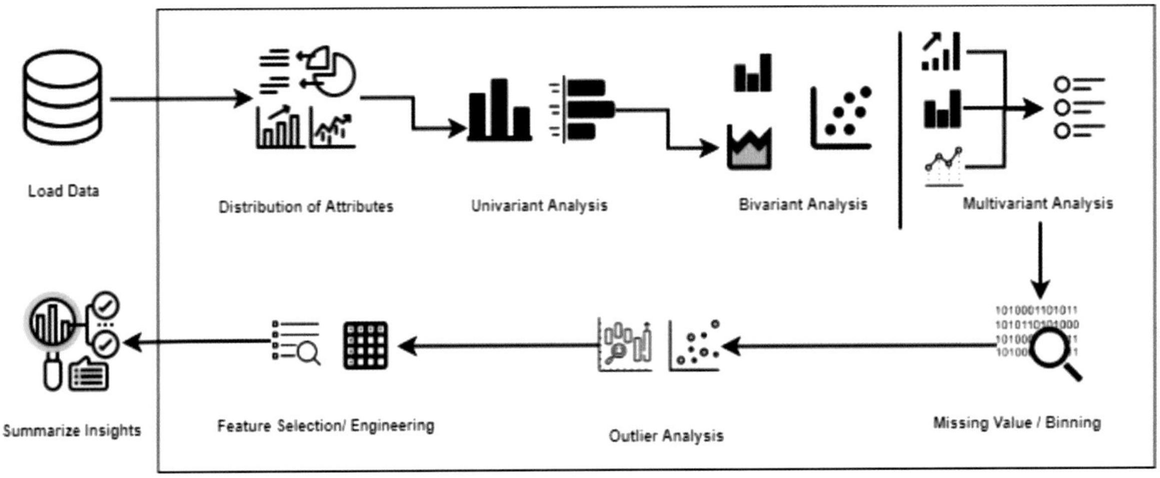

Variable Identification

As part of this step, we identify each variable by determining its type. Datatypes of variables can be changed based on our needs. Different categories of variables have been defined: First, determine the input variables (predictor variables) and the output variables (target variables). The next step is to determine the type and category of the variables. Figure 6 shows the types and categories of the variables.

Figure 6. Types and Categories of Variables

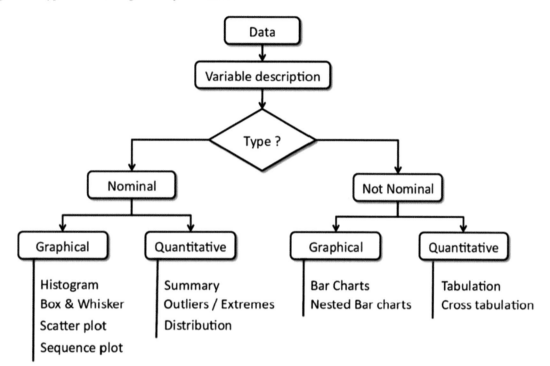

Univariate Analysis

Analyzing statistical data with a univariate approach is a fundamental technique in data analysis. It is not necessary to consider the cause or effect relationship in this case since only one variable is included and the data contains only one variable. For example, consider a student survey conducted in a classroom. Analysts are likely to count how many boys and girls are in the room. Here we have one variable, along with a variable quantity, explaining the number. A univariate analysis' main objective is to describe the data so that patterns can be found. The means, modes, medians, standard deviations, and dispersion are examined in this manner. There is a difference in the methodology for performing univariate analysis based on whether the variable being analysed is categorical or continuous. To illustrate the difference between categorical and continuous variables, here are some examples:

A continuous variable can be thought of as an item with a central tendency and a distribution. We can understand continuous variables by understanding these two concepts. Moreover, we can also use univariate analyses in order to highlight missing values as well as outliers.

For categorical variables, frequency tables can be used to interpret their distribution so that you are aware of the distribution. The percentages can also be interpreted as percentages of the individual categories. In terms of measuring it, we will use two metrics, counting and counting percentages for each category. You can visualize the data through the use of bar charts. Figure 7 shows types of graphs used in various variables.

Figure 7. Types of graphs for variables.

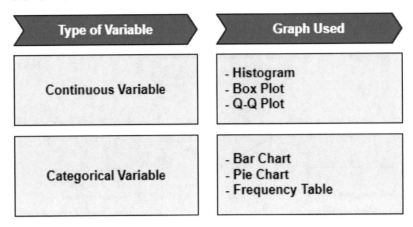

Univariate analysis can be practiced in a number of different ways, because they are all mostly descriptive in nature, as they can be carried out a variety of ways. In order to serve as a reference, I have created the following Frequency Distribution Table, Frequency Polygon, Histogram, Bar Chart, and Pie Chart.

There are several methods for analysing data; however, the one based on univariate methods is the simplest. As in the case of any analysis of data in statistics, the analysis can be both descriptive and inferential in nature. In terms of univariate analysis, one of the most important things to keep in mind is that we are only dealing with one set of data, which means that you can rest assured that we are only dealing with one set. There is no doubt that univariate analysis is an easy method to analyze and is also not complex, but there may be times when this method ends up providing false information especially if there are an increasing number of variables involved. There may be instances in this case where you will find the need to move to a multivariate or bivariate analysis which can help you analyze the data more effectively.

Bivariate / Multivariate Analysis

By using bivariate analysis, one examines the variation between variables that may be continuous-categorical, continuous-continuous, or categorical-categorical. Among other things, bivariate analysis is defined as the study of two variables and the investigation of whether there is a correlation between them. As a result, we explore associations and disassociations between variables at a predefined level of significance. There is no restriction on which variables we can analyse bivariate, and they can be categorical or continuous. You can choose any combination of categorical and categorical, categorical and continuous, or continuous and continuous. During the analysis process, different methods will be used to handle the combinations as described above.

Continuous and Continuous: The scatterplot is the best way to visualize bivariate analysis between continuous variables. By using scatter plots, we will be able to determine which variable is correlated with another variable. Scatter plot patterns provide us with information about the relationships between variables. The linearity or non-linearity of the model will depend on the relationship between the variables.

Despite the fact that scatter plots provide a visual representation of the relationship between two variables, they do not provide a way to gauge the strength of that relationship. There is a correlation between two variables, which can provide the best insight as to the strength of their relationship. The correlation is a measure of a relationship between two variables, ranging from -1 to 1.

- If the correlation is -1, then the variables are not connected.
- If the correlation is +1, then the variables are perfectly linearly related.
- A correlation of 0 suggests no correlation.

Correlation is determined by identifying the correlation between variables by using various tools. Pearson correlation values are returned by these functions to identify the relationship between two variables.

Categorical and Categorical: Finding correlations is achieved by examining two categorical variables from different perspectives to determine the relationship between them. It is necessary to create a two-way table to begin our analysis of this relationship since both the number of cases and the count percentage must be shown simultaneously. It is a matrix in which one variable is associated with each row and the other variable with each column. Observations for each combination of row and column categories are displayed in terms of number or percentage.

The Chi-Square test was designed to determine the significance of a relationship between two variables so that its relationship can be measured. As a general purpose, the overall intent of the study is to determine if there is enough evidence in the sample to conclude that the relationship holds true for a larger group of the population as a whole. As a general rule, the Chi-Square value refers to the difference between the expectation and the observed frequency in one or more categories of the two-way table in relation to the Chi-Square. We will be able to determine the probability associated with the Chi-square distribution, by using this function, because the degree of freedom of the function is the parameter that determines the probability associated with it.

Categorical and Continuous: To visualize the relationship between continuous and categorical variables, box plots can be generated to visualize the relationship between them for every level of categorical variables. Alternatively, when the number of levels is relatively few, one cannot determine the significance of the relationship. In order to indicate the significance of the results, tests such as z-tests, t-tests, and ANOVA can be applied.

Missing Values Treatment

In case that data is missing from a data set, we are likely to reduce the power/fit of the model, or we may end up with a biased model that may be our fault when we did not analyze the relationship between the different variables and their behaviour correctly. As a consequence, there is a possibility that the predictions we make or the classifications we make could be incorrect. In the left scenario, we have not dealt with the missing data, but in the right scenario, we have dealt with the missing data. The outcome of the study carried out shows that while females have the opportunity to play cricket, males have the chance to play it more frequently as a result of the study. Taking a look at the data after the missing values have been removed (based on gender) in the second set, we are able to conclude that women are far more likely to be involved in cricket than men are if we examine the data after removing missing values (based on gender). Several elements contribute to the absence of these values, and these elements need to be identified in order to solve the problem.

Outlier Treatment

Data scientists and analysts use the term "outlier" extensively, as it is one of those risks that must be carefully monitored in order not to cause wildly inaccurate estimations. Outliers are observations that diverge from the overall pattern of a sample and appear to be far from the average. Outliers can be classified as either univariate or multivariate. When we examine the distribution of a single variable, we will be able to find these outliers (*Outlier - an Overview | ScienceDirect Topics*, n.d.). Multivariate outliers are also referred to as n-dimensional outliers, and they are outliers that occur within a multivariate space. If we are going to have a better understanding of the way distributions work, we have to take a look at them in a wide variety of dimensions. Finding out what causes the outliers that occur in the data is the best way to have the ability to move past them once they appear in the data. It is important to remember that every time they happen, you need to determine how to deal with them based on the reason why they occurred in the first place. In general, outliers are generally caused by the following factors:

Type 1: Global Outliers

The value of a data point within a dataset that has a significant difference from the entire dataset it is part of is considered to be a global outlier.

Type 2: Contextual Outliers

A "data point" that has a value that is significantly different from the norm, in the same context, is considered an outlier. In the event that the same value is observed in a different context, an outlier is no longer considered. It is almost always the case when discussing only a time-series dataset, that the "context" is a chronological one since these data are records of a specific quantity over time. Therefore, it should not come as a surprise that outliers are often found in time series data due to contextual factors.

Type 3: Collective Outliers

An individual dataset or subset of data points may be categorized using either category if the deviation of their values from the overall values of the dataset is significant, but not if their individual values are abnormal in either a contextual or a global sense. There are a number of ways in which time-series data can be characterized as anomalous. Examples of abnormal results include normal peaks and valleys observed outside of a timeframe out of phase with the normal seasonal pattern, or the occurrence of a grouping of series that are out of phase with the existing trend (Khan et al., 2014; Kotu& Deshpande, 2019).

Feature Engineering

In order to carry out feature engineering, the first five steps through the data exploration process must be completed - Variable Identification, Analysis of Univariable, Analysis of Bivariate Data, Imputed Missing Values, Outlier Treatment. There are many different elements that go into the process of Data Science/Machine Learning. In order to make sense of the data given to us, it is necessary to transform it into a sensible form that can be used for interpretation. In order for the Machine Learning Model to understand the data, the data needs to be changed into something that can be understood by the Model.

We are currently working on making further improvements to the model by incorporating new features (Max-dependency, 2005; Theodoridis &Koutroumbas, 2009). This can be accomplished by separating the feature engineering process into two steps:

Transformation of Variables

Transform refers to the process of changing an attribute by substituting a function, and that is what most variables undergo when they are transformed. Variables can be transformed with their square or cube roots, logarithms, or log bases. In the simplest sense, transformation implies the altering of the distribution or relationship of an independent variable with an independent variable (Beigi et al., 2014). Typical situations in which variable transformation is necessary to include the following:

- Changing the scale or standardizing the numerical value of a variable can help us gain a deeper understanding of it. Transforming data of different scales is a crucial task, but the distribution of the variables stays the same regardless of the transformation
- When linear relationships are derived from non-linear relationships, the non-linear relationships become linear relationships. Relationships that is linear, as opposed to those that are curved or non-linear, are preferable to understand. In the case of non-linear relationships, transformation can be used in order to make them linear. A scatter plot is a useful tool for identifying relationships between continuous variables. This type of transformation also enhances the ability of the scatter plot to predict. For instance, in the calculation of correlation coefficients, the log transformation is commonly used.
- Rather than skewed distributions, asymmetric distributions make sense due to their easy interpretation. Some variables should have a normal distribution, depending on the type of modeling technique being used. When looking at a skewed distribution, in addition to trying to use transformations to improve the distribution, we can also try to reduce the amount of skewness. When analyzing skewed distributions, for example, we can take the square roots, cube roots, logarithms, or square roots of the distribution while when studying left-skewed distributions, we can take the square roots, cube roots, and exponential roots of the distribution.
- From a human perspective, there is also a variable transformation done from the standpoint of implementation (Human involvement). Let's talk about this in more detail. My research on employee performance shows that age is associated directly with the performance of an employee. That is to say, the older the employee, the better the performance. It is true that launching a program depending on the age of a person poses some challenges from a perspective of implementation. As a judicious practice, it would be prudent to categorize sales representatives into three age groups - those under 35 years old, those 35 to 50 years old, and those over 50 years old, and then formulate three different strategies depending on which group each sales representative falls into. The process of binning variables is called Binning of Variables when this categorization is employed.

There are a number of methods that can be used to transform variables. The study described a variety of statistical methods for analysing the data, such as square root, cube root, logarithmic, bidding, reciprocal, etc. (Gopika & Meena Kowshalaya, 2018). For the purpose of evaluating each method, it is important to point out its advantages and disadvantages, underlining their respective pros and cons.

- **Logarithm**: It is important to understand that the logarithm of a variable can change the shape of a distribution plot by altering its logarithmic coefficient. In order to reduce right-handed skewness, it is frequently used to reduce the difference between variables. In order to perform the operation, the value must be a positive number or a zero.

- **Square or Cube root**: There is an interesting phenomenon with square and cube roots that are greatly affecting the distribution of variables, and which has a substantial impact on their distributions. The distribution of these variables is more influenced by the logarithmic transformations as compared to logarithmic transformations. A further advantage of using cube roots over logarithmic transformations is the fact that they are based on square roots. Because they can handle negative numbers, including the zero digit, they are a suitable alternative to logarithms, since they can handle negative numbers as well as zero. This formula can also be used to determine the Square Root of positive numbers such as 0 and 1.

- **Binning**: It represents a categorization of variables. Binning may be performed based on original values, percentiles, or frequencies. Business understanding will determine the most appropriate categorization technique. If we categorize income, for instance, we can categorize it into three different categories, such as high, average, and low. In addition to multivariate binning, a co-variate binning approach can also be carried out, which depends on more than one variable.

Variable Creation

A new variable or feature is created based on the data that is currently available in the database. This is part of the continuous process of developing features and variables. As an example, let us take the variable "date" for instance as an input into a data set, with the values "dd-mm-yy". In addition to the target variable, you may be able to discover a number of additional variables that are intimately related to it, such as day, month, year, week, or day of the week. (Al-Kandari & Jolliffe, 2005). New features can be created through various methods. Listed here are a few common methods:

- **Create derived variables:**Basically, this relates to a method of generating new variables that are based on applying the existing variables to a set of functions or methods. There are missing values for the variable age in this set of data. It is suggested that a new variable be created to identify missing values through the salutation of the name (Master, Mr, Miss, Mrs) of the individual. From this information, how can we select the most appropriate variable? Analysts will have to be able to do what they have to do based on their knowledge about the business, their curiosity, and the hypotheses they have when faced with the issue. In addition to creating new variables using these techniques, it is also possible to transform existing variables in other ways, such as taking the logarithm of a variable, dividing it, and even segmenting it.

- **Creating dummy variables:**Several ways can be used to create a dummy variable. Converting categorical variables into numerical variables is one of the most common applications of this technique. Also known as dummy variables, indicator variables also can be referred to as dummy variables. Categorical variables can be used as predictor variables when building statistical models with categorical variables. Categorical variables can be categorized into three different types: zero, one or between zero and one hundred. A sample of a categorical variable, "gender", will serve as an example. The data set will be divided into two variables: one for the men and one for the women, while in the other variable, the reverse is true. It is also possible to create dummy variables for categorical variables with more than two categories, either by creating x or y dummy variables.

CONCLUSION

It is imperative that the EDA stage is done before engaging in machine learning or statistical modelling, as it provides the context necessary for the development of an appropriate model for the problem, as well as the interpretation of the results. Data scientists have a valuable role to play in this process as it ensures that the results, they produce are accurate, properly interpreted, and relevant to the business context in question. Data analysts and researchers have the ability to validate previously established assumptions by performing various statistical operations, such as these, which allow them to identify patterns that are useful in allowing them to better understand the particular problem at hand and choosing the most appropriate statistical model. Thus, researchers can ensure that their data analysis meets a high standard, as well as confirm that the data collected and arranged in a particular manner is what they intended.

In order to study exploratory data sets (EDA), a data set has to be analysed using graphics and visualizations in order to identify and interpret the data. Rather than simply verifying statistical hypotheses, the purpose of this study is to explore, investigate, and learn, not just confirm them. Data analysis generally aims to determine what information data can provide beyond formal modelling and hypothesis testing, and to gain a deeper understanding of how variables in a dataset are related. When an exploratory analysis is conducted to determine the significance of specific features in a dataset, lightweight modelling approaches are often used. Thus, the procedure you are considering for data analysis can be determined if it is appropriate or not.

REFERENCES

Al-Kandari, N. M., & Jolliffe, I. T. (2005). Variable selection and interpretation in correlation principal components. *Environmetrics*, *16*(6), 659–672. doi:10.1002/env.728

Becher, J. D., Berkhin, P., & Freeman, E. (2000). Automating exploratory data analysis for efficient data mining. *Proceeding of the Sixth ACM SIGKDD International Conference on Knowledge Discovery and Data Mining*, 424–429. 10.1145/347090.347179

Beigi, E. B., Jazi, H., Stakhanova, N., & Ghorbani, A. A. (2014). *Towards Effective Feature Selection in Machine Learning-Based Botnet Detection Approaches*. doi:10.1109/CNS.2014.6997492

Bezerra, A., Silva, I., Guedes, L. A., Silva, D., Leitão, G., & Saito, K. (2019). Extracting value from industrial alarms and events: A data-driven approach based on exploratory data analysis. *Sensors (Switzerland)*, *19*(12), 2772. Advance online publication. doi:10.339019122772 PMID:31226811

Cleff, T. (2014). *Exploratory Data Analysis in Business and Economics*. doi:10.1007/978-3-319-01517-0

Dibia, V., & Demiralp, Ç. (2019). Data2Vis: Automatic Generation of Data Visualizations Using Sequence-to-Sequence Recurrent Neural Networks. *IEEE Computer Graphics and Applications*, *39*(5), 33–46. doi:10.1109/MCG.2019.2924636 PMID:31247545

Eda, W. (2006). 1. Exploratory Data Analysis 1. Exploratory Data Analysis - Detailed Table of Contents. *Analysis*, *1*(4), 5728–5731. https://www.ncbi.nlm.nih.gov/pubmed/21097328

El, O. B., Milo, T., & Somech, A. (2020). Towards Autonomous, Hands-Free Data Exploration. *Cidr*. https://www.tableau.com

Gopika, N., & Meena Kowshalaya, A. E. A. (2018). Correlation Based Feature Selection Algorithm for Machine Learning. *Proceedings of the 3rd International Conference on Communication and Electronics Systems, ICCES 2018, Icces*, 692–695. 10.1109/CESYS.2018.8723980

Khan, M. A., Pradhan, S. K., & Khaleel, M. A. (2014). Outlier Detection for Business Intelligence using Data Mining Techniques. *International Journal of Computers and Applications*, *106*(2), 975–8887.

Kotu, V., & Deshpande, B. (2019). Anomaly Detection. *Data Science*, 447–465. doi:10.1016/B978-0-12-814761-0.00013-7

Matchev, K. T., Matcheva, K., & Roman, A. (2022). *Unsupervised Machine Learning for Exploratory Data Analysis of Exoplanet Transmission Spectra*. https://arxiv.org/abs/2201.02696

Max-dependency, C. (2005). *Feature Selection Based on Mutual Information*. Academic Press.

Outlier - an overview | ScienceDirect Topics. (n.d.). Retrieved April 13, 2022, from https://www.sciencedirect.com/topics/computer-science/outlier

Rao, A. S., Vardhan, B. V., & Shaik, H. (2021). Role of Exploratory Data Analysis in Data Science. *Proceedings of the 6th International Conference on Communication and Electronics Systems, ICCES 2021*, 1457–1461. 10.1109/ICCES51350.2021.9488986

Theodoridis, S., & Koutroumbas, K. (2009). Feature Selection. *Pattern Recognition*, 261–322. doi:10.1016/B978-1-59749-272-0.50007-4

Tukey, J. W. (1977a). *Exploratory Data Analysis*. doi:10.1007/978-1-4419-7976-6

Tukey, J. W. (1977b). Exploratory Data Analysis by John W. Tukey. In *Biometrics* (Vol. 33, p. 768). https://www.jstor.org/stable/2529486

Verbeeck, N., Caprioli, R. M., & van de Plas, R. (2020). Unsupervised machine learning for exploratory data analysis in imaging mass spectrometry. *Mass Spectrometry Reviews*, *39*(3), 245–291. doi:10.1002/mas.21602 PMID:31602691

Wasay, A., Athanassoulis, M., & Idreos, S. (2015). Queriosity: Automated Data Exploration; Queriosity: Automated Data Exploration. *2015 IEEE International Congress on Big Data*. 10.1109/BigDataCongress.2015.116

Chapter 17
Technological Interventions for Biological Fluid Flow Analysis

Priyadharshini P.
Department of Mathematics, PSG College of Arts and Science, Coimbatore, India

Vanitha Archana M.
Department of Mathematics, PSG College of Arts and Science, Coimbatore, India

Karthikeyan M. P.
https://orcid.org/0000-0002-2346-0283
School of Computer Science and IT, Bengaluru, India

ABSTRACT

The thermal and mechanical effects of human tissues and physics that governs biological processes has been developed by applying fundamental engineering principles in the investigation of numerous heat and mass transfer applications in biology and medicine. An incompressible magnetohydrodynamic nanofluid flow passing over a stretched surface along with the effect of viscous dissipation is analyzed numerically. In order to create a nonlinear transformed model in terms of ordinary differential equations, suitable similarity transformations are used and solved by employing a Mathematica algorithm. Furthermore, a minimal case comparison standard has been provided to validate the current methodology. The machine learning method is built through very important parameters. Simulations and machine learning approaches could work together to reveal new and fortunate prospects in computational science and engineering problems. The performance of the parameters in terms of heat and mass transfer is presented with an aid of graph to demonstrate the applicability of the current model.

INTRODUCTION

Thermal transfer within living organisms, bioheat transport, is a crucial biological and therapeutic problem that incorporates distinctive features in thermal therapies, cryobiology, burn injuries, illness diagnostics, and thermal comfort evaluations. The thermal side impact of different treatments is a crucial problem

DOI: 10.4018/978-1-6684-4580-8.ch017

in bioheat research, such as bone drilling (Davidson, 2003), temperature increase in knee replacement (Sawyer, 2003), and laser eye surgery ((Amara, 1995), (Chua, 2005), (Scott, 1988)). Many researchers are interested in looking at the effects of heat and mass transport on biofluids from both a theoretical and practical or clinical perspective.

The heat transfer phenomenon is caused by a temperature difference between two different types of bodies. Transportation of heat and mass has a significant impact on crystal growth, polyethylene and paper formation, cooling of metallic sheets in cooling baths, metal castings, latent heat storage, and many others. The procedure of heat and mass transfer passing through a stretching sheet is examined in many other sectors, such as glass fiber manufacture, aerodynamic extrusion of plastic sheets, and glass blowing. In all of these applications, the quality of the received product is determined by the rate of heat transfer at the stretching surfaces. Many authors examined heat and mass transport and its uses ((Bhatti, 2017), (Devi, 2009),(Raju, 2016)). There are some other related studies ((Gorla, 1994), (Hassani, 2011)) to the articles mentioned above.

A nanofluid is a fluid in which solid nanoparticles with length scales of 1–100 nm are embedded in a fundamental heat transfer fluid. It has been known that inserting highly conductive particles into basic pure fluids can effectively enhance heat conductivity. Choi et al. (Choi, 1995)analyzed the enhancing thermal conductivity of fluids with nanoparticles. Das et al. (Das, 2007)constructed an introduction to nanofluids and their properties. Kakac et al. (Kakac, 2009)considered nanofluids to offer significant advantages over heat transfer fluids. Buongiorno (Buongiorno, 2006)employed an analytical model for convective transport in nanofluids by the consideration of Brownian motion and thermophoresis. Below Figure 1 shows Schematic Diagram of the Proposed Research Model

Figure 1. Schematic diagram of the proposed research model

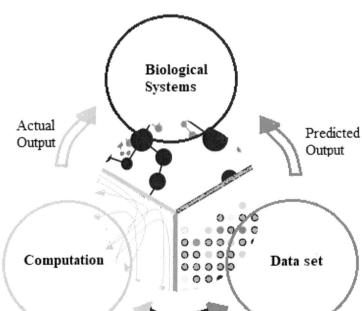

Internal friction in a viscous flow causes viscous dissipation, which is known as the continuous process of mechanical energy transmuted to thermal energy. It is only influential if the fluid has an expanded velocity and viscosity. An influence of viscous dissipation on mixed convective boundary layer heat transfer from an exponentially stretching surface was investigated by Partha et al. (Partha M. K., 2005). Makinde et al. (Makinde, 2014) evaluated the effects of viscous dissipation and Ohmic heating on thermal boundary layer flow over a heated plate. In the field of internal heat generation/absorption, infusion, and viscous dissipation on thermophoretic nanofluid flow over an exponentially stretched sheet inserted in porous medium is depicted by Naramgari et al. (Naramgari, 2016). Beg et al. (Beg, 2014) presented a numerical study of insecure MHD boundary layer flow of a nanofluid over a stretched surface in a porous medium. The magnetohydrodynamic boundary layer flow with the impact of thermal radiation across a stretching surface with convective boundary condition is researched by Nadeem et al. (Nadeem, 2014). Below figure 2 shows Flow Chart of Computational Flow Analysis.

Figure 2. Flow chart of computational flow analysis

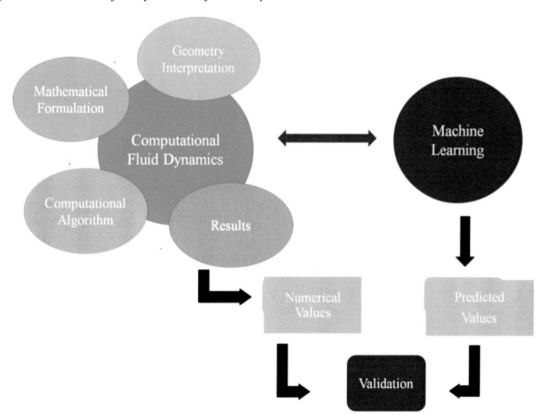

This paper studies the prospect of predicting physical quantities with the aid of Machine Learning approaches (Brenner, 2019), encouraged by the recent trend of incorporating algorithms in physics-related problems. Due to the endless great new applications, this modern work will entice a large number of other researchers to evaluate the existing effort. The various studies on machine learning approaches are applications of wind energy ((Clifton, 2013), (Heinermann, 2016), (Mostafa Rushdi, 2021), (Rushdi), (Ti,

2020), (Treiber, 2016)), solar energy ((Sharma, 2011), (Voyant, 2017)), and renewable energy systems in general (Kalogirou, 2007). Before proceeding with the machine learning approach, it is insightful to review the theoretical and computational fluid dynamics techniques. The perceptron devised by Rosenblatt (Rosenblatt, 1958) to emulate the human brain ability to perceive a separation hyperplane that splits the training data linearly. The proposed research model is displayed in Figure 1.

The entire manuscript is divided into four portions. In that, the mathematical model statement of the physical system is described in the first section. The second section discussed the methodology of the numerical and predicted solutions. The third section includes graphical and tabular representations of the temperature and concentration profiles against a broad range of pertinent parameters. The conclusion of the entire parametric investigation has been made in section 4. Below figure 3 shows Diagram of Physical Configuration.

Figure 3. Diagram of physical configuration

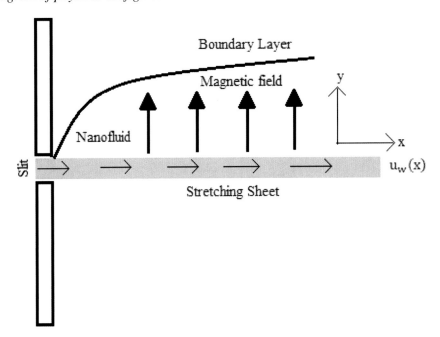

MATHEMATICAL FORMULATION

The heat and mass transfer of a two-dimensional boundary layer flow, viscous and incompressible nanofluid flow over a plate in a porous medium, is considered. The fluid is presumed to flow above and along the x-axis, with the y-axis perpendicular to the fluid movement. Stretching the sheet generates two equal and competing forces. The sheet is stretched to the point where the velocity is proportionate to the distance from the origin (x = 0). As displayed in Figure 3, the fluid is moving due to the magnetic field. The equations of continuity, momentum, energy and mass transfer are utilized to describe the flow as follows:

$$\frac{\partial u}{\partial x} + \frac{\partial v}{\partial y} = 0, \tag{1}$$

$$u\frac{\partial u}{\partial x} + v\frac{\partial u}{\partial y} = -\frac{1}{\rho_f}\frac{\partial p}{\partial y} + v\left(\frac{\partial^2 u}{\partial x^2} + \frac{\partial^2 u}{\partial y^2}\right) - \frac{\sigma B^2}{\rho_f}u, \tag{2}$$

$$u\frac{\partial T}{\partial x} + v\frac{\partial T}{\partial y} = \alpha\left(\frac{\partial^2 T}{\partial y^2}\right) + \tau\left\{D_B\left(\frac{\partial C}{\partial y}\frac{\partial T}{\partial y}\right) + \frac{D_T}{T_\infty}\left(\frac{\partial T}{\partial y}\right)^2\right\} + \frac{\mu}{\rho_p}\left[\left(\frac{\partial u}{\partial y}\right)^2\right], \tag{3}$$

$$u\frac{\partial C}{\partial x} + v\frac{\partial C}{\partial y} = D_B\left(\frac{\partial^2 C}{\partial y^2}\right) + \frac{D_T}{T_\infty}\left(\frac{\partial^2 T}{\partial y^2}\right). \tag{4}$$

For the above system of equations, the corresponding boundary conditions are,

$$u = U_w(x), \ v = 0, \ T = T_w, \ C = C_w \ at \ y = 0; \tag{5}$$

$$u = v = 0, \ T = T_\infty, \ C = C_\infty, \ at \ y \to \infty. \tag{6}$$

The velocity components in the x and y-axis are u and v, respectively. Where p is the fluid pressure, v is the kinematic viscosity, σ is the electrical conductivity, B is the magnetic induction, and ρf is the fluid density. The fluid temperature is T. and the ratio of the nanoparticle materials efficient heat range to the base fluids efficient heat range is τ, T¥ i_s ambient temperature, α is the thermal diffusivity, C is the nanoparticle concentration particles, C¥ is the free stream concentration, DB is the Brownian diffusion coefficient, and DT is the thermophoresis coefficient.

The equations (2)-(4) and the boundary conditions (5) have been converted from dimensional to dimensionless form employing the subsequent similarity transformations.

$$\begin{cases} \eta = \left(\frac{c}{v}\right)^{\frac{1}{2}}y, \qquad \psi(x,y) = (cv)^{\frac{1}{2}}xf(\eta), \\ \theta(\eta) = \frac{T - T_\infty}{T_w - T_\infty}, \quad \psi(\eta) = \frac{C - C_\infty}{C_w - C_\infty} \end{cases} \tag{7}$$

The resulting equations can be constructed by applying the boundary-layer premises and similarity transforms to the equations. (2)-(4):

$$f'''(\eta) + f(\eta)f''(\eta) - f'(\eta)^2 - Mf'(\eta) = 0, \tag{8}$$

$$\theta''(\eta) + Pr\left[f(\eta)\theta'(\eta) + Nb\theta'(\eta)\phi'(\eta) + Nt(\theta'(\eta))^2 + Ecf''(\eta)^2\right] = 0, \tag{9}$$

$$\phi''(\eta) + Lef(\eta)\phi'(\eta) + \frac{Nt}{Nb}\theta''(\eta) = 0. \tag{10}$$

Subject to the following constraints:

$$f(0) = 0, \; f'(0) = 1, \; \theta(0) = 1, \; \phi(0) = 1; \tag{11}$$

$$f'(\infty) \to 0, \; \theta(\infty) \to 0, \; \phi(\infty) \to 0. \tag{12}$$

Differentiation with respect to η is denoted by primes. The magnetic parameter M, Prandtl number Pr, Brownian motion parameter Nb, thermophoresis parameter Nt, Eckert number Ec, and Lewis number Le are described by

$$M = \frac{\sigma B^2}{(\rho c)_f}, \; \mathrm{Pr} = \frac{v}{\alpha}, \; Nb = \frac{(\rho c)_p D_B (C_w - C_\infty)}{v(\rho c)_f},$$

$$Nt = \frac{(\rho c)_p D_T (T_w - T_\infty)}{vT_\infty (\rho c)_f}, \; Ec = \frac{u_w^2}{\left[(c_p)_f (T_w - T_\infty)\right]}, \; Le = \frac{\alpha}{D_B}.$$

The Skin friction coefficient C_f, local Nusselt number Nu_x, and local Sherwood number Sh_x are,

$$C_{fx} = \frac{\tau_w}{\frac{1}{2}\rho U^2}, \; Nu_x = \frac{xq_w}{K(T_w - T_\infty)}, \; Sh_x = \frac{xq_m}{D_B(C_w - C_\infty)} \tag{13}$$

Where the Skin friction on flat plate is τw, the heat flux is qw, and the wall mass flux is qm are given by,

$$\tau_w = \left(\mu_B + \frac{p_y}{\sqrt{2\pi_c}}\right)\left(\frac{\partial u}{\partial y}\right)_{y=0}, \; q_w = -k\left(\frac{\partial T}{\partial y}\right)_{y=0}, \; q_m = -D_B\left(\frac{\partial T}{\partial y}\right)_{y=0} \tag{14}$$

Using stated similarity transforms in Equation (14) becomes,

$$\frac{C_f}{\text{Re}_x^{-\frac{1}{2}}} = f''(0), \frac{Nu_x}{\text{Re}_x^{\frac{1}{2}}} = -\theta'(0), \frac{Sh_x}{\text{Re}_x^{\frac{1}{2}}} = -\phi'(0) \tag{15}$$

Here, $Re_x = ax^2$ is the local Reynolds number.

Below Table 1 shows the Comparision result of Nusselt number for various values of Prandtl number when Nb=Nt=M=Ec=0

Table 1. Comparison result of Nusselt number for various values of Prandtl number when Nb=Nt=M=Ec=0

Pr	Hamad(Hamad, 2011)	Khan and Pop (Khan, 2010)	Nogherhabadi (Noghrehabadadi, 2012)	Wang (Wang, 1989)	Present Results
2	0.91136	0.9113	0.911358	0.9114	0.911668
7	1.89540	1.8954	1.895404	1.8954	1.89046
20	3.35390	3.3539	3.353917	3.3539	3.34994
70	6.46220	6.4621	6.462290	6.4622	6.45872

SOLUTION TECHNIQUE

The numerical treatment of the modified nondimensional equations are handled by Mathematica algorithm. This technique has the advantage of automatically selecting the proper algorithm and tracking any potential errors. Furthermore, such a process produces better computing results, with only (3–4) minutes of CPU time for each evaluation. By using this technique, complex solution formulations are avoided and graphical descriptions are directly presented. The proposed computational flow analysis is displayed in Figure 2.

Machine Learning

Machine Learning is a set of methodologies that allows computers to automate data-driven model development and build algorithms using statistical approaches to generate predictions in available data. The inferred algorithms work by developing a model from example inputs, going through a decision process, and making predictions, which are usually confirmed by the same input dataset. Gradient descent algorithm (Jiawei Zhang, 2019) is a sort of supervised learning in machine learning that involves estimating an outcome from a given dataset. Learning is the process of fine-tuning the parameters of a model so that it can generate the most precise forecasts based on the data.

If $y_{\{pred\}}$, x, h, and w are the predicted variable, input variable, bias term, and weight of the variable in a simple regression model, then:

$$y_{\{pred\}} = wx + b$$

The resulting mathematical forms are evaluated for mean square error.

$$MSE = \frac{1}{N}\sum_{i=1}^{N}(y - \widehat{y_i})^2$$

where N denotes the total number of data points in the training dataset, y denotes the dependent variable, and $\widehat{y_i}$ denotes the predicted function. The best fit will also be evaluated for each function.

Below table 2 shows Actual and predicted values of testing data

Table 2. Actual and predicted values of testing data

Physical quantities	Parameter Values		Actual Value	Predicted Value
C_f	Nb=Nt=0.1, Pr=Le=10.0, Ec=0	M=0	-1.01435	-0.92169
		M=0.5	-1.06415	-1.07052
		M=1	-1.19635	-1.21914
		M=2	-1.42899	-1.51700
Nu_x	Nb=Nt=0.1, M=Ec=0, Le=10.0	Pr=2	0.71725	0.42540
		Pr=5	0.93520	0.70768
		Pr=7	0.96713	0.89586
		Pr=10	0.95118	1.17813
Sh_x	Pr=Le=10.0, M=Ec=0, Nt=0.1	Nb=0.1	2.12051	2.19440
		Nb=0.2	2.37483	2.28650
		Nb=0.3	2.4037	2.37859
		Nb=0.4	2.4307	2.47069

Below figure 4 shows Impact of (a) Nb on temperature profile (b) Nt on concentration profile.

Figure 4. Impact of (a) Nb on temperature profile (b) Nt on concentration profile.

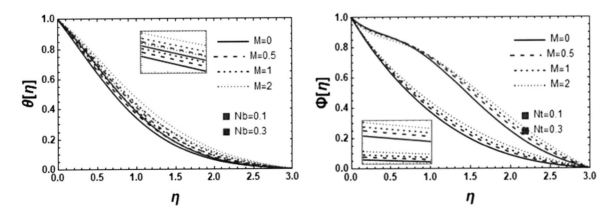

Below figure 5 shows Impact of Ec on (a) temperature profile (b) concentration profile.

Below figure 6 shows Error plot of (a) Skin friction coefficient against M (b) Nusselt number against Pr (c) Sherwood number against Nb.

Figure 5. Impact of Ec on (a) temperature profile (b) concentration profile.

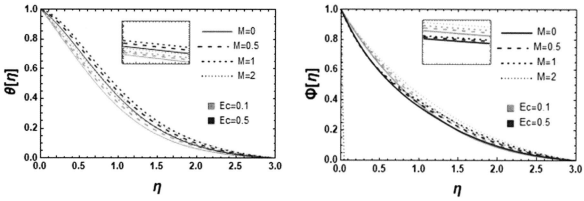

Figure 6. Error plot of (a) Skin friction coefficient against M (b) Nusselt number against Pr (c) Sherwood number against Nb.

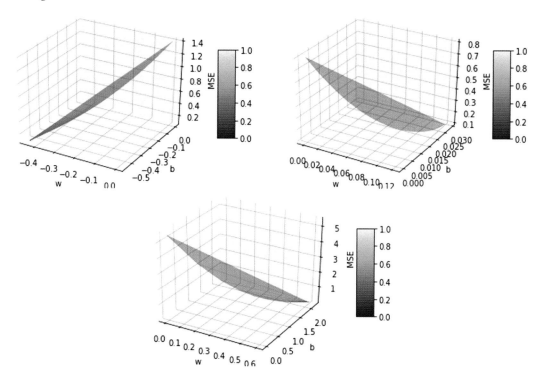

NUMERICAL FINDINGS AND DISCUSSION

The major goal of this section is to investigate the effects of various ranges of magnetic parameters and some relevant parameters on the temperature and concentration fields, such as Brownian motion parameter, thermophoresis parameter, and Eckert number. The default values are Nb=0.1, Nt=0.1, Ec=0.3, Pr=10.0, and Le=10.0, and all graphs use these values unless otherwise stated on the graph. Table 1 compares the obtained findings corresponding to the Prandtl number Pr with the available literature to validate the accuracy of the proposed computational approach.

Figures 4(a), 4(b), 5(a) and 5(b) illustrates the impact of magnetic parameter M on temperature and concentration distributions. The thickness of the boundary layer grows as the magnetic parameter gains, as seen in the figures. It is because of the Lorentz force, which is formed when a magnetic field is applied to a conducting fluid. Lorentz force has a propensity to slow down the flow, which validates the current findings. The resistance of the fluid particles raises by applying a magnetic field, which results in a temperature rise.

Figures 4(a) and 4(b) reflects the impact of the Brownian motion parameter and thermophoresis parameter on temperature and concentration profiles when the magnetic parameter of M is changed. The temperature rises with an increase in the Brownian motion parameter. Similarly, raising the thermophoresis parameter increase the distribution of concentration. Thermophoresis is a mechanism that transports tiny materials from a heated layer to a colder one. When Nb and Nt are comparably high, the magnetic field also has substantial influences on the areas far from the wall.

The Eckert number is used to define the influence of the self-heating of a fluid as a consequence of viscous dissipation effects because it describes the ratio of kinetic energy to the enthalpy difference of fluid. The influence of Eckert number Ec on the energy and mass transfer profiles is elucidated in Figures 5(a) and 5(b). It is noticed that both the energy and mass transfer profiles rise when the Eckert number is raised. Because of the increasing values of the Eckert number, heat energy is retained due to friction, resulting in an intensification of the temperature and concentration distributions. The physical reason seems to be that an enhancement in dissipation increases the thermal conductivity of the fluid, which produces an expansion in the thermal boundary layer.

MSE in checking phases of Skin friction coefficient, local Nusselt number, and local Sherwood number for wide ranges of magnetic parameter M, Prandtl number Pr, and Brownian motion parameter Nb are described in Figure 6. The errors convergence and lowest value shown in the graph. The technology interventions predicted the characteristics of the body system well through Skin friction coefficient, local Nusselt number, and local Sherwood number. The numerical values and estimated model values of several testing data sets are shown in Table 2. The expected outcomes fit the numerical data very well. Hence, the constructed model can accurately forecast the physical quantities of the considered flow.

CONCLUSION

The magnetohydrodynamic nanofluid flow over a stretched surface along with the effect of viscous dissipation is analyzed. The Wolfram Language algorithm is used to estimate the numerical outcomes. The impact of pertinent parameters are studied and compared. These parameters were effectively applied to the analysis of biological systems, yielding significant results. It is found that the heat and mass transport across porous medium is useful for the manufacture of osteoinductive material, the blood flow of tumors and muscles simulation, and modeling blood flow when fatty plaques of cholesterol and artery-clogging clots accumulate in the lumen.

REFERENCES

Amara, E. H. (1995). Numerical investigations on thermal effects of laser-ocular mediainteraction. *International Journal of Heat and Mass Transfer*, *38*(13), 2479–2488. doi:10.1016/0017-9310(94)00353-W

Beg, O. A., Khan, M. S., Karim, I., Alam, M. M., & Ferdows, M. (2014). Explicit numerical study of unsteady hydromagnetic mixed convective nanofluid flow from an exponentially stretching sheet in porous media. *Applied Nanoscience*, *4*(8), 943–957. doi:10.100713204-013-0275-0

Bhatti, M. M., & Rashidi, M. M. (2017). Study of heat and mass transfer with joule heating on magnetohydrodynamic (MHD) peristaltic blood flow under the influence of hall effect. *Propulsion and Power Research*, *6*(3), 177–185. doi:10.1016/j.jppr.2017.07.006

Brenner, M. P., Eldredge, J. D., & Freund, J. B. (2019). Perspective on machine learning for advancing fluid mechanics. *Physical Review Fluids*, *4*(10), 100501. doi:10.1103/PhysRevFluids.4.100501

Buongiorno, J. (2006). Convective transport in nanofluids. *Journal of Heat Transfer*, *128*(3), 240–250. doi:10.1115/1.2150834

Choi, S. U. S., & Eastman, J. A. (1995). *Enhancing thermal conductivity of fluids with nanoparticles (No. ANL/MSD/CP-84938; CONF-951135-29)*. Argonne National Lab.

Chua, K. J., Ho, J. C., Chou, S. K., & Islam, M. R. (2005). On the study of the temperature distribution within a human eye subjected to a laser source. *International Communications in Heat and Mass Transfer*, *32*(8), 1057–1065. doi:10.1016/j.icheatmasstransfer.2004.10.030

Clifton, A., Kilcher, L., Lundquist, J. K., & Fleming, P. (2013). Using machine learning to predict wind turbine power output. *Environmental Research Letters*, *8*(2), 024009. doi:10.1088/1748-9326/8/2/024009

Das, S. K., Choi, S. U., Yu, W., & Pradeep, T. (2007). *Nanofluids: Science and Technology*. Willey. doi:10.1002/9780470180693

Davidson, S. R. H., & James, D. F. (2003). Drilling in bone: Modeling heat generation and temperature distribution. *Journal of Biomechanical Engineering*, *125*(3), 305–314. doi:10.1115/1.1535190 PMID:12929234

Devi, S. A., & Ganga, B. (2009). Effects of viscous and Joules dissipation on MHD flow, heat and mass transfer past a stretching porous surface embedded in a porous medium. *Nonlinear Analysis (Vilnius)*, *14*(3), 303–314. doi:10.15388/NA.2009.14.3.14497

Gorla, R. S. R., & Sidawi, I. (1994). Free Convection on a Vertical Stretching Surface with Suction and Blowing. *Applied Scientific Research*, *52*(3), 247–258. doi:10.1007/BF00853952

Hamad, M. A. A. (2011). Analytical Solution of Natural Convection Flow of a Nanofluid over a Linearly Stretching Sheet in the Presence of Magnetic Field. *International Communications in Heat and Mass Transfer*, *38*(4), 487–492. doi:10.1016/j.icheatmasstransfer.2010.12.042

Hassani, M., Mohammad Tabar, M., Nemati, H., Domairry, G., & Noori, F. (2011). An Analytical Solution for Boundary Layer Flow of a Nanofluid Past a Stretching Sheet. *International Journal of Thermal Sciences*, *50*(11), 2256–2263. doi:10.1016/j.ijthermalsci.2011.05.015

Heinermann, J., & Kramer, O. (2016). Machine learning ensembles for wind power prediction. *Renewable Energy*, *89*, 671–679. doi:10.1016/j.renene.2015.11.073

Kakac, S., & Pramuanjaroenkij, A. (2009). Review of convective heat transfer enhancement with nanofluids. *International Journal of Heat and Mass Transfer*, *52*(13-14), 3187–3196. doi:10.1016/j.ijheatmasstransfer.2009.02.006

Kalogirou, S. (2007). *Artificial Intelligence in Energy and Renewable Energy Systems*. Nova Publishers.

Khan, W. A., & Pop, I. (2010). Boundary-Layer Flow of a Nanofluid Past a Stretching Sheet. *International Journal of Heat and Mass Transfer*, *53*(11-12), 2477–2483. doi:10.1016/j.ijheatmasstransfer.2010.01.032

Makinde, O. D., & Mutuku, W. N. (2014). Hydromagnetic thermal boundary layer of nanofluids over a convectively heated at plate with viscous dissipation and Ohmic heating. *Universitatea Politecnica Bucuresti Scientific Bulletin Series A*, *76*(2), 181–192.

Mostafa Rushdi, A. (2021). Machine learning approaches for thermal updraft prediction in wind solar tower systems. *Renewable Energy*, *177*, 1001–1013. doi:10.1016/j.renene.2021.06.033

Nadeem, S., & Haq, R. U. (2014). Effect of thermal radiation for magnetohydrodynamic boundary layer flow of a nanofluid past a stretching sheet with convective boundary conditions. *Journal of Computational and Theoretical Nanoscience*, *11*(1), 32–40. doi:10.1166/jctn.2014.3313

Naramgari, S., & Sulochana, C. (2016). Dual solutions of radiative MHD nanofluid flow over an exponentially stretching sheet with heat generation/absorption. *Applied Nanoscience*, *6*(1), 131–139. doi:10.100713204-015-0420-z

Noghrehabadadi, A., Ghalambaz, M., & Ghanbarzadeh, A. (2012). Heat transfer of magnetohydrodynamic viscous nanofluids over an isothermal stretching sheet. *Journal of Thermophysics and Heat Transfer*, *26*(4), 686–689. doi:10.2514/1.T3866

Partha, M. K., Murthy, P. V. S. N., & Rajasekhar, G. P. (2005). Effect of viscous dissipation on the mixed convection heat transfer from an exponentially stretching surface. *Heat and Mass Transfer*, *41*(4), 360–366. doi:10.100700231-004-0552-2

Raju, C. S. K., Sandeep, N., Sugunamma, V., Babu, M. J., & Reddy, J. R. (2016). Heat and mass transfer in magnetohydrodynamic casson fluid over an exponentially permeable stretching surface, *Engineering Science and Technology*. *International Journal (Toronto, Ont.)*, *19*(1), 45–52.

Rosenblatt, F. (1958). The perceptron: A probabilistic model for information storage and organization in the brain. *Psychological Review*, *6*(6), 386–408. doi:10.1037/h0042519 PMID:13602029

Rushdi, M. A., Rushdi, A. A., Dief, T. N., Halawa, A. M., Yoshida, S., & Schmehl, R. (2020, May 09). Power prediction of airborne wind energy systems using multivariate machine learning. *Energies*, *13*(9), 2367. doi:10.3390/en13092367

Sawyer, W. G., Hamilton, M. A., Fregly, B. J., & Banks, S. A. (2003). Temperature modeling in a total knee joint replacement using patient-specific kinematics. *Tribology Letters*, *15*(4), 343–351. doi:10.1023/B:TRIL.0000003057.60259.71

Scott, J. A. (1988). The computation of temperature rises in the human eye induced by infrared radiation. *Physics in Medicine and Biology*, *33*(2), 243–257. doi:10.1088/0031-9155/33/2/004 PMID:3362967

Sharma, N., Sharma, P., Irwin, D., & Shenoy, P. (2011). Predicting solar generation from weather forecasts using machine learning. *2011 IEEE International Conference on Smart Grid Communications (SmartGridComm)*, 528-533. 10.1109/SmartGridComm.2011.6102379

Ti, Z., Deng, X. W., & Yang, H. (2020). Wake modeling of wind turbines using machine learning. *Applied Energy*, *257*, 114025. doi:10.1016/j.apenergy.2019.114025

Treiber, N. A., Heinermann, J., & Kramer, O. (2016). Wind power prediction with machine learning. In *Computational Sustainability* (pp. 13–29). Springer. doi:10.1007/978-3-319-31858-5_2

Voyant, C., Notton, G., Kalogirou, S., Nivet, M. L., Paoli, C., Motte, F., & Fouilloy, A. (2017). Machine learning methods for solar radiation forecasting: A review. *Renewable Energy*, *105*, 569–582. doi:10.1016/j.renene.2016.12.095

Wang, C. Y. (1989). Free Convection on a Vertical Stretching Surface. *ZAMM. Journal of Applied Mathematics and Mechanics*, *69*(11), 418–420.

Zhang. (2019). *Gradient Descent based Optimization algorithms for Deep Learning Models training*. Academic Press.

Chapter 18
Predictive Analysis of Diabetes Using Machine Learning Algorithms

Nijatullah Mansoor
CHRIST University (Deemed), India

Ramesh Chandra Poonia
CHRIST University (Deemed), India

Debabrata Samanta
🆔 https://orcid.org/0000-0003-4118-2480
CHRIST University (Deemed), India

ABSTRACT

Diabetes is a very harmful disease that causes high blood sugar levels and occurs when the blood glucose level is high. Diabetes causes numerous diseases in humans: congestive heart failure, stroke, kidney and eye problems, dental issues, nerve damage, and foot problems. With the recent development in the machine learning concept, it is easy to analyze and predict whether a person is diabetic or not. This research mainly focuses on using several prediction algorithms of machine learning. The algorithms used in this research are k-nearest neighbor, logistic regression, SVM (support vector machine), Gaussian naive Bayes, decision tree, multilayer perceptron, random forest, XGBoost, and AdaBoost. Among these algorithms, the XGBoost performed better than the other algorithms achieving an accuracy of 90%, and the f1 score and Jaccard score were 91% and 86%, respectively. The primary goal of this research is to apply numerous machine learning algorithms to diabetic datasets, analyze their results, and select the best one that performs well.

DOI: 10.4018/978-1-6684-4580-8.ch018

INTRODUCTION

Diabetes is a chronic disease that happens when the quantity of glucose is immoderate. The main source of energy is blood glucose which is gained from the food we consume. Lack of insulin which is a hormone produced by the pancreas for the breakdown of glucose causes the rise of glucose in the body. There are numerous causes of diabetes, for example, genetic mutations, hormonal disease, consumption of medicines, pregnancy, age, BMI, overweight, alteration of the pancreas, and other diseases which can harm the pancreas. The most common types of diabetes are type 1, type 2, and gestational diabetes and each of them has their own symptoms and causes. The major symptoms include an increase in thirst, urination, hunger, blurred vision, weight loss, and sores that do not heal. Diabetes can cause heart attack, stroke, coma, heart failure, and coma. These issues can lead to human death. The statistics of diabetes for the year 2021, show that nearly 537 million adults between the age range of 20 to 79 years are suffering from this disease. These trends show that the total number of people suffering from this disease is likely to rise from 643 million in 2030 to 783 million in 2045. Machine learning (ML) is a subcategory of AI, where algorithms process huge amounts of datasets to discover patterns and perform tasks autonomously without being guided on exactly how to address the challenges. In the last few years, the extensive availability of vigorous hardware and cloud computing has resulted in broader adoption of ML in different parts of human lives, for instance, social networking, commute estimation, email intelligence, personal smart assistants, banking, personal finance, medical diagnosis, and healthcare. Machine learning plays a vital role in healthcare, for example accurately detecting disease at an earlier stage, discovering and developing new drugs, helps to analyze huge amounts of data in a short time and suggest outcomes, medical image diagnosis, outbreak prediction, smart health records, etc. Machine learning and AI-based technologies are being used in monitoring and predicting epidemics around the globe. With the constant rise of data that is being generated by modern technology in the healthcare sector, it is important to use machine learning, which can help to use this data and predict or diagnose a disease at an earlier stage. This paper depicts the use of different machine learning algorithms on the "Pima Indians diabetes dataset" to predict the diabetes disease based on symptoms for the patient. The dependent variable is the outcome to show whether a particular patient has diabetes or not. In this comparative analysis we have used various machine learning algorithms and applied them to the Pima Indians diabetes dataset, to see which model performs well, and accurately predict if patients in the dataset have diabetes or not. The motive of this work is to compare the performance of machine learning algorithms, which are used to predict diabetes disease. Algorithms used for the dataset to predict diabetes are, k-nearest neighbour, logistic regression, SVM (Support Vector Machine), Gaussian naive Bayes, Decision tree, Multilayer Perceptron, Random Forest, XGBoost, AdaBoost. According to the obtained results, it is discovered that XGBoost performs better than other algorithms, by achieving an accuracy score of 91% (Althar, R. R et al., 2022).

The rest of the paper is arranged as follows: the second section delves literature review, the third section illustrates the proposed methodology, section four includes the flowcharts of the model, section five discusses the algorithms and major findings, and finally section six concludes the research work.

LITERATURE REVIEW

Over the past few years, many research workers around the world worked in big data analytics and predictive analytics in the healthcare sector and other domains, to analyze, predict and forecast the present and future challenges in healthcare. The analysis of relevant works gives results on various healthcare datasets, where analysis and predictions were obtained using several methods and techniques. The paper focuses on the application of LR and RF-based ideas to analyze the dataset of Diabetes mellitus using Machine Learning. Machine Learning System has been used to determine the risk division for the classification of the patients into two different divisions of people for example diabetic patients and controlled patients. Moreover, the proposed pair of ideas gave a higher rate of accuracy in reading the data for the K10 protocol. Also, a comparative study has been presented on four different classifier experiments. They have also provided future prospects for using the same combination for other diseases as well(Bondada, P, et al., 2022). The paper aims at providing sufficient results on the application of the Gaussian Process-based model for analysis of diabetes data showing that the model increases the accuracy of the reading. Various performance aspects have been studied like ACC, SE, SP, PVV curve which shows that a GP-based model with RBF kernel gives the best results among all other classifiers for diabetes analysis in terms of medical information. In this study they have arbitrarily chosen 68994 healthy people and diabetic patients. they have used Principal component analysis (PCA) and Minimum redundancy Maximum relevance mRMR for dimensionality reduction. They have found that prediction with Random Forest could reach the utmost accuracy of 80% when all the attributes were used. During this research, they have observed that using PCA did not perform well in using all the features while using mRMR has the superior outcome. Furthermore, they have compared the result of three classification models. They find that there is not much difference among the random forest, decision tree, and neural network. However, random forest performs better compared to other classifiers in some methods. In this paper, they have used six different classifiers on the diabetes dataset. They have used accuracy, F1-score, recall, precision, and AUC for the performance measurement. AdaBoost performed well among the other algorithms, with an accuracy of 83%. And they have selected AdaBoost as the proposed model for prediction. In this study, they have applied ten ML algorithms on the Frankfurt hospital German diabetes dataset. They have applied an effective data preprocessing method 5-fold cross-validation, to obtain stable accuracy. In the resultamong these ten algorithms, three algorithms, GP, RF, and ANN perform very well, where Gaussian Process gives an accuracy of 98.25%, the random forest gives an accuracy of 97.25% and Neural Network gives an accuracy of 96.5%(Eapen, N. G. et al., 2022).

Figure 1. Model flow chart

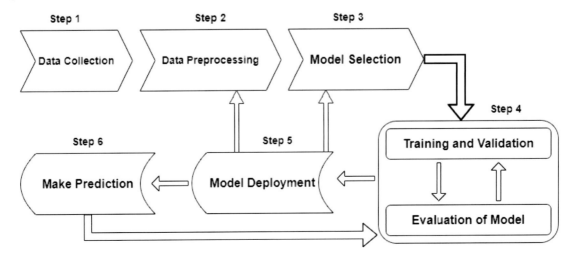

MATERIALS AND METHODS

The dataset's goal is to diagnose whether or not a patient has diabetes using particular diagnostic metrics provided in the collection. Various constraints were placed on the selection of these attributes from a big database while producing this dataset. All of the patients in this study are females aged 21 and up, according to the data. The datasets contain one target variable, outcome, and one independent variable, medical predictor variables (dependent variable). The patient's age, BMI, insulin, glucose, blood pressure, skin thickness, and other independent variables or predictors are among the independent variables or predictors. The dependent variable is the result that indicates whether a patient has diabetes or not(Guha, A, et al., 2022). There are 500 non-diabetic patients and 268 diabetes patients in this dataset, each with eight different metrics. The descriptions of the parameters and brief statistical summary are shown in the table 1 below.

Table 1. Statistical summary of the data set.

	count	mean	std	25%	50%	75%	max
Pregnancies	768	3.845052083	3.369578063	1	3	6	17
Glucose	768	120.8945313	31.9726182	99	117	140.25	199
BloodPressure	768	69.10546875	19.35580717	62	72	80	122
SkinThickness	768	20.53645833	15.95221757	0	23	32	99
Insulin	768	79.79947917	115.2440024	0	30.5	127.25	846
BMI	768	31.99257812	7.88416032	27.3	32	36.6	67.1
DiabetesPedigreeFunction	768	0.471876302	0.331328595	0.24375	0.3725	0.62625	2.42
Age	768	33.24088542	11.76023154	24	29	41	81
Outcome	768	0.348958333	0.476951377	0	0	1	1

Diabetes Pedigree Function is one of the parameters in PIDD. It includes information on diabetes illness history in the family, relatives, and the patient's hereditary relationship with those relatives. This genetic influence measurement offered us an insight of the hereditary risk of developing diabetes condition(Gupta, R. D et al., 2022). Body mass index, or BMI, is another metric that may be determined using a person's weight and height.

$BMI = kg / m^2$
Kg = person weight in kilograms
M^2 = person height in meters squared.

We used Jupyter Notebook in this work, which is an open-source web application programme that allows us to create and share documents that include live code, equations, computational output, visualisation, and other multimedia elements, as well as explanatory prose, all in one document. Jupyter Notebook is a user-friendly environment that can be used in any setting and on any platform. We utilised Python, an open-source, interpreted high-level programming language, for the programming. It is one of the most popular languages for data scientists to employ in a variety of data science projects and applications. Python has a lot of features for dealing with arithmetic, statistics, and scientific functions(Kumar, G et al., 2022). Python has a lot of features that help us solve mathematical, statistical, and scientific problems.

DATA PREPROCESSING

While creating a Machine learning model the first and most important step is data pre-processing. Real-world data is not always clean and format it is consist of noise, missing values, and sometimes the format of the data is also bad and cannot be used. Before doing any operation on data, it is essential to clean the data and put it in a formatted form, which can be easily interpreted and used by the ML model. Clean data can also increase the efficiency and accuracy of the ML model. To achieve clean and formatted data, we need to perform some operations on the data, this whole process is called data pre-processing(Hegde, D. S et al., 2022).

MISSING VALUE

It is necessary to remove missing values from the dataset because many ML algorithms will not perform if the dataset includesmissing values. Although, some algorithms like k-nearest and Naïve Bayes support data with missing values. In this study, we got missing values in the datasheet using python shown in the below table(M. Lu et al., 2020). There are many ways to handle missing values depending on the application; here we replace the missing values with the corresponding mean value. Below table 2 shows the details of missing values in the dataset.

Table 2. Missing values in the dataset.

Pregnancies	0
Glucose	5
BloodPressure	35
SkinThickness	227
Insulin	374
BMI	11
DiabetesPedigreeFunction	0
Age	0
Outcome	0

FEATURE SELECTION

We used Pearson's correlation, which is one of the most used methods, to locate and choose the most appropriate characteristics from the dataset. The correlation coefficient, which corresponds with the output and input attributes, is determined using this method. The value of the coefficient remains between 1 and -1(N. Reamaroon et al., 2019). If the value is greater than or equal to 0.5, there is a significant correlation; if the value is zero, there is no association. The correlation coefficient was calculated using the correlation function in Python, and the results and visual representation of the correlation are provided in table 3 and figure. We utilised 0.1 as a cut-off for relevant variables in this investigation. As a result, the features of BloodPressure and SkinThickness have been eliminated. Our most important six input attributes are pregnancies, glucose, BMI, insulin, diabetesPedigreeFunction, and age.

CORRELATION

Correlation is any statistical relationship, among two random attributes. It is a statistical measure that expresses the extent to which twoattributes are linearly related to each other, for example, the more time you spend studying the more information you will get, or as the temperature goes up the sales of cold soft drinks will also go up. In the correlation table, each random attribute (Ai) is correlated with earth of the other values in the table (Bi). With the help of the correlation table, we can see which pairs have the highest correlation(Nagavelli, U et al., 2022). Below table 3 show statistical summary of data after feature selection which we will be using for the models training.

Table 3. Statistical summary of data after feature selection which we will be using for the models training.

	count	mean	std	min	25%	50%	75%	max
Pregnancies	768	3.845052083	3.369578063	0	1	3	6	17
Glucose	768	121.6770833	30.46416059	44	99.75	117	140.25	199
Insulin	768	141.7539063	89.10084664	14	102.5	102.5	169.5	846
BMI	768	32.43463542	6.880497797	18.2	27.5	32.05	36.6	67.1
DiabetesPedigreeFunction	768	0.471876302	0.331328595	0.078	0.24375	0.3725	0.62625	2.42
Age	768	33.24088542	11.76023154	21	24	29	41	81
Outcome	768	0.348958333	0.476951377	0	0	0	1	1

Below figure 2 show Heatmap of the dataset.

Table 4 show the most correlated attributes with the outcome. Thecorrelation between the attribute and the outcome which are bigger than the cut of values, are pregnancies, glucose, insulin, BMI, DiabetesPedigreeFunction, and age. Among these attributes, Glucose has the highest correlation with the outcome which is 0.47, and insulin is the lowest correlation which is 0.13(P. K. Mallapragada et al., 2009).

Figure 2. Heatmap of the dataset.

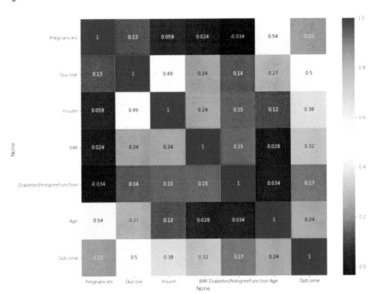

Table 4. The most correlated attributes with the outcome.

Attributes	Correlation coefficient with the outcome
Pregnancies	0.221898153
Glucose	0.466581398
Insulin	0.130547955
BMI	0.292694663
DiabetesPedigreeFunction	0.173844066
Age	0.238355983
Outcome	1

NORMALIZATION

Normalization in ML is the procedure of transforming data into the range of 0 and 1, or it can be any other range. Normalization can help ML algorithms to accelerate the training process, it basically improves model accuracy. Normalization gives equal importance to each attribute/parameter so that no single attribute drives model performance in one direction just because they are bigger values. There are numerous methods from sklearn that we can use to normalize, scale, and standardized our dataset. For example, MinMaxScaler, RobustScaler, StandardScaler, and Normalizer. In this study, we have used StandardScaler (*, copy=True, with_mean=True, with_std=True) to normalize the data(Piri, J et al., 2022). This method standardizes features by removing the mean and scaling to unit variance. The standard score of sample x is achieved as:

$$Z = (x-u) / s$$

In the above relation, u represent the mean of the training samples or zero if with_mean = False and s represent, the standard deviation of the training sample or one if with_std = False.

SPLIT THE DATASET INTO TRAIN AND TEST

The test accuracy is the percentage of right predictions that the model makes on the data that the model has not been trained on. If we do the train and test on the equivalent dataset, it will most likely have low out-of-test accuracy, because of the probability of our model overfitting. It is vital that our model has high, out-of-test accuracy, in light of the fact that the reason for any model, obviously, is to make the right forecasts on obscure data. for this reason, how can we enhance out-of-test accuracy? One way is to utilize an evaluation approach called Train/Test split, this method includes splitting the dataset into training and testing sets respectively, which are totally unrelated. After this, we train our model with the training set and test our model with testing sets. This will give a more exact assessment of out-of-test accuracy because the testing dataset is not been a part of the dataset that the model has been trained on it. this is more reasonable for real-world problems(Q. Xiao et al., 2019).

sklearn.model_selection.train_test_split(*arrays, test_size=None, train_size=None, random_state=None, shuffle=True, stratify=None)

test size This parameter's value should be between 0.0 and 1.0 if it is floating, and it basically specifies the fraction of the dataset to include in the test split. This argument can also take an int value, which specifies the test sample's absolute number. If the value of this option is None, the complement of the train size is used(Raghavendra Rao et al., 2022).

Train size if the parameter is float, the value should be between 0.0 and 1.0. It essentially shows the percentage of the dataset that is included in the train split. This argument can also take an int value, which specifies the train set's absolute number. If this parameter's value is set to None, the value is automatically set to the test size's complement.

This option regulates the shuffling used to the data before performing the split, and the value of the parameter might be int or None by default(S. Ertekin et al., 2011).

In this study, we have set the test_size = 0.2, which is 20%, our whole dataset which is 154 samples, and the remaining 80% which is 614 samples, we have used for training the models. and the random_state = 4. In our dataset "Pima Indians Diabetes Dataset" We have a total of 768 total samples, with the help of the above method we split our data into a Train/Test dataset. The shape of Train/Test data is shown below.

Train set: (614, 6) (614,)
Test set: (154, 6) (154,)

Our data set is ready, now we can train the model with this data. In this study, we will be using the same data, for all the machine learning models (S. Gibson et al., 2020).

IMPLEMENTATION OF THE MACHINE LEARNING MODEL

In this study, we have done a predictive analysis of diabetes using machine learning, the different machine learning algorithms, are k-nearest neighbor, logistic regression, SVM (Support Vector Machine), Gaussian naive Bayes, Decision tree, Multilayer Perceptron, Random Forest, XGBoost, AdaBoost(S. Hussein et al., 2019). For the implementation of these models, we follow the flow chart. Out of these 9 algorithms, we discussed the top 3 which achieve better performance. These three algorithms are XGBoost, Random Forest, AdaBoost.

Xgboost

XGBoost's full form is "Extreme Gradient Boosting" [2]. it is an optimized distributed gradient boosting library, intended to be exceptionally effective, adaptable, and versatile. It implements ML models under the gradient boosting framework. Boosting is an ensemble learning strategy to fabricate a solid classifier from a few weak classifiers in a series. Fundamentally, XGBoost is an extension of gradient boosted decision trees and is intended to further develop speed and performance. XGBoost have some feature for instance regularized learning, this term help to smooth the last learned weights and abstain from over-fitting. Another feature of XGBoost is gradient tree boosting, this implies that the tree ensemble model can't be streamlined using conventional optimization strategies in the Euclidean space, instead the model is trained in an added substance way. One more significant feature of XGBoost is shrinkage and column subsampling, these two techniques help the model to stay away from overfitting. Shrinkage scales newly added weights by a factor of η after each step of tree boosting. Shrinkage decreases the impact of each tree and passes on space for the future tree to work on the model to improve its performance. This second technique is column subsampling, this technique is used in a random forest, which can prevent over-fitting even more so than the customary row sub-sampling. The use of column sub-samples likewise accelerates computations of the parallel algorithm(S. Mirzaei et al., 2019).

While implementing the XGBClassifier () model, we have used the number of boosting rounds "n_estimator = 100", and random number seed random_state = 4. We give different values to this parameter but the result in these values was very good compared to others. We split our dataset 80% for training the model, and 20% for testing the model. The train set accuracy was 0.98%, and the test set accuracy was 0.91% this result was the highest accuracy among other models. the rest of the analysis of this model is done in the upcoming Result section(Samanta, D et al., 2022).

Adaboost

AdaBoost stands for Adaptive Boosting, it was the first boosting model which is developed for binary classification. Additionally, it is the best beginning stage for understanding boosting algorithms. This algorithm is sensitive to noisy data and anomalies AdaBoost created a single composite strong learner after a series of iterations. A new weak learner is added to the ensemble during each training period, and a weighting vector is adjusted in line with instances that were misclassified in previous rounds. As a result, the classifier is more accurate than the weak learner classifier. This approach creates a model and distributes the burden evenly among all data points. It then assigns heavier loads to the points that were classified incorrectly. In the following model, all points with greater weights are now assigned more relevance. It will keep training models until it achieves a reduced error rate(Samanta, D et al., 2022).

Implementation of this model AdaBoostClassifier (n_estimators=100, learning_rate=1, random_state=4) we have set n_estimators as 100 which represent the maximum number of estimators at which boosting is terminated. By default, it is 50 but accuracy we less if we set the n_estimators as 100 accuracy is much better than n_estimator = 50. The learning_rate shrinks the contribution of each classifier by learning_rate. And the random_state which controls the random seed given at each 'base_estimator' to 4. We have trained the model in 70% of the data and tested the model on 30% of the data. The accuracy score for the train set was 0.95, and the accuracy score for the test set was 0.89. in the case of splitting the dataset into 80% for training and 20% for testing the train set accuracy score was 0.92, and the test set accuracy was 0.86. which did not perform well as comparedto the previous state. The rest of the comparison is done in the upcoming section Result(Saritha, K et al., 2022). Below figure 3 shows Process of ensemble learning.

*Figure 3. **P**rocess of ensemble learning*

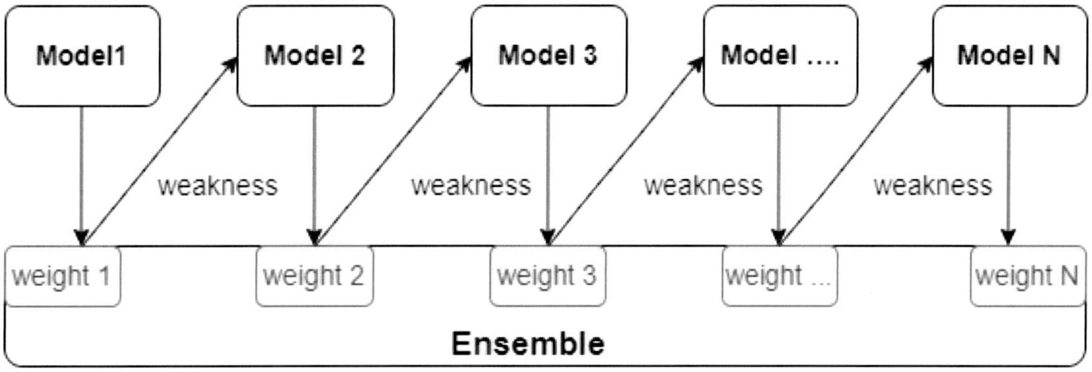

Random Forest

Random Forest, as the name implies, is made up of a large number of separate decision trees that work together. Every tree in the random forest emits a class forecast, and the class with the highest votes becomes the prediction of our model. It has a number of decision trees that each reflect a different way of classifying data that is fed into the random forest.

RandomForestClassifier(n_estimators=100, random_state=4) n_estimators = 100 which represent the number of tree in the forest. We have set different values for this attribute but we got the heist accuracy with n_estimators = 100. Another parameter is random_state = 4, this parameter Controls both the randomness of the bootstrapping of the samples used, when building trees. We have trained the model with 80% of our data and tested the model with 20% of our data. The training set accuracy was 0.97%, and the testing set accuracy was 0.89%. the rest of the analysis is done in the Result section(X. Deng et al., 2022).

MAJOR FINDING AND RESULT

To find the accuracy of the ML model, different strategies can be utilized. In this study, we have used a confusion matrix which is the most famous technique. A confusion matrix is a vital tool that helps us evaluate our ML model's performance(Tavares, J. M. R. S et al., 2022). As the name suggests it is a matrix of size n x n. where 'n' is the number of class labels in our problem.If we want to see the performance of the classification model confusion matrix the easiest way to achieve this objective(Singh, D et al., 2022). This will give us a clear image of model performance and the sort of mistake delivered by the model.Four types of outcomes are possible while evaluating a classification model performance. Table 5 shows summary of confusion matrix of all models which are predicted by models.

Table 5. Summary of confusion matrix of all models which are predicted by models.

Model	True Positives(TP)	True Negatives(TN)	False Positives(FP)	False Negatives(FN)
XGBoost	91	49	11	3
Random forest	89	48	13	4
AdaBoost	89	44	13	8
SVM (Support Vector Machines)	89	42	13	10
Multi layer Perceptron	87	44	15	8
Decision Tree	90	40	12	12
KNN	91	38	11	14
Logistic Regression	88	34	14	18
Gaussian Naïve Bayes	88	33	14	19

There are 4 main matrices that are commonly used for evaluating model performance. These are accuracy, precision, recall, and f1_score. In the study, we have used 9 different machine learning algorithms. the result of the accuracy scores, how each model performed on the data is shown in below the table 6 in the visual representation also shown in the below figure 4.

Table 6. Models accuracy

Model	Accuracy score
XGBoost	0.909090909
Random forest	0.889610390
AdaBoost	0.863636364
SVM (Support Vector Machines)	0.850649351
Multi layer Perceptron	0.850649351
Decision Tree	0.844155844
KNN	0.837662338
Logistic Regression	0.792207792
Gaussian Naïve Bayes	0.785714286

Figure 4. Models accuracy scores

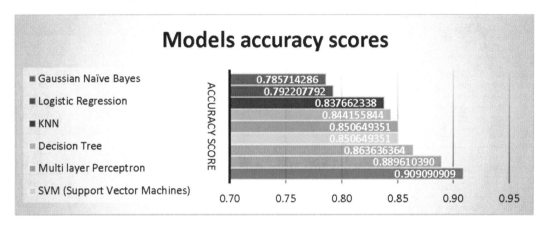

From the above result, we can see that XGBoost was the best classifier among others with an accuracy score of 90% secondly Random Forest was the best classifier among the others. Gaussian Naive Bayes performs very badly with an accuracy score of 78%.

Recall

The recall is defined as the fraction of examples that were anticipated to belong to a class with respect to all of the examples that truly belong in the class. The denominator (TP + FN) here is the actual number of positive instances present in the dataset.

Recall = TP / (TP + FN)

The below table 7, table 8 and table 9 shows the recall value for all the models. The best highest recall value was for XGBoost and KNN models. Below figure 5 show visual representation of Models train set accuracy

Table 7. Models precision scores

Model	Precision (1) diabetic	Precision (0) non-diabetic
XGBoost	0.97	0.82
Random forest	0.96	0.79
AdaBoost	0.92	0.77
Multi layer Perceptron	0.92	0.75
SVM (Support Vector Machines)	0.90	0.76
Decision Tree	0.88	0.77
KNN	0.87	0.78
Logistic Regression	0.83	0.71
Gaussian Naïve Bayes	0.82	0.7

Table 8. Models recall scores

Model	recall (1)	recall (0)
XGBoost	0.89	0.94
KNN	0.89	0.75
Decision Tree	0.88	0.77
Random forest	0.87	0.92
AdaBoost	0.87	0.85
SVM (Support Vector Machines)	0.87	0.81
Logistic Regression	0.86	0.65
Gaussian Naïve Bayes	0.86	0.63
Multi layer Perceptron	0.85	0.85

Table 9. F1_score of the models performance

Model	f1_score
XGBoost	0.910482375
Random forest	0.891458983
AdaBoost	0.865050859
SVM (Support Vector Machines)	0.851628494
Multi layer Perceptron	0.852705167
Decision Tree	0.844155844
KNN	0.836427742
Logistic Regression	0.790049950
Gaussian Naïve Bayes	0.782866257

Figure 5. Models train set accuracy

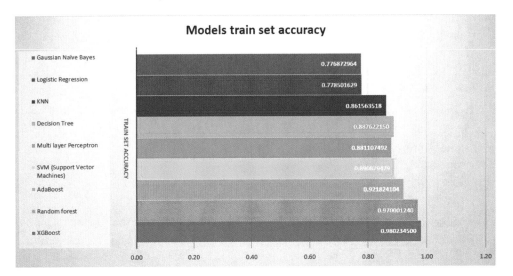

CONCLUSION

The biggest challenge in the healthcare sector is to detect diseases at an early stage. Diabetes is one of the life-threatening diseases, which case the death of thousands of people each year. It is very important to predict diabetes, at an early stage. In this study, we have applied various machine learning algorithms on the Pima Indians diabetes datasets, and predict whether a person will have diabetes or not in the dataset. The various algorithms are k-nearest neighbor, logistic regression, SVM (Support Vector Machine), Gaussian naive Bayes, Decision tree, Multilayer Perceptron, Random Forest, XGBoost, AdaBoost. Among these algorithms, the XGBoost performed better than the other algorithms achieving an accuracy of 91%. With the train set accuracy score of 98% and the test set accuracy score was 91%. The second model which performs better was the Random Forest, which gives the train set an accuracy score of a 97%, and the test set an accuracy score of 89%. The poorest performance was achieved by the Gaussian Naïve Bayes classifier with an accuracy score of 78%. Further, this study can be extended to find how likely a non-diabetic person can have diabetes in the future or in the next few years. Further, these models can be adopted for another chronic disease.

REFERENCES

Althar, R. R., Alahmadi, A., Samanta, D., Khan, M. Z., & Alahmadi, A. H. (2022). Mathematical foundations based statistical modeling of software source code for software system evolution. *Mathematical Biosciences and Engineering*, 19(4), 3701–3719. doi:10.3934/mbe.2022170 PMID:35341270

Bondada, P., Samanta, D., Kaur, M., & Lee, H.-N. (2022). Data Security-Based Routing in MANETs Using Key Management Mechanism. *Applied Sciences (Basel, Switzerland)*, 12(3), 1041. doi:10.3390/app12031041

Deng, X., Sun, T., Liu, F., & Li, D. (2022, February). SignGD with error feedback meets lazily aggregated technique: Communication-efficient algorithms for distributed learning. *Tsinghua Science and Technology*, 27(1), 174–185. doi:10.26599/TST.2021.9010045

Eapen, N. G., Rao, A. R., Samanta, D., Robert, N. R., Krishnamoorthy, R., & Lokesh, G. H. (2022). *Security Aspects for Mutation Testing in Mobile Applications. Στο Cyber Intelligence and Information Retrieval*. Springer.

Ertekin, S., Bottou, L., & Giles, C. L. (2011, February). Nonconvex Online Support Vector Machines. *IEEE Transactions on Pattern Analysis and Machine Intelligence*, 33(2), 368–381. doi:10.1109/TPA-MI.2010.109 PMID:20513924

Gibson, S., Issac, B., Zhang, L., & Jacob, S. M. (2020). Detecting Spam Email With Machine Learning Optimized With Bio-Inspired Metaheuristic Algorithms. *IEEE Access: Practical Innovations, Open Solutions*, 8, 187914–187932. doi:10.1109/ACCESS.2020.3030751

Guha, A., Alahmadi, A., Samanta, D., Khan, M. Z., & Alahmadi, A. H. (2022). A Multi-Modal Approach to Digital Document Stream Segmentation for Title Insurance Domain. *IEEE Access: Practical Innovations, Open Solutions*, 10, 11341–11353. doi:10.1109/ACCESS.2022.3144185

Gupta, R. D., Samanta, D., & Joseph, N. P. (2022). *Rendering View of Kitchen Design Using Autodesk 3Ds Max. Στο Micro-Electronics and Telecommunication Engineering*. Springer.

Hegde, D. S., Samanta, D., & Dutta, S. (2022). *Classification framework for fraud detection using hidden markov model. Στο Cyber Intelligence and Information Retrieval*. Springer.

Hussein, S., Kandel, P., Bolan, C. W., Wallace, M. B., & Bagci, U. (2019, August). Lung and Pancreatic Tumor Characterization in the Deep Learning Era: Novel Supervised and Unsupervised Learning Approaches. *IEEE Transactions on Medical Imaging*, 38(8), 1777–1787. doi:10.1109/TMI.2019.2894349 PMID:30676950

Kumar, G., & Samanta, D. (2022). *Effective View of Swimming Pool Using Autodesk 3ds Max: 3D Modelling and Rendering. Στο Internet of Things and Its Applications*. Springer.

Lu & Li. (2020). Survey on lie group machine learning. *Big Data Mining and Analytics, 3*(4), 235-258. . doi:10.26599/BDMA.2020.9020011

Mallapragada, P. K., Jin, R., Jain, A. K., & Liu, Y. (2009, November). SemiBoost: Boosting for Semi-Supervised Learning. *IEEE Transactions on Pattern Analysis and Machine Intelligence, 31*(11), 2000–2014. doi:10.1109/TPAMI.2008.235 PMID:19762927

Mirzaei, Sidi, Keasar, & Crivelli. (2019). Purely Structural Protein Scoring Functions Using Support Vector Machine and Ensemble Learning. *IEEE/ACM Transactions on Computational Biology and Bioinformatics, 16*(5), 1515-1523. . doi:10.1109/TCBB.2016.2602269

Nagavelli, U., Samanta, D., & Chakraborty, P. (2022). Machine Learning Technology-Based Heart Disease Detection Models. *Journal of Healthcare Engineering, 2022,* 2022. doi:10.1155/2022/7351061 PMID:35265303

Piri, J., Mohapatra, P., Singh, D., Samanta, D., Singh, D., Kaur, M., & Lee, H.-N. (2022). Mining and Interpretation of Critical Aspects of Infant Health Status Using Multi-Objective Evolutionary Feature Selection Approaches. *IEEE Access: Practical Innovations, Open Solutions, 10,* 32622–32638. doi:10.1109/ACCESS.2022.3161154

Raghavendra Rao, A., & Samanta, D. (2022). *A Real-Time Approach with Deep Learning for Pandemic Management. Στο Healthcare Informatics for Fighting COVID-19 and Future Epidemics.* Springer.

Reamaroon, N., Sjoding, M. W., Lin, K., Iwashyna, T. J., & Najarian, K. (2019, January). Accounting for Label Uncertainty in Machine Learning for Detection of Acute Respiratory Distress Syndrome. *IEEE Journal of Biomedical and Health Informatics, 23*(1), 407–415. doi:10.1109/JBHI.2018.2810820 PMID:29994592

Samanta, D., Dutta, S., Galety, M. G., & Pramanik, S. (2022). *A Novel Approach for Web Mining Taxonomy for High-Performance Computing. Στο Cyber Intelligence and Information Retrieval.* Springer.

Samanta, D., Karthikeyan, M. P., Agarwal, D., Biswas, A., Acharyya, A., & Banerjee, A. (2022). Trends in terahertz biomedical applications. *Generation, Detection and Processing of Terahertz Signals,* 285–299.

Saritha, K., Devi, B. M., Kurni, M., Samanta, D., & Joseph, N. P. (2022). *Controlling Node Failure Localization in Data Networks Using Probing Mechanisms. Στο Micro-Electronics and Telecommunication Engineering.* Springer.

Singh, D., Biswal, A. K., Samanta, D., Singh, D., & Lee, H.-N. (2022). Juice Jacking: Security Issues and Improvements in USB Technology. *Sustainability, 14*(2), 939. doi:10.3390u14020939

Tavares, J. M. R. S., Dutta, P., Dutta, S., & Samanta, D. (2022). Cyber Intelligence and Information Retrieval. In *Proceedings of CIIR 2021.* Springer.

Xiao, Q., Li, C., Tang, Y., & Chen, X. (2021, April). Energy Efficiency Modeling for Configuration-Dependent Machining via Machine Learning: A Comparative Study. *IEEE Transactions on Automation Science and Engineering, 18*(2), 717–730. doi:10.1109/TASE.2019.2961714

Chapter 19
Face Recognition System for Medical Information Modeling Using Machine Learning

Ramesh Chandra Poonia
CHRIST University (Deemed), India

Linesh Raja
iD https://orcid.org/0000-0002-3663-1184
Manipal University Jaipur, India

Ankit Kumar
iD https://orcid.org/0000-0002-7945-4616
GLA University, Mathura, India

Vaibhav Bhatnagar
Manipal University Jaipur, India

ABSTRACT

Face-recognition systems must be capable of identifying patient faces in an uncontrollable situation. Facial detection is a distinct problem from facial recognition in that it needs to report the location and size of all of the faces in a given image, which is not possible with face recognition. There are numerous changes in the images of the same face, which makes it a difficult problem to solve because of their general likeness in appearance. Face recognition is a very difficult procedure to do in an uncontrolled environment, since the lighting and angle of the face, as well as the quality of the image to be recognized, all have a considerable influence on the outcome of the process. This chapter provides information regarding the various face recognition machine learning models. The performance of the models is compared on the basis of values derived for FAR, FRR, TSR, and ERR.

DOI: 10.4018/978-1-6684-4580-8.ch019

INTRODUCTION

Background

When a person is identified based on their behavioural or physiological traits, biometrics is the technique of choice at the moment. Since the beginning of the twenty-first century, the physical and individual interface has played an important part in essential daily activities. However, we have been reluctant to continue this trend in the present day. A programmed society is more frequent than a private society, with mechanical representations, unsigned clients, and electronic sources of internet-related information being more common than their private counterparts. Face recognition has been related to mobile recognition systems because of the large range of visible benefits it has over traditional diagnostic techniques, which have been shown. The technology of face recognition has received a great deal of interest lately, particularly in the United States. It is utilized to draw attention to a person's individuality. As a result, facial recognition technology has depended on the human face for its accuracy. It is unknown to the general public that this facial recognition technology is capable of acting as an instantaneous fingerprint scanner. Unlike other biometric technologies like as iris recognition and central belief, facial recognition obtains images after entering a specified area on the subjects' faces. It is difficult to use computer recognition in facial recognition since the outer layer of a human face does not change much(Akbar et al., 2019).

Face Recognition System

In its most basic form, a picture is a movie, but in the context of statistics, a picture is much more than a still photograph. Two-dimensional function (x, y) in the calculation may be used to represent the coherence and amplitude of the plane f (x, y) power or the grey level of an image in the plane f (x, y). When the amplitudes of the X, Y, and NOC curves are all equal, an electronic digital image will be generated on the computer screen. A specific location and value are assigned to each element in an electronic image. An electronic picture is made up of discrete parts that may be counted. Graphic pixels, often known as elements, relate to the limited number of components in a graphic. A pixel is the smallest unit of visual representation. In a single photo, there are a colossal number of pixels.

Because of the increased interest in biometric security measures, facial recognition is a particularly profitable area of research. Facial recognition is a vital biometrics approach that is now in use. The ability to see faces with high precision is required in order to conduct research into facial recognition technology, which is now underway. Following that, we'll go through the principles of the facial recognition programme. The only thing that can be seen in a picture of someone's face are their facial traits. To put it another way, it suggests that we should only pay attention to the sections of the picture where a face could seem to be posing for the camera. In this localization procedure, it is possible to acquire inaccurate results because of a lack of quality in the picture that is used as an input or because of a variation in the expressions employed. The figure 1provides the information regarding the face localization.

It is necessary to fix the face and guarantee that each facial feature is observed in isolation in order to detect the location of the subject. Some of the methods that are utilized in the normalization process include trimming, scaling, and rotating. Normalization requires consistent image dimensions, continuous eyesight, and frontal orientation, all of which must be maintained. The same is shown in figure 2.

Figure 1. Localization of face

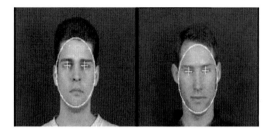

Figure 2. Normalization of face

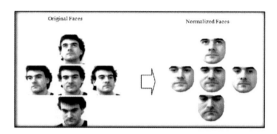

As far as decorative components are concerned, this is considered to be the first and most essential step in the extraction process. It is possible to eliminate a variety of features from the mouth, including those of the nose, eyes, lips, and ears, using this drain. This phase is prioritized at the top of the priority list by the vast majority of software. Mathematics-based strategies, colour segmentation-based approaches, and template-based approaches are just a few of the methodologies that have been used in this instance. The last stage would be to carry out a verification process. During this stage, it is checked to see whether the extracted characteristics and the stored database are connected in any way. Connection to the database is not just accomplished via facial recognition. There are a variety of other methods for assessing relevance in terms of face ability, including the use of a pre-existing template.

When it comes to recognizingpatient information, biometric technology has been widely used to do this. Facial recognition is predicted to surpass other biometric data in the near future, such as fingerprints, iris recognition, and other biometric data. This is according to current forecasts. Now, let's take a deeper look at some of the most popular face recognition technologies and applications available today. The figure 3 shows the extraction of facial features.

Figure 3. Extraction of facial features

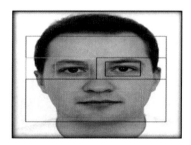

Face Recognition Technologies

Facial recognition is one of the applications that may be used as a first step in a variety of programmes and systems. Face-recognition algorithms can be divided into two broad categories:

- The feature-based technique, which tests several aspects by identifying a link between them and includes essential tactics such as the analysis of crucial components, linear discriminant analysis, and others

- The object-based technique, which tests a single aspect by identifying a link between it and other objects. This feature-based approach makes use of elastic bunch graph matching, which is a kind of graph matching.

Feature-Based Face Detection

Following the processing of an image to improve its quality (as well as quantifying its odd facial faculties such as eyes, noses, mouths, and so on), feature-based procedures work out precisely the geometric relationship between one of these decorative points, hammering an image to some vectors with geometric faculties, as shown in the following example. The use of typical statistical pattern recognition algorithms when confronted with these dimensions.

Figure 4. Face recognition by the geometric approach

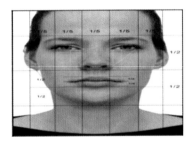

A technique for matching elastic cluster graphics is a feature-based approach that is really unique (Akbar et al., 2019). This strategy is based on the dynamic structure of the link as its foundation. A significant advantage of feature-based algorithms is that they anticipate an end-to-end investigation to adapt the image to a celebrity, and this is because the extraction of feature points predicts an end-to-end investigation to adapt the picture to the celebrity. In order to successfully apply at least one of these strategies, which entails rapid and responsive changes in mood or behavior, it is necessary to make judgements about which characteristics are important and which are not. Figure 4 shows the face recognition by the geometric approach.

Holistic Based Face Detection

To distinguish between faces, holistic perspective uses worldwide the activity of accurately identifying the position of a border or boundary, i.e., clarity based on the whole image rather than simply the local characteristic of your face, to separate them. Statistical and artificial intelligence approaches are divided into two tabs on the left side of the screen. Images are provided as a 2D matrix of relevant values, and the identification of each image is directly related with the input to the rest of the database (Chakraborty et al., 2012). In artificial intelligence operations, facial recognition may be accomplished via the use of neural networks and machine learning algorithms.

Knowledge Based Methods

As described by Liu (2004) in his knowledge-based methodologies, human cognition codes to detect how different facial features combine to make a recognized face. You may take advantage of the link between the traits of the face by using these approaches. One of its key duties is to ensure that the faces are aligned. Or, to put it another way, the face is discovered in the photograph taken by the camera during this process.

REVIEW OF LITERATURE

An overview of many face-recognition approaches for medical patients is presented in this chapter, which also contains a selection procedure for learning about the techniques' backstories and other significant ideas and concepts. A substantial amount of research has been done on the subject of Automated Facial Recognition (AFR). AFR research has had a significant impact on a broad variety of domains, including computer interfaces and theoretical problems, as a result of which its presence is readily apparent. As an added bonus, this chapter analyses several machine learning algorithms for a broad classification issue, with a particular emphasis on medical patient facial recognition. This chapter offers a review of data feature type techniques and performance metrics, as well as a discussion of how this classification version performs in comparison to other classification versions. The figure 5 identifies the FER system components.

Figure 5. FER system components

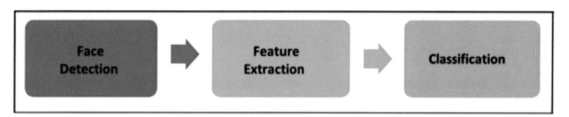

Facial Expression Recognition System Components

Face Recognition methods may be used to provide a foundation for future study. As shown in Figure 2.1 Methods, there are three high-tech components that are employed to develop Face Recognition. Face detection, feature extraction, and further classification are all performed as part of this procedure. In the below sub section feature extraction mechanism is discussed in detail.

Feature Extraction

Daugman (1980) For precisely recognizing faces, PCA is a very dependable approach. According to this research, principal component analysis (PCA) and maybe a face image are the most efficient methods to describe data. With the help of this procedure, we may shrink the image's size and dimensions significantly. The strategy described here does more than only take use of geometrical benefits. It also has other advantages. The publication has devised a real-time human head tracking programme that would follow the movement of the subject's head. Using a Pentium 4 Core Processor with a clock speed of 1.4GHz, the calculations were performed. With an accuracy rate of more than 92 percent, this face-detection technology is very accurate in its work. It makes no difference from whatever perspective you look at it: from the front, from the side, or even from the rear.

Lanitis et al. (1997) Here is a link to a paper titled "A Recognition System Using a 7-State HMM Combined with SVD Coefficients." A 99 percent success rate has been achieved on one-half of all pictures in the Olivetti Research Laboratory (ORL) database of interest as a consequence of continual training provided by the Olivetti Research Laboratory (ORL). The success percentage of the YALE database is 97.7percent. It has been decided to add two more parts to the book. The use of quantized SVD coefficients as features for characterizing facial image cubes was carried out with the use of a bare minimum of these coefficients in order to reduce computational costs. In the pre-processing system, an order statistic filter was utilized to filter out the noise. An investigation was carried out on a top-down chain of co-occurring sub-image Cubes that seemed to be connected. When employing quantized SVD coefficients of the cubes' SVD coefficients, HMM may be applied to each face of the cube. The table 1 compares the results of the different images sizes of ORL.

Table 1. Comparing the results of the different image size of ORL (Lanitiset al., 1997)

Image size	64x64	32x32
# Of train Image (s)	5	5
Training Time per image (second)	0.63	0.46
Reorganization Time per image	0.28	0.15
# of symbols	1260	960
Recognition (%)	99	92.5

At the same time figure 2 provide the information regarding the computational costs and recognition results of some of the other methods as reported by the respective authors on the ORL face database. Table 2 compares the results of comparative computational costs and recognition results of some of the other methods as reported by the respective authors on the ORL face database

Table 2. Comparative computational costs and recognition results of some of the other methods as reported by the respective authors on the ORL face database (Lanitiset al., 1997)

Method	% Recognition	Training time per image	Recognition time per image(sec)
Pseudo-2D HMM (Baudat and Anouar, 2000)	95	NA	240
DCT-HMM (Georghiadeset al., 2000)	99.5	23.5 sec.	3.5
DHMM + Wavelet (Guo et al., 2001)	100	1.13 sec	0.3
PDBNN (Xu and Deng, 2008)	96	20 min.	<= 0.1
n-Tuple	86	0.9 sec.	0.025
DHMM + SVD (Sato et al., 2013).	99	0.63 sec.	0.28

Eventually, they developed a method that has the fastest identification speed when the number of training photos is much more than five. While LDA normally outperforms the suggested strategy for ORL D B, the proposed approach beat LDA by a large margin in this instance. Yale's face D B has a resolution of 231231 pixels. A high-speed approach is developed by cutting the face graphics background, which has image dimensions of 6 4 6 4, to make a 6 4 6 4 picture.

YALE Face database Face Recognition

Table 3 provide the experimental results of YALE face database.

Table 3. Experiments on YALE face database

Number of train Image(s)	MRF	LDA	PCA	NN	1DHMM+ SVD
1	81.6	NA	60	68.31	78
2	93.11	91.23	75.2	80.49	82.22
3	95.2	98.2	79	83.5	90.83
4	95,9	99.41	79.8	84	94.29
5	96.11	99.69	81.1	83.51	97.78
6	96.67	99.87	81.1	82.8	100
7	98.67	99.97	81.9	82.63	100
8	97.33	100	81.2	81.6	100
9	97.33	100	81.7	82.2	100
10	99.33	100	81.7	83.07	100

Gabor-Wavelets Based Feature Extraction

Edwards *et al.* (2001): Methods of extraction that are related with each of these groupings are listed below. His findings indicate that the efficacy of appearance-based procedures outperforms that of version-based approaches, and that they are on par with that of motion-based practices. Motion-based systems, which employ lighting normalized graphic sequences as the foundation for their appearance, need a more athletic approach based on statistical methods and a greater focus on static images than other types of systems. In terms of appearance-based techniques, the community binary patterns (LBP) and Gabor wavelets were compared to one another. LBP has been selected as the preferable technique of choice for Gabor-wavelets due to the complexity and basic requirements of the wavelets.

Heisele*et al.* (2003): Consider estimating the vector parameters for any assessment graphic in comparison to the majority of model squares estimation, as well as decision rules developed in favour of this category having estimation. This method is used to classify the subspace that is closest to the user. In fact, as shown by the results of the LRC, performance is often insufficient even when simple improvements are made. Because of this, advanced main component regression classification (IPCRC) was proposed as a potential solution to the problem at hand. In addition to managing, it is essential that you have a straightforward demeanour. In the studies, there were 25 images of the face and another 25 shots of the skin on the face. The database is used in order to assign the noise reduction work. Following the discovery of the epidermis, the goal is to identify the complexion area by analyzing the components and pores present in the skin's surface. The Y-value of each pit and crevice is measured in order to determine the properties of the face. The face is the component of the body that is associated with the feature gender that was spoken.

Xu and Deng (2008): The YALE DB to 6 4 x 6 4 jpeg face graphics at a resolution of 231x195 pixels was created using the YALE DB. Other than cropping and desktop trimming, no other changes were done to the image. Many newspapers utilized this D B to test their own systems, and it was widely used in the industry. In order to accommodate the limited number of train recorded graphics that were imprisoned, they quantized their first feature (W11) into 8 levels, their second feature (W11) into 6 levels, and their third feature (U11) into 20 levels. As a result, they changed their approach from one image into ten graphics for training with 960 logos to one image into ten graphics for training with 960 logos.

Chakraborty *et al.* (2012): What the study presented here demonstrates is something that can be acquired. When comparing a person's face to a well-known one from the rectal perspective, it is feasible to tell the difference between their facial form and the well-known one. It is possible to handle the issue of face and lighting alignment in preprocessed graphics by using encapsulation techniques. Face recognition was achieved in this study with the use of the Eigenface solution from Eigenface. The right face of an image's covariance matrix contains a vector that represents the distance between the picture and the observer. In practically every new facial photograph, a linear combination of faces may be identified. Face recognition gets easier to do as you implement this method, owing to the use of two specialized images that are employed throughout the process.

Using this method, the data obtained is more than 95 percent accurate. The experiment is carried out in a one-of-a-kind manner. Each of the 105 photographs is included inside three different datasets. In this investigation, tests were carried out on a series of images for new and familiar faces in their three states, with the faces being new or familiar (daylight, deficient, middle, and equal histograms). There are few instances in which faces have been put in the face unknown, but the database faces are not there in those instances. We discovered that the average distance between well-known visuals is almost non-existent. As a consequence, only the database image may be recognized by a pair of training graphics when a pair of training graphics is used. For anonymous photographs, an average distance between database visuals and a training collection of graphics is calculated, indicating that the input images are not recognized by anybody in the database. It's a respectable task considering the circumstances. It can accurately identify both known and unknown drawings in the database, and it does it with 100 percent accuracy.

FACE RECOGNIZATION APPROACH

General Structure for the Face Recognition System

The most important parts of this assessment are the individual faces and their placement in the image as a whole. In the input photo, you can see the expected results in all of your face characteristics, including your smile. It is also possible to utilize object identification to determine the position and size of the majority of the objects in a photograph. Face detection may be useful in a variety of applications such as area of interest identification, object discovery, photo and video classification, and so on.

Feature Extraction

During this time period, human facial scars are removed from the photos in order to increase the accuracy of face recognition. Because human faces are recognised based on geometric features like the nose, eyes, and lips (among others), the mouth region has excellent facial identification skills. Those organs have gaps in their structure, form, and arrangement, allowing the faces to be identified in a variety of ways based on their differences. For the purpose of isolating facial characteristics, one well-known strategy is to first separate the facial features depending on the size and distance of the limbs from one another. Figure 6detect features from face and figure 7 shows the feature extraction.

Figure 6. Detect features from face

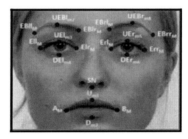

Figure 7. Extraction of feature and representation of feature vector

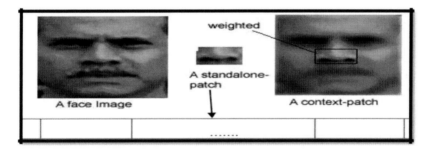

Face Recognition

Lastly, the extraction of facial features and presentation of the vector of features take place in the last step. In order to achieve intuitive understanding, a face database is required. The face database contains a range of images as well as information on the personalities of the individuals who appear in it. Face detection and feature extraction will begin as soon as an image is loaded into the programme. Run a comparison on each attribute value in the database to see whether or not they are the same. Facial recognition technology is used to identify and authenticate the identification of a person in the vast majority of instances (Yaman et al., 2018). Using a facial image to detect whether or not a person is face-to-face, the computer will be able to tell whether or not they are. The steps of face recognition system are given in the figure 8.

Figure 8. Steps in the face recognition system

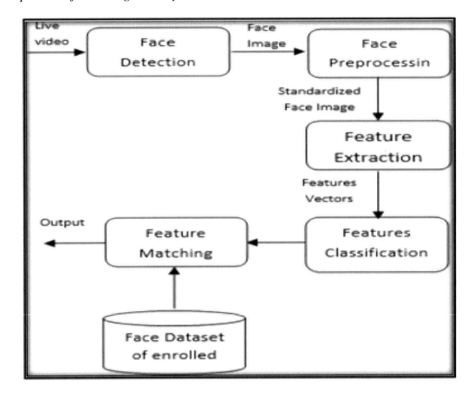

SVM Classifier

The information is included inside a multiclass or two-type issue. It will be necessary in this research to separate seed plant data sets from the United States and South America into two separate groups using two distinct labels. As a result, we will be forced to cope with a two-class situation. Many applications have been developed, including the supply of species and the detection of potential mineral resources. In the field of regression and classification, heuristic methods established by statistical learning theory are used to address issues.

mx + b>= +1 mx
  + b>= -1

The hyperplane can also be represented mathematically by (Perkins, 1975).

$$f(x) = sgn(mx + b)$$

Where () Sign functions are represented by the following equation in mathematics.

$$(x) = \begin{cases} 1, & \text{if } x > 0 \\ 0, & \text{if } x = 0 \\ -1, & \text{if } x < 0 \end{cases}$$

Figure 9. Distance of the nearest data vectors from the hyperplane

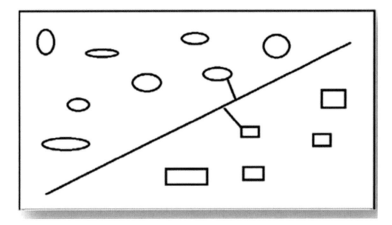

The figure 9 shows the distance of the nearest data vectors from the hyperplane. When x is a data point, the equation expresses mathematically how far it is away from the hyperplane. It is necessary to pick a hyperplane with the most distantly created connecting points in order to carry out the classifications that have been stated. SVM may be used to solve problems involving several classes and classes. When faced with categorization issues involving a large number of classes, a variety of ways may be utilized to overcome them. One possibility is to move the data vectors to a different distance from one another, in order to linearize the current situation. Another option is to break down the multi-class problem into a series of two-class questions to simplify the process (Lades et al., 1993). The voting method pulls together the services provided by each two-class issue in order to discover a solution to the initial multi-level problem that was presented to the participants. This SVM is represented by a formula that has psychedelic elements (Breiman, 2001).

The aim is to increase the size of the perimeter while decreasing the amount of error in the measurements. The information sample files from your practice data collection are included in the input collection (Bianconi and Fernández, 2011). A certain set of features is shared by all of these information vectors, and these qualities are specified by the classification model. Because of this mix of features, it is hypothesized that a feature distance is created. SVM takes advantage of this radial basis kernel work in order to function with a less amount of input space (Bartlett et al., 2002). The output of this kernel work is that you are able to do classification based on the input area rather than complex feature distances as a consequence of your effort. Most other classification approaches do not allow for the construction of classification models from a limited number of features, which is true for supervised learning. This is achievable with the help of SVM (Krishnapriya and Hemanth, 2013). Individual photo data's facial skin may be categorizedutilizing a hybrid approach, which may increase the overall efficacy and accuracy of the standard classification strategy. It is necessary to employ the data sets in order to construct a classification version, which can then be tested against an evaluation data collection and used in the future (Mahmoudi et al., 2003). Because the classification tags associated with data sets are well established, this method should be referred to as supervised classification. Because the information about the group tags is unknown, clustering is sometimes referred to as unsupervised classification. Identical attributes exist for each data vector in the data set, and these properties may be used to categories the data in the classification version of the data set. It is necessary to divide the data distance into two distinct zones in order to categories their input data space in order to use it (Sodhi and Lal, 2013). The figure 10 shows the SVM classification technique.

Figure 10. SVM classification

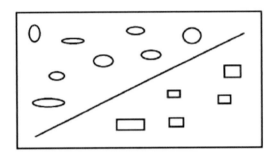

The table 4 provides the information regarding the algorithm 1.

Table 4. Classification using linear kernel-based SVM classifier

Input
Input: I: Input data (Input Data)
Output
Output: V: Support vectors set(SVM data Set)
Procedure Begin
• Split The specified dataset into two sets of data items having different category labels assigned to them // Divide the specified data set into two sets of information items
• Insert Them to encourage vector set V
• Loop Divided n info items
• In case A data item isn't assigned someone of these category tags you can put in it to place squat
• Break If insufficient data items are found
• end Loop
• Train Utilizing the derived SVM classifier model and test to validate within the Data items
• End

Random Forest Classifier

The first subset has two-thirds of the information points, whereas the second subset contains one-third of them. On the other hand, we have a subset that contains one-third of the information points. All of the data points are utilized to construct type trees, with two-thirds of the data points being used to generate (OOB) instances of the types trees generated. (1973). It is possible to estimate instructional data collection indicators for a broad variety of educational applications. When evaluating an important aspect, the parameters for Gini index reduction and OOB error estimate may be employed together. When the range of qualities is broad and the relative significance comes to prominence as a result, calculating the relative value of components is a useful technique in investigations (Moore, 1987). When it comes to bias and fluctuation, the RF technique is quite exact (Brunelli and Poggio, 1993). When RF assigns a rating to a factor, it considers the factor's categorization accuracy as well as other data collection criteria. There may be a hint of importance in this particular site. The comparison of each component is what is utilized to establish the categorization of the component(Zhang, T et al., 2007) (Zhou, S. K et al., 2006). The importance of a factor may be assessed by averaging the classification trees that have been developed by the organization. When it comes to categorization, the bigger the significance of an indication, the greater the significance of a variable. It is referred to as the Z-score when the significance index of a given element is divided by the probability of making an ordinary error. There is no truncation applied to any of the classes in Shrub. There is no doubt that the RF classification trees (Chellappa et al., 1995) that were used are the finest available. It is eventually discovered that the output of each category tree serves as a vote in determining the result of this clothing classifier, i.e., the assignment of an item-specific class tag, by the clothes classifier. Belhumeur and his associates Data classification requires an ensemble of classifiers, or it may be able to gather all classifiers in a single collection. As a consequence, they surpass human classifiers when it comes to accuracy in classification. A nice example of a costume classifier is the one used in random forests, which can be found here. The RF classification approach, as well as other anti-inflammatory classification modelling strategies, may be utilized in combination to deal with misleading data. There are no restrictions on the number of classification trees that may be constructed, or on the amount of data or variable samples that can be used to construct classification trees (roughly two-thirds of the data or samples are utilized) (Kalocsai et al., 2000). This, as well as a slew of other ensemble strategies, is incorrect (Geurts et al., 2005). When SVM and RF are used together, it is possible to produce significantly more accurate classification results than previously possible. Comparing our hybrid system to a human-classification technique, our hybrid system is more noise-resistant (Fogel, 2006).

While random woods continue to expand, the location of the features will remain the same. The evaluation set is used in RF to validate the classification result and to call the category tags for unlabeled data once the classification version has been prepared and is ready to be used. This tool allows you to compare classification trees inside your organization(Wiskott, L. et al., 1997) (Xu, Q et al., 2008). A data value sample was used to cross-certify the outside, and the results were published. Therefore, it has a higher likelihood of being correct and less likelihood of suffering from erroneous classifications than human classification trees, among other advantages (Fogel, 2006). Because the random woodlands outfit selects two-thirds of the input criteria for each classification tree at random, there is very little link between the countless trees in the woods due to the randomness of the selection process. An individual may choose to limit the number of variables that split a parent node at the classification tree in order to lower the number of connections between trees in their database. In the event of large datasets, the random woodlands classification strategy is more successful than the other techniques(Sodhi, K. S et al., 2013). Combining the advantages of random forests with those of support vector machines and nurturing is possible in this thesis classification technique(Sato, W. et al., 2013)(Sim, R et al., 2009). In applications such as remote sensing picture classification and credit analysis, the RF approach is less likely to be employed than other methods. When evaluating classification, it is also important to consider the distance between the two samples being evaluated. If the amount classification trees for the two data sets finish up at the same node, this is a good indication that they are close. It may be easier to find outliers in data if they are organized into trees(Yaman, M. A et al., 2018) (Zahoor, E et al., 2013). As a result of the large number of sample recordings and classification trees used in this calculation, a significant quantity of storage space is required (Sato et al., 2013). In this section, you can get a pseudocode reference for the random forest approach (Liu and Kehtarnavaz, 2013). The table 5 provides the information regarding the algorithm 2.

Table 5. Classification based on Random Forest Classifier

Input **Input:** Training sample a: number of input instance to be used to generate classification tree UT: Total number of classification trees in random forest OT: Classification Output from each tree T
Output Output: V: Random Forest Classification set
Procedure Begin • OT is empty • For i=1 to T • Db = Form random sample subsets after selecting 2/3rd instances randomly from D. /* For every tree this sample would be randomly selected*/ • Cb = Build classification trees using random subsets Db • Validate the classifier Cb using remaining 1/3rdinstances //Refer Step 3. • OT=store classification outputs of classification trees • Next i • Apply voting mechanism to derive output ORT of the random forest (ensemble of classification trees) • Return ORT

RESULT DISCUSSION

Image Matching

Images may be used to gather information about people's faces, which can then be utilized as a standard for constructing a face arrangement. Because they are all in such strong contrast, it is able to easily see the connection between each of the photos in the box portions. For example, it is conceivable for non-facial sites to be of low relevance while facial parts are of great importance. Following that, the less important boxes are no longer visible(Sujay, S, N. et al., 2017) (Wiskott, L. et al., 1999). There are no constraints on the size of the boxes; the attribute is saved in pixels up to 220 at a scale of 1 pixel per pixel (pixels per inch) (boxes are square boxes). For face creation assessments, square photos of 100x100 pixels are accepted. Refer figure 11 for sample database images used for tanning.

Figure 11. Sample database images used for tanning

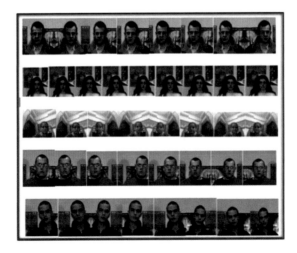

There have been several instances of faces being discovered in their identical place, as well as instances of non-facial surface material being mistaken for a face. It was 100 percent successful after adding colour to the background. It has also been tried out on a different image as an experiment. Everyone is presented with a one-of-a-kind identification number(Naseem, I. et al., 2010)(Nefian, A.V. et al., 1998). High-contrast photos (the vast majority of which were under the category of skin colour) led to incorrect assumptions being drawn. The filter co-efficient was rectified, and the range of the filter was changed in order to get a better result. Refer figure 12.

Figure 12. Out of identified face with their label

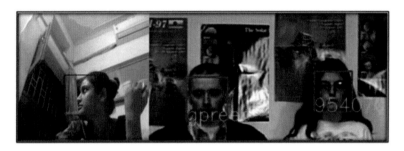

Comparative Performance Evaluation

False Accept Rate (FAR): Frequency that the system makes false accepts.Example: FAR of 0.1% system will make 1 false except for every 1000 fake attempt. The comparative analysis of FAR parameters in face recognition is given in figure 13.

Figure 13. Comparative analysis of FAR parameters in face recognition

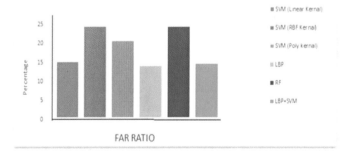

False Reject Rate (FRR): In the event that a bad image is supplied for face recognition, how often does the system reject it as a faulty image with no matching data in the dataset(Paul, L. C et al., 2012) (Perkins, D et al., 1975). The comparative analysis of FRR parameters in face recognition system is given in figure 14.

Figure 14. Comparative analysis of FRR parameters in face recognition system

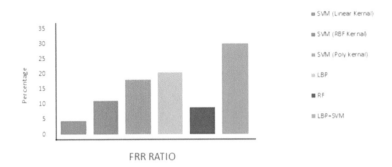

True Success Rate (TSR): A person's accurate match rate is defined as the ratio of the total number of people properly matched in the database to the total number of people. The comparative analysis of TSR parameters in face recognition system is given in figure 15.

Figure 15. Comparative analysis of TSR parameters in face recognition system

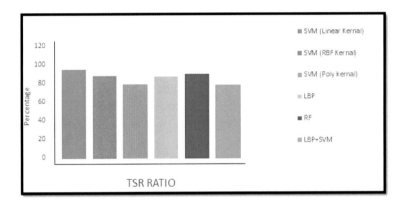

Error Rate (ERR): The Comparative analysis of ERR parameters in face recognition system is given in figure 16.

Figure 16. Comparative analysis of ERR parameters in face recognition system

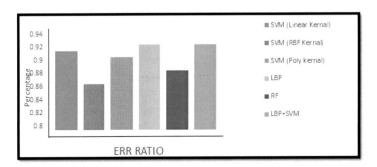

400 photos were subjected to testing, with the results divided into five groups for further examination. A subset is created by selecting ten images of two patients from which to choose. Only four patientfeatures in the second batch of 40 images, which totals 40 in total. Subset 3 has 70 photos, each of which depicts a different patient from the rest of the set(Phillips, P.J et al., 1998)(Salhi, A. l et al., 2012). There are a total of 10 photographs for each patient. Subset 4 has 120 images, while subset 5 contains 150 photographs, both of which have 1-2 themes. The results of recognition testing, as well as the rate period of tests, are displayed in the table6:

Table 6. Result comparison

Approach Used	Mean Recognition Rate
• **Optimized SVM/ RF** • **RF** • **SVM(linear kernel)** • **SVM(rbf kernel)**	• **96.05%** • **94.73%** • **96.05%** • **94.73%**
• **LBP+SVM** Face Recognition Using ExtendedLBP Features and Multilevel SVM Classifier	93%
• **LBP** Face Description with Local Binary Patterns: Application to Face Recognition	94.6%
• **RF** Fast and efficient face recognition system using Random Forest and Histograms of OrientedGradients	92.6%

The final comparative analysis of recognition rate is given in figure 17.

Figure 17. Comparative analysis of recognition rate

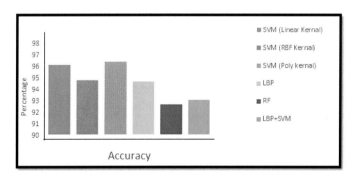

CONCLUSION

The chapter studied the performance of the multiple machine learning model for the face recognition of the medical patient. On the basis of the same the comparative analysis of the recognition rate of the existing models are derived. The same is mentioned the table 6 and graphically represented in figure 17. On the basis of the derived recognition rate, it can be concluded that there is a requirement of hybrid model which can enhance the recognition rate of patient identification through their images.

REFERENCES

Ahonen, T., Hadid, A., & Pietikainen, M. (2006). Face recognition by independent component analysis. *IEEE Transactions on Pattern Analysis and Machine Intelligence, 28,* 2037-2041.

Akbar, T. A., Hassan, Q. K., Ishaq, S., Batool, M., Butt, H. J., & Jabbar, H. (2019). Investigative Spatial Distribution and Modelling of Existing and Future Urban Land Changes and Its Impact on Urbanization and Economy. *Remote Sensing, 11*(2), 105–115. doi:10.3390/rs11020105

Arora, R., & Doegar, A. (2016). An Effective Approach for Face Recognition using PCA and LDA on Visible and IR images. *International Journal of Computer Trends and Technology, 32*(1), 44–48. doi:10.14445/22312803/IJCTT-V32P108

Bartlett, M. S., Movellan, J. R., & Sejnowski, T. J. (2002). Face recognition by independent component analysis. *IEEE Transactions on Neural Networks, 13*(6), 1450–1464. doi:10.1109/TNN.2002.804287 PMID:18244540

Baudat, G., & Anouar, F. (2000). Generalized Discriminant Analysis Using a Kernel Approach. *Neural Computation, 12*(10), 2385–2404. doi:10.1162/089976600300014980 PMID:11032039

Belhumeur, P. N., Hespanha, J. P., & Kriegman, D. J. (1997). Eigenfaces vs. Fisherfaces: Recognition using class specific linear projection. *IEEE Transactions on Pattern Analysis and Machine Intelligence, 19*(7), 711–720. doi:10.1109/34.598228

Bianconi, F., & Fernández, A. (2011). On the Occurrence Probability of Local Binary Patterns: A Theoretical Study. *Journal of Mathematical Imaging and Vision, 40*(3), 259–268. doi:10.100710851-011-0261-7

Breiman, L. (2001). Random forests. *Machine Learning, 45*(1), 5–32. doi:10.1023/A:1010933404324

Brunelli, R., & Poggio, T. (1993). Face recognition: Features versus templates. *IEEE Transactions on Pattern Analysis and Machine Intelligence, 15*(10), 1042–1052. doi:10.1109/34.254061

Chakraborty, D., Saha, S. K., & Bhuiyan, M. A. (2012). Face Recognition using Eigenvector and Principle Component Analysis. *International Journal of Computers and Applications, 50*(10), 42–49. doi:10.5120/7811-0947

Chellappa, R., Wilson, C. L., & Sirohey, S. (1995). Human and machine recognition of faces: A survey. *Proceedings of the IEEE, 83*(5), 705–741. doi:10.1109/5.381842

Chitaliya, N. G., & Trivedi, A. L. (2010). An Efficient Method for Face Feature Extraction and Recognition based on Contourlet Transform and Principal Component Analysis using Neural Network. *International Journal of Computers and Applications, 6*(4), 28–34. doi:10.5120/1066-1260

Daugman, J. (2016). Information theory and the iriscode. *IEEE Transactions on Information Forensics and Security, 11*(2), 400–409. doi:10.1109/TIFS.2015.2500196

Daugman, J. G. (1980). Two-dimensional spectral analysis of cortical receptive field profiles. *Vision Research, 20*(10), 847–856. doi:10.1016/0042-6989(80)90065-6 PMID:7467139

Duc, B., Fischer, S., & Bign, J. (1999). Face Authentication with Gabor Information on Deformable Graphs. *IEEE Transactions on Image Processing*, *8*(4), 504–516. doi:10.1109/83.753738 PMID:18262894

Edwards, J., Pattision, E. P., Jackson, H. J., & Wales, R. J. (2001). Facial affect and affective prosody recognition in first-episode schizophrenia. *Schizophrenia Research*, *48*(2-3), 235–253. doi:10.1016/S0920-9964(00)00099-2 PMID:11295377

Eleccion, M. (1973). Automatic fingerprint identification. *IEEE Spectrum*, *10*(9), 36–45. doi:10.1109/MSPEC.1973.5212832

Farokhi, S., Shamsuddin, S. M., Flusser, J., Sheikh, U. U., Khansari, M., & Jafari-Khouzani, K. (2013). Rotation and noise invariant near-infrared face recognition by means of Zernike moments and spectral regression discriminant analysis. *Journal of Electronic Imaging*, *22*(1), 1–11. doi:10.1117/1.JEI.22.1.013030

Fasel, I. R., Bartlett, M. S., & Movellan, J. R. (2002). A comparison of Gabor filter methods for automatic detection of facial landmarks. *Proceedings of Fifth IEEE international conference on automatic face gesture recognition*, 1-5. 10.1109/AFGR.2002.1004161

Fogel, G. B. (2005). IEEE symposium on computational intelligence in bioinformatics and computational biology (IEEE CIBCB 2005). *IEEE Computational Intelligence Magazine*, *1*(2), 43–44. doi:10.1109/MCI.2006.1626495

Georghiades, A. S., Belhumeur, P. N., & Kriegman, D. J. (2000). From few to many: Generative models for recognition under variable pose and illumination. *Proceedings of Fourth IEEE international conference on automatic face and gesture recognition*, 1-8.

Geurts, P., Ernst, D., & Wehenkel, L. (2006). Extremely randomized trees. *Machine Learning*, *63*(1), 3–42. doi:10.100710994-006-6226-1

Geurts, P., Fillet, M., de Seny, D. D., Meuwis, M. A., Malaise, M., Merville, M. P., & Wehenkel, L. (2005). Proteomic mass spectra classification using decision tree based ensemble methods. *Bioinformatics (Oxford, England)*, *21*(14), 3138–3145. doi:10.1093/bioinformatics/bti494 PMID:15890743

Grudin, M. A. (2000). On internal representations in face recognition systems. *Pattern Recognition*, *33*(7), 1161–1177. doi:10.1016/S0031-3203(99)00104-1

Guo, G., Li, S. Z., & Chan, K. L. (2001). Support vector machines for face recognition. *Image and Vision Computing*, *19*(9-10), 631–638. doi:10.1016/S0262-8856(01)00046-4

Heisele, B., Ho, P., Wu, J., & Poggio, T. (2003). Face recognition: Component-based versus global approaches. *Computer Vision and Image Understanding*, *91*(1-2), 6–21. doi:10.1016/S1077-3142(03)00073-0

Ho, T. K. (1995). Random Decision Forests. *Proceedings of the 3rd International Conference on Document Analysis and Recognition*, 278 282.

Ho, T. K. (2002). A Data Complexity Analysis of Comparative Advantages of Decision Forest Constructors. *Pattern Analysis & Applications*, *5*(2), 102–112. doi:10.1007100440200009

Howell, A. J., & Buxton, H. (1995). Invariance in radial basis function neural networks in human face classification. *Neural Processing Letters*, *2*(3), 26–30. doi:10.1007/BF02311576

Hussain, A., & Saini, H. K. (2018). A Novel Approach for Enhancing the Face Recognition Accuracy using SIFT with Multiple LDA-PCA Techniques. *International Journal for Research in Applied Science and Engineering Technology*, *6*(5), 2588–2594. doi:10.22214/ijraset.2018.5423

Kalocsai, P., Malsburg, C. V. D., & Horn, J. (2000). Face recognition by statistical analysis of feature detectors. *Image and Vision Computing*, *18*(4), 273–278. doi:10.1016/S0262-8856(99)00051-7

Kirby, M., & Sirovich, L. (1990). Application of the Karhunen-Loeve procedure for the characterization of human faces. *IEEE Transactions on Pattern Analysis and Machine Intelligence, 12,* 103-108.

Kouzani, A. Z., Nahavandi, S., & Koshmanesh, K. (2007). Face classification by a random forest. Proceeding TENCON 2007 - 2007 IEEE Region 10 Conference, 1–4. doi:10.1109/TENCON.2007.4428937

Kremic, E., & Subasi, A. (2016). Performance of random forest and SVM in face recognition. *International Arab Journal of Information Technology, 13,* 87-293.

Lades, M., Vorbruggen, J. C., Buhmann, J., Lange, J., Malsburg, C. V. D., Wurtz, R. P., & Konen, W. (1993). Distortion invariant object recognition in the dynamic link architecture. *IEEE Transactions on Computers*, *42*(3), 300–311. doi:10.1109/12.210173

Lanitis, A., Taylor, C. J., & Cootes, T. F. (1997). Automatic interpretation and coding of face images using flexible models. *IEEE Transactions on Pattern Analysis and Machine Intelligence*, *19*(7), 743–756. doi:10.1109/34.598231

Lee, T. S. (1996). Image representation using 2D Gabor wavelets. *IEEE Transactions on Pattern Analysis and Machine Intelligence*, *18*(10), 959–971. doi:10.1109/34.541406

Liu, C. (2004). Gabor-based kernel pca with fractional power polynomial models for face recognition. *IEEE Transactions on Pattern Analysis and Machine Intelligence*, *26*(5), 572–581. doi:10.1109/TPAMI.2004.1273927 PMID:15460279

Liu, K., & Kehtarnavaz, N. (2013). Real-time robust vision-based hand gesture recognition using stereo images. *Journal of Real-Time Image Processing*, *11*(1), 201–209. doi:10.100711554-013-0333-6

Mahmoudi, F., Shanbehzadeh, J., Moghadam, A. M. E., & Zadeh, S. H. (2003). Image retrieval based on shape similarity by edge orientation autocorrelogram. *Pattern Recognition*, *36*(8), 1725–1736. doi:10.1016/S0031-3203(03)00010-4

Matas, J., Jonsson, K., & Kittler, J. (1999). Fast face localisation and verification. *Image and Vision Computing*, *17*(8), 575–581. doi:10.1016/S0262-8856(98)00176-0

Moore, D. (1987). Classification and regression trees. *Cytometry*, *8*(5), 534–535. doi:10.1002/cyto.990080516

Naseem, I., Togneri, R., & Bennamoun, M. (2010). Linear Regression for Face Recognition. *IEEE Transactions on Pattern Analysis and Machine Intelligence*, *32*(11), 2106–2112. doi:10.1109/TPAMI.2010.128 PMID:20603520

Nefian, A. V., & Hayes, M. H. (1998). Hidden Markow models for face recognition. *Proceedings of the 1998 IEEE International Conference on Acoustics, Speech and Signal Processing*, 2721-2724.

Paul, L. C., & Sumam, A. A. (2012). Face Recognition Using Principal Component Analysis Method. *International Journal of Advanced Research in Computer Engineering and Technology*, *1*, 135–139.

Perkins, D. (1975). A Definition of Caricature and Caricature and Recognition. *Studies In Visual Communications*, *2*(1), 1–24. doi:10.1525/var.1975.2.1.1

Phillips, P. J., Wechsler, H., Huang, J., & Rauss, P. (1998). The FERET database and evaluation procedure for face-recognition algorithms. *Image and Vision Computing*, *16*(5), 295–306. doi:10.1016/S0262-8856(97)00070-X

Salhi, A. l., Kardouchi, M., & Belacel, N. (2012). Fast and efficient face recognition system using random forest and histograms of oriented gradients. *Proceedings of the International Conference of Biometrics Special Interest (BIOSIG) Group*, 1-12.

Sato, W., Fujimura, T., Kochiyama, T., & Suzuki, N. (2013). Relationships among facial mimicry, emotional experience, and emotion recognition. *PLoS One*, *8*(3), 1–8. doi:10.1371/journal.pone.0057889 PMID:23536774

Sim, R., Mori, G., & Rekleitis, Y. (2009). Second and Third Canadian Conferences on Computer and Robot Vision. *Image and Vision Computing*, *27*(1-2), 1–2. doi:10.1016/j.imavis.2008.09.002

Sodhi, K. S., & Lal, M. (2013). Comparative Analysis of PCA-based Face Recognition System using different Distance Classifiers. *International Journal of Application or Innovation in Engineering & Management.*, *2*, 341–348.

Sujay, S. N., Reddy, H. S. M., & Ravi, J. (2017). Face recognition using extended LBP features and multilayer SVM classifier. Proceedings International Conference on Electrical, Electronics, Communication, Computer, and Optimization Techniques, 713-716.

Wiskott, L. (1999). The role of topographical constraints in face recognition. *Pattern Recognition Letters*, *20*(1), 89–96. doi:10.1016/S0167-8655(98)00122-6

Wiskott, L., Fellous, J. M., Krüger, N., & Malsburg, C. V. D. (1997). Face recognition by elastic bunch graph matching. *Proceedings of International Conference on Image Processing held at Santa Barbara during*, 129-132. 10.1109/ICIP.1997.647401

Xu, Q., & Deng, W. (2008). Adaptively weighted 2DPCA based on local feature for face recognition. *Fourth International Conference on Natural Computation*, 76-79.

Yaman, M. A., Subasi, A., & Rattay, F. (2018). Comparison of Random Subspace and Voting Ensemble Machine Learning Methods for Face Recognition. *Symmetry*, *10*(11), 1–19. doi:10.3390ym10110651

Zahoor, E., Munir, K., Perrin, O., & Godart, C. (2013). An event-based approach for declarative, integrated and self-healing web service composition. *International Journal of Services Computing, 1,* 13-24.

Zhang, T., Yang, J., Zhao, D., & Ge, X. (2007). Linear local tangent space alignment and application to face recognition. *Neurocomputing*, *70*(7-9), 1547–1553. doi:10.1016/j.neucom.2006.11.007

Zhou, S. K., Chellappa, R., & Zhao, W. (2006). Unconstrained face recognition. *Neurocomputing*, *45*, 478–493.

Chapter 20

A Social Ecological Model (SEM) to Manage Methadone Programmes in Prisons

Rita Komalasari

https://orcid.org/0000-0001-9963-2363

Yarsi University, Indonesia

ABSTRACT

This chapter presents findings for managing methadone programs in prisons. For the first time, the findings presented in this chapter contribute to socio-cultural and ecological approaches to solving problems, as well as providing policy alternatives for managing methadone programs in prisons. The social ecological model (SEM) is used in this research to examine the interaction of public policy, community, institutional, interpersonal, and intrapersonal elements. The findings presented in this chapter will have an impact on efforts to improve organizational, interpersonal, and intrapersonal factors.

INTRODUCTION

OAT treatment has been connected to decreased drug use, injecting drug use, and sharing of injecting equipment among those receiving treatment, as well as enhanced antiretroviral therapy adherence (ART) (Altice et al, 2016). As a result, the OAT program in prisons serves a critical role in reducing dangerous injecting practices, which helps in order to decrease the spread of HIV and the hepatitis C virus (Asher 2013). Despite its effectiveness, however, the jail OAT program's availability and coverage remain limited. Only 80 nations with reported injecting drug users had established OAT programs in 2016. The use of OAT in prisons is considerably less common. In 2008, just 29 countries offered such a program.

The Social-Ecological Model (SEM) is used in this research to examine the interaction of public policy, community, institutional, interpersonal, and intrapersonal elements (Ritchie et al, 2014). Research on HIV risk behavior among injecting drug users has previously used this model because it emphasizes the necessity of understanding intrapersonal, interpersonal, and social structure aspects. Using this ap-

DOI: 10.4018/978-1-6684-4580-8.ch020

proach, it is possible to explore the numerous aspects that contribute to complex circumstances and to suggest possible strategies for improvement in these contexts (Azbel 2016). The SEM model is used in this study to combine multilevel analysis as well as assess what kinds of interventions may be put in place in prisons to make it easier for OAT programs to be implemented.

METHODS

Participants in each jail were selected through random samples with the support of the facility's main security and health staff members. In order to reduce participant selection bias, snowball sampling was also used. From December 2015 and March 2016, the data for this research was acquired via in-depth face-to-face interviews. Both methadone and non-methadone inmates, as well as the prison's governor and a variety of security and medical professionals, were interviewed.

During the interviews, participants were able to relax in a private room or somewhere they felt at ease. All interviews were conducted in Bahasa, the primary language. In order to make comparisons between prisons and sub-groups, the study's overarching premise led to the creation of four subject guides. The guide was translated from Bahasa to English and then from English back to Indonesian by the researcher (and the guide's primary author). Except for one interview with a detainee and one with a staff member, all interviews were recorded digitally. In this scenario, handwritten notes are used. The interviews lasted anywhere from 30 minutes to almost an hour. More than 50 people were interviewed, including three prison governors, nine security staff, 10 health workers (including psychologists, nurses, and doctors), 19 non-methadone detainees, and 16 methadone inmates. At the Methadone Narcotics Prison, there are 17 inmates; there are 12 inmates at the Methadone General Prison, and six inmates at the Non-Methadone General Prison.

Anonymous transcriptions and translations of interview tapes into English were performed. Nvivo 11 was used to code and analyze the transcripts. Although additional themes were analyzed, this study relied on a framework analysis because it was more transparent. Identifying core concerns, concepts, and themes establishes an initial thematic framework. The process of analysis starts with the creation of a narrative description of how the program functions across the system and aims to discover similarities and variations in both individual cases and prisons. As a further step, you'll look for additional explanations by mapping the relationship between searching and categories throughout the complete set of data for other explanations. As a result of the social ecology model, it was possible to categorize the obstacles and enablers to the OAT program's implementation in prisons.

The University of Stirling's Campus Research Ethics Committee gave its blessing to this investigation. The Indonesian Ministry of Law and Human Rights does not have a process for approving research ethics. A letter of reference from the Ministry of Home Affairs must first be obtained and given to each jail that is being considered for investigation in order to gain access to services. Every single one of the study prison's three governors signed the authorization letter.

Prior to the interview, each participant provided written and verbal agreement for study participation. Nothing is offered in return for participation. The study's participants' and inmates' privacy are top priorities. As a result, no personal information about the inmate or the institution is released to the public or anybody else, not even the inmates themselves.

RESULTS

Prisoners' Opinions on the OAT Program's Advantages

The OAT program was well-received by both prison personnel and inmates at all three facilities. A drop in the number of convicts who inject heroin on a regular basis, as well as better management of prisoners, are some of the benefits of this approach. Prisoners no longer need heroin because we provide them with methadone. According to my understanding, heroin users are less likely to contract HIV due to the usage of unsterilized needles and syringes, which reduces the risk of HIV transmission. "(Lapas Methadone Narcotics, Prison officials were late in their response.)

People in their twenties have a hard time relating to other people because of their dependence on drugs. They are less uptight because they are taking methadone. "(Methadone Narcotics Prison, Prison officer, mid-20s)

It is believed that the OAT program, which is supported by both methadone and non-methadone convicts, may boost the health of methadone inmates by lowering the use of injection devices and increasing their overall well-being in terms of their physical, social, financial, and emotional health. They used to exchange needles that transmitted HIV. Before, I was apprehensive about stepping on needles. I was surprised to see no syringes in this place. The fact that they're HIV-positive doesn't bother me, and I feel more at ease and secure with them. " [Mid-30s Non-Methadone Inmates in a Narcotics Treatment Facility].

According to a methadone prison prisoner, "I've discovered that methadone has positive consequences for my life—physically and mentally—so there is no reason why I should reject methadone" (Methadone General Prison, Methadone Prisoners, late 30s).

"I used to be hated by my family, but now we're incredibly tight as a unit." Mid-30s Methadone Narcotics Prison inmates: "We can develop stronger family relationships.

Execution of the Government

As a rule, clinics in general methadone prisons are open from 8:45 am to 9:15 am and close 30 minutes later. On most days, the clinic at the Methadone Narcotics Prison opens at 10:00 WIB. Before administering methadone, the staff urges all methadone patients to meet together. Anxieties over early start times are common among metabolites at the General Methadone Prison:

"The clinic was closed because my pal overslept and couldn't receive methadone." Non-Methadone inmates in their mid-20s at the General Methadone Prison

For people with specific health needs, such as those infected with HIV or TB, the early start time of 8.30 or 9.00 am has caused worry in the Methadone Narcotics Prison. When I wake up, I'm unwell because I'm taking ART. " In the early 30s, (Methadone Narcotics Prison).

Inmates at both prisons with methadone programs are also concerned about weekend closing times. On weekends, the health professionals are sometimes late. A methadone detainee from the general methadone jail claimed that the methadone clinic opened at 11 a.m. instead of 9 a.m. (General Methadone Prison, Methadone Prisoners, mid-20s).

In most cases, medical professionals do not consider these characteristics to be an issue. Only one member of the general methadone prison's health care team admitted that these issues might have contributed to the program's low absorption.

Most of the methadone users [in this jail] are referred by the methadone program at the Detention Center; just a small number of them are inmates at the facility themselves. I don't know if it's the hours of operation or the attitude of the employees, other than that, "(General methadone prison, health staff, female, early 30s).

The clinic is a daily annoyance for both methadone inmates and those who have chosen not to participate in the program. A methadone general prison inmate complained of boredom and a desire to earn more money:

I'd had enough of the clinic visits every day and had to stand in line for long periods to acquire methadone because of everyone else. I'm a drug addict who keeps being arrested, and no one gives me any financial assistance. I have to put all of my efforts towards earning money (early 30s, methadone prisoners in general).

Even if the practice of delivering methadone is not controlled according to the requirements of those receiving it, methadone convicts say that being late for their sessions has repercussions. Among the punishments they face are chores that are unpleasant and nasty, as well as delays in their urine and methadone drug tests. Inmates from the Methadone General Prison stated that "if we arrived at 09.01 instead of 09.00, we were told to clean the toilet." In the early '30s, (Methadone General Prison, Methadone detainees), "as a kind of punishment, methadone is provided to convicts in the afternoon so that pre-dose methadone withdrawal symptoms are possible" (General Methadone Prison, Methadone Prisoners, mid-30s).

According to a fellow Methadone Narcotics Prison inmate, "I get it." As a result of our tardiness, my acquaintance was subjected to questioning and a possible urine test. I opted not to use methadone that day because I was terrified, "says a Methadone Narcotics Prison inmate in his early 30s" (Methadone Narcotics Prison, Methadone Prisoners, early 30s).

According to convicts, there are numerous impediments to methadone distribution in jails.

Resources are Limited

Staffing levels are low, and there is a shortage of education and health training, as well as psychological and basic support services for patients in Indonesian prisons, which have been blamed by many inmates for further harm to methadone programs in Indonesian jails. Problems with program delivery in understaffed settings, such as a lack of medical personnel dispensing methadone on weekends in both Methadone Prisons, are a common occurrence. Inmates at Methadone Narcotics Prisons are "fighting for simple things like getting the treatment they applied for," a Methadone Narcotics Prisons medical staff member said. Because I was the only woman at the clinic during the weekend, I closed the door and called the police (Methadone Narcotics Prison, Health Staff, female, early 30s).

As a non-methadone general jail officer put it, "At night, there is no medical personnel to treat the patients." Due to a lack of care, numerous inmates have perished in this facility. There is nothing we can do about it because we don't know how to deal with inmates who are trying to kick their drug habit "(General of non-methadone prisons, Prison Officers, early 30s).

In addition, there is a problem with methadone being diverted. It's common for inmates and prison personnel alike to complain about the absence of medical supervision staff: When he had finished taking his methadone, he walked into the clinic's bathroom to vomit it up. Because no one on the staff is watching us, you're free to pull stunts like this (Metropolitan Narcotics Correctional Facility (MNC), Methadone Inmates, about 1940).

One of the medical staff members described it this way: "Even though we have guidelines, such as "after detainees consume methadone, it's important to check in with them to see whether they've taken it in, but sometimes the staff forgets," officers are often bored and negligent, even though we have rules. (A doctor, female, at Methadone Narcotics Prison).

A Scarcity of Knowledge and Experience

As a result of this lack of training, prison officers at all three jails expressed their dissatisfaction. For more details, we spoke with a methadone narcotics officer who said "no TB or HIV education sessions were provided by the Ministry of Health. Only prison officials or other inmates were allowed to discuss HIV-related problems. " (Methadone Narcotics Prison, Lapas Officer, late 20s)

According to information gleaned from discussions with others, the Ministry of Health offers health-related training to some jail staff on a yearly or annual basis. Convicts may not be able or willing to attend the prison officer training courses that are held every month by the health care workers in all three prisons.

"That would be a problem if the health workers here were responsible for training in prisons." Because of our other responsibilities, we (the Lapas officers) may be reluctant to attend (Methadone General Prison, Prison Officer, late 20s).

For inmates who already knew they had HIV, the information about methadone was merely given as a supplement.

While I'm here, I attended two HIV education seminars. Methadone was briefly discussed as well, but I was left in the dark as to its intended use. A group of non-Methadone inmates in their early 30s (General Methadone Prison).

Services for Mental Health and Well-Being

There is little support for drug-abusing detainees, compared to HIV-positive inmates. As a healthcare worker in a general methamphetamine jail, I believe these issues are minor and that we [healthcare workers] are not the right people to help those in need:

Many methadone-inmates use illegal drugs to deal with personal problems, but this happens only a few times a year, and most of them (Methadone General Prison, Doctor, male) are afraid to talk about it with us.

When it comes to coping with past trauma, methadone inmates know they need these programs.

"I needed to talk about this subject since I had the horrible experience of witnessing the deaths of friends and family members as a result of methadone withdrawal" (Methadone General Prison, Methadone Prisoners, early 30s).

Inmates' Fundamental Needs are Not Being Met

Some methadone convicts may not be able to take a shower because of a scarcity of water in their quarters, a subject that has been brought up by many inmates in all three institutions. "I wish they would pay more attention to the quality of our cells," says one inmate from the Methadone Narcotics Prison. For example, there was hardly any space to move on our old bed. For example, there was no water in our toilets, so we had to fetch water from the faucet outside our cells every day. (Convicts in their late twenties are among the non-methadone offenders.)

DISCUSSION

It's the first time we've heard of anyone talking about how to make the prison methadone program work in Indonesian jails, and it's one of the few times this topic has been discussed at all. With the use of a socio-ecological model, it's easy to see what helps and hinders the delivery of services (SEM). Inmates, guards, medical personnel, and the prison governor all participated in the study.

According to our findings, prison employees and inmates alike have benefited from the methadone program in Indonesian jails. Another study found a decrease in drug-related risk behaviors and an increase in overall mental well-being (financial, social, and physical) among convicts when the program was implemented. This finding is in accordance with those others.

Most prison staff, including medical personnel at the three facilities under investigation, believed that the spread of HIV was no longer an issue in prisons, according to the findings of the current study. According to the findings of a recent study, because convicts use injection equipment more often in jails, HIV transmission is more probable. It's worth noting that this correlation has been seen in both high- and middle-income nations, like Indonesia, in jails.

Similar to previous studies(Baral 2013), prison officials and inmates in all three research prisons were found to have significant misconceptions about the implementation of the methadone program as part of an HIV harm reduction strategy. Certain health care workers and prison authorities in all three jails have the belief that methadone is merely a form of unlawful medication (Greer et al, 2016). Based on prior prison-related studies, prison workers and officials concluded that methadone programs were not fit for use in prisons (Grella et al, 2020). In contrast, past research has shown a link between less institutional resistance to prison-based methadone programs and a greater understanding of methadone programs (Izenberg et al, 2013).

Both Methadone prison inmates expressed a deep fear of methadone detox. In their opinion, it's significantly more harmful than heroin withdrawal, and it might be fatal. There is a significant barrier to participation in this program based on this belief. There are many public displays of death in Indonesian culture. It's no secret that many inmates find it upsetting that bodies are often left in jail clinic corridors due to a lack of funding. The trauma of seeing other prisoners' deaths and their families' anguish and comparing it to one's own mortality was a common theme among inmates in all three study prisons. Previous investigations have found similar results (Larney et al, 2017).

Greater treatment process adaptability is in line with work in "risk contexts," which can improve OAT program accessibility and engagement by inmates (Moradi et al, 2015). However, the Methadone Narcotics Prison illustrates the difficulty of obtaining the OAT program, with the restriction that offenders must first receive approval from their families. Many drug users' families may be unaware of their loved ones' drug use history. Many inmates who take drugs have personal hardships, and this rule shows a lack of respect for their circumstances. According to the research, limited clinic time was also found to be a factor in methadone switching and other high-risk behaviors. Non-attendance to the clinic means that other methadone prisoners or illicit substances may be used, which could lead to a methadone overdose.

Clinic opening hours and daily attendance requirements have been the subject of prior research, which this study confirms. This inflexibility might exacerbate mental health issues such as worry and insomnia. Especially when clinic and work schedules collide, this can be an issue. Prisoners who have little or no support from their families need to earn money through employment more than others. In other research, this conclusion hasn't been reported, but it's critical for understanding what happens to convicts in nations with low or middle incomes.

The development of programs and the improvement of prisoner participation and program effectiveness in Indonesia may be greatly assisted by family support and education. This can be done by educating family members about the OAT program and asking them to give their assent, monetary assistance, and assistance. While incarcerated, convicts preserve their drug-free status. For example, Participation may also be limited by the way the assessment is done, which asks about risky behavior and urine drug tests.

Any harm reduction plan must take into account all relevant institutional elements. Methadone diversion is also exacerbated by a lack of jail workers, most notably, individuals who are knowledgeable about drug abuse and addiction. Prisoners' anxiety over methadone withdrawal is exacerbated by a lack of medical personnel available after hours.

It is recommended that the OAT program include psychosocial assistance and instruction, particularly on how to deal with withdrawal symptoms. A number of studies have found that OAT participants are negatively impacted by a lack of psychosocial support. As a result of these negative consequences, people may be less motivated to modify their habits, have more difficulty cutting back or quitting drugs, and suffer from worsened physical and mental health. People who work in the healthcare field need special training to better understand the evidence for substitution therapy and how to treat drug addiction and mental health problems (Friedmann et al, 2012). There is a link between low satisfaction with OAT and not knowing about the methadone program in Vietnam, which is in the middle-income group.

Some studies have shown that the lack of health care in low-income prisons increases one's chances of contracting HIV, such as in Malaysia (Mukherjee et al, 2016). An increase in measures to establish a healthy environment for convicts and to safeguard their human rights has long been linked with the better administration of prison facilities.

CONCLUSION AND POLICY RECOMMENDATIONS

Compiling data on methadone program facilitators and barriers have never been done before using a social ecology approach. This approach emphasizes the significance of intrapersonal, organizational, and interpersonal aspects. In low- and middle-income nations, socio-structural elements, as our research reveals, are particularly crucial in the introduction and delivery of methadone programs. It's also worth noting that these factors are interrelated. Overall, there were more obstacles than advantages. They also need to be dealt with at the interpersonal, interpersonal, and organizational levels, as outlined by the SEM model.

There are three basic ways to improve: inmates' educational programs, as well as a thorough training program for all prison employees, including health care workers and top management. ii,) re-examination of methadone delivery procedures, for example, in order to better understand the role of harm reduction programs (acceptance, administration practices). Harm reduction strategies in correctional facilities will be reviewed, as well as the role of families and the role they play in promoting prisoner participation, such that harm reduction measures may be taught to all members of the family. Correctional procedures will be changed to support methadone programs, including the provision of psychological support for those who use them.

REFERENCES

Altice, F., Azbel, L., Stone, J., Brooks-Pollock, E., Smyrnov, P., & Dvoriak, S. (2016). In Eastern Europe and Central Asia, incarceration and a high-risk environment combine to perpetuate HIV, hepatitis C virus, and tuberculosis transmission. *Lancet*, *388*(10050), 1228–1248. doi:10.1016/S0140-6736(16)30856-X PMID:27427455

Asher, H. (2013). Methadone is prescribed in local prisons in England. *Drugs and Alcohol Today*, *13*(4), 234–243. doi:10.1108/DAT-04-2013-0018

Azbel, L., Wegman, M., Polonsky, M., Bachireddy, C., Meyer, J., Shumskaya, N., Kurmanalieva, A., Dvoryak, S., & Altice, F. L. (2018). Drug injection within the prison in Kyrgyzstan: Elevated HIV risk and implications for scaling up opioid agonist treatments. *International Journal of Prisoner Health*, *14*(3), 175–187. doi:10.1108/IJPH-03-2017-0016 PMID:30274558

Baral, S., Logie, C., Grosso, A., Wirtz, A., & Beyrer, C. (2013). Modified social-ecological model: A tool for guiding the assessment of HIV epidemic risks and risk contexts. *BMC Public Health*, *13*(1). Advance online publication. doi:10.1186/1471-2458-13-482

Friedmann, P., Hoskinson, R. Jr, Gordon, M., Schwartz, R., Kinlock, T., Knight, K., Flynn, P. M., Welsh, W. N., Stein, L. A. R., Sacks, S., O'Connell, D. J., Knudsen, H. K., Shafer, M. S., Hall, E., & Frisman, L. K.for the MAT Working Group of CJ-DAT. (2012). Medication-Assisted Treatment in Criminal Justice Agencies Affiliated with the Criminal Justice-Drug Abuse Treatment Studies (CJ-DATS): Availability, Barriers, and Intentions. *Substance Abuse*, *33*(1), 9–18. doi:10.1080/08897077.2011.611 460 PMID:22263709

Greer, A., Hu, S., Amlani, A., Morehart, S., Sampson, O., & Buxton, J. (2016). Patient perspectives on methadone formulation change in British Columbia, Canada: outcomes of a provincial survey. *Treatment, Prevention, and Policy in Substance Abuse*, *11*(1).

Grella, C., Ostile, E., Scott, C., Dennis, M., & Carnavale, J. (2020). A Scoping Review of Barriers and Facilitators to the Implementation of Medications for the Treatment of Opioid Use Disorder within the Criminal Justice System. *International Journal of Drug Policy*.

Izenberg, J., Bachireddy, C., Wickersham, J., Soule, M., Kiriazov, T., & Dvorak, S. (2014). Within-prison drug injection among HIV-infected Ukrainian prisoners: Prevalence and correlates of extremely high-risk behavior. *The International Journal on Drug Policy*, *25*(5), 845–852. doi:10.1016/j.drugpo.2014.02.010 PMID:24951025

Larney, S., Peacock, A., Leung, J., College, S., Hickman, M., & Vickerman, P. (2017). Global, regional, and country-level coverage of interventions to prevent and manage HIV and hepatitis C among people who inject drugs: A systematic review. *The Lancet. Global Health*, *5*(12), e1208–e1220. doi:10.1016/ S2214-109X(17)30373-X PMID:29074410

Moradi, G., Farnia, M., Shokoohi, M., Shahbazi, M., Moazen, B., & Rahmani, K. (2015). A qualitative study in Iran explored methadone maintenance treatment programs in prisons from the perspective of medical and non-medical prison staff. *International Journal of Health Policy and Management, 4*(9), 583–589. doi:10.15171/ijhpm.2015.60 PMID:26340487

Mukherjee, T., Wickersham, J., Desai, M., Pillai, V., Kamarulzaman, A., & Altice, F. (2016). Factors associated with interest in receiving prison-based methadone maintenance therapy in Malaysia. *Drug and Alcohol Dependence, 164*, 120–127. doi:10.1016/j.drugalcdep.2016.04.037 PMID:27207155

Ritchie, J., Lewis, J., Nicholls, C. M., & Ormston, R. (2014). *Qualitative research practises a guide for social science students and researchers.* Sage.

Chapter 21

Application Placement in Fog-Enabled Internet of Things (IoT) Healthcare System Using Body Sensor Networks

Hemant Kumar Apat

National Institute of Technology, Rourkela, India

Rashmiranjan Nayak

National Institute of Technology, Rourkela, India

Bibhudatta Sahoo

 https://orcid.org/0000-0001-8273-9850

National Institute of Technology, Rourkela, India

Sagarika Mohanty

National Institute of Technology, Rourkela, India

ABSTRACT

The advancement of internet technology along with the high adoption rate of various IoT devices with various emergent IoT applications has put stringent quality of service (QoS) and quality of experience (QoE) requirements on the service provider. The existing IoT-cloud model cannot effectively and efficiently cater to the QoS and QoE requirements of these IoT applications due to low bandwidth and high propagation delay between the IoT device layer to the cloud data center. In order to meet the stringent requirement of healthcare IoT applications, it is essential to adopt a new computing paradigm that could process these latency-sensitive IoT applications. The requests generated through various sensors yield mostly random and dynamic changes; hence, finding the optimal fog resources for the processing and execution is a challenge. In this chapter, the authors have formulated an optimization model for multiple healthcare IoT application placement problems in fog computing architecture.

DOI: 10.4018/978-1-6684-4580-8.ch021

INTRODUCTION

Over the last two years the people across the globe has been facing a nobel coronavirus disease (CO-VID-19) and pandemicity of this virus significantly disrupting various sector specifically healthcare services is mostly affected. Due to this covid-19 outbreak, many people suffering from different diseases like diabetics and cardiovascular patients staying in the home are regularly monitored through telephonic and video conferencing to break the covid-19 epidemic (Brogi, A.et al. 2017) (Gia, T. N. et al.2017). The shortage of nurses and beds leads to the development of various real-time health monitoring applications. The projected growth of wireless healthcare is expected to reach USD 337.55 billion by 2026. Similarly, in some other report released by Cisco, there are nearly 7.1 million patients are using connected medical devices, and the global wireless healthcare market is expected to reach USD110B by 2020. Healthcare IoT services put many stringent requirements to the service provider in terms resource utilization efficiency and bandwidth efficiency. The traditional computing paradigm solution is not able to satisfy the IoTusers' requirements (Deng, S. et al. 2020). To combat the various issues like undesired latency, Quality of Service(QoS) parameters like average response time, deadline satisfaction ratio, accuracy, etc. various extension of cloud computing is proposed like Mobile Cloud Computing, Edge Computing, Fog Computing, Mist Computing and Serverless computing to meet the demand of large scale IoT applications e.g. Smart healthcare, Smart City, Intelligent Transport System, Virtual Reality and Augmented Reality application (Chang, C. et al.2017) (Alam, M. F.et al. 2017).The Internet of Things (IoT) is a revolutionary communication technology capable of connecting different physical things tothe network through different long-range and short-range communication protocols. The rapid development of IoT devices supporting various smart city applications with various applications is increasing at a very rapid rate. A recent report by different organizations like International Data Corporation(IDC) and Gartner Inc. projected that the growth rate of various types of sensors will increase 50 million by 2025 and correspondingly, the devices will be increasing in the range of 50 billion to 1 trillion. Due to this ever-growing number of IoT devices, it makes possible to connect 7.1 million patients using medical sensor devices attached to the human body to sense the physiological data continuously. The above growth of wireless healthcare products tends to the development of various smart healthcare IoT applications through which a patient can be monitored remotely. Each sensor device attached into the body is uniquely identified by the UID, or MAC, or IP connected to the gateway (Barik, R. K.et al.2018) (Aydin, M. E. et al.2004). The large number of sensor devices manufactured by different vendors are used in healthcare that results into high volume of data. To analyze, pre-processing and storing these large volume and varieties of IoT data cloud computing has been used earlier on a large scale. The IoT-Cloud paradigm was the only solution for healthcare IoT devices (Bajeh, A. O. et al. 2011). The sensor devices continuously sense and forward environmental and physiological data to the cloud server for execution and analysis. The IoT-Cloud paradigm enables on-demand network and computational resources like server, storage, application, and services that an IoT user can use with minimal effort and pay per use basis in different form like IaaS, PaaS, and SaaS. Despite these wonderful benefits, the desired (QoS) requirement of various real-time IoT applications cannot meet by the cloud service provider. The delay that occurred due to centralized processing of IoT tasks may lead to a serious problem if a patient is waiting for some result. The other limitations of cloud computing are low bandwidth, energy consumption, etc.. In recent years, smart healthcare has become an emerging IoT application (Baker, S. B.et al. 2017).A smart healthcare system consisting of various wearable sensors, body area networks, etc.,is used by medical professionals to monitor the status of health in real-time. Most importantly, smart healthcare and body sensor network assist early detection of disease and their safety provision. To meet the desired QoS requirement of various real-time IoT applications such as Intelligent Healthcare, Intelligent traffic monitoring, Smart Home, and with many more real-time applications in a smart city, the pioneer of networking system CISCO proposed Fog computing model to support the ultra-low latency requirement of various mission-critical IoT applications with various other characteristics like mobility support and geographical location support.

Recently Open Fog Consortium proposed Open Fog Reference Architecture for the different communities, whether from a business or developer point of view, unlocked many questions. The scalability, security, and elasticity are still open challenges in current architecture (Eden Estopace et al.2019).

Fog computing paradigm is the extension of the existing cloud computing framework used to handle emergency cases using the fog gateway with a minimum delay. The basic idea behind Fog computing is to inherit the physical resources from the cloud data center to the fog nodes that empower service delivery on time with consistency and minimize the delay (Mahmud, R. et al.2018). Despite the numerous benefits of adopting the Fog paradigm, several questions are still unanswerable, such as what are the different parameters needs to consider for efficient resource management of Fog landscape, providing efficient service delivery to the end-users by considering privacy and security as the important factor, and under which technique optimal placement of IoT services/applications on Fog devices can be done (Tsai, W. T. et al.2010) (Tuli, S. et al.2020). Few existing studies suggested various methods such as service placement in fog computing, service discovery, resource scheduling,etc., attempt to address such questions, but could not address service discovery mechanism by various IoT applications, what types of services are initially required for initiating an IoT application so that some services could be provisioned in advance in order to minimize the latency of various latency-sensitivehealthcareIoT applications (Tong, L. et al.2016).

Now a days the smart healthcare applications come up with various latency-sensitive and accuracy-sensitive IoT data that need to be computed with minimum processing time. The patients attached with wearable sensor device sends the physiological data and other health rawdata like the temperature of the body, insulin level, glucose level, and heart bit rate in continuous form. The raw data is aggregated by different gateway like smart e-health gateway was implemented in. Fog computing offers various healthcare services like data processing, data analysis, and real-time analysis with temporary storage of the processed data. If any abnormal condition is happening, then detection and analysis of disease are performed by distributed Fog devices where a large number of doctors and specialists are involved in monitoring and prescribing the medicine (Mutlag, A. A. et al.2019) (Naranjo, P. G. V. et al.2019). Despite of these wonderful benefits of adopting Fog computing at the edge of the network,it's very critical to identify the type of IoT applications and their requirements. The generic Fog computing architecture need not be able to address these questions. The problem of mapping the healthcare IoT data to the available resources is one of the challenges when a certain quality of service is required. The IoT application placement problem has been studied by many authors has already been proved as an NP-complete problem. This implies that the IoT application placement problem has no unique solution,i.e., it has multiple solutions as well as multiple objective functions. For effective mapping of these IoT applications, a controller is required to take the decision of various IoT tasks generated by the Body Sensor Network to the available Fog device in a particular cluster. We have designed and listed the functionality of this controller as Fog Control Manager(FCM).QoS requirement of Various Healthcare Service is shown in below Table 1.

Table 1. QoS requirement of various healthcare service

Healthcare Service	Data rate	Delay	Packet loss
Audio	4-25 kbps	150-400 ms	3%
Video	32-384 kbps	150-400 ms	1%
Electrocardiogram (ECC)	1-20kbps	Max 1 sec	0
File Transfer	N/A	N/A	0

In this article, we have proposedthree-layer Fog computing architecture along with the functionality of each device presented in Section 2. In Section 5, we have discussed real-time healthcare IoT application Continuous Glucose Monitoring (CGM) as a use case. In Section 5.2 mathematical model of healthcare IoT application is presented along with a possible task model is presented in Sections 5.3 and 5.4.The available resource is presented as Fog resource model and Cloud resource model in sections5.5 and 5.6. In Section 6, the mathematical significance of the IoT application placement problem is discussed in terms of the cartesian product of two sets. The complexity analysis is done in Section 6.1, with a lemma and theorem discussed in Sections 6.2 and 6.3. In Section 7, we have discussed the solution methodology for IoT application placement problems; specifically, optimization problem taxonomy is depicted in Figure 10. We have presented taxonomy for various parameters that could be treated as the objective function is presented in section 7.2. Finally, a single optimization problem formulation is presented with response time as an objective function followed by a conclusion.

FOG COMPUTING ARCHITECTURE

Fog computing architecture is a highly distributed virtualized environment consisting of various networking devices like switches, routers, base stations, etc., to process the latency-sensitive IoTapplications. The conventional fog computing model concists of three layernamed as IoT device layer, Fog computing layer, and cloud computing layer.TheIoT device layer consists of various geographically distributed IoT devices(healthcare IoT devices) capable of sending incoming sensor data from the patients. These IoT devices have the capability to execute different healthcare applications like measuring the oxygen saturation through the oxymeter, measuring the pulse through pulse meter etc. Each application hasafinite number of tasks (Cisco. et al.2019) (DadashiGavaber, M. et al.2021) (Datta, S. K. et al. 2014). These tasks can be executed independently in different computing nodes to achieve the common goal. In the proposed architecture, these IoT devices are connected wireless through the Smart e-health Gatewayto the next layer called as Fog Computing Layer layer. Fog Computing consistsof Fog device in a Fog-Cluster (FC) where each cluster is managed by a control node termed as Fog Control Manager(FCM). Each FCM has a finite number of Fog devices supporting advanced networking concepts like Network Function Virtualization (NFV) to analyze incoming task requests. Also, these Fog devices support virtualization to create multiple copies of Virtual Machine(VM) to support heterogeneity tasks of an IoT application capable of executing multiple tasks. These Fog clusters are connected with a centralized cloud server through the Fog-Cloud gateway to support resource-intensive IoT applications (Mehran, N. et al.2019) (Mell, P. et al.2011) (Minh, Q. T. et al.2017). A single cloud data center with multiple clouds is considered in our architecture to process a large number of resource-intensive IoT applications. A detailed illustration is provided in the next section of each layer. The mathematical model of various resource configurations is presented in the mathematical model section. Below figure 1 shows Fog computing architecture.

Figure 1. Fog computing architecture

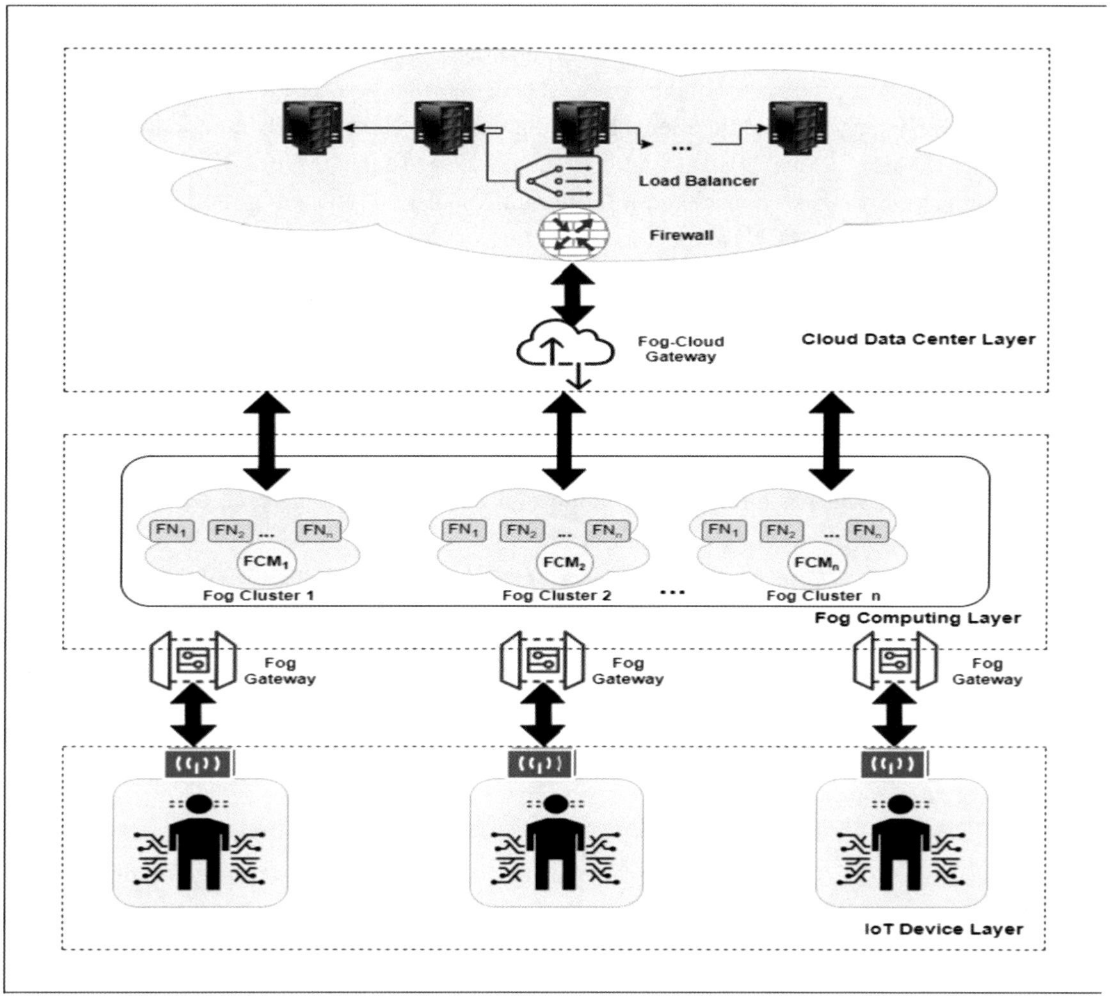

Body Sensor Network

A body sensor network is a network of body sensors connected through a centralized gateway responsible for data aggregation and analysis. The data generated through the sensor device are non-homogenous in nature. It consists of different type of medical devices such as wearbaleIoT is attached to the patients body for acquiring the data from the body or environment. The limited computational resources in these IoT devices offloads some sensor data to the centralized server for processing and execution. The devices used in this layer are accountable for sensing, transmitting, and sensory processing data to the upper layer.

Fog Computing Layer

The Fog computing layer is an intermediate layer between the body sensor network and cloud computing layer. The hetrogenous Fog devices are placed at the edge of the network, these devices includes gateways, switches, access points, base station and micro data centers. The fog node may be static at a fixed location or non-static, i.e., they can move from one location to another location like smartphones and smart vehicles, etc. The IoT devices can easily be connected with these Fog devices to take the different services. Fog devices are also resource-constrained. So, processing of the latency-sensitive IoT application improves the performance of the Fog device. In case of non-availability of sufficient resources to execute resource-intensiveIoTapplications, these fog devices process partly and offload to the cloud computing layer (Saurez, E. et al.2016) (Shukla, S. et al.2019) (Taneja, M. et al. 2017).

In our architecture, we have considered a finite number of Fog devices in the Fog layer. One will act as Fog Control Manager (FCN) among the finite Fog devices in a particular geographical location represented as Fog Cluster 1. Similarly, we can create multiple Custer to provide scalable features. Every FCM has its own local queue to store the task arrives. FCM of one cluster can easily communicate with another cluster.

Cloud Computing Layer

The cloud computing layer has a large finite number of heterogeneous physical servers or hosts with large resources capacity. A single cloud data center with multiple clouds consists of different high-performance computing servers, data storage servers, and other resources in our architecture. These servers can execute a very large task from different IoT applications. When the request received by the Fog layer does not sufficiently execute the task, then the request is forwarded to the cloud layer if there is no deadline requirement. However, some data analytics, data prepossessing, data cleansing activities can be performed in the Fog layer to relieve the heavy computation burden to the cloud data center.

Fog Control Manager (FCM)

Fog Control Manager (FCM) is designed as a controller node for one cluster very similar to Fog Orchestrator Node. The FCN is a centralized component responsible for planning, deploying execution plans, managing the resource, andIoT applications. Each FCM communicates with other devices in the cluster to know the current status of a resource in the system (i.e., free or occupied), the frequency of IoT application request in a particular instant of time, the characteristics of each IoT application, whether they belong to latency-sensitive or resource-intensive, etc. Our model assumes that FCM consists of the following modules: Data Management, Resource Management, QoS management, Device Management, and Security Management. The optimal location of FCM is assumed to be fixed where a large number of Fog devices could be connected easily, and the delay between the FCM and Fog devices is considered as negligible (Uchechukwu, A. et al.2014) (Velasquez, K. et al.2017) (White, G. et al. 2018). FCM is also responsible for scheduling the resource and resource provisioning for resource-intensive IoT applications. FCM receives the IoT data from the devices or sensors and forwards it to the cloud for future use.The functionality of Fog Control Manager is shown in below figure 2.

Figure 2. The functionality of fog control manager

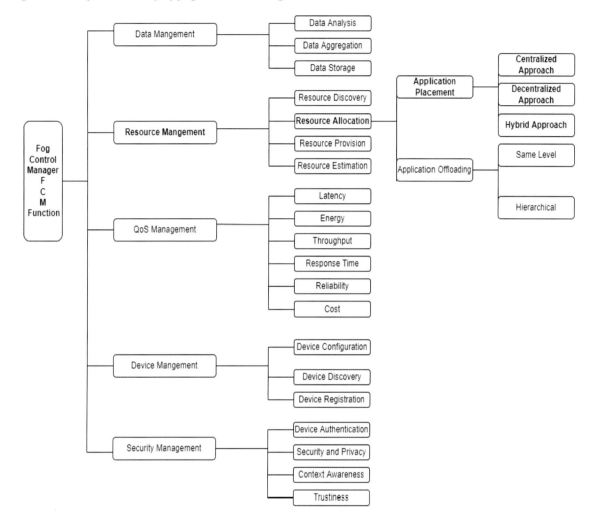

LITERATURE SURVEY

In this section, we have conducted a survey from different literature specifically for IoT healthcare with cloud and edge computing. The advantage and disadvantages of both paradigms have been analyzed critically. However,adopting the edge computing paradigm, specifically the Fog computing model in healthcare, has numerous benefits to support the ultra-low latency requirement of various healthcare IoT applications. Among different challenges in Fog computing, we have considered only Healthcare IoT application placement in Fog computing that primarily aims to map the latency-sensitive IoT application to the Fog layer for minimizing the latency and other parameters like resource utilization and energy consumption. We have surveyed various works proposed by numerous authors, more specificallyopti- mizing the QoS parameters basically used in a diverse range of IoT applications. We have considered the work related to resource allocation methodology in Fog computing and Edge computing paradigm. Our survey categorized the QoS parameters along with the application domain and the framework they used for evaluation in the table 2.

A Fog-Cloud architecture named as Health-Fog at the edge of the network is proposed to analyze various latency-sensitive IoT healthcare applications.Various performance metrics parameters accuracy, response time, network bandwidth, and energy consumption.are used to validate the proposed model.

In (Doukas, C. et al. 2012) authors proposed a heuristic approach to place the applications module on the available virtualized fog resource. A fuzzy rule is incorporated to classify the type of IoT application based on their characteristics. Cost and resource usage is considered as the performance metrics for evaluating the proposed scheme. The IoT application placement problem is formulated using Mixed Integer Linear Programming (MILP). The priority of an IoT application is predicted on the basis of IoT application request, deadline, and length of the task. The authors have not discussed other performance parameters like energy and response time of an IoT application.

A Multi Fog Placement (MFP) approach has been proposed for the placement of the application module. Distributed Data Flow(DDF) is considered for IoT applications (Benedetti, P.et al.2021). In DDF, an IoT application consists of modules, and module placement is the goal of the application placement problem. The proposed methodology is validated by considering two different use cases: Microbenchmark and EEG tractor game proposed. In this work, authors consider only dependent modules, i.e., DAG-based IoT applications, which is not applicable in the case of practical IoT applications,andthere may exist some independent modules. Independent module of an IoT application is lacking. The performance parameters considered in this work are latency and energy consumption. However, there are other parameters that need to validate.

In (Binh, H. T. T.et al. 2018)authors proposed resource aware placement policy for various IoT applications in fog computing architecture. A generic three layer fog computing architecture is used by the authors to validate the result. The IoTapplications module are represented through the Distributed Data Flow model. Each IoT application is modeled as a Directed Acyclic Graph(DAG) where the vertices represent the module and the edges represent the data dependencies between the two modules.

In (Dorigo, M. et al. 1996) authors proposed a distributed Deep Reinforcement Learning(DDRL) approach to place the tasks of IoT applications in fog/edge computing layer. A cost optimization model is formulated based on IoT devices' execution time and energy consumption. They have a model IoT application as Directed Acyclic Graph (DAG) to conduct the experiment. The authors have not discussed the independent task model of an IoT application. Further, (Imai, S. et al.2018) describe the optimal application placement for microservice-based applications. The objective function is considered as the cost depends on the computation and storage cost (Pham, D. et al.2012). Table 2 shows the difference in Literature for various IoT applications.

HEALTHCARE IOT APPLICATIONS

A Healthcare IoT application is a pre-built software as a service(SaaS) capable of extracting and analyzing the data from the body sensor network as described in section application program interface(API) by the user in order to get a meaningful and useful result. By executing the tasks associated with. For better understanding, the IoT healthcare application uses cases for continuous glucose monitoring inFigure3. Remote patients care is one of the IoT healthcare applications that facilitates different services remotely by using IoT devices. In most of the country, the residents live miles away from the hospital, and it takes an hour journey to reach the healthcare facilities. IoT promises to support remote patients care services at a low cost. The IoT applications used in these contexts extract the contextual data from the patient's

Table 2. Literature for various IoT applications

Reference	IoT application	Performance metrics	Advantage	Disadvantage	Evaluation Tools
Rahmaniet al. [2017][14]	Smart Healthcare	ECG Signal &Bio signals and Contextual data	Reducing the service latency for Notification	Only an ECG sensor has been implemented. Other sensors are not implemented.	Prototype
Mutgalet al. [2019][22]	IoT Healthcare	Computation offloading, Load balancing, Interoperability	Resource Management in fog layer is discussed &	IoT healthcare Application model has not been discussed	Review
Elmiseryet al. [2019][23]	IoT Healthcare	Privacy and Confidentiality	Trust of the gateway is calculated	Health care application is not categorized well	Python
Goudarziet al. [2020] [24]	Multiple IoT applications	Cost	Cost is considered as executing time	Only the DAG model is used	ifogsim
Denget al. [2020] [25]	Microservice based IoT Application	Cost	Both Computation and Storage cost is included as a cost metric	The proposed algorithm has not been validated for real-time IoT tasks.	Matlab2018b
Fan et al. [2018] [26]	IoT Application	Response Time	The modular approach is used to divide the problem into two parts first part is the assignment of tasks and the second part is allocation of workload to the cloudlets	QoS criteria of each applicationare different need to model the different applications not clearly understood the QoS	MATLAB 2018b

body and send the data to the mobile device (Elmisery, A. M. et al.2019) (Fan, Q. et al.2018) (Gaur, A. et al.2015). The device sends the application request to the nearest server for execution of the application. The healthcare professional analyzes the data and sends appropriate action in the form of the audio stream, video stream, or text data to the user through the actuator. Similarly,another application of IoT healthcare is Emergency care. In case of emergency, the health care service provider receives the sensor data and then sends the advice in the form of an audio stream or video stream to the end-user through the actuators. Similarly, other use cases of IoT application are Continuous Glucose Monitoring (CGM) used explicitly by diabetic patients remotely to monitor the glucose level of the patients in critical condition. A patienthas normally implanted a CGM sensor inside the skin to measure the blood sugar level. The transmitter in the sensor is responsible for sending the blood sugar data to the smartphone (Ness, M. M. et al.2021) (Perera, C. et al.2014). The CGM IoT applications continuously check the blood sugar count by executing other tasks depicted in Figure-3 for self-decision or doctors' decisions. Other related sensors are Brain Swelling Sensor that continuously monitors the pressure level of the brain in case of any injury to avoid the major complication of the brain. Smart Video Pills is a medical IoT application that allows the smart pill to move through the patient's body to take different pictures oftheintestinal tract and send the collected information to the smart wearable IoT devices, and finally, an IoT application is executed. Below figure 3 shows A sample of CGM IoT Application.

Figure 3. A sample of CGM IoT application

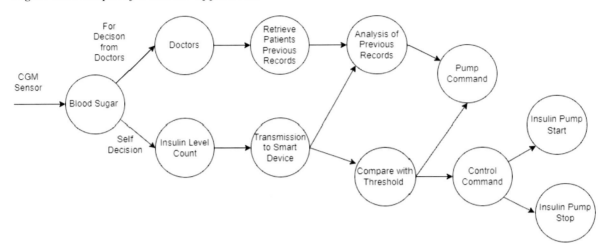

IoT Application Offloading

IoT Application offloading is a method of shifting the processing to execute the IoT application to other available resources in case of non-availability of resources in a particular resource. As the Fog devices also have resource-constrained, it is not advisable to execute all the tasks in a single fog device; hence, a decision is to be made where to execute some tasks so that objective remains satisfied. Application offloading is seemed a multi-criterion decision problem in which the controller node takesthedecision for partial execution. The resource may be computation, communication, or storage (Rahmani, A. M. et al. 2018) (Ray, P. P. et al.2019). When an IoT device sends a request to the edge layer for processing and execution, the edge layer executes some parts while other parts execute in the cloud layer.

IoT Service Deployment

The IoT service deployment means deploying the various services to the computing layer so that when an IoT application sends a request, it can execute and send the result through the actuator in minimum time. The services may be computation, infrastructure, or platform depending on the IoT application services are deployed over the computing paradigm to execute an IoT application. The situation may arise when multiple IoT applications demand an atomic service; in this case, which one is to execute is a challenging problem if all the tasks are high priority. Therefore, optimal service deployment is multi criterion decision problem edge computing for handling multiple IoT applications simultaneously (Tavousi, F. et al.2021).

Energy Consumption

IoT healthcare devices mostly have inbuilt-ed low energy battery to support for a long time. The life of an IoT device can be determined through the energy consumption usage of the device. Hence processing the IoT data by itself seeks maximum energy consumption. In order to save the power capcityofIoT devices, they offload compute-intensive tasks to the edge layer or cloud layer. However, some preprocessing tasks could be performed by the IoT device (Mordor-intelligence et al.2021). Various heterogeneous edge devices are available at the edge layer with varying power consumption rates. The energy consumption issue is a genuine issue for all client-server models. There is a critical need to quantify the power consumption of each edge device in a busy and idle state to minimize the energy consumption of edge layer,.

Availability

Availability is one of the major challenges in IoT as the request generated by the IoT devices are mostly un-schedule, and the demand for resources is highly heterogeneous. It requires different resources like computation, communication, and storage. The computing framework should have enough resources to get the result quickly (Mahmud, R. et al.2019).

Quality of Service(QoS)

QoS is a major issue, especially in the context of IoT applications. Most of the studies listed some conventional QoS parameters for IoT applications (Lo'ai, A. T. et al.2016). However, there must be some procedure to categorize the QoS parameters for various IoT applicationsscenarios (different traffic patterns, varied communication protocol), including time sensitive, I/O intensive, resource intensive, etc.

Privacy and Security

IoT is constantly growing due to the emergence of various forms of wireless technology RFID, WSN, and cloud services. The IoT devices connected through the gateway continuously send the sensor data to the gateway for analysis. The sensor data may include some private data related to health or financial data that needs to be encrypted to be safe. Different types of threats are possible in IoT related to hardware, network, and communication (Goudarzi, M. et al.2020).

SYSTEM MODEL

In this section, various IoT healthcare applications and resource models are modeled.

Body Area Sensor Network

Consider a finite set of medical sensor devices are attached in the patient's body represented $S= \{S_1, S_2, S_3, S_4, S_5, S_6\}$.

Each sensor is responsible for acquiring different data required to initiate a healthcare IoT application. A healthcare IoT applications may may take one sensor data or it can take all the sensor data. We also consider that each sensor device is responsible for sensing the environment or physiological data from the patients, the data received from the sensor attached is further analyzed by the set of tasks for executing number of applications. An application may required one sensor data or combination of all sensor data. The total possible number of combination is 26-1represenetd as the power set of the set represented by S. The possible combination of data is represented bythe power set denoted as $\{S_1\}$, $\{S_2\}$, $\{S_3\}$, $\{S_4\}$, $\{S_5\}$, $\{S_6\}$ … $\{S_1, S_2, S_3, S_4, S_5, S_6\}$.

Healthcare IoT Application Model

Consider a finite set of healthcare IoT applications are generated through the geo-distributed IoT devices represented as $A = \{A_1, A_2, A_3, ..., A_n\}$. A generic IoT application can be defined as a Finite State Machine(FSM) consisting of six-tuple represented as $A = \{\xi, \acute{O}, \psi, data, deadline, \phi\}$ where ξ represent the set of non-empty tasks represented as a $T_i = \bigcup_{j=1}^{j=k} t_i^j$ where i and j represent the application index and task index, respectively. $\acute{O}$ represents the set of all possible data generated through the sensor device, ψ is transition function defined by $\Psi: \xi \times \Sigma \rightarrow \xi \times \Sigma$ where $\Psi(t_i^j, data_j) = \Psi(t_i^{j+1}, data_{j+1})$ represent the output of the data item $data_u$ sing the task t_i^j producing a new data item $data_{j+1}$, *data* represent the sensor data, *deadline* represent the deadline of application if any is assigned by the application developer, and ϕ represent the period of occurrence of IoT application (Jin, J. et al.2014).

Periodic IoT Application- AnIoT application that occurs after a certain period is said to be as periodic IoT application. In this case, the value of ϕ is non zero number.

Aperiodic- If the occurrence of IoTapplications is random in nature, we say that the nature of occurrence is said to be Aperiodic. In this case, the value of ϕ is zero.

Deadline- A deadline-based application has some predefined deadline assigned by the application developer so that they need to be prioritized before execution starts. Less deadline application needs to be executed first,whereas average deadline or high deadline-based IoT applications need to be executed later. Further,thedeadline can be categorized into three parts High, Medium and Low deadline.

Task(or Services)- Each IoT application hasafinite number of tasks. The response time of an IoT application can be calculated by executing all the tasks. However, there may be some cases when there is a dependency between the two tasks, and there is no dependency in other cases. In this section, we have modeled two types of task models first one is Bag of Tasks (BoT) represented as a finite non-empty set, and the execution of one task does not affect the execution of another task. The second one is the Dependent task model represented through a Directed Acyclic Graph (DAG). The execution of one task initiates the execution of other tasks, or we can say that execution may be affected by ordering. Here, the execution of one task does not affect the execution of other tasks. The second type is the dependency task model, also referred to as DAG workflow or IoT application workflow. In DAG workflow, the tasks of an IoT application is represented in the form of Directed Acyclic Graph $G=(V,E)$ where V represent the set of tasks and E represent the set of edge representing the dependency between two tasks.

A. DependentTask model

An IoT application where the tasks are dependent is called as dependent task model. The dependent task model can be represented through a DAG called as IoT workflow. Consider an IoT application represented by a DAG Graph $G=(T,E)$ where T represents the set of tasks and E represents the communication link between the two tasks. Each task $T_i = \{t_i^1, t_i^2, t_i^3 ... t_i^k\}$ a where each t_i^k representskth task of ithapplication. Each task t_i^k has specific requirements such as t_i^{cpu} CPU(MIPS), memory(MB), size(MI) denoted by t_i^{cpu}, t_i^{memory}, t_i^{size} and E represent the link between the two tasks $E = \{e_{ij} : t_i^j, t_i^k \in E\}$. A Sample IoT workflow of 10 tasks is depicted in Figure-4.

Figure 4. Sample of DAG IoT workflow

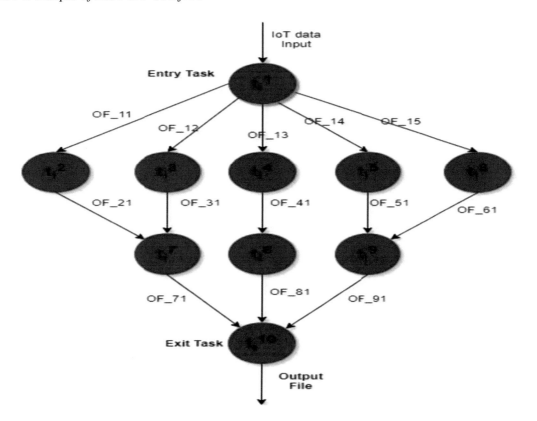

Figure 4 is represented as a DAG consisting of dependent tasks bounded by some precedence constraints, i.e., the execution of these tasks depends on the execution of other dependent tasks. The first node whose parent node is empty is called the entry node responsible for sensing the environment and sending the sensors data to the successor node. The last node or exit node is that node whose successor node is empty, i.e., the exit node has no further successor node. Here we have assumed that there is one entry task and one exit task (1:1); however, there may be other possible combinations of entry task and exit task represented as (1:M), (M:M), and (M:1), respectively. where (1:M) represents the one entry task and many exit task, (M:M) represent many entry tasks and many exit task, and (M:1) represent many entry tasks to one exit task represented in Figure-5.

Independent Task Model

In this case, the tasks of an IoT application are represented by a non-empty finite set. The execution of one task does not affect the execution of another task. The independent task model is also referred as the Bag of Task (BoT) model. Consider a set of healthcare IoT Applications generated by the body sensor network devices in any instance of time is represented $A = \{A_1, A_2, A_3, \ldots, A_n\}$ where each A_i where $i \in 1$ ton represent by a finite set of tasks represented as $A = T_i = t_i^1, t_i^2, t_i^3, t_i^1, \ldots, t_i^\alpha$ where each t_i^β where $\beta \in 1$ to α is an indivisible task execute independently.

Figure 5. Possible DAG model for different IoT applications

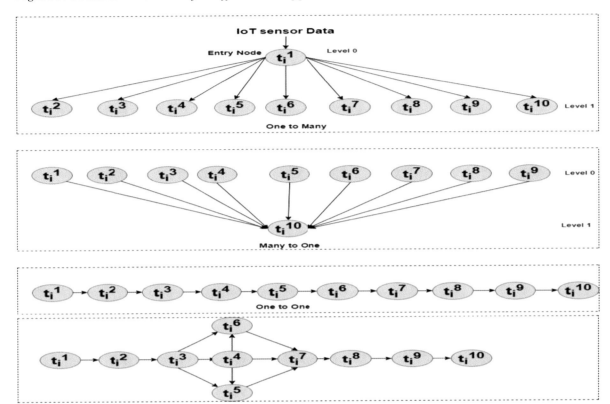

Figure 6. Independent task model of an IoT application

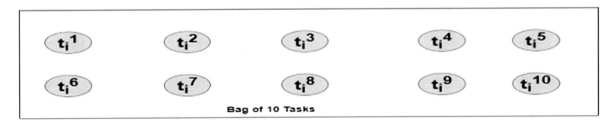

Fog Resource Model

Consider a set of heterogeneous fog devices $F = F_1, F_2, F_3, ..., F_k$ capable of executing the IoT tasks. Each F_i where $1 \leq i \leq k$ consists of various physical and virtual resources managed by the controller devices named as Fog Control Manager (FCM). The whole Fog layer is divided into the various cluster as per the IoT request rate, FCM can create a new instance of a fog device or delete a fog device. Two or more fog clusters can easily communicate using CoAP and MQTT protocol to send and receive data. A Fog device is defined as 5 tuple $[F_{id}, F_{Hardware}, F_{Software}, FCM_{id}, F_{device}]$ where F_{id} represent the Fog device identifier $F_{Hardware}$ represent the hardware capacity, i.e., RAM and ROM capacity. $F_{Software}$ represent the software available to run and execute IoT tasks (Gupta, H. et al.2017) (He, S. et al.2017).

Cloud Computing Resource Model

A cloud computing layer consists of cloud data center consists of various cloud servers represented by $C = C_1, C_2, C_3, \ldots, C_j$, where each cloud hosts C_p where $1 \leq p \leq j$ is capable to run and execute multiple IoT tasks whether they are latency sensitive or resource-intensive. Each of the cloud server can be modeled as 4 tuple represented by $[R_P^{CPU}, R_P^{RAM}, R_P^{STORAGE}]$ where R_P^{CPU} represent the CPU capacity measured in Million Instruction Per Cycle(MIPS), R_P^{RAM} represent the RAM capacity measured in Megabytes(MB) and $R_P^{STORAGE}$ represent the storage capacity measured in Gigabytes(GB). All the cloud servers are controlled by the Software Defined Control(SDN) enabled to switch to enable On/OFF dynamically based on the input task request.

IOT APPLICATION PLACEMENT PROBLEM

An IoT Application Placement problem aims to find the best computing device for the processing and execution of various dependent and independent tasks. Mathematically finding the best computing is node is equivalent to finding the set of range from a set of input domains such that some specific objective must be satisfied. We define a function $f_{placement}: A \rightarrow R$ where A is the set of IoT application A_i represented as $T_i = \bigcup_{j=1}^{\alpha} t_i^j$ consists of various dependent or independent tasks, R is the set of computing devices(resource) from both layer Fog and Cloud Computing. The total number of possible combinations is the power set of all possible subsets of resources i.e, if R^f and R^c denotes the fog and cloud resources, respectively, then finding the best map for a set of IoT applications is non-polynomial time complexity i.e. $2^{(R^f \cup R^c)}$. We need to check each of the possible solutions to find out the best map from this large solution space. However, finding the best map is not the solution in most cases for e.g., if the tasks of an IoT application mostly deal with latency-sensitive tasks like healthcare IoT data, then mapping the tasks to those computing devices which are capable of executing the tasks in minimum computation time is not only the objective so again we have to apply the brute force method to find the best computing node that satisfies the application constraints like accuracy and security. Similarly, other possible constraints like the deadline, bandwidth, uplink capacity, downlink capacity, etc., must be satisfied when an IoT device sends an application request. Sometimes, mapping the IoT tasks to cloud server might be an intelligent idea when we have a large set of heterogeneous IoT applications with computation-intensive or I/O intensive tasks. Hence, there are two possible places where an IoT application can get executed one is Fog layer, and the other is Cloud layer (Klas, G. I et al.2015). Figure 7 shows Sequence diagram of IoT application placement problem.

Complexity Analysis of IoT Application Placement Problem

Lemma-1

The time complexity for finding the number of functions between two non-empty finite sets *A* and *B* with cardinality m and n respectively is $O(n^m)$

Figure 7. Sequence diagram of IoT application placement problem

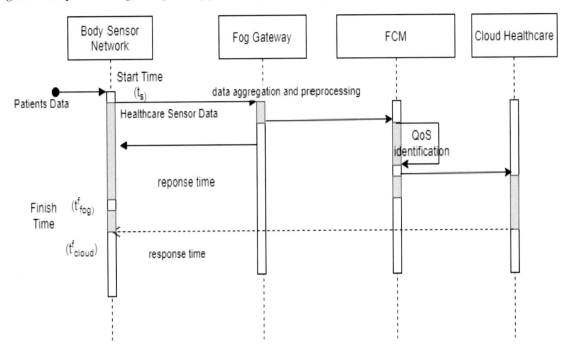

Proof:

To prove, we have given two non-empty finite sets A and B. A function $f: A \rightarrow B$ is the assignment of each element of set B to each element of set A. Moreover if x_1, x_2 are the elements of set A then $f(x_1)$ and $f(x_2)$ represent the elements in set B. We also assume that the cardinality of set A is more than the cardinality of set B. The possible mapping between the two sets and the total number of possible functions is depicted in Figure 8 and Figure 9, respectively.

Figure 8. Mapping of domain and range between two non-empty finite sets

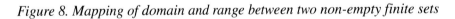

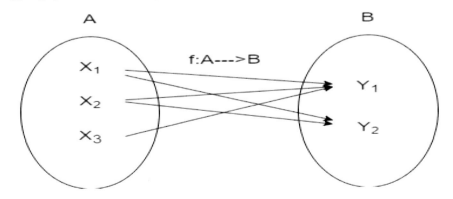

Figure 9. Possible Combination of a mapping problem

No of Function	X_1	X_2	X_3
f_1	Y_1	Y_1	Y_1
f_2	Y_2	Y_2	Y_2
f_3	Y_1	Y_1	Y_2
f_4	Y_1	Y_2	Y_1
f_5	Y_2	Y_1	Y_1
f_6	Y_1	Y_2	Y_2
f_7	Y_2	Y_1	Y_1
f_8	Y_2	Y_2	Y_1

From Figure 8 and Figure 9, we conclude that the total number of possible functions between the two non-empty finite sets consisting of 3 members in set A and 2 members in set A is 8, i.e., 2^3. In this case, we have assumed that the cardinality of set A is more than the cardinality of set B. Similarly, if we have the cardinality of set A is m and cardinality of set B is n, the possible number of functions from A to B is n^m. This proves our lemma.

Theorem-1: *IoT Application Placement Problem is a NP class problem*

Proof:

To proveIoT Application Placement problem is NP class, we have to assume the number of tasks as a finite set of an IoT application represented by the set $A = T_i = \bigcup_{j=1}^{\alpha} t_i^j$ where i and j denote the application and task indices, respectively. Similarly, the available computing resources where these tasks will be mapped for execution are represented by $= F \cup C$. A Function $\partial : A \to 2^{(F \cup C)}$ gives the total number of possible combinations,i.e., a non-polynomial time complexity.

SOLUTION APPROACH

Optimization

Optimization is the process of finding the best solution (global optima) among the set of possible solutions (local optima). The set of possible solutionsis referred as a feasible solution, whereas the best is called as an optimal solution. The quality of the solution depends on the problem formulation as well as the number of constraints; hence we can say that the best solution is relative to some other solution, i.e., there exists more than one solution to the optimization problem. To find the solution to an optimization problem, we need to compute the objective function, which needs to be optimized, and characterize the constraints of the problem. The objective function may be linear or nonlinear depending on the nature of the problem bounded by some linear or nonlinear constraints that must satisfy the objective function. The various categorization of the optimization problem is discussed in Figure 10.

Figure10. Taxonomy of optimization problem

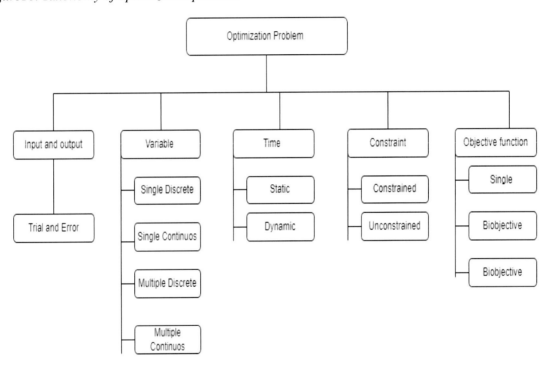

1. Trial and Error Optimization

In this case, the output depends on adjusting the input variable. Theoretically, trial and error methods lead to the optimal solution, but this seems to be unuseful in a practical situation.

2. Single vs. Multi-Dimensional Optimization

In this case, a single variable is used in the objective function, and the constraint is also in a single variable. Similarly, an optimization problem may consist of more than one variable, referred as a multi-dimensional optimization problem. As we move for a greater number of variables in the optimization model, the complexity of finding the solution increases.

3. Static vs. Dynamic Optimization

The output of the optimization problem may be dependent on time or independent of time. Suppose the output of an optimization problem produces the result is independent of time. In that case, the problem is said to be static optimization. However, if the output of an optimization problem depends on time, it is said to be a dynamic optimization problem. For example, finding the best path between the two cities where multiple roads are connected is a static optimization whereas finding the fastest route between the two cities in a road network is a dynamic optimization problem.

IoT Application Optimization Objective

The IoT Application Placement in the context of Fog computing is mapping the set of IoT tasks of an healthcare application to the available computing resources among the Fog and cloud. The Placement plan is executed periodically and performed by a specific computing node FCM. In order to execute the placement plan for a set of IoT tasks, FCM has to wait until the global queue is full. The global queue is maintained by the FCM dividing the placement authority into three sections. Centralized Placement deals with one central authority that performs placement schedules forIoT tasks. However,a centralized placement policy does not always give a better result in a distributed hierarchical Fog architecture. Hence, the Decentralized placement approach has been considered as the intelligent approach towards the placement plan for an IoT application. Similarly, in some contexts, both centralized and decentralized approaches are mixed up, know hybrid approaches are preferred. As the IoT application placement problem is an NP class problem,various QoS parameters need to be optimized. The most important part of the application placement problem is validating the algorithm proposed and estimating the time complexity and optimization of the various resource utilization factors like execution time, response time, and other delaysthatoccurred during the transmission like queuing latency, etc. The non-polynomial time complexity of the various algorithm used to find the optimal solution of application placement tends us to find the sub-optimal solution. In this, we have categorized various optimization categories in order to solve the problem. The optimization problem deals with finding the best solution from a set of feasible solutions. Further,theOptimization problem can be divided into two types exact and approximate. An exact optimization problem gives the optimal solution, while approximate optimization may give or may not give an optimal solution. The former method takes significant time to produce the optimal solution while the latter one gives a sub-optimal solution in a reasonable time. The approximate optimization is further divided into various categories. The first is heuristic method includes local search algorithm, Divide and Conquer, Branch and Bound, Dynamic Programing, Cut & Plane, etc. However,metaheuristics approach is used in the literature are nature-inspired or physic inspired methods includes, including Genetic Algorithm (GA), Simulated Annealing (SA), Particle Swarm Optimization (PSO), Ant Colony Optimization (ACO), Grey Wolf Optimization (GWO), and many more [47] [48] [49] [50]. In order to solve the optimization problem, we have to set an objective function. The IoT application Placement problem can be solved using different heuristic and meta-heuristic approaches, as depicted in Figure 11.

Figure 11. Taxonomy of IoT Application Placement Problem

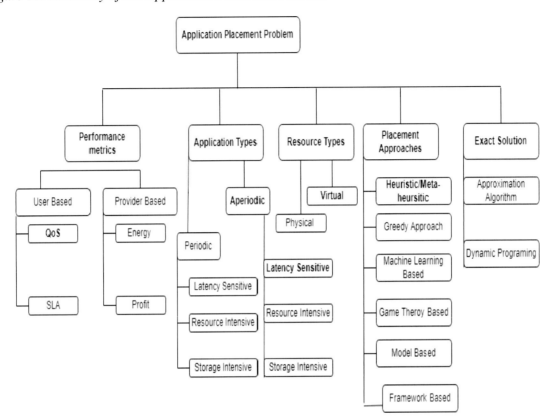

Healthcare IoT Application Placement Problem

Given a set of healthcare IoT application requests generated by heterogeneous Body sensor network devices represented as $A = \bigcup_{i=1}^{n} A_i$, where each application A_i consists of a finite set of independent tasks $T_i = \bigcup_{j=1}^{\alpha} t_i^j$ where i and j denote the application and task indices respectively associated with a fixed deadline λ_d, with a set of all computing devices in fog and cloud layer represented by R= {R_1, R_2, R_3, ..., R_m} where $R = F \cup Cand\,(n >> m)$. Our aim is to find an optimal mapping between the tasks and resources such that, application requests have a minimum response time.

subject to satisfy the following constraints

1. No Application should miss the deadline i.e $R_{A_k} \leq D_{A_k} \forall A_k$, $1 \leq k \leq n$
2. Number of tasks deployed in the fog layer is maximum.
3. Resource requirements must be less than the resource available.

let us consider three binary decision variables $x_{i,j}$ and $y_{i,k}$ and $z_{i,l}$

defined as given below

1. $x_{ij} = \begin{cases} 1, & \text{if task is placed in fog device} \\ 0, & \text{otherwise} \end{cases}$

2. $y_{ik} = \begin{cases} 1, & \text{if task is placed in neighbour fog device} \\ 0, & \text{otherwise} \end{cases}$

3. $z_{il} = \begin{cases} 1, & \text{if task is placed in cloud server} \\ 0, & \text{otherwise} \end{cases}$

Average Response Time

The average response time of an healthcare IoT application is the total elapsed time between the IoT application request by the wearable healthcare IoT devices from the Body Sensor Network to the time it receives the result. The response time can be calculated by adding the propagation time, processing time, and queuing delay. We assume that queuing latency is zero.

$$R_{A_i} = D_T + D_{Proc} + D_Q + D_{Prop}$$

Where R_{A_i} is the response time of a healthcare IoT application D_T is the delay that occurred during the transmission of IoT data from the body sensor network to the fog layer or cloud computing layer, D_{Proc} is the delay occur during the processing of IoT tasks, D_Q is the queuing delay occurred and D_{Prop} is the propagation latency occurred. The average response time of an IoT application can be calculated using the equation

1. $\dfrac{1}{n} \sum R_{A_i}$

2. $Minimize \left(\acute{O} \dfrac{1}{n} R_{A_i} \right)$

Subject to the constraints

1. $\displaystyle\sum_{j=1}^{F^c} x_{ij} + \sum_{k=1}^{F^n} y_{ik} + \sum_{l=1}^{C} z_{il} = 1, \forall i \in T_i$

2. $\displaystyle\sum_{i=1}^{n} x_{ij}.T_i^{Mem} \le F_j^{Mem}, \forall j \in F^c$

3. $\displaystyle\sum_{i=1}^{n} y_{ik}.T_i^{Mem} \le F_j^{Mem}, \forall j \in F^n$

4. $\displaystyle\sum_{i=1}^{n} z_{il}.T_i^{Mem} \le C_l^{Mem}, \forall l \in C$

Equation (vi) is the objective function, i.e., the aim of the problem is to minimize the average response time of a healthcare IoT application by executing all the independent tasks of an IoT application. The constraints of the optimization problem are represented as the Equation (vii), which means the task should be placed on either fog device or neighbor fog device, or cloud server. Equation (viii) represents the resource requirement of tasks must be less than the task available in fog device similarly, Equation (ix) and (x) represent the resource requirement of a task is less than the neighbor fog cluster and cloud server, respectively.

CONCLUSION

The main objective of this work is to present and evaluate the IoT application placement problem as an optimization problem that deals with various performance parameters as an objective function.From the literature survey, we concludedthattheIoT application placement problem is considered as one of the challenges when heterogeneity and dynamicity are imposed on the network side or clientside. In order to find an effective and efficient solution for IoT application placement, there is a need to figure out the objective function. The user's requirement some time varies from time to time in terms of more than one objective function criterion. In such cases, a multi-objective optimization model is required to find an effective solution. There is a critical need to analyze the tradeoff when both objectives are conflict in nature like minimizing the energy consumption and minimizing the cost, etc. For a better perspective of IoT application problems, we need to study other nature-inspired algorithms, Deep Learning based solutions, Game-theoretic models for solving multi-criterion decision problemsthat provide sub-optimal solutions in a reasonable time. In this article, we have assumed that the fog devices in the fog computing layer can run various applications by running the hypervisor to create different instances of the virtual machine. There is further scope of improving the virtualization model by incorporating Docker engine and Serverless computing model at the edge layer, i.e., in Fog computing layer.

REFERENCES

Alam, M. F., Katsikas, S., Beltramello, O., & Hadjiefthymiades, S. (2017). Augmented and virtual reality based monitoring and safety system: A prototype IoT platform. *Journal of Network and Computer Applications*, *89*, 109–119. doi:10.1016/j.jnca.2017.03.022

Aydin, M. E., & Fogarty, T. C. (2004). A distributed evolutionary simulated annealing algorithm for combinatorial optimisation problems. *Journal of Heuristics*, *10*(3), 269–292. doi:10.1023/B:HEUR.0000026896.44360.f9

Bajeh, A. O., & Abolarinwa, K. O. (2011). Optimization: A comparative study of genetic and tabu search algorithms. *International Journal of Computers and Applications*, *31*(5), 43–48.

Baker, S. B., Xiang, W., & Atkinson, I. (2017). Internet of things for smart healthcare: Technologies, challenges, and opportunities. *IEEE Access: Practical Innovations, Open Solutions*, *5*, 26521–26544. doi:10.1109/ACCESS.2017.2775180

Barik, R. K., Dubey, A. C., Tripathi, A., Pratik, T., Sasane, S., Lenka, R. K., Dubey, H., Mankodiya, K., & Kumar, V. (2018). Mist data: Leveraging mist computing for secure and scalable architecture for smart and connected health. *Procedia Computer Science*, *125*, 647–653. doi:10.1016/j.procs.2017.12.083

Benedetti, P., Femminella, M., Reali, G., & Steenhaut, K. (2021). Experimental analysis of the application of serverless computing to IoT platforms. *Sensors (Basel)*, *21*(3), 928. doi:10.339021030928 PMID:33573209

Binh, H. T. T., Anh, T. T., Son, D. B., Duc, P. A., & Nguyen, B. M. (2018, December). An evolutionary algorithm for solving task scheduling problem in cloud-fog computing environment. In *Proceedings of the ninth international symposium on information and communication technology* (pp. 397-404). 10.1145/3287921.3287984

Brogi, A., & Forti, S. (2017). QoS-aware deployment of IoT applications through the fog. *IEEE Internet of Things Journal*, *4*(5), 1185–1192. doi:10.1109/JIOT.2017.2701408

Chang, C., Srirama, S. N., & Buyya, R. (2017). Indie fog: An efficient fog-computing infrastructure for the internet of things. *Computer*, *50*(9), 92–98. doi:10.1109/MC.2017.3571049

Cisco. (2019). *Role of IoT healthcare. HIMSS Analytics Infrastructure Adoption Model (INFRAM) At-a-Glance*. cisco.com

Dadashi Gavaber, M., & Rajabzadeh, A. (2021). MFP: An approach to delay and energy-efficient module placement in IoT applications based on multi-fog. *Journal of Ambient Intelligence and Humanized Computing*, *12*(7), 7965–7981. doi:10.100712652-020-02525-7

Datta, S. K., Bonnet, C., & Nikaein, N. (2014, March). An IoT gateway centric architecture to provide novel M2M services. In *2014 IEEE World Forum on Internet of Things (WF-IoT)* (pp. 514-519). IEEE.

Deng, S., Xiang, Z., Taheri, J., Khoshkholghi, M. A., Yin, J., Zomaya, A. Y., & Dustdar, S. (2020). Optimal application deployment in resource constrained distributed edges. *IEEE Transactions on Mobile Computing*, *20*(5), 1907–1923. doi:10.1109/TMC.2020.2970698

Dorigo, M., Maniezzo, V., & Colorni, A. (1996). Ant system: Optimization by a colony of cooperating agents. *IEEE Transactions on Systems, Man, and Cybernetics. Part B, Cybernetics*, *26*(1), 29–41. doi:10.1109/3477.484436 PMID:18263004

Doukas, C., & Maglogiannis, I. (2012, July). Bringing IoT and cloud computing towards pervasive healthcare. In *2012 Sixth International Conference on Innovative Mobile and Internet Services in Ubiquitous Computing* (pp. 922-926). IEEE. 10.1109/IMIS.2012.26

Eden Estopace.(2019). *Growth of IoT devices IDC forecasts connected IoT devices to generate 79.4ZB of data in 2025 – FutureIoT*. Author.

Elmisery, A. M., Rho, S., & Aborizka, M. (2019). A new computing environment for collective privacy protection from constrained healthcare devices to IoT cloud services. *Cluster Computing*, *22*(1), 1611–1638. doi:10.100710586-017-1298-1

Fan, Q., & Ansari, N. (2018). Application aware workload allocation for edge computing-based IoT. *IEEE Internet of Things Journal*, *5*(3), 2146–2153. doi:10.1109/JIOT.2018.2826006

Gaur, A., Scotney, B., Parr, G., & McClean, S. (2015). Smart city architecture and its applications based on IoT. *Procedia Computer Science*, *52*, 1089–1094. doi:10.1016/j.procs.2015.05.122

Gia, T. N., Jiang, M., Sarker, V. K., Rahmani, A. M., Westerlund, T., Liljeberg, P., & Tenhunen, H. (2017, June). Low-cost fog-assisted healthcare IoT system with energy-efficient sensor nodes. In *2017 13th international wireless communications and mobile computing conference (IWCMC)* (pp. 1765-1770). IEEE.

Goudarzi, M., Wu, H., Palaniswami, M., & Buyya, R. (2020). An application placement technique for concurrent IoT applications in edge and fog computing environments. *IEEE Transactions on Mobile Computing, 20*(4), 1298–1311. doi:10.1109/TMC.2020.2967041

Gupta, H., VahidDastjerdi, A., Ghosh, S. K., & Buyya, R. (2017). iFogSim: A toolkit for modeling and simulation of resource management techniques in the Internet of Things, Edge and Fog computing environments. *Software: Practice and Experience, 47*(9), 1275-1296.

He, S., Cheng, B., Wang, H., Huang, Y., & Chen, J. (2017). Proactive personalized services through fog-cloud computing in large-scale IoT-based healthcare application. *China Communications, 14*(11), 1–16. doi:10.1109/CC.2017.8233646

Imai, S., Varela, C. A., & Patterson, S. (2018, December). A performance study of geo-distributed IoT data aggregation for fog computing. In *2018 IEEE/ACM International Conference on Utility and Cloud Computing Companion (UCC Companion)* (pp. 278-283). IEEE. 10.1109/UCC-Companion.2018.00068

Jin, J., Gubbi, J., Marusic, S., & Palaniswami, M. (2014). An information framework for creating a smart city through internet of things. *IEEE Internet of Things Journal, 1*(2), 112–121. doi:10.1109/JIOT.2013.2296516

Klas, G. I. (2015). Fog computing and mobile edge cloud gain momentum open fog consortium, etsimec and cloudlets. *Google Scholar, 1*(1), 1–13.

Lo'ai, A. T., Mehmood, R., Benkhlifa, E., & Song, H. (2016). Mobile cloud computing model and big data analysis for healthcare applications. *IEEE Access: Practical Innovations, Open Solutions, 4*, 6171–6180. doi:10.1109/ACCESS.2016.2613278

Mahmud, R., Ramamohanarao, K., & Buyya, R. (2018). Latency-aware application module management for fog computing environments. *ACM Transactions on Internet Technology, 19*(1), 1–21. doi:10.1145/3186592

Mahmud, R., Srirama, S. N., Ramamohanarao, K., & Buyya, R. (2019). Quality of Experience (QoE)-aware placement of applications in Fog computing environments. *Journal of Parallel and Distributed Computing, 132*, 190–203. doi:10.1016/j.jpdc.2018.03.004

Mehran, N., Kimovski, D., & Prodan, R. (2019, October). MAPO: a multi-objective model for IoT application placement in a fog environment. In *Proceedings of the 9th International Conference on the Internet of Things* (pp. 1-8). 10.1145/3365871.3365892

Mell, P., & Grance, T. (2011). *The NIST definition of cloud computing.* Academic Press.

Minh, Q. T., Nguyen, D. T., Van Le, A., Nguyen, H. D., & Truong, A. (2017, November). Toward service placement on fog computing landscape. In *2017 4th NAFOSTED conference on information and computer science* (pp. 291-296). IEEE. 10.1109/NAFOSTED.2017.8108080

Mordor-intelligence. (2021). *Impact of global covid 19 and smart healthcare Healthcare Facilities Management Market | Growth, Trends, COVID-19 Impact, and Forecasts (2022 - 27).* mordorintelligence.com

Mutlag, A. A., Abd Ghani, M. K., Arunkumar, N., Mohammed, M. A., & Mohd, O. (2019). Enabling technologies for fog computing in healthcare IoT systems. *Future Generation Computer Systems*, *90*, 62–78. doi:10.1016/j.future.2018.07.049

Naranjo, P. G. V., Pooranian, Z., Shojafar, M., Conti, M., & Buyya, R. (2019). FOCAN: A Fog-supported smart city network architecture for management of applications in the Internet of Everything environments. *Journal of Parallel and Distributed Computing*, *132*, 274–283. doi:10.1016/j.jpdc.2018.07.003

Ness, M. M., Saylor, J., Di Fusco, L. A., & Evans, K. (2021). Healthcare providers' challenges during the coronavirus disease (COVID-19) pandemic: A qualitative approach. *Nursing & Health Sciences*.

Perera, C., Jayaraman, P. P., Zaslavsky, A., Christen, P., & Georgakopoulos, D. (2014, January). Mosden: An internet of things middleware for resource constrained mobile devices. In *2014 47Th hawaii international conference on system sciences* (pp. 1053-1062). IEEE.

Pham, D., & Karaboga, D. (2012). *Intelligent optimisation techniques: genetic algorithms, tabu search, simulated annealing and neural networks*. Springer Science & Business Media.

Rahmani, A. M., Gia, T. N., Negash, B., Anzanpour, A., Azimi, I., Jiang, M., & Liljeberg, P. (2018). Exploiting smart e-Health gateways at the edge of healthcare Internet-of-Things: A fog computing approach. *Future Generation Computer Systems*, *78*, 641–658. doi:10.1016/j.future.2017.02.014

Ray, P. P., Dash, D., & De, D. (2019). Edge computing for Internet of Things: A survey, e-healthcare case study and future direction. *Journal of Network and Computer Applications*, *140*, 1–22. doi:10.1016/j.jnca.2019.05.005

Saurez, E., Hong, K., Lillethun, D., Ramachandran, U., & Ottenwälder, B. (2016, June). Incremental deployment and migration of geo-distributed situation awareness applications in the fog. In *Proceedings of the 10th ACM International Conference on Distributed and Event-based Systems* (pp. 258-269). 10.1145/2933267.2933317

Shukla, S., Hassan, M. F., Khan, M. K., Jung, L. T., & Awang, A. (2019). An analytical model to minimize the latency in healthcare internet-of-things in fog computing environment. *PLoS One*, *14*(11), e0224934. doi:10.1371/journal.pone.0224934 PMID:31721807

Taneja, M., & Davy, A. (2017, May). Resource aware placement of IoT application modules in Fog-Cloud Computing Paradigm. In *2017 IFIP/IEEE Symposium on Integrated Network and Service Management (IM)* (pp. 1222-1228). IEEE. 10.23919/INM.2017.7987464

Tavousi, F., Azizi, S., & Ghaderzadeh, A. (2021). A fuzzy approach for optimal placement of IoT applications in fog-cloud computing. *Cluster Computing*, 1–18.

Tong, L., Li, Y., & Gao, W. (2016, April). A hierarchical edge cloud architecture for mobile computing. In *IEEE INFOCOM 2016-The 35th Annual IEEE International Conference on Computer Communications* (pp. 1-9). IEEE. 10.1109/INFOCOM.2016.7524340

Tsai, W. T., Sun, X., & Balasooriya, J. (2010, April). Service-oriented cloud computing architecture. In *2010 seventh international conference on information technology: New generations* (pp. 684-689). IEEE. 10.1109/ITNG.2010.214

Tuli, S., Basumatary, N., Gill, S. S., Kahani, M., Arya, R. C., Wander, G. S., & Buyya, R. (2020). HealthFog: An ensemble deep learning based Smart Healthcare System for Automatic Diagnosis of Heart Diseases in integrated IoT and fog computing environments. *Future Generation Computer Systems, 104,* 187–200. doi:10.1016/j.future.2019.10.043

Uchechukwu, A., Li, K., &Shen, Y. (2014). Energy consumption in cloud computing data centers. *International Journal of Cloud Computing and Services Science (IJ-CLOSER), 3*(3), 31-48.

Velasquez, K., Abreu, D. P., Curado, M., & Monteiro, E. (2017). Service placement for latency reduction in the internet of things. *Annales des Télécommunications, 72*(1-2), 105–115. doi:10.100712243-016-0524-9

White, G., Cabrera, C., Palade, A., & Clarke, S. (2018, November). Augmented reality in IoT. In *International Conference on Service-Oriented Computing* (pp. 149-160). Springer.

Chapter 22
Scaling Up of Software Development With Algorithm–Based Agile Methodologies

Somesh Kumar Sahu

 https://orcid.org/0000-0003-2171-0338
LTI, India

Kiran Muloor
LTI, India

Shreeya Bajpai
CHRIST University (Deemed), India

ABSTRACT

The organization spends a significant part of its investment on operations and implementing projects. Project managers often face challenges regarding project management. Project managers face many challenges that get in the way of completing tasks, including poor communication. Setbacks and failures must be constantly analyzed and applied. Agile project management involves managing software development projects iteratively under continuous release cycles and incorporating customer feedback at each stage.

INTRODUCTION

Each year, technology occupies a larger and more prominent place in our lives and businesses. The software industry's many products and services are globalized, causing constant and rapid change. Software development, quality assurance, and testing require expert project management expertise as a highly specialized industry. The primary environmental variables for companies' success in market competitiveness through the implementation of projects are personnel, technology, resources, management, market, and projects(Olekh et al., 2013). Managing projects requires decision-making. With the help of data mining and machine learning techniques, better decisions can be made, and some project

DOI: 10.4018/978-1-6684-4580-8.ch022

problems can be resolved using selected or analyzed project data. Any organization relies heavily on data. Managers and executives can use analytics to correct any slippages in budgets, costs, and timelines. Analyzing data allows you to advance the skills of your team members and optimize your project management implementation. Every project gets delayed because tasks get delayed. Of course, that's an obvious point. However, when you consider the repercussions of a delayed charge, another team will have less time to complete their studies since the dependent job is late or necessary data has not been provided. Automating data consolidation, integration, and restructuring can simplify the budget formulation process. Project managers should analyze data contributing to operational planning decisions to drive budgets. But in many data science projects, data scientists cannot use developments from previous projects since they haven't tackled similar problems before.

Machine learning initiatives are more experimental than standard software engineering projects. As a result, data science teams struggle to predict the scope of work, time frames, and prices required to attain the required accuracy and results. The pandemic is an example of a worldwide tragedy that makes it impossible to sustain work and duties, but it has also given rise to the concept of distant and hybrid working cultures.(Mahfoodh et al., 2021). Agile is a project management approach that originated in the software sector and has lately been applied to other industries. This approach has encouraged the usage and development of several techniques to reduce project-related risks(Anes et al., 2020). When confronted with many fast-paced difficulties in an uncertain and dynamic environment, professionals are compelled to employ agile methodologies in various settings, resulting in hybrid project management models. (Bianchi et al., 2021). A hybrid method is more popular than elegant with IT teams, which combines waterfall and elegance, creating a more flexible yet structured process that can lend itself to IT projects.

After becoming dissatisfied with complex methodologies that would not scale, seventeen software engineers gathered in Snowbird, Utah, in February 2001 to examine lightweight alternatives to modify and deliver on-time feedback. Martin Fowler, Jim Highsmith, Jon Kern, Jeff Sutherland, Ken Schwaber, and Bob Martin were among others who spoke on fast-tracking development to get innovative software to market. In the meeting, they primarily discussed ways to simplify or come up with a lightweight concept that would be able to be converted based on project requirements, thereby helping us build software by having a quick understanding of what the client needs, which will have minimal impacts on the project documentation and needed planning. By achieving this goal, they recognized two critical opportunities in resolving the product-market fit and development graveyard by speeding up the delivery of benefits to users. Users' feedback on new software quickly helps confirm its usefulness and improve it accordingly.

Uncertainty has become a barrier in project management throughout the covid -19 phase. Agile project management is viewed as a solution to this problem since project management requires a more flexible and dynamic approach(al Maamzi& Tawfik, 2022). Agile methods and mindset have altered software development. It addresses some of the flaws of waterfall techniques' excessively linear system. The ultimate outputs of waterfall development and outcomes-driven analytics development are similar in that they are anticipated to meet well-defined goals. However, because analytics development is an exploratory process, precise requirements cannot be specified with certainty. The details of the end-state analytics models become apparent only when the findings satisfy the company's needs. They are affected by data analytics. Agile analytics aims to balance creating value from data, and it's time to get there. Three key factors are fueling the transition to agile software development.

In software development, human considerations are essential—the nature of complex systems and cost and risk considerations(Grady et al., 2017; Marnada et al., 2021). In addition, using Agile techniques alongside a waterfall method during a project is advised to boost efficiency. As a result of this growth, new hybrid practices mixing waterfall and Agile approaches have emerged(Baijens et al., 2020). In agile development, the technique and efficiency of decision-making are crucial, yet they are little understood. The decisions made during the four stages of the sprint cycle, Sprint Planning, Sprint Execution, Sprint Review, and Sprint Retrospective, are critical in making the sprint cycle successful. Decisions (Drury et al., 2011). As a result, determine what talents are necessary to accomplish the specific activities required to create and implement extensive data analytics systems.

Discrete works with data, such as data management, data processing systems, data analytics, and so on, and is frequently referred to as a data scientist. The talents necessary for these various duties, however, vary substantially. As data science becomes more popular and teams get more prominent, specialization within the group becomes more natural. Giving the phrase "data scientist" more definition and specificity would aid in the training and hiring individuals with the necessary abilities(Saltz& Grady, 2017). The transition from data analysis to data science, data science concepts, a big picture of the data science era, significant challenges and directions in data innovation, the nature of data analytics, new industrialization and service opportunities in the data economy, data education's profession and competency, and the future of data science(Cao, 2017).

While this meeting did not lead to the Agile methodology we know today, it was a crucial milestone in the history of Agile since speed to market, rapid feedback, and continuous improvement are hallmarks of the Agile methodology. Any organization can adopt Agile, but to lay the foundations for its adoption, it must understand why it is embracing it in the first place. After answering that question, organizations can determine how and when to embrace it. Creating new roles, such as Leadership, Sponsor, and Advisor, within your organization to use skills across functional areas will help transform your business. Over 71% of organizations already use some form of agile approach, making elegant design the go-to business operational model of the future. If you wish to remain competitive, you must now implement and develop these agile practices.

AGILE MANIFESTO

Companies focus on the wrong things and spend time and money on the bad stuff. It was essential to create a modern, inventive technique that could swiftly adjust to changing conditions and provide project teams some leeway to improve their performance and efficiency—the waterfall paradigm aided in meeting the technical requirements of software projects. The Agile Manifesto was created to meet this requirement as the pace of technology intensified. On the other hand, the Agile Manifesto is designed to be a set of ideas rather than standards for establishing norms and formal processes. The idea is for a person or people to declare what they are enthusiastic about publicly or to make known what they believe. Its specific values are given simply and without more explanation, allowing each project to build its own best practices based on these minimum principles. The four Agile manifesto ideals encourage high-quality software development. They accomplish this by developing software that satisfies the needs and aspirations of their clients. It tells us to prioritize people and connections compared to processes and equipment.

1. Four Agile Manifesto values are
   a. Individuals and Interactions over Processes and Tools
       Communication is an essential value of the Agile manifesto. There are several things a client may want to ask, and it is the team's responsibility to ensure that their queries and suggestions are promptly addressed.
   b. Working Software over Comprehensive Documentation
       Before Agile, project teams would spend more time documenting every component of the project, which would impact the project's ultimate delivery. According to Agile ideals, the project team's first and primary responsibility is to accomplish the final deliverable.
   c. Customer Collaboration over Contract Negotiation
       Traditional techniques only allow for client involvement before and after the project. This used to be a waste of both time and money. Customers must be involved throughout the process for agile principles to be followed. Team members can assure a satisfying result if the client is continuously informed throughout the development process.
   d. Responding to Change over Following a Plan
       As opposed to management methods of the past, Agile values do not have elaborate plans before the start of a project, and they do not stick to them no matter what. Situations change, and even customers can demand extra features in the end product that may change the course of the project. To meet these expectations manager and technical development team must adjust fast to provide a quality product and assure complete client satisfaction.

2. Agile Principles
   Agile principles clustered as Customer Satisfaction, Quality, Teamwork, and Project Management taken from part of the Agile Manifesto.It would be helpful if you remembered the twelve concepts that applying all of these principles isn't as simple as reciting them and that mastering them requires time and dedication to Agile.
   a. Customer Satisfaction: Agile methodologies strive to communicate and regularly adapt to changing customer needs, bringing value to the customer.
   b. Welcome Changes: By doing this, the team stays aware of any changes in requirements and can be more flexible with the design instead of preplanning and going through formal change control procedures each time the scope of work changes.
   c. Frequent delivery: The purpose of anticipated delivery is to generate something useable as soon as possible and as frequently as possible. Many techniques and frameworks are designed to function with short iterations. Delivering regular increments entails paying a useable increment in a short period that the consumer values.
   d. Collocated teams: Collocated teams are familiar with agile project management approaches. Meeting at least once throughout each iteration, if feasible, is the most successful technique for distant or virtual team members.
   e. Self-motivated Individuals: Teams are self-organized and self-managed, and their members attend because they want to. When a team is demotivated, it cannot develop effective working increments or focus on generating value.
   f. In-person contact: Agile project management is strongly reliant on communication. Face-to-face communication is an essential component of verbal communication. Every day people discuss their views and opinions whenever they get the opportunity. It is a typical kind of

informational communication. Communication and collocation at all organizational levels are critical to team dynamics.

g. Useable Software: It is vital to focus on generating a usable increment of software that works rather than spending too much time developing software that does not. Feedback, testing, and evaluations are undertaken regularly to determine what adjustments might be made.

h. Constant/Sustainable Pace: Maintain a 40-hour workweek and avoid overtime if possible.

i. Continuous Focus: Each team member is always looking for ways to enhance the quality, design, and overall project process.

j. Simplicity: Try to keep things as simple as possible. Don't include any extraneous features.

k. Self-Organization: The team decides what it can and cannot do and works together to find answers.

l. Consistent Reflection: The team is always looking back to go forward more successfully.

3. Agile Methodology

The Agile Alliance recognized that requirements and solutions needed to evolve via cooperation and self-organizing, cross-functional teams, allowing the evolution of company value and the development of a hybrid knowledge of the team's results. Even when the vision changes, everyone is aware of it.

Agile methodology reduces the risk of losing a significant amount of time if required changes. Teams can work directly with clients rather than coordinate with other groups. As a result, a defined result can achieve a clearly defined objective step by step. With agile software development, requirements and solutions evolve through team engagement, continuous planning, and continual learning. Flexibility focuses on reducing conventional barriers between employees and their goals to make your organization versatile and practical. Breakdown of work means that projects are required to divide into short cycles. Collaboration is vital where team members work closely together and are clear about their responsibilities. Enhancements iteratively where teamwork is done during a cycle are frequently reassessed to improve outcomes. Client collaboration is essential where clients are actively involved in the development process and can amend requirements or accept recommendations made by the team. Figure1 shows the Agile development Life cycle.

Figure 1. Agile development life cycle

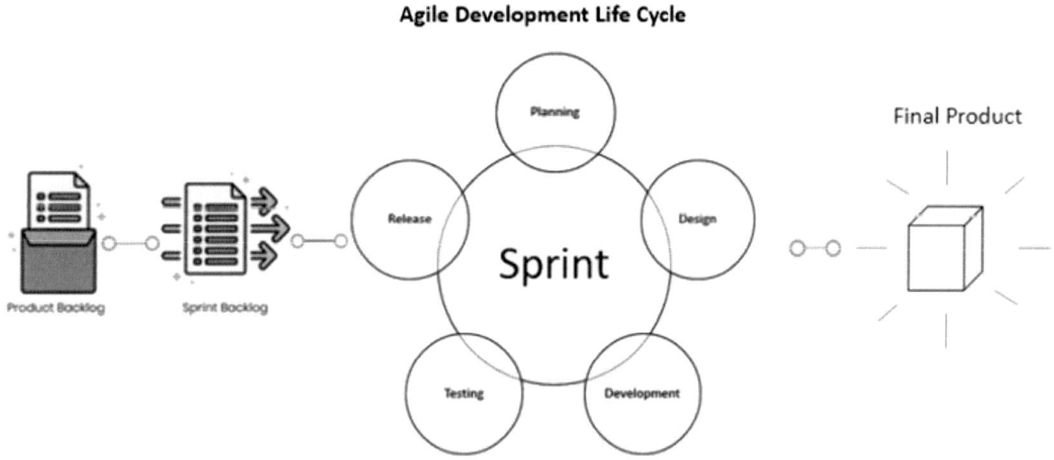

The agile development lifecycle is all about the development cycle constantly developing and evolving. In the agile development lifecycle, a large portion of work, Product Backlog, is divided into several small sprints or iterations as Sprint Backlog. The agile lifecycle is based on continual learning via these iterations in the form of Sprint. The developers deliver the client and other stakeholders with a functional product that includes all of the customer's features after the iteration as a Final Product. Each iteration in the Sprint usually lasts from one to four weeks and provides planning, design, development, testing, and release phases from the software development life cycle. Every project has a backlog and stages for design, development, testing, and deployment, all within a pre-defined scope of work. Each Sprint comes to a close with a possibly shippable product increment. As a result, new features are added to the product with each iteration, leading to a continuous project expansion. You repeat the process until all of the items in the product backlog are finished. In contrast to a linear method, there is a cyclical process. The sequence is seen on the Agile software development life cycle diagram.

Several iterations will occur during the Agile software development lifecycle, each with its unique methodology. Consumers and business stakeholders must be aware that they and business stakeholders share feedback throughout an iteration to verify that the features have developed. They need to share feedback throughout an iteration to confirm that the parts are designed to meet their requirements. Figure 2 shows the Agile project information flow.

Figure 2. Agile project information flow

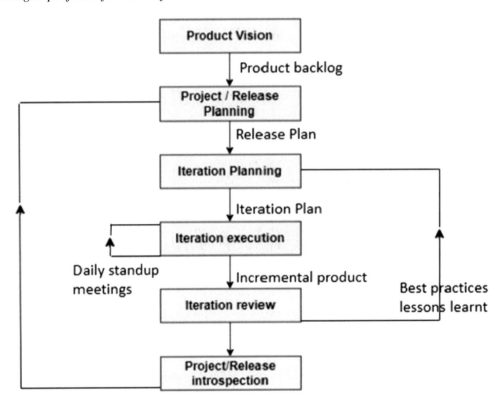

A streamlined life cycle for agile information flow flows between scrum events and a product vision, which facilitates securing commitments from all stakeholders involved in the product's creation by outlining the cost/time associated with each stage of the iteration cycle. The Product vision shares inputs in accumulating the product backlog, which helps in release planning where teams create release plans, scope-boxed, and time-boxed. It is followed by daily stand-ups, sprint planning, sprint reviews, and finally, a retrospective that concludes with lessons learned and practices to incorporate in the next iteration. Agile Software Development is a technique for creating more efficient software. The emphasis of this strategy is on people and results.

What Makes Agile Different?

When fixing time, budget, and quality, Agile teams maintain the integrity of their plans, maintain their means, and avoid the burnout, drama, and dysfunction that have traditionally characterized the industry. We continuously analyze, design, code, and test an Agile project, which is a continuous process. Feature building and delivery activities continue as long as there are features to build.

Figure 3 shows the Iterative **nature of agile in** development.

Figure 3. Iterative model

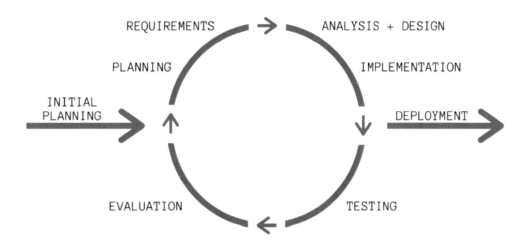

Iterative involves starting with something straightforward and building incrementally. By constantly refining and tweaking your product, you'll evolve the architecture, accept that your requirements may change, and optimize your product as you grow. Adaptive planning is essential. It is easier for agilest to alter their plans when reality disagrees with their projects is called adaptive planning. Changes to programs happen in many ways, but flexing the scope is preferred. Changing roles is typical. Parts tend to blur on Agile projects. Working in an Agile team is like working in a mini-start-up when done right. Regardless of position or title, everyone pitches to make the project successful.

People still have core competencies, and they generally stick to what they know better. The traditional roles of analyst, programmer, and tester do not exist on an agile project - at least not in the conventional sense. The project scope can be flexible.It solves the age-old dilemma of having too many tasks and not enough time to meet them. Agile teams stick to their goals, operate within their means, and avoid the fatigue, drama, and dysfunction that is so frequent in our sector by focusing on schedule, money, and quality while being flexible on the scope. The specifications are adaptable. Late in the game, it has a sizeable perceived cost.

On the other hand, Agile rejects this assumption, claiming that the change charge might be pretty cheap. Through current software engineering principles and transparent, honest planning, agility accommodates changes even late in the delivery process. The fundamental metric of success is functional software. Productivity is measured by how quickly their teams can transform their clients' requests into helpful software.The project plans, test plans, and analysis artifacts are all good, but Agilists recognize that they are useless to the client. The agile development approach incorporates the Scrum concept from rugby, employing a scrum framework to organize product development. A team works as a cohesive unit toward a single objective.

COMPARATIVE STUDY ON DIFFERENT TYPES OF SHORTEST-PATH ALGORITHMS

Shortest path algorithms are a set of problem-solving operations that aim to find an optimal path that connects the nodes in a network such that efforts and costs are minimized. The varied applications of shortest path algorithms in communication, transportation, and electronics, have made these algorithms an integral part of today's world.

Types of shortest path algorithms. There exist various algorithms to solve four categories of shortest path problems:

1. Single pair shortest path problem
2. Single source shortest path problem
3. Single destination shortest path problem
4. All pair's shortest path problem

The single pair shortest path problem deals with finding the optimal path between a given pair of nodes. The A* algorithm is the handiest solution for finding the fastestwayto this problem.

The single-source shortest path problem requires the user to compute the optimal path from a chosen 'source' node to other nodes. Dijkstra's and Bellman-Ford's algorithms are famous for solving this problem.

The single destination shortest path problem deals with finding the optimal path from all nodes in a graph to a chosen 'destination' node. Dijkstra's algorithm can be optimized and adapted to solve this problem efficiently.

All pair's shortest path problem requires the user to compute the optimal path between any two nodes from the set of all nodes in a network. Johnsons' and Floyd-Warshall algorithms are employed to solve this problem.

Routing

A primary real-life application of shortest-path algorithms in computer technology is routing. Routing is selecting an optimal path or route for the flow of information traffic in a network or across many networks. The principles of graph theory and shortest path algorithms are applied to construct a graph wherein each node represents a router, and each edge represents the communication link between two routers. The most straightforward path calculationminimizes one or more metrics (such as distance, time, bandwidth, traffic, cost, delay).

A* Algorithm

This algorithm is employed to solve the single pair shortest path problem. It has three parameters:

g – the cost of traversing from the initial node to the current node
h – the estimated cost of traveling from the current node to the destination node (also known as heuristic value)
f – the sum of g and h (f=g+h)

This algorithm starts from the initial node and selects the minor f-valued node till it reaches the final node.

Pseudocode

```
create array A[] that contains only the starting node
create empty array B[]
while (node != lastnode)
        node = choose node with lowest f value in A[]
        if (node == lastnode)
                return
        else
                place node in B[] and check its neighbors
                for-each neighbor of node
                        if (g of neighbor< g of node &&neighbor is in B[])
                                g of neighbor = new g value
                                neighbor's parent = node
                        else if (g of node < g of neighbor&&neighbor is in
A[])

                                g of neighbor = new g value
                                neighbor's parent = node
                        else if (neighbor does not belong to A[] or B[])
                                add neighbor to A[] and set g value
```

The time complexity depends on the heuristic. In the case of an unbounded search space, complexity is $O(b^d)$ where b is the branching factor.

DIJKSTRA'S ALGORITHM

This algorithm solves the single-source shortest path problem and the single destination most straightforward path problem. It has a greedy approach, and the shortest path it provides does not necessarily have to traverse every node in the network.

In Dijkstra's, we overestimate the distance of each node from the starting node. Then we visit each node and its neighboring nodes to find the shortest sub-path to those neighbors. We try to find the following local optimal solution to find the optimal global solution for the entire graph in the end.

Pseudocode

```
create array distance[] of size = no. of nodes
set distance[s] = 0
set distance[u] = ¥     //u is a node in graph G, except s
create array Q[]          //contains all nodes in G
create array S[]          //contains all visited nodes
while (Q[] is not empty)
       remove u from Q[]       //u is node having smallest distance[u] && u is
not in S[]
                                      //if it is the first run, distance[s] is
removed
       insert u in S[]
       for-each node v that is adjacent to u
               if (distance[u] = weight(u-v) < distance[v]) then
                       distance[v] = distance[u] + weight(u-v)
distance[] contains the optimal shortest paths
```

The worst-case time complexity is O(E log V)

BELLMAN-FORD ALGORITHM

This algorithm is used to solve single source shortest path problems. Its advantage over Dijkstra's algorithm is that it can detect negative cycles and provide an optimal solution despite them, although this algorithm is comparatively slower than Dijkstra's.

The rule of this algorithm is that we relax all edges (n-1) times, where n is the total number of nodes.

Pseudocode

```
create array distance[] of size n, n = no. of nodes
set all values of array as ¥
set distance[s] = 0
for i =0 to n
       if (distance[v] > (distance[u] + weight(u-v), then
```

```
                        distance[v] = distance[u] + weight(u-v)
distance[] contains the optimal shortest paths from s to every node v
```

The worst-case time complexity of this algorithm is O(V*E).

FLOYD-WARSHALL ALGORITHM

This algorithm is used to solve all-pairs shortest path problems in weighted graphs. It employs the concepts of dynamic programming to generate different matrices, the last of which contains the optimal paths from each node to every node. This algorithm is more effective for dense graphs.

Pseudocode

```
create matrix A of size n x n, n = no. of nodes
for i = 1 to n, do
        for j =1 to n, do
                for k =1  to n
                        Ai[j, k] = min(Ai-1[j, k], Ai-1[j, i] + Ai-1[i, k])
return matrix A, which contains all optimal shortest paths
```

The worst-case time complexity of this algorithm is O(n3).

JOHNSON'S ALGORITHM

We use Johnson's algorithm for graphs with directed edges and weights for those edges. It employs two shortest path algorithms – Dijkstra's and Bellman-Ford, as subroutines to calculate the paths. It uses the technique of reweighing edges (using the Bellman-Ford algorithm) of the original graph to eliminate any opposing edges and avoid negative cycles. Dijkstra's algorithm is applied to this reweighed graph to calculate the optimal shortest paths between all pairs. The output that is obtained appliesto the original chart as well.

Pseudocode

```
create function bellmanFord() to implement Bellman-Ford Algorithm
create function dijkstra() to implement Dijkstra's Algorithm
for qraph G, create G' such that
G'.V = G.V + {p}
G'.E = G.E + ((p, u) for u in G.V
weight(p,u) = 0 in G.V
if (bellmanFord(p) == false)
        return "Error! Negative cycle exists"
else
```

```
for v in G.V
        t(v) = distance(p, v)    //computed by bellmanFord
for edge(u, v) in G'.E
        w(u, v) = weight(u, v) + t(u) - t(v)
create matrix M with values initialized to ¥
for u in G.V
        dijkstra(G, w, u)        //to compute distance(u, v) for all v
        for-each v in G.V
                D(u, v) = distance(u, v) + t(v) - t(u)
return D
```

INDUSTRY-LEVEL APPLICATIONS OF DIJKSTRA'S ALGORITHMS

Dijkstra's Algorithm is a greedy algorithm used to solve shortest path problems. It provides an optimal path that minimizes metrics to build an efficient network.

Since its invention in 1956 by Dutch physicist Edsger Dijkstra, numerous industry-level applications have been found for Dijkstra's algorithm. Some of them are listed below:

1. Routing
    A significant application of the algorithm, network routing, is selecting the best path or route for traffic flow inside or across many networks. Dijkstra's algorithm is applied to decide how to ensure the data packets efficiently reach their destination nodes.

2. Mapping
    Dijkstra's algorithm is employed to find the shortest path between two points in a graph. Logistics departments of companies use this mapping technique to calculate the best route to transport goods from warehouses to destinations. Fire departments use it to calculate the most time-efficient path from a fire station to any burning building. Food-delivery companies use it to deliver food under tight deadlines while ensuring the driver's safety. It is also used by digital mapping services that use GPS to suggest the shortest road routes between cities.

3. Networks in civil planning
    It is imperative to find an optimal way of putting up telephone or internet cables in residential areas that use the most petite length of lines while connecting every house in a network to the central station. This is where Dijkstra's algorithm comes in. It provides an optimal connection that does not compromise the bandwidth.

4. Computer networks
    Dijkstra's algorithm is used in Local Area Network (LAN) to ensure the least number of 'hops' required to be made by a file that has to be transferred from the server to a client machine.

5. Social networking applications
    Social networking sites employ Dijkstra's algorithm to suggest people the user might know. This is done by calculating the shortest 'path' between two users. This path is based on the number of connections or 'handshakes' required for one user to reach another.

6. Artificial Intelligence (AI)
    Automated drones and robotic servers in restaurants use Dijkstra's algorithm to find an efficient path between the source and the destination. This is done to ensure the delivery of a package in the least amount of time by calculating an optimal way to be taken by the robot.

INDUSTRY APPLICATIONS FOR DIVIDE AND CONQUER ALGORITHMS

The divide and Conquer approach involves picking one big complex problem and dividing it into smaller, simpler subproblems, which are then solved. Their solutions are combined to find the final solution for the initial complex problem. The divide-and-conquer approach is utilized in many algorithms such as – Binary Search, Merge Sort, Quick Sort, Strassen's Method, and Karatsuba Algorithm.

1. **Binary Search**: It has many industrial applications such as searching for a particular element in an array, debugging a code snippet, in semiconductor testing, finding the resource requirements for any system (e.g.,the minimum number of CPUs required for a set load), and finding solutions to equations.
2. **Merge Sort**: Its most significant application is to sort linked lists or arrays without the need to allocate any extra space. It is also used to count the total number of inversions in a list and is applied in external sorting.
3. **Quick Sort**: Apart from its regular application of sorting elements due to its cache-friendly nature, quicksort is also applied in operational research, numerical computations, commercial computing, and event-driven simulation. It is also used in tail-call optimizations due to its tail-recursive nature or to find out the k-largest or smallest element.
4. **Strassen's Method**: It is used in matrix multiplication due to better complexity when compared to the O(N3) naïve method.
5. **Karatsuba Algorithm**: It is beneficial for faster integer multiplications of any base and can also be used to multiply polynomials.

INDUSTRY PERSPECTIVE FOR GREEDY ALGORITHM WITH DYNAMIC PROGRAMMING

One industry perspective could be the Knapsack problem faced during the transportation of goods. The knapsack problem is a linear problem with only one constraint – the total weight that can be carried in the knapsack. The ideal solution is identified by checking the many possible solutions and seeking the best solution. Hence it follows a combinatorial optimization approach. This problem can be solved by using a greedy method or dynamic programming.

The greedy approach first sorts the data based on the density of the goods. Then it fills the knapsack by inserting one element after another till the weight limit is reached. The dynamic programming approach starts by getting an idea of the basic structure of the problem,i.e., it counts the total number of objects to be inserted. Next, it determines the optimum profit for each object by considering the weights and postage, using the recursive forward procedure (from the 1st object to the last thing). Finally, a recursive equation is generated to maximize the optimal profit. These are then inserted into the knapsack for transportation.

Thus, upon taking an arbitrary set of weights for objects, the solution obtained by dynamic programming is better than the solution obtained by a greedy algorithm. This is because the greedy algorithm simply takes the weights into account, whereas, through dynamic programming, we optimize the profits for each object using recursive equations and then insert them into the knapsack.

THE ORIGINS OF THE SCRUM FRAMEWORK

SCRUM began long before the Agile Manifesto was published. We need to go back to 1986 to understand its origins. Japanese industries, such as Toyota, Honda, Takeuchi Hiroyuki, and Nogami Yujiro, profoundly influenced agile thinking. As a result of the above research and inspiration from software projects worldwide, Jeff Sutherland first defined Scrum for the software development industry in 1993 at Easel and began implementing it(Schwaber, 1997).Figure 4 shows the Scrum Framework

Figure 4. Scrum Framework

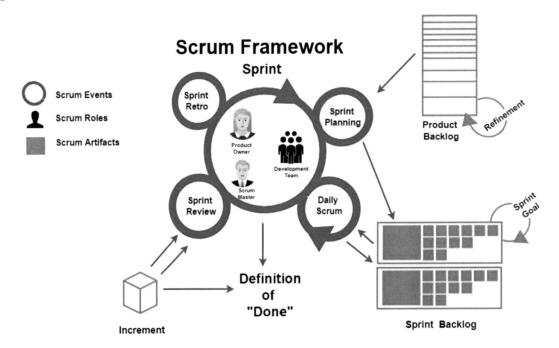

Scrum framework works to clarify responsibilities; organize your job into manageable parts. Allow for effective prioritization allow for greater efficiency in completing tasks.

Ken Schwaber and Jeff Sutherland created Scrum. They used empirical process control to determine the most acceptable Scrum procedures, with the Agile Manifesto as the driving principle(Schwaber, 1997). Scrum's three pillars are likewise the three essential features of empirical process control. The Scrum Framework has three pillars and five ideals.

Empirical Process Control, or Empiricism, is made up of three fundamental notions that serve as the three pillars of Scrum(Bang, 2007):

1. Transparency: This includes the procedure itself and all communications.
2. Inspection: It is vital to conduct frequent product, service, or outcome reviews and assessments.
3. Adaptation: None of the previous will be completely effective until there is an adaptation, which is the capacity to accept ambiguity and change while managing risks appropriately.

Transparency using everyday language and shared standards. With the help of Artifacts, Meetings, and Information radiators team can be more transparent in the activities(Schwaber, 1997). Figure 5 shows Scrum Artifacts

Figure 5. Scrum artifacts

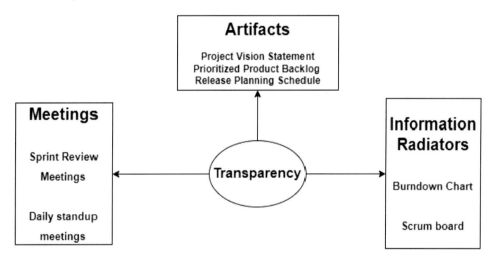

Transparency allows anybody to witness all aspects of any Scrum process. Transparency encourages the free and open flow of information and fosters an open work culture.

Inspection means in Scrum artifacts and progress toward Sprint Goal using frequent feedback and review(Schwaber, 1997). Figure 6 shows the Scrum inspection.

Scrum inspection is portrayed using a shared Scrum board and other information radiators that indicate progress, feedback collection, review, and approval of deliverables by the Product Owner and the customer.

Adaptation helps achieve improvements and adjustments to minimize deviations using agile events(Schwaber, 1997). Figure 7 shows the Scrum adaptation.

Adaptation occurs as the Scrum Core Team and Stakeholders learn via transparency and inspection and then adjust by improving their work.

Figure 6. Scrum Inspection

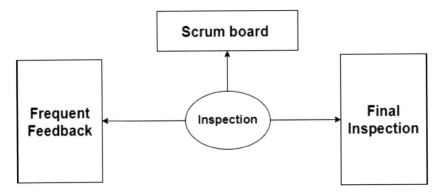

Figure 7. Scrum Adaptation

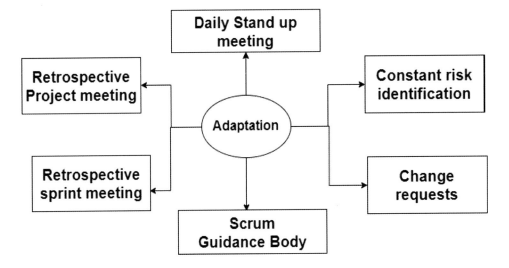

SCRUM VALUES

Scrum emphasizes the following ideals to be lived by each Scrum Team to support these three pillars:

1. Commitment in Scrum Teams to achieving goals.
2. Courage to face challenges and do what's right
3. Focuses on activities, the Sprint, and the goals.
4. Openness is availability to talk about problems with the rest of the team.
5. Respect each Scrum Team member is capable and independent.

Scrum Roles

For the effective adoption of Agile Scrum Methodology for product development and project delivery, the Scrum Body of Knowledge Guide (SBOK Guide) clearly defines Scrum roles. The figure above shows how the Scrum Roles formed and how they appear in a real-world Scrum implementation.

Product Owner

The Product Owner is essentially the Product's C.E.O., who is accountable for the product's success and responsible for maximizing the product's value. Because of the complexities of the zone's requirements, this job falls to a single person. The Product Owner is in charge of the Product Backlog's expectations and chances to provide value. Product Backlog management comprises clarifying and clearly expressing high-level Product Backlog items. Ordering of product backlog items depending on goals. They are increasing the worth of the Development Team's efforts. Everyone can see, understand, and appreciate the product backlog. Ensure that the items in the Product Backlog are ready for the next Sprint. Working along with the Development Team,A Product Owner is similar to a Movie Director. They grasp the primary narrative, goal, audience, needs, artists' abilities, budgetary constraints, latest trends, go-to-market techniques, and when to release their movie. Product owners determine and tell everyone about what will be delivered first by discussing everyone before deciding. He also delegated decision-making, but he is ultimately responsible for the consequences.

Scrum Master

Scrum Masters make sure that the team adheres to agreed-upon protocols. By removing impediments and diverting the group from its goals, the Scrum Master facilitates the team's success. This individual serves as the Scrum team's point of contact with individuals or teams outside of Scrum. A Scrum Master's responsibilities include primarily mentoring team members to ensure that they have received sufficient training and understand Agile practices. Set up daily stand-up meetings: Holds 15-minute daily stand-up meetings during which each team member responds to the following questions: What did you do the day before? What are your plans for today? What's keeping you from taking the next step? When the product owner is in charge of developing and maintaining the product backlog, offer assistance. The product backlog is a list of tasks that the team must complete. The Scrum Master uses information acquired during daily stand-up meetings to support the product owner in improving and managing the product backlog.The Scrum master's primary role is to eliminate roadblocks, which he accomplishes by detecting distractions and bottlenecks that impede the team from concentrating on the work being done in each iteration. Scrum masters must act as mentors and trainers for new staff to keep work going; therefore, teaching Scrum methods and principles is vital.Table1 shows a Comparison of roles between the Product Owner and Scrum Master.

There is a noticeable difference between the responsibilities of the Scrum Master and Product Owner in the above figure. Scrum Masters and Product Owners play crucial roles in the processes. They both aim to produce a viable product using Scrum's best practices. In some ways, their skillsets overlap even though they are working on different aspects of the job.

Table 1. Comparison of roles between product owner and scrum master.

	Product Owner		**Scrum Master**
Vision	Communicate Vision / Strategy	Team	Effective Collaboration
	Value Proposition		Realistic commitments
	Business Goals, Product Release, and Goals		Product Work Environment
Product	Maintain product Backlog	Organization	Educate the stakeholders
	Direction and Prioritization		Resolve Conflicts
	Collect Feedback Available		Organizational changes required by Scrum
Collaboration	But, in the process	Product Owner	Helps with tools and techniques
	Manage the Stakeholders		Support in decision making and empowerment issues
	Be available		Help establish Agile practices in Enterprise.

Scrum Development Team

Each scrum team member does their utmost to fulfill a defined job (Bang, 2007). When a player cannot execute, teammates are expected to step in. Scrum Teams in Agile must support and empower one another. This necessitates regular communication, realistic goal setting, and dedication to the team. Scrum development teams are self-organizing, cross-functional teams of individuals at their heart. They are in charge of developing product increments and meeting sprint objectives. Scrum's success is strongly reliant on the development team's performance. During the Sprint, the development team is in charge of several duties.Scrum development teams consist of self-organizing, cross-functional teams of individuals at their core. They are responsible for creating the product increments and achieving sprint goals. Scrum's success depends heavily on the performance of the development team. The development team is responsible for a variety of tasks during the Sprint. We will examine how these duties contribute to a successful sprint in depth.

SPRINT EXECUTION

The development team spends the majority of their time. Following the Sprint planning meeting, the team receives a Sprint backlog and a Sprint objective. The development team plans and manages this work together. It entails creating a possibly shippable product by designing, constructing, integrating, and testing sprint backlog items. Every day, meet your sprint goals - The Scrum model's flexibility to adjust daily is one of its distinguishing features. The Scrum team jointly assesses the sprint goal's progress in the daily scrum meeting. As a result, the unit modifies its day-to-day approach. As a result, there will be no shocks following the Sprint.

Organize the Product Backlog - In addition to completing the sprint backlog, the development team must also spend some time grooming the backlog. The product owner is in charge of managing the backlog. On the other side, the development team assists him in refining, estimating, and prioritizing backlog items. This effort consumed just 10% of the development team's resources. Sprint planning - At the beginning of each sprint, the development team, the product owner, and the Scrum Master convene for a Sprint Planning meeting. During the meeting, the development team contributes to the determination of the Sprint objective.

Furthermore, they assess how much work they can finish to meet the Sprint target. It is often accomplished by giving points to each story and comparing them to the number of issues previously earned by the development team in a Sprint. Whenever the development team doubts a need, it will seek clarification from the product owner. Adapt Product and Process - At the end of each Sprint, development teams have two opportunities to examine and adapt. The Development Team is one of the Scrum Team's tasks. They are specialists who complete the task! The Development Team oversees creating the product increment. They have communal responsibility and determine how to construct it!

SCRUM EVENTS

A sprint is a limited-time iteration used in agile development. Iterations are commonly referred to as 'iterations' in agile development. Depending on the Scrum team and project, sprints or iterations may differ in their timeframe; however, the shorter the Sprint, the more feedback a Scrum team gets to review and change their product and procedures. Sprints are rarely very long, with 1-2 weeks being the norm, and in some cases even as little as a single day. Figure 8 shows Scrum Events, and the Table2 shows a Comparison of Scrum events.

Figure 8. Scrum events

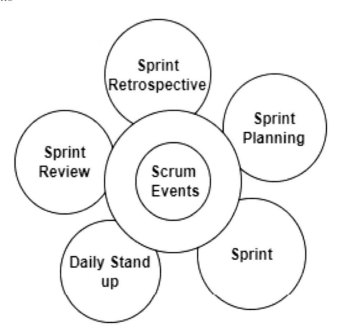

Table 2. Comparisons of Scrum events.

	Sprint Planning	**Daily Scrum**	**Sprint Review**	**Sprint Retrospective**
Goal	Create the sprint goal and Sprint Backlog (Plan to reach the goal)	Inspect and adapt towards sprint goal and Plan for the day	Inspect and Adapt on Product increment developed	Inspect and Adapt to be Effective / Efficient and Continuous Improvement
Input	Ready Product Backlog Items	The current state of the work	Product increment that is developed during the Sprint	Observations, Patterns, Ideas, Metrics & Issues
Output	Sprint Goal and Sprint Backlog	Plan for the day and Identification of impediments	Acceptance and Feedback on product increment, Forecast for the future of the product	Actions for being the Scrum Team to be Effective and Efficient
Duration	Max of 8 hrs / 4 Week sprint	Max 15 minutes / day	Max 4 hrs / 4 wk sprint	Max 3 hrs / 4 wk sprint
Who	Scrum Team	Development team (SM - Facilitate f needed and PO - Optional / Clarify requirements)	Scrum Team + Stakeholders and anyone interested	Scrum Team
When	First Day of the Sprint	Every Day	Last day of the Sprint	Last day of the Sprint

Scrum describes several activities (often referred to as ceremonies) within a sprint: sprint planning, daily Scrum, sprint review, and sprint retrospective. Each of these activities has a time limit. After the goal is met or the timer expires, it should end.

Sprint Plan

Before the Sprint begins, there is a sprint planning meeting. It aims to finalize our sprint strategy and set a deadline. The sprint plan has two phases. During the first session, the product owner analyzes the list of features and decides what needs to be developed during the next Sprint. The following session identifies the activities that need to be completed to complete the build. A sprint planning meeting should result in sprint targets and a backlog. Sprint planning's goal is after defining and committing to an immediate objective; the scrum team determines requirements that support that goal through user stories and supporting tasks that fully meet the team's Definition of Done. Scrum team in sprint planning meeting takes new work according to the capacity of the team and historical data, pulls items from the product backlog, and works out "how*" to meet sprint goals. Identify high-level design approaches, low-level designs, test scenarios, and other functional implementation areas and new assumptions, risks, and dependencies. To self-organize and manage their work & reach sprint goals, create a sprint backlog. The Development Team forecasts the functionality developed during the Sprint. Product backlog items should be broken down into tasks and estimates, which helps in capacity-based planning. It should explain to the Product Owner and Scrum Master how it plans to operate as a self-organizing team which allows them to meet the Sprint Goal and generate the planned increment. The product owner is responsible for presenting "what to do" / "goal" using the product backlog items.

Provide clarity on acceptance criteria by answering questions and resolving misunderstandings. Make trade-offs and negotiates with the development team on the feasible outcome and sprint goal. Scrum Master helps in facilitating events as required. He participates in all circumstances and ensures that attendees understand why they are there and keep the team's focus on the sprint planning goal.

Teach tools/techniques and strategies that help the Scrum Team keep it within the time box. Ensure the development team & product owner have open discussions and plan effectively. Sprint Planning's Results allow Scrum Team to be confident in the goal and has identified user stories to support it. The product owner verifies that the sprint plan is consistent with the vision, roadmap, and release target. It is thoroughly documented on the team's task board or agile tool. Create a burndown chart. When the meeting is over, each member of the Dev Team knows what needs to work.

Daily Stand-up

The team holds a daily scrum meeting on each Sprint called a "daily scrum." Meetings are usually held at the same place and time every day. The best time to have a daily scrum meeting is in the morning since it sets the tone for the day's activities. Scrum meetings are only allowed to last 15 minutes. It keeps the conversation relevant and moving. In the daily Scrum, team members answer the following three questions: What did you do the day before? What are your plans for today? Are there any roadblocks on your path? Scrum Team needs to focus on the Sprint Goal & Sprint Backlog. Keep monitoring the progress toward completing the sprint backlog. Adapt to optimize their plans for the next 24 hours, to work together towards the sprint goal. Meet after the Daily Scrum for detailed discussions or to adapt, or replan, the rest of Sprint's work. Can decide on any format, time, or place, and use the 3-question form if required. Product Owner is optional, but be a quiet observer and don't disturb the team if present. He clarifies acceptance criteria by answering questions & resolving conflicts; if asked by the development team and the response is short, discuss after Daily Scrum. Scrum Master is the individual who facilitates the activity as required to make sure the Development Team meets regularly. Teach tools/techniques and strategies that help the development team keep it within the 15 min time-box. Even ensure the development team plan effectively for the day and external people do not disrupt the meeting.

Sprint Review

Sprint Review is an important event for the Product Owner. It allows both the Scrum Team and stakeholders/customers to examine what was provided, discuss progress toward the Product Goal, and change accordingly. Even though a demo may be on the agenda, the Sprint Review is not merely a demo. An inspection and adaptation event assists the Product Owner in updating the Product Backlog and Product Forecast using feedback gathered during the event. Getting ready for the Sprint Review requires events that are the product's goal where product Owners are responsible for Product Goals. A team may only concentrate on one Product Goal at a time—an Increment in development, where a product is the total of all Increments provided by Developers per Sprint. Sprints are intended to create a completed, useable increment. Backlog of products where openness and accessibility are essential to the Product Backlog, indicating what the Scrum Team will work on next. The definition of Done outlines how much work must be finished from the product backlog to be deemed done. The Scrum Team uses the Definition of Done to identify what position to push into each Sprint and Product Owners and stakeholders to assist them in understanding how much effort has gone into each Product Backlog Item before its discussion at the Sprint Review meeting. The Sprint is part of the Sprint Review meeting; the Sprint Goal and Product Backlog Items are vital inputs. The forecast shows when the product will be delivered or released. Changes in the market Weakness product Owner should gather any market changes before the Sprint Review could impact the development.

What Happens in Sprint Review?

The Scrum Team and stakeholders hold a Sprint Review meeting to discuss how the Sprint was completed. In assessing the work done and the changes made to the Product Backlog, the group determines the following steps to maximize software value at the Sprint Review. All attendees collaborate on the next steps based on this information. The Sprint Review should not be viewed as a presentation or a team-building activity but as a working session. Agenda for Sprint Review is where the product's goal helps keep the team on track, including during the Sprint Review. Plans for the Sprint, which allows the Scrum Team to create a Sprint Goal as part of the Sprint Planning meeting for each Sprint, describe WHY the Sprint is being delivered. Review the market changes during the Sprint Review meeting; any market changes that may impact the product should be discussed. Describe what was done and what was not done by the Scrum Team, who can emphasize transparency by describing which items from the Product Backlog were initial. Completed - or not - by the Sprint's end. Demonstrate working software (or an increment) by the team who will decide to demonstrate or present the done increment of software development products to stakeholders to provide feedback when the time comes. Gather input for newer groups, an integral part of the Sprint Review, is often skipped. A forecast review, which discusses the Product Forecast, might conclude the Sprint review. Sprint Review Results are shared after the Sprint Review meeting ends with feedback; the Product Owner will update the Product Backlog (including detailed orders) and the forecast.

Sprint Retrospective

Retrospectives are recurring meetings held at the end of sprints to discuss what went well and what could be improved. The Agile sprint retrospective is a critical component of the Scrum framework for developing, delivering, and managing complex projects. Scrum sprint retrospectives occur after the sprint review and before sprint planning. Their purpose is to explore how the just-completed Sprint went beyond performance, relationships, processes, and tools. Identify and order what worked. Analyze what didn't work. Identify ways to improve. Create a plan for improving how the Scrum team works. Scrum retrospectives ensure the team's weakness understands and implements needed changes before burying all the ongoing work at the end of each Sprint. Each team member can identify how they can improve what they contributed to the Sprint by asking: In this Sprint, what was done well? How could it be improved? How can we improve?

During each Agile sprint retrospective, the development team focuses on improving work processes or adapting the definition of "done," which may differ among Scrum teams. The entire team must share the same understanding of "done" to assess when work has met expectations. Scrum teams will gain more experience developing defining "done" standards that demand higher quality results.

When managing small projects is challenging enough, putting together many teams to work on a single product might be a nightmare. A group of 50-200 professionals has many of the same obstacles as smaller groups, but the intensity of the problems is significantly greater. Big enterprises confront various challenges while transitioning from a linear and traditional project management style to an Agile framework; huge organizations encounter multiple challenges. The reality of continually changing customer expectations, the requirement for a short time to market, and the need to develop creative techniques to achieve a competitive edge are compelling reasons to adopt today's Lean-Agile frameworks. Culture transformation and high Scrum Maturity are required in all SAFe, LeSS, and Nexus organizations.

SAFE: LEADING FRAMEWORK FOR SCALING AGILE ACROSS THE ENTERPRISE

Imagine the following scenario: your team grows to 150 members. What communication methods will you use? Is it possible to keep up with the team members? Such situations are suitable for SAFe. Safe is an Agile framework designed to coordinate big Agile teams and projects, which has helped some of the world's largest enterprises find a new way to develop software and deliver value(Berntzen et al., 2022).

SAFe has the following principles

1. Use systems thinking
   to anticipate variability while preserving options
   by building incrementally and learning quickly
2. Establish milestones based on the delivery of functional systems
3. Minimize batch sizes, track and restrict work-in-process, and manage queues
4. by applying cadence and synchronizing with cross-domain planning
5. enables knowledge workers to be intrinsically motivated
6. while decentralizing decision-making

The SAFe architecture proved to be quite effective, yielding excellent outcomes.:

1. Reduced time to market by 30-75%
2. 10-50% increase in employee engagement
3. 25-75% improvement in productivity
4. 20-50% enhancement in quality

The following prerequisites will ensure its successful implementation as a leader among Agile scaling framework is an agile management style with an agile mindset. An agile process is a development framework based on user stories. The team should be flexible, make rapid choices, and have clearly defined user stories with approval criteria. In SAFe, there are three degrees of collaboration.

1. Portfolios comprise investment themes and budgets for each topic.
2. An Agile Release Train (ART) program element reflects numerous teams working on the same business result.
3. There is a Product Owner, a Scrum Master, and a Development Team.

LEARN MORE ABOUT LESS: AN AGILE FRAMEWORK FOR CONTINUOUS IMPROVEMENT

Figure 9 shows an Overview of the LeSS Framework, which says what can be done to ensure that the team emphasizes the product rather than just a part of it? LeSS is here to help! The LeSS framework complements Scrum by looking at the objective of one-team Scrum parts and finding ways to achieve the same goals while staying within Scrum's framework-specific constraints. LeSS is an Agile framework that provides product teams with principles for testing and figuring out what works best in different scenarios. The LeSS frameworks extend Scrum up to 10 units: LeSS (up to eight teams) and LeSS Huge (up to ten teams) (up to several thousand people on one project).

Figure 9. Overview of LeSS framework

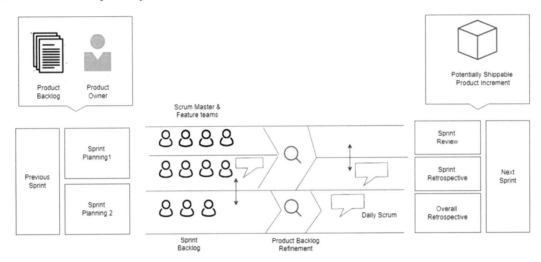

The LeSS principles are

1. Scrum at a large scale is Scrum
2. As an empirical process control
3. Model with transparency
4. To achieve more with less
5. Focus on the whole product
6. Being customer-centric
7. With continuous improvement
8. Based on systems thinking
9. Built on lean principles
10. Based on queueing theory

With LeSS, each team is led by a full-time Scrum Master who assists its members in maintaining a holistic view of the product. The Product Owner is accountable for prioritizing and clarifying items in the backlog. The Development Team consistsof a cross-functional and self-organized building unit with two to eight teams. All groups must attend Sprint Planning One and Two events, Product Backlog Refinement (PBR), Daily Scrum, Sprint Review, Retrospective, and Overall Retrospective, according to LeSS. Each team's sprint backlog will be combined to create a single Product Backlog.(The LesSS Company B.V., 2016).

LeSS Huge is the right solution for bigger teams.

The Huge Roles of LeSS:

1. A single PO owns the whole product
2. POD Product Owner: one PO for each requirement
3. Each team contains one scrum master
4. No more than three development teams per product area

The Huge artifacts created by LeSS:

1. Work to be done on the Product Backlog
2. Product Backlog based on a requirement from the client, in which activities are broken down, defined and prioritized separately
3. In a sprint backlog, the team identifies the activities it needs to perform to complete the selected sprint Backlog Items

LeSS offers the following benefits:

1. Delivers benefits to the business every Sprint by scaling up Scrum patterns
2. That organize teams around features
3. Coordinates multiple product teams
4. Prioritizes customer collaboration over contract negotiations
5. Encourages cross-team cooperation and learning

SCRUM TEAMS CAN SCALE AGILE FRAMEWORKS WITH NEXUS

Figure 10 shows the Nexus A Process for Scaling Agile framework

Scrum teams of 3 to 9 members work together on a single Product Backlog in the Nexus framework(Guide et al., 2021).Nexus differs from other previous frameworks in terms of its organization process.The Nexus Team consists of the Nexus Integration Team, which comprises Product Owners, Scrum Masters, and Nexus Integration Team Members. Its Scrum Teams has 3 to 9 team members.

How does the workflow work in Nexus?

1. Refining the Product Backlog by identifying and minimizing/removing dependencies.
2. During Nexus Sprint Planning, representatives from each Scrum Team evaluate the Product Backlog.
3. Planned testing: integrating all work into a shared testing environment
4. Daily meetings: members from each development team
5. Over the Sprint, an integrated increment is developed, and the Nexus Sprint Review offers input on it
6. Nexus Sprint Retrospective: a discussion of common difficulties among the Nexus Scrum teams. Individual sprint retrospectives are held following the Nexus Sprint Retrospective.
7. Nexus and its related components: roles, events, artifacts, and rules are created by Scrum Teams.

Figure 10. Nexus framework

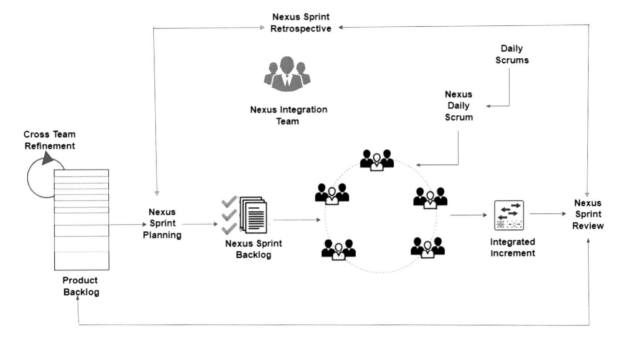

The Nexus Events are:

1. Identify cross-team dependencies to improve the Product Backlog: a forecast of which team will deliver each item
2. Nexus Sprint Planning: coordination of all Sprint activities across all Scrum teams.
3. Nexus Sprint Goals: establishing the Sprint's objectives
4. Nexus Daily Scrum: Reviewing the current status of the integrated increment to identify integration issues and cross-team dependencies/impacts.
5. We collect input on the incremental improvements achieved during the sprint cycle in Nexus Sprint Review.
6. A Nexus Sprint Retrospective is a meeting to evaluate the previous Sprint and make changes for the next one, guaranteeing continual improvement.

In addition to Nexus, Artifacts provide the opportunity for inspection and adaptation, which is crucial to ensuring transparency.

Artifacts from the Nexus

1. The Product Owner manages Nexus Scrum Product Backlog for all Nexus Scrum Teams.
2. Nexus Sprint Backlog: a grouping of Product Backlog entries from several Sprint Backlogs (Scrum teams)
3. Nexus Sprint Review: an examination of the integrated work after the Sprint.

Nexus has the following advantages:

1. High levels of productivity
2. By making the best use of available team members and resources.
3. Improved developer self-organization
4. Detection of productivity abnormalities through the optimization of all efforts
5. intended to handle issues that may occur in huge groups

What are the Advantages of Agile Methodologies in Remote Working?

The trend towards remote work and the subsequent rise in distributed teams has been the most noticeable development in the past year. Only 3% of developers and IT professionals plan to return to the office in the foreseeable future. After COVID-19, 25% of respondents said they would remain utterly virtual, and 56% said they would prefer a hybrid approach that includes regular visits but not daily.

Digital.ai Agility (70%) and Atlassian Jira (81%) are the most common tools used and recommended in the State of Agile Report. Among scaling frameworks, the Scaled Agile Framework is the most popular. This basis was cited most often by 37% of respondents.

Scrumban (9%), the closest scaling method, performs significantly better than SAFe. Relevant considers SAFe to be the most suitable solution for large enterprises managing the long lifecycles of multiple products on a large scale. The following other agile methods and practices can use in software product development services:

1. Daily stand-ups – 87%
2. Retrospectives – 83%
3. Iteration / Sprint Planning – 83%
4. Kanban boards – 77%
5. Quest Boards – 67%
6. Flexible planning tables – 66%

THE TRANSFORMATION FROM TRADITIONAL PRACTICES TO AGILE PRACTICES.

Agile transformation improves organizations' long-term viability and growth by changing how they function and perform. This transformation aims to replace traditional business models with a new approach that allows companies to adapt to change more easily(Alsari et al., 2020). The rapid transition has become much more critical now that COVID-19 requires agility to sustain operations. Organizations can change their skill by becoming adaptive, flexible, collaborative, self-organizing, and capable of adapting to fast-changing environments. As the Agile Manifesto does not only apply to development teams, its values and principles can be taught, practiced, and spread throughout any organization. Figure 11 shows Transformation into agile.

Figure 11. Transformation to Agile

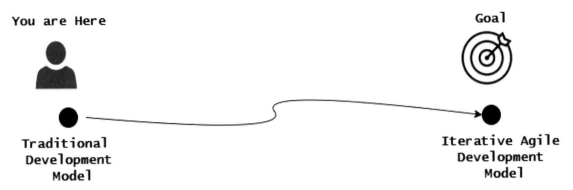

Individual team members accomplish Agile transformation when they intuitively and voluntarily adopt the values, principles, and Agile methodologies to finish the job at hand rather than being pushed or directed to do so. To reap the rewards of achieving accurate, healthy agility, the entirety of the organization needs to understand the definition and value of agile transformation(Ganesh &Thangasamy, 2012). To achieve self-organization and collaboration, the culture and organizational mindset must change. Following are the best practices performed by champions in agile who can be either Scrum Master or Agile coaches. Organizations increasingly adopt agile methodologies to realize they need to respond fast and efficiently in a constantly changing world.

The best practices that teams will use will help them transform into Agile methodology.

1. Identify the organization's goals and objectives for Agile Transformation
2. Compile a list of all the pain points that management/organization faces
3. Inspect the system by performing a Gemba walk
4. Discussion with leaders and management of the organization regarding observations and critical points
5. Analyze the root causes and point out the problems.
6. Create mutually agreed upon pain points, goals, and objectives
7. Decide what measurements to use and what KPIs to set
8. Announcing objectives and changes to all teams and departing from the organization
9. If any team members have concerns about the change, set up a system to voice them.
10. Identify champions with a positive attitude toward change and understand the objectives.
11. Make sure the management team is accountable for change
12. Coaching/mentoring champions on how their contributions will add value
13. Setup a system for advocates to talk/discuss with team members
14. Design changes to the organization's structure, process, tools, techniques, and strategies
15. Create teams based on a new design
16. Educating people about the framework, new changes, tools, and techniques
17. The new framework and practices required to be practiced and implemented
18. Coaching and mentoring the team in the implementation of the new practices
19. Analyze the results against the initially agreed KPIs and criteria
20. Planning for continuous improvement

21. Keeps track of the progress
22. Share the progress we are making towards achieving our goal
23. Continue to improve continuously.

CONCLUSION

To consistently generate high-quality software deliverables, software engineers must adhere to the software design life cycle as a regular practice. This traditional strategy has certain drawbacks. We must address project management's weaknesses. Another way is known as agile methodology, which is far more efficient and enhances product quality if team members adhere to the agile ideals. As a result, established methods will be phased out in favor of agile processes. The most challenging task for the organization is shifting the team's thinking from a waterfall paradigm to an elegant thought pattern. Implementing agile software development entails adapting to changing demands or requirements and serving the client's expectations rather than adhering to fixed rules and norms. These projects should not have inflexible and unwilling people to change their ways. The article describes how agile methods were used in one project. Agility leaders should adapt to the changing demands of their teams rather than following a preset plan or set of rules when using a flexible approach. It's more about meeting the consumer's needs than following a set of processes.

REFERENCES

al Maamzi, J. J., & Tawfik, T. (2022). The effectiveness of agile management on traditional projects within public organizations. *IOP Conference Series. Materials Science and Engineering, 1218*(1), 012037. doi:10.1088/1757-899X/1218/1/012037

Alsari, A., Qureshi, R., & Algarni, A. (2020). Agile Framework to Transform Traditional Team. *Proceedings - Frontiers in Education Conference, FIE.* 10.1109/FIE44824.2020.9274240

Anes, V., Abreu, A., & Santos, R. (2020). A new risk assessment approach for agile projects. *Proceedings - 2020 International Young Engineers Forum, YEF-ECE 2020*, 67–72. 10.1109/YEF-ECE49388.2020.9171808

Baijens, J., Helms, R., & Iren, D. (2020). Applying Scrum in Data Science Projects. *Proceedings - 2020 IEEE 22nd Conference on Business Informatics, CBI 2020, 1*, 30–38. 10.1109/CBI49978.2020.00011

Bang, T. J. (2007). An agile approach to requirement specification. Lecture Notes in Computer Science, 4536. doi:10.1007/978-3-540-73101-6_35

Berntzen, M., Hoda, R., Moe, N. B., & Stray, V. (2022). A Taxonomy of Inter Team Coordination Mechanisms in Large-Scale Agile. IEEE Transactions on Software Engineering. doi:10.1109/TSE.2022.3160873

Bianchi, M. J., Conforto, E. C., Rebentisch, E., Amaral, D. C., Rezende, S. O., & de Padua, R. (2021). Recommendation of Project Management Practices: A Contribution to Hybrid Models. *IEEE Transactions on Engineering Management, 00*(X), 1–14. doi:10.1109/TEM.2021.3101179

Cao, L. (2017). Data science: A comprehensive overview. *ACM Computing Surveys*, *50*(3), 1–42. Advance online publication. doi:10.1145/3076253

Drury, M., Conboy, K., & Power, K. (2011). Decision making in agile development: A focus group study of decisions & obstacles. *Proceedings - 2011 Agile Conference, Agile 2011*, 39–47. 10.1109/AGILE.2011.27

Ganesh, N., & Thangasamy, S. (2012). Lessons learned in transforming from traditional to agile development. *Journal of Computational Science*, *8*(3), 389–392. doi:10.3844/jcssp.2012.389.392

Grady, N. W., Payne, J. A., & Parker, H. (2017). Agile big data analytics: AnalyticsOps for data science. *Proceedings - 2017 IEEE International Conference on Big Data, Big Data 2017*, 2331–2339. 10.1109/BigData.2017.8258187

Guide, T. D., Scrum, S., & January, N. (2021). *The Nexus ™ Guide*. Academic Press.

Mahfoodh, H., Aleid, K., Bahzad, A., Matar, S., Shubbar, Z. S., & Mattar, E. (2021). Sustaining Work Continuity through Hybrid Work Environments: Tracking Systems. *2021 International Conference on Innovation and Intelligence for Informatics, Computing, and Technologies, 3ICT 2021*, 677–684. 10.1109/3ICT53449.2021.9581371

Marnada, P., Raharjo, T., Hardian, B., & Prasetyo, A. (2021). Agile project management challenge in handling scope and change: A systematic literature review. *Procedia Computer Science*, *197*, 290–300. doi:10.1016/j.procs.2021.12.143

Olekh, T. M., Vlasenko, O. V., Kolesnikova, K., & Lukianov, D. (2013). *Markov's model in Project Management Communications in Organizational and Technscal System*. Unpublished. doi:10.13140/rg.2.1.5015.0484

Saltz, J. S., & Grady, N. W. (2017). The ambiguity of data science team roles and the need for a data science workforce framework. *Proceedings - 2017 IEEE International Conference on Big Data, Big Data 2017*, 2355–2361. 10.1109/BigData.2017.8258190

Schwaber, K. (1997). SCRUM Development Process. *Business Object Design and Implementation*, 117–134. doi:10.1007/978-1-4471-0947-1_11

The LesSS Company B.V. (2016). LeSS Framework. *LeSS*, 1–2. https://less.works/less/framework/index.html

Compilation of References

Aazam, M., Zeadally, S., & Flushing, E. F. (2021). Task offloading in edge computing for machine learning-based smart healthcare. *Computer Networks*, *191*, 108019. doi:10.1016/j.comnet.2021.108019

Abate, A. F., Nappi, M., & Ricciardi, S. (2016, October). Smartphone enabled person authentication based on ear biometrics and arm gesture. *2016 IEEE International Conference on Systems, Man, and Cybernetics (SMC)*. 10.1109/SMC.2016.7844812

Abd El-Latif, A. A. (2020). Secret Images Transfer in Cloud System Based on Investigating Quantum Walks in Steganography Approaches. *Physica A: Statistical Mechanics and Its Applications, 541*. . doi:10.1016/j.physa.2019.123687

Abdellatif, A. A. (2019). Edge-based compression and classification for smart healthcare systems: Concept, implementation and evaluation. *Expert Systems with Applications*, *117*, 1–14. doi:10.1016/j.eswa.2018.09.019

Abdulkudhur & Al Saffar. (2021). LSB Based Image Steganography Using McEliece Cryptosystem. *Materials Today: Proceedings*. . doi:10.1016/j.matpr.2021.07.182

Abdullatif, Akram, Chebil, & Gunawan. (2013). Properties of Digital Image Watermarking. *Proceedings of the IEEE 9th International Colloquium on Signal Processing and its Applications*, 235–240. 10.1109/CSPA.2013.6530048

Abdurrahman, U. A., Kaiiali, M., & Muhammad, J. (2013, November). A new mobile-based multi-factor authentication scheme using pre-shared number, GPS location and time stamp. *2013 International Conference on Electronics, Computer and Computation (ICECCO)*. 10.1109/ICECCO.2013.6718286

Abhishek, K., Roshan, S., Kumar, P., & Ranjan, R. (2013). A comprehensive study on multifactor authentication schemes. In *Advances in Computing and Information Technology* (pp. 561–568). Springer Berlin Heidelberg. doi:10.1007/978-3-642-31552-7_57

Abie, H., & Balasingham, I. (2012). Risk-Based Adaptive Security for Smart IoT in eHealth. *Proceedings of the 7th International Conference on Body Area Networks*. 10.4108/icst.bodynets.2012.250235

Abraham, J. (2011). Digital Image Watermarking: An Overview. *National Seminar on Modern Trends in EC & SP*, 36–42.

Abraham, J., & Paul, V. (2019). An imperceptible spatial domain color image watermarking scheme. *Journal of King Saud University-Computer and Information Sciences*, *31*(1), 125–133. doi:10.1016/j.jksuci.2016.12.004

Abu Bakar, K. A., & Haron, G. R. (2014, August). Adaptive authentication based on analysis of user behavior. *2014 Science and Information Conference*. 10.1109/SAI.2014.6918248

Acar, A., Liu, W., Beyah, R., Akkaya, K., & Uluagac, A. S. (2019). A privacy-preserving multifactor authentication system. *Security and Privacy*, *2*(6). Advance online publication. doi:10.1002py2.94

Acter, T., Uddin, N., Das, J., Akhter, A., Choudhury, T. R., & Kim, S. (2020). Evolution of severe acute respiratory syndrome coronavirus 2 (SARS-CoV-2) as coronavirus disease 2019 (COVID-19) pandemic: A global health emergency. *The Science of the Total Environment, 730*, 138996. doi:10.1016/j.scitotenv.2020.138996 PMID:32371230

Adzic, G., & Chatley, R. (2017). Serverless computing: economic and architectural impact. *Proceedings of the 2017 11th joint meeting on foundations of software engineering*, 884–889. 10.1145/3106237.3117767

Agadakos, I., Hallgren, P., Damopoulos, D., Sabelfeld, A., & Portokalidis, G. (2016, December 5). Location-enhanced authentication using the IoT. *Proceedings of the 32nd Annual Conference on Computer Security Applications.* 10.1145/2991079.2991090

Agarwal, H., Raman, B., & Venkat, I. (2015). Blind reliable invisible watermarking method in wavelet domain for face image watermark. *Multimedia Tools and Applications, 74*(17), 6897–6935. doi:10.100711042-014-1934-1

Agarwal, N., Singh, A. K., & Singh, P. K. (2019). Survey of robust and imperceptible watermarking. *Multimedia Tools and Applications, 78*(7), 8603–8633. doi:10.100711042-018-7128-5

Agarwal, R., Baghel, N., & Khan, M. A. (2020). Load balancing in cloud computing using mutation based particle swarm optimization. In *2020 International Conference on Contemporary Computing and Applications (IC3A)*. IEEE.

Agrawal, R., Haas, P. J., & Kiernan, J. (2003). Watermarking relational data: Framework, algorithms and analysis. *The VLDB Journal-The International Journal on Very Large Data Bases, 12*(2), 157–169. doi:10.100700778-003-0097-x

Ahmed, F., & Moskowitz, I. S. (2016). A Semi-Reversible Watermark for Medical Image Authentication. *Proceedings of the 1st Transdisciplinary Conference on Distributed Diagnosis and Home Healthcare*, 59–62. 10.1109/DDHH.2006.1624797

Ahmed, S. (2012). Applications of Graph Coloring in Modern Computer Science. *International Journal of Computer and Information Technology, 3*(2), 1–7.

Ahonen, T., Hadid, A., & Pietikainen, M. (2006). Face recognition by independent component analysis. *IEEE Transactions on Pattern Analysis and Machine Intelligence, 28*, 2037-2041.

Aickelin, U., Chapman, W. W., & Hart, G. K. (2019). *Health Informatics—ambitions and purpose.* Frontiers in Digital Health.

Akbar, T. A., Hassan, Q. K., Ishaq, S., Batool, M., Butt, H. J., & Jabbar, H. (2019). Investigative Spatial Distribution and Modelling of Existing and Future Urban Land Changes and Its Impact on Urbanization and Economy. *Remote Sensing, 11*(2), 105–115. doi:10.3390/rs11020105

Akhtar, Z., & Khan, E. (2016). Identifying high quality jpeg compressed images through exhaustive recompression technique. *Proceedings of the International conference on advances in computing, communications and informatics (ICACCI)*, 652–656. 10.1109/ICACCI.2016.7732120

Akmandor, A. O., & Jha, N. K. (2017). Keep the stress away with SoDA: Stress detection and alleviation system. *IEEE Transactions on Multi-Scale Computing Systems, 3*(4), 269–282.

Akpakwu, G. A., Silva, B. J., Hancke, G. P., & Abu-Mahfouz, A. M. (2017). A survey on 5G networks for the Internet of Things: Communication technologies and challenges. *IEEE Access: Practical Innovations, Open Solutions, 6*, 3619–3647. doi:10.1109/ACCESS.2017.2779844

al Maamzi, J. J., & Tawfik, T. (2022). The effectiveness of agile management on traditional projects within public organizations. *IOP Conference Series. Materials Science and Engineering, 1218*(1), 012037. doi:10.1088/1757-899X/1218/1/012037

Al Nuaimi, E., Al Neyadi, H., Mohamed, N., & Al-Jaroodi, J. (2015). Applications of big data to smart cities. *Journal of Internet Services and Applications*, *6*(1), 1–15. doi:10.118613174-015-0041-5

Ala-Kitula, A., Talvitie-Lamberg, T., Tyrväinen, P., & Silvennoinen, M. (2017). Developing Solutions for Healthcare-Deploying Artificial Intelligence to an Evolving Target. *International Conference on Computational Science and Computational Intelligence (CSCI)*, 1637-1642. 10.1109/CSCI.2017.285

Al-Ameen, M. N., Wright, M., & Scielzo, S. (2015, April 18). Towards making random passwords memorable. *Proceedings of the 33rd Annual ACM Conference on Human Factors in Computing Systems*. http://dx.doi.org/10.1145/2702123.2702241

Alam, M. F., Katsikas, S., Beltramello, O., & Hadjiefthymiades, S. (2017). Augmented and virtual reality based monitoring and safety system: A prototype IoT platform. *Journal of Network and Computer Applications*, *89*, 109–119. doi:10.1016/j.jnca.2017.03.022

Al-Azzam, M. K., Alazzam, M. B., & Al-Manasra, M. K. (2019). MHealth for decision making support: A case study of EHealth in the public sector. *International Journal of Advanced Computer Science and Applications*, *10*(5), 381–387.

Ali Fahmi, P. N., Kodirov, E., Choi, D.-J., & Lee, G.-S., MohdFikriAzli, A., & Sayeed, S. (2012, October). Implicit authentication based on ear shape biometrics using smartphone camera during a call. *2012 IEEE International Conference on Systems, Man, and Cybernetics (SMC)*. 10.1109/ICSMC.2012.6378079

Alim, M., Ye, G. H., Guan, P., Huang, D. S., Zhou, B. S., & Wu, W. (2020). Comparison of ARIMA model and XG-Boost model for prediction of human brucellosis in mainland China: A time-series study. *BMJ Open*, *10*(12), e039676.

Ali, R., & Pal, A. K. (2017). An efficient three factor-based authentication scheme in multiserver environment using ECC. *International Journal of Communication Systems*, *31*(4), e3484. doi:10.1002/dac.3484

Ali, Z., Imran, M., Alsulaiman, M., Zia, T., & Shoaib, M. (2018). A zero-watermarking algorithm for privacy protection in biomedical signals. *Future Generation Computer Systems*, *82*, 290–303. doi:10.1016/j.future.2017.12.007

Alizadeh, A. A., Eisen, M. B., Davis, R. E., Ma, C., Lossos, I. S., Rosenwald, A., Boldrick, J. C., Sabet, H., Tran, T., Yu, X., Powell, J. I., Yang, L., Marti, G. E., Moore, T., Hudson, J. Jr, Lu, L., Lewis, D. B., Tibshirani, R., Sherlock, G., ... Staudt, L. M. (2000). Distinct types of diffuse large B-cell lymphoma identified by gene expression profiling. *Nature*, *403*(6769), 503–511. doi:10.1038/35000501 PMID:10676951

Al-Kandari, N. M., & Jolliffe, I. T. (2005). Variable selection and interpretation in correlation principal components. *Environmetrics*, *16*(6), 659–672. doi:10.1002/env.728

Alkawaz, M. H., Sulong, G., Saba, T., Almazyad, A. S., & Rehman, A. (2016). Concise analysis of current text automation and watermarking approaches. *Security and Communication Networks*, *9*(18), 6365–6378. doi:10.1002ec.1738

AlKhodaidi & Gutub. (2021). Refining Image Steganography Distribution for Higher Security Multimedia Counting-Based Secret-Sharing. *Multimedia Tools and Applications, 80*(1), 1143–73. . doi:10.1007/s11042-020-09720-w

Allani, O., Zghal, H. B., Mellouli, N., & Akdag, H. (2016). A knowledge-based image retrieval system integrating semantic and visual features. *Procedia Computer Science*, *96*, 1428–1436.

Allhoff, F. (2009). The coming era of nanomedicine. *The American Journal of Bioethics*, *9*(10), 3–11.

Alliance, N. (2014). *5g white paper-executive version.* White Paper.

Al-Masri, E., Diabate, I., Jain, R., Lam, M. H., & Nathala, S. R. (2018). A serverless IoT architecture for smart waste management systems. *2018 IEEE International Conference on Industrial Internet (ICII)*, 179–180. 10.1109/ICII.2018.00034

Almuairfi, S., Veeraraghavan, P., & Chilamkurti, N. (2013). A novel image-based implicit password authentication system (IPAS) for mobile and non-mobile devices. *Mathematical and Computer Modelling*, *58*(1–2), 108–116. doi:10.1016/j.mcm.2012.07.005

Almulhem, A. (2011, February). A graphical password authentication system. *2011 World Congress on Internet Security (WorldCIS-2011)*. 10.1109/WorldCIS17046.2011.5749855

AlRashidi, M. R., & El-Hawary, M. E. (2008). A survey of particle swarm optimization applications in electric power systems. *IEEE Transactions on Evolutionary Computation*, *13*(4), 913–918. doi:10.1109/TEVC.2006.880326

Al-Roomi, M., Al-Ebrahim, S., Buqrais, S., & Ahmad, I. (2013). Cloud computing pricing models: A survey. *International Journal of Grid and Distributed Computing*, *6*(5), 93–106. doi:10.14257/ijgdc.2013.6.5.09

Alsari, A., Qureshi, R., & Algarni, A. (2020). Agile Framework to Transform Traditional Team. *Proceedings - Frontiers in Education Conference, FIE*. 10.1109/FIE44824.2020.9274240

Alsulaiman, F. A., & El Saddik, A. (2008). Three-Dimensional password for more secure authentication. *IEEE Transactions on Instrumentation and Measurement*, *57*(9), 1929–1938. doi:10.1109/TIM.2008.919905

Altaa, A. A. J., Sahib, S. B., & Zamani, M. (2012). An Introduction to Image Steganography Techniques. *Proceedings of the 2012 International Conference on Advanced Computer Science Applications and Technologies (ACSAT)*, 122–126. 10.1109/ACSAT.2012.25

Althar, R. R., Alahmadi, A., Samanta, D., Khan, M. Z., & Alahmadi, A. H. (2022). Mathematical foundations based statistical modeling of software source code for software system evolution. *Mathematical Biosciences and Engineering*, *19*(4), 3701–3719. doi:10.3934/mbe.2022170 PMID:35341270

Altice, F., Azbel, L., Stone, J., Brooks-Pollock, E., Smyrnov, P., & Dvoriak, S. (2016). In Eastern Europe and Central Asia, incarceration and a high-risk environment combine to perpetuate HIV, hepatitis C virus, and tuberculosis transmission. *Lancet*, *388*(10050), 1228–1248. doi:10.1016/S0140-6736(16)30856-X PMID:27427455

Amanda, J. W. (2019). Design Thinking for a User-Centered Approach to Artificial Intelligence. *She Ji: The Journal of Design, Economics, and Innovation*, *5*(4), 394-396. doi:10.1016/j.sheji.2019.11.015

Amara, E. H. (1995). Numerical investigations on thermal effects of laser-ocular mediainteraction. *International Journal of Heat and Mass Transfer*, *38*(13), 2479–2488. doi:10.1016/0017-9310(94)00353-W

Amazon, E. C. (2015). *Amazon web services*. Available in: Error! Hyperlink reference not valid.

Amin, R., Islam, S. H., Biswas, G. P., Khan, M. K., & Kumar, N. (2015). An Efficient and Practical Smart Card Based Anonymity Preserving User Authentication Scheme for TMIS using Elliptic Curve Cryptography. *Journal of Medical Systems*, *39*(11), 180. Advance online publication. doi:10.100710916-015-0351-y PMID:26433889

Anand, A., & Singh, A. K. (2020). An improved DWT-SVD domain watermarking for medical information security. *Computer Communications*, *152*, 72–80. doi:10.1016/j.comcom.2020.01.038

Andreu-Perez, J. (2015). From wearable sensors to smart implants--toward pervasive and personalized healthcare. *IEEE Transactions on Biomedical Engineering*, *62*(12), 2750–2762.

Aneiros, G., Cao, R., Fraiman, R., Genest, C., & Vieu, P. (2019). Recent advances in functional data analysis and high-dimensional statistics. *Journal of Multivariate Analysis*, *170*, 3–9. doi:10.1016/j.jmva.2018.11.007

Anes, V., Abreu, A., & Santos, R. (2020). A new risk assessment approach for agile projects. *Proceedings - 2020 International Young Engineers Forum, YEF-ECE 2020*, 67–72. 10.1109/YEF-ECE49388.2020.9171808

An, J., Zhang, X., Zhou, H., Feng, J., & Jiao, L. (2018, July). Patch Tensor-Based Sparse and Low-Rank Graph for Hyperspectral Images Dimensionality Reduction. *IEEE Journal of Selected Topics in Applied Earth Observations and Remote Sensing, 11*(7), 2513–2527. doi:10.1109/JSTARS.2018.2833886

Ansari, A. S., Mohammadi, M. S., & Parvez, M. T. (2020). A Multiple-Format Steganography Algorithm for Color Images. *IEEE Access: Practical Innovations, Open Solutions, 8,* 83926–83939. doi:10.1109/ACCESS.2020.2991130

Apostolopoulos, I. D., & Mpesiana, T. A. (2020). *Covid-19: automatic detection from x-ray images utilizing transfer learning with convolutional neural networks.* Physical and Engineering Sciences in Medicine.

Aronowitz, H., Li, M., Toledo-Ronen, O., Harary, S., Geva, A., Ben-David, S., Rendel, A., Hoory, R., Ratha, N., Pankanti, S., & Nahamoo, D. (2014, September). Multi-modal biometrics for mobile authentication. *IEEE International Joint Conference on Biometrics.* 10.1109/BTAS.2014.6996269

Arora, R., & Doegar, A. (2016). An Effective Approach for Face Recognition using PCA and LDA on Visible and IR images. *International Journal of Computer Trends and Technology, 32*(1), 44–48. doi:10.14445/22312803/IJCTT-V32P108

Arulkumar, V., & Bhalaji, N. (2021). Performance analysis of nature inspired load balancing algorithm in cloud environment. *Journal of Ambient Intelligence and Humanized Computing, 12*(3), 3735–3742.

Asher, H. (2013). Methadone is prescribed in local prisons in England. *Drugs and Alcohol Today, 13*(4), 234–243. doi:10.1108/DAT-04-2013-0018

Ashibani, Y., & Mahmoud, Q. H. (2019). A behavior-based proactive user authentication model utilizing mobile application usage patterns. In *Advances in Artificial Intelligence* (pp. 284–295). Springer International Publishing. doi:10.1007/978-3-030-18305-9_23

Ashibani, Y., & Mahmoud, Q. H. (2020, October 11). An intelligent risk-based authentication approach for smartphone applications. *2020 IEEE International Conference on Systems, Man, and Cybernetics (SMC).* 10.1109/SMC42975.2020.9283267

Ashraf, Z. (2020). Interval Type-2 Fuzzy Logic System Based Similarity Evaluation for Image Steganography. *Heliyon, 6*(5). . doi:10.1016/j.heliyon.2020.e03771

Atanasssov, K. (1989). Intuitionistic fuzzy sets. *Fuzzy Sets and Systems, 20*(1), 87–96. doi:10.1016/S0165-0114(86)80034-3

Atique, S., Bautista, J. R., Block, L. J., Lee, J. J., Lozada-Perezmitre, E., Nibber, R., O'Connor, S., Peltonen, L.-M., Ronquillo, C., Tayaben, J., Thilo, F. J. S., & Topaz, M. (2020). A nursing informatics response to COVID-19: Perspectives from five regions of the world. *Journal of Advanced Nursing, 76*(10), 2462–2468. doi:10.1111/jan.14417 PMID:32420652

Atlam, H. F., Alenezi, A., Walters, R. J., Wills, G. B., & Daniel, J. (2017, June). Developing an adaptive risk-based access control model for the internet of things. *2017 IEEE International Conference on Internet of Things (IThings) and IEEE Green Computing and Communications (GreenCom) and IEEE Cyber, Physical and Social Computing (CPSCom) and IEEE Smart Data (SmartData).* http://dx.doi.org/10.1109/ithings-greencom-cpscom-smartdata.2017.103

Aydin, M. E., & Fogarty, T. C. (2004). A distributed evolutionary simulated annealing algorithm for combinatorial optimisation problems. *Journal of Heuristics, 10*(3), 269–292. doi:10.1023/B:HEUR.0000026896.44360.f9

Azbel, L., Wegman, M., Polonsky, M., Bachireddy, C., Meyer, J., Shumskaya, N., Kurmanalieva, A., Dvoryak, S., & Altice, F. L. (2018). Drug injection within the prison in Kyrgyzstan: Elevated HIV risk and implications for scaling up opioid agonist treatments. *International Journal of Prisoner Health, 14*(3), 175–187. doi:10.1108/IJPH-03-2017-0016 PMID:30274558

Bae, S. H., Sarkis, J., & Yoo, C. S. (2011). Greening transportation fleets: Insights from a two-stage game theoretic model. *Transportation Research Part E, Logistics and Transportation Review, 47*(6), 793–807. doi:10.1016/j.tre.2011.05.015

Bahri, S., Kdayem, M., & Zoghlami, N. (2020, December). Deep Learning for COVID-19 prediction. In *2020 4th International Conference on Advanced Systems and Emergent Technologies (IC_ASET)* (pp. 406-411). IEEE.

Baijens, J., Helms, R., & Iren, D. (2020). Applying Scrum in Data Science Projects. *Proceedings - 2020 IEEE 22nd Conference on Business Informatics, CBI 2020, 1*, 30–38. 10.1109/CBI49978.2020.00011

Bajeh, A. O., & Abolarinwa, K. O. (2011). Optimization: A comparative study of genetic and tabu search algorithms. *International Journal of Computers and Applications, 31*(5), 43–48.

Baker, S. B., Xiang, W., & Atkinson, I. (2017). Internet of things for smart healthcare: Technologies, challenges, and opportunities. *IEEE Access: Practical Innovations, Open Solutions, 5*, 26521–26544. doi:10.1109/ACCESS.2017.2775180

Bakkar, N. (2018). Artificial intelligence in neurodegenerative disease research: Use of IBM Watson to identify additional RNA-binding proteins altered in amyotrophic lateral sclerosis. *Acta Neuropathologica, 135*(2), 227–247.

Baldini, I., Castro, P., Chang, K., Cheng, P., Fink, S., & Ishakian, V. (2017). Serverless computing: Current trends and open problems. In Research Advances in Cloud Computing (pp. 1–20). Springer.

Bang, T. J. (2007). An agile approach to requirement specification. Lecture Notes in Computer Science, 4536. doi:10.1007/978-3-540-73101-6_35

Baral, S., Logie, C., Grosso, A., Wirtz, A., & Beyrer, C. (2013). Modified social-ecological model: A tool for guiding the assessment of HIV epidemic risks and risk contexts. *BMC Public Health, 13*(1). Advance online publication. doi:10.1186/1471-2458-13-482

Barik, R. K., Dubey, A. C., Tripathi, A., Pratik, T., Sasane, S., Lenka, R. K., Dubey, H., Mankodiya, K., & Kumar, V. (2018). Mist data: Leveraging mist computing for secure and scalable architecture for smart and connected health. *Procedia Computer Science, 125*, 647–653. doi:10.1016/j.procs.2017.12.083

Bartlett, M. S., Movellan, J. R., & Sejnowski, T. J. (2002). Face recognition by independent component analysis. *IEEE Transactions on Neural Networks, 13*(6), 1450–1464. doi:10.1109/TNN.2002.804287 PMID:18244540

Baudat, G., & Anouar, F. (2000). Generalized Discriminant Analysis Using a Kernel Approach. *Neural Computation, 12*(10), 2385–2404. doi:10.1162/089976600300014980 PMID:11032039

Becher, J. D., Berkhin, P., & Freeman, E. (2000). Automating exploratory data analysis for efficient data mining. *Proceeding of the Sixth ACM SIGKDD International Conference on Knowledge Discovery and Data Mining*, 424–429. 10.1145/347090.347179

Beer, D. G., Kardia, S. L. R., Huang, C.-C., Giordano, T. J., Levin, A. M., Misek, D. E., Lin, L., Chen, G., Gharib, T. G., Thomas, D. G., Lizyness, M. L., Kuick, R., Hayasaka, S., Taylor, J. M. G., Iannettoni, M. D., Orringer, M. B., & Hanash, S. (2002). Gene-expression Profiles Predict Survival of Patients with Lung Adenocarcinoma. *Nature Medicine, 8*(8), 816–823. doi:10.1038/nm733 PMID:12118244

Beez, U., Humm, B. G., & Walsh, P. (2015). Electronic health records. *2015 International Conference on Computational Science and Computational Intelligence (CSCI).*

Beg, O. A., Khan, M. S., Karim, I., Alam, M. M., & Ferdows, M. (2014). Explicit numerical study of unsteady hydromagnetic mixed convective nanofluid flow from an exponentially stretching sheet in porous media. *Applied Nanoscience, 4*(8), 943–957. doi:10.100713204-013-0275-0

Behera, R. K., & Rath, S. K. (2016). An efficient modularity-based algorithm for community detection in social network. *Internet of Things and Applications (IOTA), International Conference on*, 162–167. 10.1109/IOTA.2016.7562715

Behera, R. K., Jena, M., Rath, S. K., & Misra, S. (2021). Co-LSTM: Convolutional LSTM model for sentiment analysis in social big data. *Information Processing & Management*, *58*(1), 102435. doi:10.1016/j.ipm.2020.102435

Behera, R. K., Sahoo, K. S., Mahapatra, S., Rath, S. K., & Sahoo, B. (2018). Security issues in distributed computation for big data analytics. In *Handbook of e-Business Security* (pp. 167–190). Auerbach Publications. doi:10.1201/9780429468254-7

Behera, R. K., Sahoo, K. S., Naik, D., Rath, S. K., & Sahoo, B. (2021). Structural Mining for Link Prediction Using Various Machine Learning Algorithms. *International Journal of Social Ecology and Sustainable Development*, *12*(3), 66–78. doi:10.4018/IJSESD.2021070105

Beigi, E. B., Jazi, H., Stakhanova, N., & Ghorbani, A. A. (2014). *Towards Effective Feature Selection in Machine Learning-Based Botnet Detection Approaches*. doi:10.1109/CNS.2014.6997492

Belgacem, A., Beghdad-Bey, K., & Nacer, H. (2018). Task scheduling in cloud computing environment: A comprehensive analysis. In *International Conference on Computer Science and its Applications*. Springer.

Belhumeur, P. N., Hespanha, J. P., & Kriegman, D. J. (1997). Eigenfaces vs. Fisherfaces: Recognition using class specific linear projection. *IEEE Transactions on Pattern Analysis and Machine Intelligence*, *19*(7), 711–720. doi:10.1109/34.598228

Benchamardimath, B., & Hegadi, R. (2012). *Graph Theoretical Approaches for Image Segmentation*. Academic Press.

Benedetti, P., Femminella, M., Reali, G., & Steenhaut, K. (2021). Experimental analysis of the application of serverless computing to IoT platforms. *Sensors (Basel)*, *21*(3), 928. doi:10.339021030928 PMID:33573209

Benjaafar, S., Li, Y., & Daskin, M. (2013). Carbon footprint and the management of supply chains: Insights from simple models. *IEEE Transactions on Automation Science and Engineering*, *10*(1), 99–116. doi:10.1109/TASE.2012.2203304

Berkaya, S. K., Uysal, A. K., Gunal, E. S., Ergin, S., Gunal, S., & Gulmezoglu, M. B. (2018). A survey on ECG analysis. *Biomedical Signal Processing and Control*, *43*, 216–235. doi:10.1016/j.bspc.2018.03.003

Berntzen, M., Hoda, R., Moe, N. B., & Stray, V. (2022). A Taxonomy of Inter-Team Coordination Mechanisms in Large-Scale Agile. IEEE Transactions on Software Engineering. doi:10.1109/TSE.2022.3160873

Bezerra, A., Silva, I., Guedes, L. A., Silva, D., Leitão, G., & Saito, K. (2019). Extracting value from industrial alarms and events: A data-driven approach based on exploratory data analysis. *Sensors (Switzerland)*, *19*(12), 2772. Advance online publication. doi:10.339019122772 PMID:31226811

Bhanipati, J., Singh, D., Biswal, A. K., & Rout, S. K. (2021). Minimization of Collision Through Retransmission and Optimal Power Allocation in Wireless Sensor Networks (WSNs). In *Advances in Intelligent Computing and Communication* (pp. 653–665). Springer.

Bhardwaj, H., Bhatia, K., Jain, A., & Verma, N. (2021, July). IOT Based Health Monitoring System. In *2021 6th International Conference on Communication and Electronics Systems (ICCES)* (pp. 1-6). IEEE.

Bhatia. (2021). Fog Computing-inspired Smart Home Framework for Predictive Veterinary Healthcare. *Microprocessors and Microsystems*, *78*, 10322.

Bhatti, M. M., & Rashidi, M. M. (2017). Study of heat and mass transfer with joule heating on magnetohydrodynamic (MHD) peristaltic blood flow under the influence of hall effect. *Propulsion and Power Research*, *6*(3), 177–185. doi:10.1016/j.jppr.2017.07.006

Bianchi, L., Dorigo, M., Gambardella, L. M., & Gutjahr, W. J. (2009). A survey on metaheuristics for stochastic combinatorial optimization. *Natural Computing*, *8*(2), 239–287. doi:10.100711047-008-9098-4

Bianchi, M. J., Conforto, E. C., Rebentisch, E., Amaral, D. C., Rezende, S. O., & de Padua, R. (2021). Recommendation of Project Management Practices: A Contribution to Hybrid Models. *IEEE Transactions on Engineering Management*, *00*(X), 1–14. doi:10.1109/TEM.2021.3101179

Bianconi, F., & Fernández, A. (2011). On the Occurrence Probability of Local Binary Patterns: A Theoretical Study. *Journal of Mathematical Imaging and Vision*, *40*(3), 259–268. doi:10.100710851-011-0261-7

Bibiks, K., Hu, Y. F., Li, J. P., Pillai, P., & Smith, A. (2018). Improved discrete cuckoo search for the resource-constrained project scheduling problem. *Applied Soft Computing*, *69*, 493–503. doi:10.1016/j.asoc.2018.04.047

Bienko, C. D., Greenstein, M., Holt, S. E., Phillips, R. T., & ... (2015). *IBM Cloudant: Database as a Service Advanced Topics*. IBM Redbooks.

Bila, N., Dettori, P., Kanso, A., Watanabe, Y., & Youssef, A. (2017). Leveraging the serverless architecture for securing linux containers. *2017 IEEE 37th International Conference on Distributed Computing Systems Workshops (ICDCSW)*, 401–404. 10.1109/ICDCSW.2017.66

Binh, H. T. T., Anh, T. T., Son, D. B., Duc, P. A., & Nguyen, B. M. (2018, December). An evolutionary algorithm for solving task scheduling problem in cloud-fog computing environment. In *Proceedings of the ninth international symposium on information and communication technology* (pp. 397-404). 10.1145/3287921.3287984

Bin, X., Jiajun, B., Chen, C., Wang, C., Cai, D., & He, X. (2013). EMR: A scalable graph-based ranking model for content-based image retrieval. *IEEE Transactions on Knowledge and Data Engineering*, *27*(1), 102–114.

Biswal, A. K., Singh, D., & Pattanayak, B. K. (2021). IoT-Based Voice-Controlled Energy-Efficient Intelligent Traffic and Street Light Monitoring System. In *Green Technology for Smart City and Society* (pp. 43–54). Springer.

Biswal, A. K., Singh, D., Pattanayak, B. K., Samanta, D., Chaudhry, S. A., & Irshad, A. (2021). Adaptive fault-tolerant system and optimal power allocation for smart vehicles in smart cities using controller area network. *Security and Communication Networks*.

Biswal, A. K., Singh, D., Pattanayak, B. K., Samanta, D., & Yang, M. H. (2021). IoT-Based Smart Alert System for Drowsy Driver Detection. *Wireless Communications and Mobile Computing*, 2021.

Bo, C., Zhang, L., Jung, T., Han, J., Li, X.-Y., & Wang, Y. (2014, December). Continuous user identification via touch and movement behavioral biometrics. *2014 IEEE 33rd International Performance Computing and Communications Conference (IPCCC)*. http://dx.doi.org/10.1109/pccc.2014.7017067

Bo, C., Zhang, L., Li, X.-Y., Huang, Q., & Wang, Y. (2013). SilentSense. *Proceedings of the 19th Annual International Conference on Mobile Computing & Networking - MobiCom '13*. http://dx.doi.org/10.1145/2500423.2504572

Bondada, P., Samanta, D., Kaur, M., & Lee, H.-N. (2022). Data Security-Based Routing in MANETs Using Key Management Mechanism. *Applied Sciences (Basel, Switzerland)*, *12*(3), 1041. doi:10.3390/app12031041

Bonneau, J., Herley, C., van Oorschot, P. C., & Stajano, F. (2015). Passwords and the evolution of imperfect authentication. *Communications of the ACM*, *58*(7), 78–87. doi:10.1145/2699390

Bonney, M., & Jaber, M. Y. (2011). Environmentally responsible inventory models: Non-classical models for a non-classical era. *International Journal of Production Economics*, *133*(1), 43–53. doi:10.1016/j.ijpe.2009.10.033

Bontempi, G., Taieb, S. B., & Le Borgne, Y. A. (2012, July). Machine learning strategies for time series forecasting. In *European business intelligence summer school* (pp. 62–77). Springer.

Bouchery, Y., Ghaffari, A., Jemai, Z., & Dallery, Y. (2012). Including sustainability criteria into inventory models. *European Journal of Operational Research*, *222*(2), 229–240. doi:10.1016/j.ejor.2012.05.004

Boykov, Y., & Funka-Lea, G. (2006). Graph Cuts and Efficient N-D Image Segmentation. *International Journal of Computer Vision*, *70*, 109–131. https://doi.org/10.1007/s11263-006-7934-5

Breiman, L. (2001). Random forests. *Machine Learning*, *45*(1), 5–32. doi:10.1023/A:1010933404324

Brenner, M. P., Eldredge, J. D., & Freund, J. B. (2019). Perspective on machine learning for advancing fluid mechanics. *Physical Review Fluids*, *4*(10), 100501. doi:10.1103/PhysRevFluids.4.100501

Brenner, S., & Kapitza, R. (2019). Trust more, serverless. *Proceedings of the 12th ACM International Conference on Systems and Storage*, 33–43. 10.1145/3319647.3325825

Brikman, Y. (2019). *Terraform: Up & Running: Writing Infrastructure as Code*. O'Reilly Media.

Brogi, A., & Forti, S. (2017). QoS-aware deployment of IoT applications through the fog. *IEEE Internet of Things Journal*, *4*(5), 1185–1192. doi:10.1109/JIOT.2017.2701408

Brunelli, R., & Poggio, T. (1993). Face recognition: Features versus templates. *IEEE Transactions on Pattern Analysis and Machine Intelligence*, *15*(10), 1042–1052. doi:10.1109/34.254061

Buongiorno, J. (2006). Convective transport in nanofluids. *Journal of Heat Transfer*, *128*(3), 240–250. doi:10.1115/1.2150834

Buriro, A., Gupta, S., Yautsiukhin, A., & Crispo, B. (2021). Risk-Driven behavioral biometric-based one-shot-cum-continuous user authentication scheme. *Journal of Signal Processing Systems for Signal, Image, and Video Technology*, *93*(9), 989–1006. doi:10.100711265-021-01654-2

Cabarcos, P. A., & Krupitzer, C. (2017). On the Design of Distributed Adaptive Authentication Systems. *Thirteenth Symposium on Usable Privacy and Security (SOUPS 2017)*. https://www.usenix.org/conference/soups2017/workshop-program/way2017/arias-cabarcos

Cabestany, J., Rodriguez-Martín, D., Pérez, C., & Sama, A. (2018). Artificial Intelligence Contribution to eHealth applications. *2018 25th International Conference "Mixed Design of Integrated Circuits and System" (MIXDES)*. 10.23919/MIXDES.2018.8436743

California Consumer Privacy Act (CCPA). (2018, October 15). State of California - Department of Justice - Office of the Attorney General. https://oag.ca.gov/privacy/ccpa

Cao, L. (2017). Data science: A comprehensive overview. *ACM Computing Surveys*, *50*(3), 1–42. Advance online publication. doi:10.1145/3076253

Carbonell, J. G., Michalski, R. S., & Mitchell, T. M. (1983). An overview of machine learning. *Machine Learning*, 3–23.

Carreira, J., Fonseca, P., Tumanov, A., Zhang, A., & Katz, R. (2018). A case for serverless machine learning. *Workshop on Systems for ML and Open-Source Software at NeurIPS*.

Centre, N. C. S. (2019, April 15). *Cloud security guidance*. National Cyber Security Centre. https://www.ncsc.gov.uk/collection/cloud-security/implementing-the-cloud-security-principles/identity-and-authentication

Chakir, F., & Rachid, E. (2020). Machine Learning and Deep Learning applications in E-learning Systems: A Literature Survey using Topic Modeling Approach. *2020 6th IEEE Congress on Information Science and Technology (CiSt)*, 267-273. https://ieeexplore.ieee.org/xpl/conhome/9357063/proceeding

Chakkaravarthy, S. S., Sangeetha, D., & Vaidehi, V. (2019). A survey on malware analysis and mitigation techniques. *Computer Science Review, 32*, 1–23. doi:10.1016/j.cosrev.2019.01.002

Chakrabarti, T., & Chaudhuri, K. S. (1997). An EOQ model for deteriorating items with a linear trend in demand and shortages in all cycles. *International Journal of Production Economics, 49*(3), 205–213. doi:10.1016/S0925-5273(96)00015-1

Chakraborty, D., Saha, S. K., & Bhuiyan, M. A. (2012). Face Recognition using Eigenvector and Principle Component Analysis. *International Journal of Computers and Applications, 50*(10), 42–49. doi:10.5120/7811-0947

Chakraborty, M., Dhavale, S. V., & Ingole, J. (2020). Corona-nidaan: Lightweight deep convolutional neural network for chest x-ray based covid-19 infection detection. *Applied Intelligence*. Advance online publication. doi:10.100710489-020-01978-9 PMID:34764582

Chang, C., Srirama, S. N., & Buyya, R. (2017). Indie fog: An efficient fog-computing infrastructure for the internet of things. *Computer, 50*(9), 92–98. doi:10.1109/MC.2017.3571049

Chaudhuri, B., Demir, B., Chaudhuri, S., & Bruzzone, L. (2018, February). Multilabel Remote Sensing Image Retrieval Using a Semisupervised Graph-Theoretic Method. *IEEE Transactions on Geoscience and Remote Sensing, 56*(2), 1144–1158. doi:10.1109/TGRS.2017.2760909

Chauhan, A., Jakhar, S. K., & Chauhan, C. (2021). The interplay of circular economy with industry 4.0 enabled smart city drivers of healthcare waste disposal. *Journal of Cleaner Production, 279*, 123854. doi:10.1016/j.jclepro.2020.123854 PMID:32863607

Chauhan, J., Hu, Y., Seneviratne, S., Misra, A., Seneviratne, A., & Lee, Y. (2017, June 16). BreathPrint. *Proceedings of the 15th Annual International Conference on Mobile Systems, Applications, and Services*. 10.1145/3081333.3081355

Chawla, M. P. S. (2011). PCA and ICA processing methods for removal of artifacts and noise in electrocardiograms: A survey and comparison. *Applied Soft Computing, 11*(2), 2216–2226. doi:10.1016/j.asoc.2010.08.001

Chellappa, R., Wilson, C. L., & Sirohey, S. (1995). Human and machine recognition of faces: A survey. *Proceedings of the IEEE, 83*(5), 705–741. doi:10.1109/5.381842

Cheng, B., Fuerst, J., Solmaz, G., & Sanada, T. (2019). Fog function: Serverless fog computing for data intensive iot services. *2019 IEEE International Conference on Services Computing (SCC)*, 28–35. 10.1109/SCC.2019.00018

Chen, J., Ramanathan, L., & Alazab, M. (2021). Holistic big data integrated artificial intelligent modeling to improve privacy and security in data management of smart cities. *Microprocessors and Microsystems, 81*, 103722. doi:10.1016/j.micpro.2020.103722

Chen, M., Hao, Y., Hwang, K., Wang, L., & Wang, L. (2017). Disease prediction by machine learning over big data from healthcare communities. *IEEE Access: Practical Innovations, Open Solutions, 5*, 8869–8879.

Chen, Q., & Lu, Y. (2018). Construction and application effect evaluation of integrated management platform of intelligent hospital based on big data analysis. *Chin. Med. Herald., 15*(35), 161–164.

Chen, X., Benjaafar, S., & Elomri, A. (2013). The carbon-constrained EOQ. *Operations Research Letters, 41*(2), 172–179. doi:10.1016/j.orl.2012.12.003

Chen, X., Ma, M., & Liu, A. (2018). Dynamic power management and adaptive packet size selection for IoT in e-Healthcare. *Computers & Electrical Engineering, 65*, 357–375.

Chen, X., & Pan, L. (2018). A Survey of Graph Cuts/Graph Search Based Medical Image Segmentation. *IEEE Reviews in Biomedical Engineering, 11*, 112–124. doi:10.1109/RBME.2018.2798701 PMID:29994356

Chen, Y., Sun, J., Zhang, R., & Zhang, Y. (2015, April). Your song your way: Rhythm-based two-factor authentication for multi-touch mobile devices. *2015 IEEE Conference on Computer Communications (INFOCOM).* 10.1109/INFO-COM.2015.7218660

Cheung, G., Magli, E., Tanaka, Y., & Ng, M. K. (2018, May). Graph Spectral Image Processing. *Proceedings of the IEEE, 106*(5), 907–930. doi:10.1109/JPROC.2018.2799702

Chiasson, S. (2009). *Usable authentication and click-based graphical passwords.* Carleton University. http://dx.doi.org/doi:10.22215/etd/2009-06388

Chiroma, H., Herawan, T., Fister, I. Jr, Fister, I., Abdulkareem, S., Shuib, L., Hamza, M. F., Saadi, Y., & Abubakar, A. (2017). Bio-inspired computation: Recent development on the modifications of the cuckoo search algorithm. *Applied Soft Computing, 61*, 149–173. doi:10.1016/j.asoc.2017.07.053

Chitaliya, N. G., & Trivedi, A. L. (2010). An Efficient Method for Face Feature Extraction and Recognition based on Contourlet Transform and Principal Component Analysis using Neural Network. *International Journal of Computers and Applications, 6*(4), 28–34. doi:10.5120/1066-1260

Chitara, D., Niazi, K. R., Swarnkar, A., & Gupta, N. (2018). Cuckoo search optimization algorithm for designing of multimachine power system stabilizer. *IEEE Transactions on Industry Applications, 54*(4), 3056–3065. doi:10.1109/TIA.2018.2811725

Choi, S. U. S., & Eastman, J. A. (1995). *Enhancing thermal conductivity of fluids with nanoparticles (No. ANL/MSD/CP-84938; CONF-951135-29).* Argonne National Lab.

Choi, W., Seo, M., & Lee, D. H. (2018). Sound-Proximity: 2-Factor authentication against relay attack on passive keyless entry and start system. *Journal of Advanced Transportation, 2018*, 1–13. doi:10.1155/2018/1935974

Choi, Y., Lee, Y., Moon, J., & Won, D. (2017). Security enhanced multi-factor biometric authentication scheme using bio-hash function. *PLoS One, 12*(5), e0176250. doi:10.1371/journal.pone.0176250 PMID:28459867

Christoforou, A., & Andreou, A. S. (2018). An effective resource management approach in a FaaS environment. ESSCA@ UCC, 2–8.

Chua, K. J., Ho, J. C., Chou, S. K., & Islam, M. R. (2005). On the study of the temperature distribution within a human eye subjected to a laser source. *International Communications in Heat and Mass Transfer, 32*(8), 1057–1065. doi:10.1016/j.icheatmasstransfer.2004.10.030

Chung, I. M., Kim, J. K., Lee, K. J., Park, S. K., Lee, J. H., Son, N. Y., Jin, Y.-I., & Kim, S. H. (2018). Geographic authentication of Asian rice (Oryza sativa L.) using multi-elemental and stable isotopic data combined with multivariate analysis. *Food Chemistry, 240*, 840–849. doi:10.1016/j.foodchem.2017.08.023 PMID:28946350

Cisco. (2019). *Role of IoT healthcare. HIMSS Analytics Infrastructure Adoption Model (INFRAM) At-a-Glance.* cisco.com

Cleff, T. (2014). *Exploratory Data Analysis in Business and Economics.* doi:10.1007/978-3-319-01517-0

Clifton, A., Kilcher, L., Lundquist, J. K., & Fleming, P. (2013). Using machine learning to predict wind turbine power output. *Environmental Research Letters, 8*(2), 024009. doi:10.1088/1748-9326/8/2/024009

Coelho, C., Coelho, D., & Wolf, M. (2015). An IoT smart home architecture for long-term care of people with special needs. *2015 IEEE 2nd World Forum on internet of things (WF-IoT).* 10.1109/WF-IoT.2015.7389126

Coelho, L. S., Guerra, F., Batistela, N. J., & Leite, J. V. (2013). Multiobjective cuckoo search algorithm based on Duffing's oscillator applied to Jiles-Atherton vector hysteresis parameters estimation. *IEEE Transactions on Magnetics*, *49*(5), 1745–1748. doi:10.1109/TMAG.2013.2243907

Condoluci, M. (2016). Enabling the IoT machine age with 5G: Machine-type multicast services for innovative real-time applications. *IEEE Access: Practical Innovations, Open Solutions*, *4*, 5555–5569.

Conoscenti, M., Vetrò, A., & De Martin, J. C. (2017). Peer to Peer for Privacy and Decentralization in the internet of Things. *2017 IEEE/ACM 39th International Conference on Software Engineering Companion (ICSE-C)*. 10.1109/ICSE-C.2017.60

Covert, R. P., & Philip, G. C. (1973). An EOQ model for items with Weibull distribution deterioration. *AIIE Transactions*, *5*(4), 323–326. doi:10.1080/05695557308974918

Crespo-Cepeda, R., Agapito, G., Vazquez-Poletti, J. L., & Cannataro, M. (2019). Challenges and opportunities of amazon serverless lambda services in bioinformatics. *Proceedings of the 10th ACM International Conference on Bioinformatics, Computational Biology and Health Informatics*, 663–668. 10.1145/3307339.3343462

Cruz-Duarte, J. M., Garcia-Perez, A., Amaya-Contreras, I. M., Correa-Cely, C. R., Romero-Troncoso, R. J., & Avina-Cervantes, J. G. (2017). Design of microelectronic cooling systems using a thermodynamic optimization strategy based on cuckoo search. *IEEE Transactions on Components, Packaging, and Manufacturing Technology*, *7*(11), 1804–1812. doi:10.1109/TCPMT.2017.2706305

Cui, J., Zhang, P., Li, S., Zheng, L., Bao, C., Xia, J., & Li, X. (2021). Multitask Identity-Aware Image Steganography via Minimax Optimization. *IEEE Transactions on Image Processing*, *30*, 8567–8579. doi:10.1109/TIP.2021.3107999 PMID:34469298

Cusumano, M. (2010). Cloud computing and SaaS as new computing platforms. *Communications of the ACM*, *53*(4), 27–29. doi:10.1145/1721654.1721667

da Rosa Mesquita, R., Francelino Silva, L. C. Jr, Santos Santana, F. M., Farias de Oliveira, T., Campos Alcântara, R., Monteiro Arnozo, G., ... Freire de Souza, C. D. (2021). Clinical manifestations of COVID-19 in the general population: Systematic review. *Wiener Klinische Wochenschrift*, *133*(7), 377–382. doi:10.100700508-020-01760-4 PMID:33242148

Dadashi Gavaber, M., & Rajabzadeh, A. (2021). MFP: An approach to delay and energy-efficient module placement in IoT applications based on multi-fog. *Journal of Ambient Intelligence and Humanized Computing*, *12*(7), 7965–7981. doi:10.100712652-020-02525-7

Dalal & Juneja. (2021). Steganography and Steganalysis (in Digital Forensics): A Cybersecurity Guide. *Multimedia Tools and Applications, 80*(4), 5723–71. . doi:10.1007/s11042-020-09929-9

Dalbhanjan, P. (2015). *Overview of deployment options on aws*. Amazon Whitepapers.

Dalgarno, B., & Lee, M. J. (2010). What are the learning affordances of 3-D virtual environments? *British Journal of Educational Technology*, *41*(1), 10–32.

Dam, S. (2018). An ant-colony-based meta-heuristic approach for load balancing in cloud computing. In *Applied Computational Intelligence and Soft Computing in Engineering* (pp. 204–232). IGI Global.

Dananjayan & Raj. (2021). 5G in healthcare: How fast will be the transformation? *Irish Journal of Medical Science*, *190*(2), 497-501.

Das, A., Bonneau, J., Caesar, M., Borisov, N., & Wang, X. (2014). The tangled web of password reuse. *Proceedings 2014 Network and Distributed System Security Symposium*. 10.14722/ndss.2014.23357

Dasgupta, D., Roy, A., & Nag, A. (2016). Toward the design of adaptive selection strategies for multi-factor authentication. *Computers & Security, 63*, 85–116. doi:10.1016/j.cose.2016.09.004

Dash, R. (2017). A two stage grading approach for feature selection and classification of microarray data using Pareto based feature ranking techniques: A case study. *Journal of King Saud University-Computer and Information Sciences.*

Dash, R. (2018). An adaptive harmony search approach for gene selection and classification of high dimensional medical data. *Journal of King Saud University-Computer and Information Sciences.*

Dash, R., Dash, R., & Rautray, R. (2019). An evolutionary framework based microarray gene selection and classification approach using binary shuffled frog leaping algorithm. *Journal of King Saud University-Computer and Information Sciences.*

Dash, R., & Misra, B. (2017). Gene selection and classification of microarray data: A Pareto DE approach. *Intelligent Decision Technologies, 11*(1), 93–107. doi:10.3233/IDT-160280

Dash, R., & Misra, B. B. (2016). Pipelining the ranking techniques for microarray data classification: A case study. *Applied Soft Computing, 48*, 298–316. doi:10.1016/j.asoc.2016.07.006

Dash, R., & Misra, B. B. (2018). Performance analysis of clustering techniques over microarray data: A case study. *Physica A, 493*, 162–176. doi:10.1016/j.physa.2017.10.032

Das, S. K., Choi, S. U., Yu, W., & Pradeep, T. (2007). *Nanofluids: Science and Technology.* Willey. doi:10.1002/9780470180693

Datta, S. K., Bonnet, C., & Nikaein, N. (2014, March). An IoT gateway centric architecture to provide novel M2M services. In *2014 IEEE World Forum on Internet of Things (WF-IoT)* (pp. 514-519). IEEE.

Datta, T. K. (2017). Effect of a green technology investment on a production-inventory system with carbon tax. Advances in operations research, 2017. *Article ID, 4834839*, 1–12.

Daugman, J. (2016). Information theory and the iriscode. *IEEE Transactions on Information Forensics and Security, 11*(2), 400–409. doi:10.1109/TIFS.2015.2500196

Daugman, J. G. (1980). Two-dimensional spectral analysis of cortical receptive field profiles. *Vision Research, 20*(10), 847–856. doi:10.1016/0042-6989(80)90065-6 PMID:7467139

Davenport & Kalakota. (2019). The potential for artificial intelligence in healthcare. *Future Healthcare Journal, 6*(2), 94.

Davidson, S. R. H., & James, D. F. (2003). Drilling in bone: Modeling heat generation and temperature distribution. *Journal of Biomechanical Engineering, 125*(3), 305–314. doi:10.1115/1.1535190 PMID:12929234

Davis, E. A., Keating, B., Byrne, G. C., Russell, M., & Jones, T. W. (1997). Hypoglycemia: Incidence and clinical predictors in a large population-based sample of children and adolescents with IDDM. *Diabetes Care, 20*(1), 22–25. doi:10.2337/diacare.20.1.22 PMID:9028688

Dawod, Georgakopoulos, Jayaraman, & Nirmalathas. (2019). Advancements towards Global IoT devices Discovery and Integration. *2019 IEEE International Congress on Internet of Things (ICIOT).*

De Silva, H. L. S. R. P., Wittebron, D. C., Lahiru, A. M. R., Madumadhavi, K. L., Rupasinghe, L., & Abeywardena, K. Y. (2019). AuthDNA: An Adaptive Authentication Service for any Identity Server. *2019 International Conference on Advancements in Computing (ICAC)*, 369–375. 10.1109/ICAC49085.2019.9103382

Demšar, J. (2006). Statistical comparisons of classifiers over multiple data sets. *Journal of Machine Learning Research, 7*(Jan), 1–30.

Deng, S., Xiang, Z., Taheri, J., Khoshkholghi, M. A., Yin, J., Zomaya, A. Y., & Dustdar, S. (2020). Optimal application deployment in resource constrained distributed edges. *IEEE Transactions on Mobile Computing, 20*(5), 1907–1923. doi:10.1109/TMC.2020.2970698

Deng, X., Sun, T., Liu, F., & Li, D. (2022, February). SignGD with error feedback meets lazily aggregated technique: Communication-efficient algorithms for distributed learning. *Tsinghua Science and Technology, 27*(1), 174–185. doi:10.26599/TST.2021.9010045

De, S. K., & Mahata, G. (2019). A cloudy fuzzy economic order quantity model for imperfect-quality items with allowable proportionate discounts. *Journal of Industrial Engineering International, 15*(4), 571–583. doi:10.100740092-019-0310-1

Devi, S. A., & Ganga, B. (2009). Effects of viscous and Joules dissipation on MHD flow, heat and mass transfer past a stretching porous surface embedded in a porous medium. *Nonlinear Analysis (Vilnius), 14*(3), 303–314. doi:10.15388/NA.2009.14.3.14497

Dewangan, K., & Mishra, M. (2018). Internet of things for healthcare: A review. *International Journal of Advanced in Management. Technology and Engineering Sciences, 8*(3), 526–534.

Dey, J. K., Mukherjee, A., Dey, S. K., Udayat, M. P., Pramanik, A., & Giri, S. (2020). *An assessment of the efficacies and therapeutic interventions of homoeopathic medicines in combating viral disorders with implications in the treatment of SARS-CoV-2 (Covid-19), a global pandemic.* Academic Press.

Dhanwant, J. N., & Ramanathan, V. (2020). *Forecasting covid 19 growth in india using susceptible-infected-recovered (sir) model.* arXiv preprint arXiv:2004.00696.

Dhawan, S., Chakraborty, C., Frnda, J., Gupta, R., Rana, A. K., & Pani, S. K. (2021). SSII: Secured and High-Quality Steganography Using Intelligent Hybrid Optimization Algorithms for IoT. *IEEE Access: Practical Innovations, Open Solutions, 9*, 87563–87578. doi:10.1109/ACCESS.2021.3089357

Dhiman, S., & Singh, O. (2016). Analysis of Visible and Invisible Image Watermarking - A Review. *International Journal of Computers and Applications, 147*(3), 975–8887. doi:10.5120/ijca2016911055

Dibia, V., & Demiralp, Ç. (2019). Data2Vis: Automatic Generation of Data Visualizations Using Sequence-to-Sequence Recurrent Neural Networks. *IEEE Computer Graphics and Applications, 39*(5), 33–46. doi:10.1109/MCG.2019.2924636 PMID:31247545

Dickinson, S., Pelillo, M., & Zabih, R. (2001). Introduction to the special section on graph algorithms in computer vision. Pattern Analysis and Machine Intelligence. *IEEE Transactions on., 23*, 1049–1052. doi:10.1109/TPAMI.2001.954597

Ding, X., Xie, Y., Li, P., Cui, M., & Chen, J. (2020). Image Steganography Based on Artificial Immune in Mobile Edge Computing With Internet of Things. *IEEE Access: Practical Innovations, Open Solutions, 8*, 136186–136197. doi:10.1109/ACCESS.2020.3010513

Dixit, A., & Dixit, R. (2017). A Review on Digital Image Watermarking Techniques. International Journal of Image, Graphics &. *Signal Processing, 9*(4), 56–66. doi:10.5815/ijigsp.2017.04.07

Dokeroglu, T., Sevinc, E., Kucukyilmaz, T., & Cosar, A. (2019). A survey on new generation metaheuristic algorithms. *Computers & Industrial Engineering, 137*, 106040. doi:10.1016/j.cie.2019.106040

Dong, E., Du, H., & Gardner, L. (2020). An interactive web-based dashboard to track COVID-19 in real time. *The Lancet. Infectious Diseases, 20*(5), 533–534.

Dong, P., Ning, Z., Obaidat, M. S., Jiang, X., Guo, Y., Hu, X., Hu, B., & Sadoun, B. (2020, September/October). Edge Computing Based Healthcare Systems: Enabling Decentralized Health Monitoring in Internet of Medical Things. *IEEE Network, 34*(5), 254–261. doi:10.1109/MNET.011.1900636

Dorigo, M., Maniezzo, V., & Colorni, A. (1996). Ant system: Optimization by a colony of cooperating agents. *IEEE Transactions on Systems, Man, and Cybernetics. Part B, Cybernetics, 26*(1), 29–41. doi:10.1109/3477.484436 PMID:18263004

Dorota, O. (2021). *Applying Design Thinking to Artificial Intelligence. Why should you use it in your AI-based projects?* https://nexocode.com/blog/posts/applying-design-thinking-to-ai/

Dorothee, D., Reinhard, H., Julia, H., & Olga, K. (2004). Assessment of glycemic control by continuous glucose monitoring system in 50 children with type 1 diabetes starting on insulin pump therapy. *Pediatric Diabetes, 5*(3), 117–121. doi:10.1111/j.1399-543X.2004.00053.x PMID:15450005

dos Santos, D. R., Westphall, C. M., & Westphall, C. B. (2014, May). A dynamic risk-based access control architecture for cloud computing. *2014 IEEE Network Operations and Management Symposium (NOMS)*, 1-9. 10.1109/NOMS.2014.6838319

Doukas, C., & Maglogiannis, I. (2012, July). Bringing IoT and cloud computing towards pervasive healthcare. In *2012 Sixth International Conference on Innovative Mobile and Internet Services in Ubiquitous Computing* (pp. 922-926). IEEE. 10.1109/IMIS.2012.26

Dowell, D., Haegerich, T. M., & Chou, R. (2016). CDC guideline for prescribing opioids for chronic pain—United States, 2016. *Journal of the American Medical Association, 315*(15), 1624–1645.

Drury, M., Conboy, K., & Power, K. (2011). Decision making in agile development: A focus group study of decisions & obstacles. *Proceedings - 2011 Agile Conference, Agile 2011*, 39–47. 10.1109/AGILE.2011.27

Duc, B., Fischer, S., & Bign, J. (1999). Face Authentication with Gabor Information on Deformable Graphs. *IEEE Transactions on Image Processing, 8*(4), 504–516. doi:10.1109/83.753738 PMID:18262894

Eapen, N. G., Rao, A. R., Samanta, D., Robert, N. R., Krishnamoorthy, R., & Lokesh, G. H. (2022). *Security Aspects for Mutation Testing in Mobile Applications. Στο Cyber Intelligence and Information Retrieval*. Springer.

Eberhart, R., & Kennedy, J. (1995, November). Particle swarm optimization. In *Proceedings of the IEEE international conference on neural networks* (Vol. 4, pp. 1942-1948). IEEE.

Eda, W. (2006). 1. Exploratory Data Analysis 1. Exploratory Data Analysis - Detailed Table of Contents. *Analysis, 1*(4), 5728–5731. https://www.ncbi.nlm.nih.gov/pubmed/21097328

Eden Estopace.(2019). *Growth of IoT devices IDC forecasts connected IoT devices to generate 79.4ZB of data in 2025 – FutureIoT*. Author.

Edwards, J., Pattision, E. P., Jackson, H. J., & Wales, R. J. (2001). Facial affect and affective prosody recognition in first-episode schizophrenia. *Schizophrenia Research, 48*(2-3), 235–253. doi:10.1016/S0920-9964(00)00099-2 PMID:11295377

El, O. B., Milo, T., & Somech, A. (2020). Towards Autonomous, Hands-Free Data Exploration. *Cidr.* https://www.tablcau.com

Eldefrawy, M. H., Khan, M. K., Alghathbar, K., Kim, T.-H., & Elkamchouchi, H. (2011). Mobile one-time passwords: Two-factor authentication using mobile phones. *Security and Communication Networks, 5*(5), 508–516. doi:10.1002ec.340

Eleccion, M. (1973). Automatic fingerprint identification. *IEEE Spectrum, 10*(9), 36–45. doi:10.1109/MSPEC.1973.5212832

Elhoseny, M. (2018). Secure medical data transmission model for IoT-based healthcare systems. *IEEE Access: Practical Innovations, Open Solutions, 6*, 20596–20608.

El-Khamy, S. E., Korany, N. O., & Mohamed, A. G. (2020). A New Fuzzy-DNA Image Encryption and Steganography Technique. *IEEE Access: Practical Innovations, Open Solutions, 8*, 148935–148951. doi:10.1109/ACCESS.2020.3015687

Elmagzoub, M. (2021). A Survey of Swarm Intelligence Based Load Balancing Techniques in Cloud Computing Environment. *Electronics (Basel), 10*(21), 2718.

Elmisery, A. M., Rho, S., & Aborizka, M. (2019). A new computing environment for collective privacy protection from constrained healthcare devices to IoT cloud services. *Cluster Computing, 22*(1), 1611–1638. doi:10.100710586-017-1298-1

Elshoush, H. T. (2022). A New High Capacity and Secure Image Realization Steganography Based on ASCII Code Matching. *Multimedia Tools and Applications, 81*(4), 5191–237. . doi:10.1007/s11042-021-11741-y

Eremin, A., & Kogos, K. (2018). Incoming call implicit user authentication - User authentication via hand movement pattern. *Proceedings of the 4th International Conference on Information Systems Security and Privacy.* 10.5220/0006555200240029

Ernest, Y.B., & Daniel, A. (2019). A Review of the Logistic Regression Model with Emphasis on Medical Research. *Journal of Data Analysis and Information Processing*, 190-207.

Ertekin, S., Bottou, L., & Giles, C. L. (2011, February). Nonconvex Online Support Vector Machines. *IEEE Transactions on Pattern Analysis and Machine Intelligence, 33*(2), 368–381. doi:10.1109/TPAMI.2010.109 PMID:20513924

EU General Data Protection Regulation (GDPR): Regulation (EU) 2016/679 of the European Parliament and of the Council of 27 April 2016 on the protection of natural persons with regard to the processing of personal data and on the free movement of such data, and repealing Directive 95/46/EC (General Data Protection Regulation), OJ 2016 L 119/1

Eyssa, A. A. (2020). An Efficient Image Steganography Approach over Wireless Communication System. *Wireless Personal Communications, 110*(1), 321–37. . doi:10.1007/s11277-019-06730-2

Fanelli, D., & Piazza, F. (2020). Analysis and forecast of COVID-19 spreading in China, Italy and France. *Chaos, Solitons, and Fractals, 134*, 109761.

Fan, Q., & Ansari, N. (2018). Application aware workload allocation for edge computing-based IoT. *IEEE Internet of Things Journal, 5*(3), 2146–2153. doi:10.1109/JIOT.2018.2826006

Farahani, B., Firouzi, F., Chang, V., Badaroglu, M., Constant, N., & Mankodiya, K. (2018). Towards fog-driven IoT eHealth: Promises and challenges of IoT in medicine and healthcare. *Future Generation Computer Systems, 78*, 659–676. doi:10.1016/j.future.2017.04.036

Farash, M. S. (2014). An improved password-based authentication scheme for session initiation protocol using smart cards without verification table. *International Journal of Communication Systems, 30*(1), e2879. doi:10.1002/dac.2879

Fares, K., Amine, K., & Salah, E. (2020). A robust blind color image watermarking based on Fourier transform domain. *Optik (Stuttgart), 208*, 164562. Advance online publication. doi:10.1016/j.ijleo.2020.164562

Farokhi, S., Shamsuddin, S. M., Flusser, J., Sheikh, U. U., Khansari, M., & Jafari-Khouzani, K. (2013). Rotation and noise invariant near-infrared face recognition by means of Zernike moments and spectral regression discriminant analysis. *Journal of Electronic Imaging, 22*(1), 1–11. doi:10.1117/1.JEI.22.1.013030

Fasel, I. R., Bartlett, M. S., & Movellan, J. R. (2002). A comparison of Gabor filter methods for automatic detection of facial landmarks. *Proceedings of Fifth IEEE international conference on automatic face gesture recognition*, 1-5. 10.1109/AFGR.2002.1004161

Fattah, J., Ezzine, L., Aman, Z., El Moussami, H., & Lachhab, A. (2018). Forecasting of demand using ARIMA model. *International Journal of Engineering Business Management*, *10*, 1847979018808673.

Fefie, D. (2009). From data to knowledge in e-health applications: An integrated system for medical information modelling and retrieval. *Medical Informatics and the Internet in Medicine*, 231–251. PMID:14668128

Fei, J., Yong, J., Hui, Z., Yi, D., Hao, L., Sufeng, M., Yilong, W., Qiang, D., Haipeng, S., & Yongjun, W. (2017). Artificial intelligence in healthcare: Past, present and future. *SVN Stroke and Vascular Neurology, BMJ Journals*. https://svn.bmj.com/content/2/4/230

Feig, D. S., Zinman, B., Wang, X., & Hux, J. E. (2008). Risk of development of diabetes mellitus after diagnosis of gestational diabetes. *Canadian Medical Association Journal*, *179*(3), 229–234. doi:10.1503/cmaj.080012 PMID:18663202

Feng, M. Q., Leung, R. Y., & Eckersley, C. M. (2020). Non-Contact vehicle Weigh-in-Motion using computer vision. *Measurement*, *153*, 107415. doi:10.1016/j.measurement.2019.107415

Feng, S., Liming, X., Fei, S., Dijia, W., Ying, W., Huan, Y., Huiting, J., Yaozong, G., He, S., & Dinggang, S. (2021). Large-scale screening of covid-19 from community acquired pneumonia using infection size-aware classification. *Physics in Medicine and Biology*. arXiv2003.09860v1

Feng, T., Zhao, X., DeSalvo, N., Gao, Z., Wang, X., & Shi, W. (2015, April). Security after login: Identity change detection on smartphones using sensor fusion. *2015 IEEE International Symposium on Technologies for Homeland Security (HST)*. 10.1109/THS.2015.7225268

Ferrara, A. (2007). Increasing prevalence of gestational diabetes mellitus: A public health perspective. *Diabetes Care*, *30*(2), S141–S146. doi:10.2337/dc07-s206 PMID:17596462

Fertleman, C. (2018). A discussion of virtual reality as a new tool for training healthcare professionals. *Frontiers in Public Health*, *6*, 44.

Fogel, G. B. (2005). IEEE symposium on computational intelligence in bioinformatics and computational biology (IEEE CIBCB 2005). *IEEE Computational Intelligence Magazine*, *1*(2), 43–44. doi:10.1109/MCI.2006.1626495

Fox, A., Griffith, R., Joseph, A., Katz, R., Konwinski, A., & Lee, G. (2009). *Above the clouds: A Berkeley view of cloud computing*. Dept. Electrical Eng. and Comput. Sciences, University of California, Berkeley, Rep. UCB/EECS, 28, 2009.

Fracastoro, G., Thanou, D., & Frossard, P. (2020). Graph Transform Optimization with Application to Image Compression. *IEEE Transactions on Image Processing*, *29*, 419–432. doi:10.1109/TIP.2019.2932853 PMID:31403414

Franssen, J., Pagnozzi, J., & Arrillaga, G.-P. (2018). RFID Technology for Management and Tracking: e-Health Applications. *Sensors (Basel)*, *18*(8).

Frew, R., Higgs, G., Harding, J., & Langford, M. (2017). Investigating geospatial data usability from a health geography perspective using sensitivity analysis: The example of potential accessibility to primary healthcare. *Journal of Transport & Health*, *6*, 128–142. doi:10.1016/j.jth.2017.03.013

Fridman, L., Weber, S., Greenstadt, R., & Kam, M. (2017). Active authentication on mobile devices via stylometry, application usage, web browsing, and GPS location. *IEEE Systems Journal*, *11*(2), 513–521. doi:10.1109/JSYST.2015.2472579

Friedmann, P., Hoskinson, R. Jr, Gordon, M., Schwartz, R., Kinlock, T., Knight, K., Flynn, P. M., Welsh, W. N., Stein, L. A. R., Sacks, S., O'Connell, D. J., Knudsen, H. K., Shafer, M. S., Hall, E., & Frisman, L. K.for the MAT Working Group of CJ-DAT. (2012). Medication-Assisted Treatment in Criminal Justice Agencies Affiliated with the Criminal Justice-Drug Abuse Treatment Studies (CJ-DATS): Availability, Barriers, and Intentions. *Substance Abuse*, *33*(1), 9–18. doi:10.1080/08897077.2011.611460 PMID:22263709

Fu, Z. (2020). The Secure Steganography for Hiding Images via GAN. EURASIP Journal on Image and Video Processing. doi:10.118613640-020-00534-2

Gadepalli, P. K., Peach, G., Cherkasova, L., Aitken, R., & Parmer, G. (2019). Challenges and opportunities for efficient serverless computing at the edge. *2019 38th Symposium on Reliable Distributed Systems (SRDS)*, 261–2615. 10.1109/SRDS47363.2019.00036

Ganesh, N., & Thangasamy, S. (2012). Lessons learned in transforming from traditional to agile development. *Journal of Computational Science*, 8(3), 389–392. doi:10.3844/jcssp.2012.389.392

Gan, Y., Zhang, Y., Cheng, D., Shetty, A., Rathi, P., & Katarki, N. (2019). An open-source benchmark suite for microservices and their hardware-software implications for cloud & edge systems. *Proceedings of the Twenty-Fourth International Conference on Architectural Support for Programming Languages and Operating Systems*, 3–18. 10.1145/3297858.3304013

Gardašević, G., Katzis, K., Bajić, D., & Berbakov, L. (2020). Emerging wireless sensor networks and Internet of Things technologies—Foundations of smart healthcare. *Sensors (Basel)*, 20(13), 3619. doi:10.339020133619 PMID:32605071

Gaur, A., Scotney, B., Parr, G., & McClean, S. (2015). Smart city architecture and its applications based on IoT. *Procedia Computer Science*, 52, 1089–1094. doi:10.1016/j.procs.2015.05.122

Gawanmeh, A. (2016). Open issues in reliability, safety, and efficiency of connected health. *First IEEE Conference on Connected Health: Applications, Systems and Engineering Technologies*, Washington, DC. 10.1109/CHASE.2016.60

Gebrie, M. T., & Abie, H. (2017, September 11). Risk-based adaptive authentication for internet of things in smart home eHealth. *Proceedings of the 11th European Conference on Software Architecture: Companion Proceedings*. 10.1145/3129790.3129801

Gelogo, Y. E., Hwang, H. J., & Kim, H. K. (2015). Internet of things (IoT) framework for u-ealthcare system. *International Journal of Smart Home*, 9(11), 323–330. doi:10.14257/ijsh.2015.9.11.31

General Data Protection Regulation (GDPR) – official legal text. (2016, July 13). General Data Protection Regulation (GDPR). https://gdpr-info.eu

Georghiades, A. S., Belhumeur, P. N., & Kriegman, D. J. (2000). From few to many: Generative models for recognition under variable pose and illumination. *Proceedings of Fourth IEEE international conference on automatic face and gesture recognition*, 1-8.

Gertrud, S. B., Robert, H.L., Rosemary, W., & Deborah, L. (1992). Race/Ethnicity and Other Risk Factors for Gestational Diabetes. *American Journal of Epidemiology, 135*(9), 965–973. doi:10.1093/oxfordjournals.aje.a116408

Geurts, P., Ernst, D., & Wehenkel, L. (2006). Extremely randomized trees. *Machine Learning*, 63(1), 3–42. doi:10.100710994-006-6226-1

Geurts, P., Fillet, M., de Seny, D. D., Meuwis, M. A., Malaise, M., Merville, M. P., & Wehenkel, L. (2005). Proteomic mass spectra classification using decision tree based ensemble methods. *Bioinformatics (Oxford, England)*, 21(14), 3138–3145. doi:10.1093/bioinformatics/bti494 PMID:15890743

Ghare, P., & Schrader, G. (1963). A model for exponentially decaying inventories. *Journal of Industrial Engineering*, 14, 238–243.

Ghazal, T. M., Hasan, M. K., Alshurideh, M. T., Alzoubi, H. M., Ahmad, M., Akbar, S. S., Al, K. B., & Akour, I. A. (2021). IoT for Smart Cities: Machine Learning Approaches in Smart Healthcare—A Review. *Future Internet, 13*(8), 218. doi:10.3390/fi13080218

Gia, T. N., Jiang, M., Sarker, V. K., Rahmani, A. M., Westerlund, T., Liljeberg, P., & Tenhunen, H. (2017, June). Low-cost fog-assisted healthcare IoT system with energy-efficient sensor nodes. In *2017 13th international wireless communications and mobile computing conference (IWCMC)* (pp. 1765-1770). IEEE.

Gibson, S., Issac, B., Zhang, L., & Jacob, S. M. (2020). Detecting Spam Email With Machine Learning Optimized With Bio-Inspired Metaheuristic Algorithms. *IEEE Access: Practical Innovations, Open Solutions, 8*, 187914–187932. doi:10.1109/ACCESS.2020.3030751

Gobinda, G. C. (2003). Natural language processing. *Annual Review of Information Science & Technology, 37*, 51–89.

Gokhale, A. S., & Waghmare, V. S. (2016). The shoulder surfing resistant graphical password authentication technique. *Procedia Computer Science, 79*, 875–884. doi:10.1016/j.procs.2016.03.091

Golec, M., Ozturac, R., Pooranian, Z., Gill, S. S., & Buyya, R. (2021). iFaaSBus: A security and privacy based lightweight framework for serverless computing using IoT and machine learning. *IEEE Transactions on Industrial Informatics*.

Golub, T. R., Slonim, D. K., Tamayo, P., Huard, C., Gaasenbeek, M., Mesirov, J. P., Coller, H., Loh, M. L., Downing, J. R., Caligiuri, M., Bloomfield, C. D., & Lander, E. S. (1999). Molecular classification of cancer: class discovery and class prediction by gene expression monitoring. *Science, 286*(5439), 531-7.

Gong, F., & ... . (2013). Primary exploration in establishment of China's intelligent medical treatment. *Modern Hospital Management, 11*(2), 28–29.

Gonzalez-Manzano, L., Fuentes, J. M. D., & Ribagorda, A. (2019). Leveraging user-related internet of things for continuous authentication. *ACM Computing Surveys, 52*(3), 1–38. doi:10.1145/3314023

Gope, P., Amin, R., Hafizul Islam, S. K., Kumar, N., & Bhalla, V. K. (2018). Lightweight and privacy-preserving RFID authentication scheme for distributed IoT infrastructure with secure localization services for smart city environment. *Future Generation Computer Systems, 83*, 629–637. doi:10.1016/j.future.2017.06.023

Gopika, N., & Meena Kowshalaya, A. E. A. (2018). Correlation Based Feature Selection Algorithm for Machine Learning. *Proceedings of the 3rd International Conference on Communication and Electronics Systems, ICCES 2018, Icces*, 692–695. 10.1109/CESYS.2018.8723980

Gordon, G. J. (2002). Translation of Microarray Data into Clinically Relevant Cancer Diagnostic Tests Using Gege Expression Ratios in Lung Cancer And Mesothelioma. *Cancer Research, 62*, 4963–4967. PMID:12208747

Gorgal, R., Gonçalves, E., Barros, M., Namora, G., Magalhães, A., Rodrigues, T., & Montenegro, N. (2012). Gestational diabetes mellitus: A risk factor for non-elective cesarean section. *Journal of Obstetrics and Gynaecology Research, 38*(1), 154–159.

Gorla, R. S. R., & Sidawi, I. (1994). Free Convection on a Vertical Stretching Surface with Suction and Blowing. *Applied Scientific Research, 52*(3), 247–258. doi:10.1007/BF00853952

Goswami, A., & Chaudhuri, K. (1991). EOQ model for an inventory with a linear trend in demand and finite rate of replenishment considering shortages. *International Journal of Systems Science, 22*(1), 181–187. doi:10.1080/00207729108910598

Goudarzi, M., Wu, H., Palaniswami, M., & Buyya, R. (2020). An application placement technique for concurrent IoT applications in edge and fog computing environments. *IEEE Transactions on Mobile Computing, 20*(4), 1298–1311. doi:10.1109/TMC.2020.2967041

Gowda, & Shashidhara, Ramesha, & Kumar. (2021). Recent advances in graph theory and its applications. *Advances in Mathematics: Scientific Journal., 10*, 1407–1412. doi:10.37418/amsj.10.3.29

Grady, N. W., Payne, J. A., & Parker, H. (2017). Agile big data analytics: AnalyticsOps for data science. *Proceedings - 2017 IEEE International Conference on Big Data, Big Data 2017*, 2331–2339. 10.1109/BigData.2017.8258187

Gragnaniello, D., Poggi, G., Sansone, C., & Verdoliva, L. (2013, September). Fingerprint liveness detection based on Weber Local image Descriptor. *2013 IEEE Workshop on Biometric Measurements and Systems for Security and Medical Applications*. 10.1109/BIOMS.2013.6656148

Grassi, P. A., Fenton, J. L., Newton, E. M., Perlner, R. A., Regenscheid, A. R., Burr, W. E., Richer, J. P., Lefkovitz, N. B., Danker, J. M., Choong, Y.-Y., Greene, K. K., & Theofanos, M. F. (2017). *Digital identity guidelines: Authentication and lifecycle management*. National Institute of Standards and Technology. doi:10.6028/nist.sp.800-63b

Greer, A., Hu, S., Amlani, A., Morehart, S., Sampson, O., & Buxton, J. (2016). Patient perspectives on methadone formulation change in British Columbia, Canada: outcomes of a provincial survey. *Treatment, Prevention, and Policy in Substance Abuse, 11*(1).

Grella, C., Ostile, E., Scott, C., Dennis, M., & Carnavale, J. (2020). A Scoping Review of Barriers and Facilitators to the Implementation of Medications for the Treatment of Opioid Use Disorder within the Criminal Justice System. *International Journal of Drug Policy*.

Griffin, M. E., Coffey, M., Johnson, H., Scanlon, P., Foley, M., Stronge, J., O'Meara, N. M., & Firth, R. G. (2000). Universal vs. risk factor-based screening for gestational diabetes mellitus: Detection rates, gestation at diagnosis and outcome. *Diabetic Medicine, 17*(1), 26–32.

Grudin, M. A. (2000). On internal representations in face recognition systems. *Pattern Recognition, 33*(7), 1161–1177. doi:10.1016/S0031-3203(99)00104-1

Guha, A., Alahmadi, A., Samanta, D., Khan, M. Z., & Alahmadi, A. H. (2022). A Multi-Modal Approach to Digital Document Stream Segmentation for Title Insurance Domain. *IEEE Access: Practical Innovations, Open Solutions, 10*, 11341–11353. doi:10.1109/ACCESS.2022.3144185

Guide, T. D., Scrum, S., & January, N. (2021). *The Nexus ™ Guide*. Academic Press.

Gunasekaran, J. R., Mishra, C. S., Thinakaran, P., Kandemir, M. T., & Das, C. R. (2020). Implications of Public Cloud Resource Heterogeneity for Inference Serving. *Proceedings of the 2020 Sixth International Workshop on Serverless Computing*, 7–12. 10.1145/3429880.3430093

Gunson, N., Marshall, D., Morton, H., & Jack, M. (2011). User perceptions of security and usability of single-factor and two-factor authentication in automated telephone banking. *Computers & Security, 30*(4), 208–220. doi:10.1016/j.cose.2010.12.001

Guo, G., Li, S. Z., & Chan, K. L. (2001). Support vector machines for face recognition. *Image and Vision Computing, 19*(9-10), 631–638. doi:10.1016/S0262-8856(01)00046-4

Gupta, H., VahidDastjerdi, A., Ghosh, S. K., & Buyya, R. (2017). iFogSim: A toolkit for modeling and simulation of resource management techniques in the Internet of Things, Edge and Fog computing environments. *Software: Practice and Experience, 47*(9), 1275-1296.

Gupta, V., Phade, S., Courtade, T., & Ramchandran, K. (2020). *Utility-based Resource Allocation and Pricing for Serverless Computing*. arXiv preprint arXiv:2008.07793.

Gupta, P., Wee, T. K., Ramasubbu, N., Lo, D., Gao, D., & Balan, R. K. (2012, March). HuMan: Creating memorable fingerprints of mobile users. *2012 IEEE International Conference on Pervasive Computing and Communications Workshops*. 10.1109/PerComW.2012.6197540

Gupta, R. D., Samanta, D., & Joseph, N. P. (2022). *Rendering View of Kitchen Design Using Autodesk 3Ds Max. Στο Micro-Electronics and Telecommunication Engineering*. Springer.

Gupta, S., Buriro, A., & Crispo, B. (2019). DriverAuth: A risk-based multi-modal biometric-based driver authentication scheme for ride-sharing platforms. *Computers & Security*, *83*, 122–139. doi:10.1016/j.cose.2019.01.007

Gupta, V. (2018). An energy efficient fog-cloud based architecture for healthcare. *Journal of Statistics and Management Systems*, *21*(4), 529–537.

Gurav, S. M., Gawade, L. S., Rane, P. K., & Khochare, N. R. (2014, January). Graphical password authentication: Cloud securing scheme. *2014 International Conference on Electronic Systems, Signal Processing and Computing Technologies*. 10.1109/ICESC.2014.90

Gutub & Al-Ghamdi. (2020). Hiding Shares by Multimedia Image Steganography for Optimized Counting-Based Secret Sharing. *Multimedia Tools and Applications, 79*(11), 7951–85. . doi:10.1007/s11042-019-08427-x

Gutub & Al-Shaarani. (2020). Efficient Implementation of Multi-Image Secret Hiding Based on LSB and DWT Steganography Comparisons. *Arabian Journal for Science and Engineering, 45*(4), 2631–44. . doi:10.1007/s13369-020-04413-w

Haiming, L. (2018). Embedding and Extracting Digital Watermark Based on DCT Algorithm. *Journal of Computer and Communications*, *6*(11), 287–298. doi:10.4236/jcc.2018.611026

Hall, A., & Ramachandran, U. (2019). An execution model for serverless functions at the edge. *Proceedings of the International Conference on Internet of Things Design and Implementation*, 225–236. 10.1145/3302505.3310084

Hamad, M. A. A. (2011). Analytical Solution of Natural Convection Flow of a Nanofluid over a Linearly Stretching Sheet in the Presence of Magnetic Field. *International Communications in Heat and Mass Transfer*, *38*(4), 487–492. doi:10.1016/j.icheatmasstransfer.2010.12.042

Hang, A., De Luca, A., Smith, M., Richter, M., & Hussmann, H. (2015). Where have you been? using location-based security questions for fallback authentication. In *Eleventh Symposium On Usable Privacy and Security (SOUPS 2015)* (pp. 169-183). Academic Press.

Hanine, M. (2018). QoS in the Cloud Computing: A Load Balancing Approach Using Simulated Annealing Algorithm. In *International Conference on Big Data, Cloud and Applications*. Springer.

Han, W., Xu, J., Zhou, M., Tian, G., Wang, P., Shen, X., & Hou, E. (2016). Cuckoo search and particle filter-based inversing approach to estimating defects via magnetic flux leakage signals. *IEEE Transactions on Magnetics*, *52*(4), 1–11. doi:10.1109/TMAG.2015.2498119

Hartley, D. (2009). Secure ecommerce web application design principles, beyond PCI DSS. *Computer Fraud & Security*, *6*(6), 13–17. doi:10.1016/S1361-3723(09)70074-0

Hassani, M., Mohammad Tabar, M., Nemati, H., Domairry, G., & Noori, F. (2011). An Analytical Solution for Boundary Layer Flow of a Nanofluid Past a Stretching Sheet. *International Journal of Thermal Sciences*, *50*(11), 2256–2263. doi:10.1016/j.ijthermalsci.2011.05.015

Hayashi, E., Das, S., Amini, S., Hong, J., & Oakley, I. (2013). CASA. *Proceedings of the Ninth Symposium on Usable Privacy and Security - SOUPS '13*. http://dx.doi.org/10.1145/2501604.2501607

Hegde, D. S., Samanta, D., & Dutta, S. (2022). *Classification framework for fraud detection using hidden markov model. Στο Cyber Intelligence and Information Retrieval*. Springer.

Heinermann, J., & Kramer, O. (2016). Machine learning ensembles for wind power prediction. *Renewable Energy, 89,* 671–679. doi:10.1016/j.renene.2015.11.073

Heisele, B., Ho, P., Wu, J., & Poggio, T. (2003). Face recognition: Component-based versus global approaches. *Computer Vision and Image Understanding, 91*(1-2), 6–21. doi:10.1016/S1077-3142(03)00073-0

Hemdan, E., Shouman, M. A., & Karar, M. (2020). *Covidx-net: A framework of deep learning classifiers to diagnose covid-19 in x-ray images.* arXiv preprint arXiv:200311055

Hendrickson, S., Sturdevant, S., Harter, T., Venkataramani, V., Arpaci-Dusseau, A. C., & Arpaci-Dusseau, R. H. (2016). Serverless computation with openlambda. *8th USENIX Workshop on Hot Topics in Cloud Computing (HotCloud 16).*

Henricks, A., & Kettani, H. (2019, October 14). On data protection using multi-factor authentication. *Proceedings of the 2019 International Conference on Information System and System Management.* 10.1145/3394788.3394789

Hernández-Gracidas, C., & Enrique Sucar, L., & Montes-y Gómez, M. (2009). Modeling spatial relations for image retrieval by conceptual graphs. *Proceedings of the First Chilean Workshop on Pattern Recognition.*

He, S., Cheng, B., Wang, H., Huang, Y., & Chen, J. (2017). Proactive personalized services through fog-cloud computing in large-scale IoT-based healthcare application. *China Communications, 14*(11), 1–16. doi:10.1109/CC.2017.8233646

He, Z., & Tao, H. (2018). Epidemiology and ARIMA model of positive-rate of influenza viruses among children in Wuhan, China: A nine-year retrospective study. *International Journal of Infectious Diseases, 74,* 61–70.

Hintze, D., Findling, R. D., Muaaz, M., Koch, E., & Mayrhofer, R. (2015). Cormorant. *Proceedings of the 2015 ACM International Joint Conference on Pervasive and Ubiquitous Computing and Proceedings of the 2015 ACM International Symposium on Wearable Computers - UbiComp '15.* http://dx.doi.org/10.1145/2800835.2800906

Hintze, D., Koch, E., Scholz, S., & Mayrhofer, R. (2016). Location-Based Risk Assessment for Mobile Authentication. *Proceedings of the 2016 ACM International Joint Conference on Pervasive and Ubiquitous Computing: Adjunct,* 85–88. doi:10.1145/2968219.2971448

Hipaa. (2019). *Health information privacy.* Available at: www.hhs.gov/hipaa/index.html

Ho, T. K. (1995). Random Decision Forests. *Proceedings of the 3rd International Conference on Document Analysis and Recognition,* 278–282.

Ho, T. K. (2002). A Data Complexity Analysis of Comparative Advantages of Decision Forest Constructors. *Pattern Analysis & Applications, 5*(2), 102–112. doi:10.1007100440200009

Howell, A. J., & Buxton, H. (1995). Invariance in radial basis function neural networks in human face classification. *Neural Processing Letters, 2*(3), 26–30. doi:10.1007/BF02311576

Hsieh & Wang. (2022). Constructive Image Steganography Using Example-Based Weighted Color Transfer. *Journal of Information Security and Applications, 65.* . doi:10.1016/j.jisa.2022.103126

Hua, G., Cheng, T. C. E., & Wang, W. (2011). Managing carbon footprints in inventory management. *International Journal of Production Economics, 132*(2), 178–185. doi:10.1016/j.ijpe.2011.03.024

Huang, B., Chen, W., Lin, C. L., Juang, C. F., & Wang, J. (2022). MLP-BP: A novel framework for cuffless blood pressure measurement with PPG and ECG signals based on MLP-Mixer neural networks. *Biomedical Signal Processing and Control, 73,* 103404.

Huang, W., Bolton, T. A. W., Medaglia, J. D., Bassett, D. S., Ribeiro, A., & Van De Ville, D. (2018, May). A Graph Signal Processing Perspective on Functional Brain Imaging. *Proceedings of the IEEE*, *106*(5), 868–885. doi:10.1109/JPROC.2018.2798928

Huang, Z., Mi, Z., & Hua, Z. (2020). HCloud: A trusted JointCloud serverless platform for IoT systems with blockchain. *China Communications*, *17*(9), 1–10. doi:10.23919/JCC.2020.09.001

Hui, D. S., Azhar, E. I., Madani, T. A., Ntoumi, F., Kock, R., Dar, O., ... Petersen, E. (2020). The continuing 2019-nCoV epidemic threat of novel coronaviruses to global health—The latest 2019 novel coronavirus outbreak in Wuhan, China. *International Journal of Infectious Diseases*, *91*, 264–266. doi:10.1016/j.ijid.2020.01.009 PMID:31953166

Huma, N., & Sachin, A. (2020). Deep learning approach for diabetes prediction using PIMA Indian dataset. *J Diabetes Metab Disord*, 391-403. https://pubmed.ncbi.nlm.nih.gov/32550190/

Hurrah, N. N., Parah, S. A., Loan, N. A., Sheikh, J. A., Elhoseny, M., & Muhammad, K. (2019). Dual watermarking framework for privacy protection and content authentication of multimedia. *Future Generation Computer Systems*, *94*, 654–673. doi:10.1016/j.future.2018.12.036

Huseynov, E., & Seigneur, J.-M. (2017). Context-Aware multifactor authentication survey. In *Computer and Information Security Handbook* (pp. 715–726). Elsevier. doi:10.1016/B978-0-12-803843-7.00050-8

Hussain, A., & Saini, H. K. (2018). A Novel Approach for Enhancing the Face Recognition Accuracy using SIFT with Multiple LDA-PCA Techniques. *International Journal for Research in Applied Science and Engineering Technology*, *6*(5), 2588–2594. doi:10.22214/ijraset.2018.5423

Hussain, K., Salleh, M. N. M., Cheng, S., & Shi, Y. (2019). Metaheuristic research: A comprehensive survey. *Artificial Intelligence Review*, *52*(4), 2191–2233. doi:10.100710462-017-9605-z

Hussein, S., Kandel, P., Bolan, C. W., Wallace, M. B., & Bagci, U. (2019, August). Lung and Pancreatic Tumor Characterization in the Deep Learning Era: Novel Supervised and Unsupervised Learning Approaches. *IEEE Transactions on Medical Imaging*, *38*(8), 1777–1787. doi:10.1109/TMI.2019.2894349 PMID:30676950

Ilic, A., Staake, T., & Fleisch, E. (2009). Using sensor information to reduce the carbon footprint of perishable goods. *IEEE Pervasive Computing*, *8*(1), 22–29. doi:10.1109/MPRV.2009.20

Imai, S., Varela, C. A., & Patterson, S. (2018, December). A performance study of geo-distributed IoT data aggregation for fog computing. In *2018 IEEE/ACM International Conference on Utility and Cloud Computing Companion (UCC Companion)* (pp. 278-283). IEEE. 10.1109/UCC-Companion.2018.00068

Imbriaco, M., Iodice, D., Erra, P., Terlizzi, A., Di Carlo, R., Di Vito, C., & Imbimbo, C. (2011). Squamous cell carcinoma within a horseshoe kidney with associated renal stones detected by computed tomograpy and magnetic resonance imaging. *Urology*, *78*(1), 54–55. doi:10.1016/j.urology.2010.06.006 PMID:20801492

Ioannis, K., Olga, T., Athanasios, S., Nicos, M., Ioannis, V., & Ioanna, C. (2017). Machine Learning and Data Mining Methods in Diabetes Research. *Computational and Structural Biotechnology Journal*, *15*, 104–116.

Islam, M. M., Rahaman, A., & Islam, M. R. (2020). Development of smart healthcare monitoring system in IoT environment. *SN Computer Science, 1*, 1-11.

Ismagilova, E. (2020). Security, privacy and risks within smart cities: Literature review and development of a smart city interaction framework. *Information Systems Frontiers*, 1–22.

ISO/IEC 29100:2011. (2011). European Innovation Partnership - European Commission. https://ec.europa.eu/eip/ageing/standards/ict-and-communication/data/isoiec-291002011_en.html

ISO/IEC 29100:2011. (2011). ISO. Retrieved October 9, 2021, from https://www.iso.org/standard/45123.html

Ivan, C., & Josep, V. (2018). Artificial Intelligence for Diabetes Management and Decision Support: Literature Review. *Journal of Medical Internet Research, 20*(5).

Ivan, C., Vasile, R., & Dadarlat, V. (2019). Serverless computing: An investigation of deployment environments for web apis. *Computers, 8*(2), 50. doi:10.3390/computers8020050

Izenberg, J., Bachireddy, C., Wickersham, J., Soule, M., Kiriazov, T., & Dvorak, S. (2014). Within-prison drug injection among HIV-infected Ukrainian prisoners: Prevalence and correlates of extremely high-risk behavior. *The International Journal on Drug Policy, 25*(5), 845–852. doi:10.1016/j.drugpo.2014.02.010 PMID:24951025

Jaeger, S., Candemir, S., Antani, S. K., Wang, L. P., & Thoma, G. R. (2014, December 4). Two public chest X-ray datasets for computer-aided screening of pulmonary diseases. *Quantitative Imaging in Medicine and Surgery*, (6), 475–477. doi:10.3978/j.issn.2223-4292.2014.11.20 PMID:25525580

Jaggi, C. K., Pareek, S., Khanna, A., & Nidhi, N. (2016). Optimal replenishment policy for fuzzy inventory model with deteriorating items and allowable shortages under inflationary conditions. *Yugoslav Journal of Operations Research, 26*(4), 1–21. doi:10.2298/YJOR150202002Y

Jaggi, C. K., Tiwari, S., & Shafi, A. A. (2015). Effect of deterioration on two-warehouse inventory model with imperfect quality. *Computers & Industrial Engineering, 88*(C), 378–385. doi:10.1016/j.cie.2015.07.019

Jahan, N., Rashid, I. B., & Al Numan, O. (2021). Collaborative AI in Smart Healthcare System. *International IEEE Conference on Automation, Control and Mechatronics for Industry 4.0 (ACMI)*.

Jain, N., &Menache, I. (2016, September). *Resource management for cloud computing platforms*. Google Patents.

Jain, K. K. (2008). Nanomedicine: Application of nanobiotechnology in medical practice. *Medical Principles and Practice, 17*(2), 89–101.

Jain, M., Singh, V., & Rani, A. (2018). A novel nature-inspired algorithm for optimization: Squirrel search algorithm. *Swarm and Evolutionary Computation*.

Jangda, A., Pinckney, D., Brun, Y., & Guha, A. (2019). Formal foundations of serverless computing. *Proceedings of the ACM on Programming Languages, 3*, 1–26.

Javaid, M., & Haleem, A. (2020). Virtual reality applications toward medical field. *Clinical Epidemiology and Global Health, 8*(2), 600–605.

Jayamalar, T., & Radha, V. (2010). Survey on Digital Video Watermarking Techniques and Attacks on Watermarks. *International Journal of Engineering Science and Technology, 2*(12), 6963–6967.

Jayapandiyan, J. R., Kavitha, C., & Sakthivel, K. (2020). Enhanced Least Significant Bit Replacement Algorithm in Spatial Domain of Steganography Using Character Sequence Optimization. *IEEE Access: Practical Innovations, Open Solutions, 8*, 136537–136545. doi:10.1109/ACCESS.2020.3009234

Jayashree, J., & Kumar, S. A. (2019). Evolutionary correlated gravitational search algorithm (ECGS) with genetic optimized Hopfield neural network (GHNN)–A hybrid expert system for diagnosis of diabetes. *Measurement, 145*, 551–558. doi:10.1016/j.measurement.2018.12.083

Jensen, D. M., Korsholm, L., Ovesen, P., Beck, N. H., Mølsted, P. L., & Damm, P. (2008). Adverse pregnancy outcome in women with mild glucose intolerance: Is there a clinically meaningful threshold value for glucose? *Acta Obstetricia et Gynecologica Scandinavica, 87*(1), 59–62. doi:10.1080/00016340701823975 PMID:18158628

Jeong, J. S., Han, O., & You, Y. Y. (2016). A design characteristics of smart healthcare system as the IoT application. *Indian Journal of Science and Technology, 9*(37), 52. doi:10.17485/ijst/2016/v9i37/102547

Jiang, M., Luo, J., Jiang, D., Xiong, J., Song, H., & Shen, J. (2016). A cuckoo search-support vector machine model for predicting dynamic measurement errors of sensors. *IEEE Access: Practical Innovations, Open Solutions, 4*, 5030–5037. doi:10.1109/ACCESS.2016.2605041

Jiang, Q., Ma, J., Li, G., & Li, X. (2013). Improvement of robust smart-card-based password authentication scheme. *International Journal of Communication Systems, 28*(2), 383–393. doi:10.1002/dac.2644

Jiang, X., Coffee, M., Bari, A., Wang, J., Jiang, X., Huang, J., ... Huang, Y. (2020). Towards an artificial intelligence framework for data-driven prediction of coronavirus clinical severity. Computers. *Materials & Continua, 63*(1), 537–551.

Jin, J., Gubbi, J., Marusic, S., & Palaniswami, M. (2014). An information framework for creating a smart city through internet of things. *IEEE Internet of Things Journal, 1*(2), 112–121. doi:10.1109/JIOT.2013.2296516

Joana, C. (2021). *The design process of human-centered AI—part 1.* https://bootcamp.uxdesign.cc/human-centered-ai-design-process-part-1-8cf7e3ce00

Joana, C. (2021). *The design process of human-centered AI—part 2.* https://bootcamp.uxdesign.cc/human-centered-ai-design-process-part-2-empathize-hypothesis-6065db967716

Johansson, M. A., Quandelacy, T. M., Kada, S., Prasad, P. V., Steele, M., Brooks, J. T., ... Butler, J. C. (2021). SARS-CoV-2 transmission from people without COVID-19 symptoms. *JAMA Network Open, 4*(1), e2035057–e2035057.

Jonas, E., Schleier-Smith, J., Sreekanti, V., Tsai, C.-C., Khandelwal, A., & Pu, Q. (2019). *Cloud programming simplified: A berkeley view on serverless computing.* arXiv preprint arXiv:1902.03383.

José, G. B. D., Marius, R., Wayne, S. C., Teresa, E. P., Sheryl, T., Ann, F., Jane, M. P., Paul, L. D., & Paul, L. H. (2014). Effects of Age, Gender, BMI, and Anatomical Site on Skin Thickness in Children and Adults with Diabetes. *PLoS One, 9*(1), e86637. Advance online publication. doi:10.1371/journal.pone.0086637 PMID:24466182

Kacprzyk, J., & Staniewski, P. (1982). Long-term inventory policy- making through fuzzy decision-making models. *Fuzzy Sets and Systems, 8*(2), 117–132. doi:10.1016/0165-0114(82)90002-1

Kaewkasi, C. (2018). *Docker for Serverless Applications. In Containerize and orchestrate functions using OpenFaas, OpenWhisk, and Fn.* Packt Publishing Ltd.

Kaffes, K., Yadwadkar, N. J., & Kozyrakis, C. (2019). Centralized core-granular scheduling for serverless functions. *Proceedings of the ACM Symposium on Cloud Computing*, 158–164. 10.1145/3357223.3362709

Kakac, S., & Pramuanjaroenkij, A. (2009). Review of convective heat transfer enhancement with nanofluids. *International Journal of Heat and Mass Transfer, 52*(13-14), 3187–3196. doi:10.1016/j.ijheatmasstransfer.2009.02.006

Kalarthi, Z. M. (2016). A review paper on smart health care system using internet of things. *International Journal of Research in Engineering and Technology, 5*(03), 8084.

Kalocsai, P., Malsburg, C. V. D., & Horn, J. (2000). Face recognition by statistical analysis of feature detectors. *Image and Vision Computing, 18*(4), 273–278. doi:10.1016/S0262-8856(99)00051-7

Kalogirou, S. (2007). *Artificial Intelligence in Energy and Renewable Energy Systems.* Nova Publishers.

Kamaruddin, N. S., Kamsin, A., Por, L. Y., & Rahman, H. (2018). A Review of Text Watermarking: Theory, Methods, and Applications. *IEEE Access: Practical Innovations, Open Solutions, 6*, 8011–8028. doi:10.1109/ACCESS.2018.2796585

Kamoona, A. M., & Patra, J. C. (2019). A novel enhanced cuckoo search algorithm for contrast enhancement of gray scale images. *Applied Soft Computing*, *85*, 105749. doi:10.1016/j.asoc.2019.105749

Kampmann, U., Madsen, L. R., Skajaa, G. O., Iversen, D. S., Moeller, N., & Ovesen, P. (2015). Gestational diabetes: A clinical update. *World Journal of Diabetes*, *6*(8), 1065–1072. doi:10.4239/wjd.v6.i8.1065 PMID:26240703

Kang, S. H., Baek, H., Cho, J., Kim, S., Hwang, H., Lee, W., ... Suh, J. W. (2021). Management of cardiovascular disease using an mHealth tool: A randomized clinical trial. *NPJ Digital Medicine*, *4*(1), 1–7.

Karthigaiveni, M., & Indrani, B. (2019). An efficient two-factor authentication scheme with key agreement for IoT-based E-health care application using a smart card. *Journal of Ambient Intelligence and Humanized Computing*. Advance online publication. doi:10.100712652-019-01513-w

Karthikeyan, N. (2021). Assessment of Composite Materials on Encrypted Secret Message in Image Steganography Using RSA Algorithm. *Materials Today: Proceedings*. . doi:10.1016/j.matpr.2021.04.260

Katsini, C., Belk, M., Fidas, C., Avouris, N., & Samaras, G. (2016, November 10). Security and usability in knowledge-based user authentication. *Proceedings of the 20th Pan-Hellenic Conference on Informatics*. 10.1145/3003733.3003764

Kaufmann, A., & Gupta, M. M. (1991). *Introduction to fuzzy arithmetic theory and applications*. International Thomson Computer Press.

Kaur, B., & Sharma, S. (2017). Digital Watermarking and Security Techniques: A Review. *International Journal of Computer Science and Technology*, *8*(2), 44–47.

Kavishwar, B. W., Vijayraghavan, S., & Ashok, W. D. (2012). Modeling Paradigms for Medical Diagnostic Decision Support: A Survey and Future Directions. *Journal of Medical Systems*, *36*, 3029–3049. https://link.springer.com/article/10.1007/s10916-011-9780-4

Ke & Yin. (2021). On the Security and Robustness of 'Keyless Dynamic Optimal Multi-Bit Image Steganography Using Energetic Pixels.' *Multimedia Tools and Applications*, *80*(3), 3997–4005. . doi:10.1007/s11042-020-09807-4

Keeling, M. J., Hill, E. M., Gorsich, E. E., Penman, B., Guyver-Fletcher, G., Holmes, A., ... Tildesley, M. J. (2021). Predictions of COVID-19 dynamics in the UK: Short-term forecasting and analysis of potential exit strategies. *PLoS Computational Biology*, *17*(1), e1008619.

Ketu, S., & Mishra, P. K. (2021). Internet of Healthcare Things: A contemporary survey. *Journal of Network and Computer Applications*, *192*, 103179. doi:10.1016/j.jnca.2021.103179

Khadam, U., Iqbal, M. M., Azam, M. A., Khalid, S., Rho, S., & Chilamkurti, N. (2016). Digital Watermarking Technique for Text Document Protection Using Data Mining Analysis. *IEEE Access: Practical Innovations, Open Solutions*, *7*, 64955–64965. doi:10.1109/ACCESS.2019.2916674

Khaloufi. (2018). Security model for Big Healthcare Data Lifecycle. *Proceedings of the 8th International Conference on Current and Future Trends of Information and Communication Technologies in Healthcare (ICTH 2018)*, 294–301. 10.1016/j.procs.2018.10.199

Khamparia, A., Singh, P. K., Rani, P., Samanta, D., Khanna, A., & Bhushan, B. (2021). An internet of health things-driven deep learning framework for detection and classification of skin cancer using transfer learning. *Transactions on Emerging Telecommunications Technologies*, *32*(7), e3963.

Khan Mamun, M. M. R., & Alouani, A. T. (2022). Cuffless Blood Pressure Measurement Using Linear and Nonlinear Optimized Feature Selection. *Diagnostics (Basel)*, *12*(2), 408.

Khandelwal, A., Kejariwal, A., & Ramasamy, K. (2020). Le Taureau: Deconstructing the Serverless Landscape & A Look Forward. *Proceedings of the 2020 ACM SIGMOD International Conference on Management of Data*, 2641–2650. 10.1145/3318464.3383130

Khan, H., & Hengartner, U. (2014, February 26). Towards application-centric implicit authentication on smartphones. *Proceedings of the 15th Workshop on Mobile Computing Systems and Applications.* 10.1145/2565585.2565590

Khan, M. A., Pradhan, S. K., & Khaleel, M. A. (2014). Outlier Detection for Business Intelligence using Data Mining Techniques. *International Journal of Computers and Applications*, *106*(2), 975–8887.

Khan, M., Mehran, M. T., Haq, Z. U., Ullah, Z., Naqvi, S. R., Ihsan, M., & Abbass, H. (2021, December). Applications of artificial intelligence in COVID-19 pandemic: A comprehensive review. *Expert Systems with Applications*, *185*, 115695. Advance online publication. doi:10.1016/j.eswa.2021.115695 PMID:34400854

Khan, W. A., & Pop, I. (2010). Boundary-Layer Flow of a Nanofluid Past a Stretching Sheet. *International Journal of Heat and Mass Transfer*, *53*(11-12), 2477–2483. doi:10.1016/j.ijheatmasstransfer.2010.01.032

Kikuchi, H., Hattori, T., & Nakanishi, S. (2002.). User authentication with facial images. Human-friendly identification in the Internet. *Proceedings Joint 9th IFSA World Congress and 20th NAFIPS International Conference* (Cat. No. 01TH8569). http://dx.doi.org/10.1109/nafips.2001.944424

Kim, J., & Lee, K. (2019). Functionbench: A suite of workloads for serverless cloud function service. *2019 IEEE 12th International Conference on Cloud Computing (CLOUD)*, 502–504) 10.1109/CLOUD.2019.00091

Kırbaş, İ., Sözen, A., Tuncer, A. D., & Kazancıoğlu, F. Ş. (2020). Comparative analysis and forecasting of COVID-19 cases in various European countries with ARIMA, NARNN and LSTM approaches. *Chaos, Solitons, and Fractals*, *138*, 110015.

Kirby, M., & Sirovich, L. (1990). Application of the Karhunen-Loeve procedure for the characterization of human faces. *IEEE Transactions on Pattern Analysis and Machine Intelligence*, *12*, 103-108.

Kirupa Shankar, K. M. (2021). A Novel Approach For Secure & Smart Healthcare Using Internet Of Things Infrastructure. *Turkish Journal of Computer and Mathematics Education*, *12*(11), 5992–5997.

Kishor, A., & Chakraborty, C. (2021). Artificial intelligence and internet of things based healthcare 4.0 monitoring system. *Wireless Personal Communications*, 1–17.

Klas, G. I. (2015). Fog computing and mobile edge cloud gain momentum open fog consortium, etsimec and cloudlets. *Google Scholar*, *1*(1), 1–13.

Korhonen, M. (2017). *Analyzing Resource Usage on Multitenant Cloud Cluster for Invoicing.* University Of Oulu, Faculty Of Information Technology And Electrical Engineering.

Korus, P., Białas, J., & Dziech, A. (2014). A new approach to high-capacity annotation watermarking based on digital fountain codes. *Multimedia Tools and Applications*, *68*(1), 59–77. doi:10.100711042-011-0986-8

Kotu, V., & Deshpande, B. (2019). Anomaly Detection. *Data Science*, 447–465. doi:10.1016/B978-0-12-814761-0.00013-7

Kouzani, A. Z., Nahavandi, S., & Koshmanesh, K. (2007). Face classification by a random forest. Proceeding TENCON 2007 - 2007 IEEE Region 10 Conference, 1–4. doi:10.1109/TENCON.2007.4428937

Kremic, E., & Subasi, A. (2016). Performance of random forest and SVM in face recognition. *International Arab Journal of Information Technology*, *13*, 87-293.

Krollner, B., Vanstone, B. J., & Finnie, G. R. (2010, April). Financial time series forecasting with machine learning techniques: A survey. ESANN.

Kumanov, D., Hung, L.-H., Lloyd, W., & Yeung, K. Y. (2018). *Serverless computing provides on-demand high performance computing for biomedical research.* arXiv preprint arXiv:1807.11659.

Kumar, C., Singh, A. K., & Kumar, P. (2018). A recent survey on image watermarking techniques and its application in e-governance. *Multimedia Tools and Applications, 77*(3), 3597–3622. doi:10.100711042-017-5222-8

Kumar, G., & Samanta, D. (2022). *Effective View of Swimming Pool Using Autodesk 3ds Max: 3D Modelling and Rendering. Στο Internet of Things and Its Applications.* Springer.

Kumari, A., Behera, R. K., Sahoo, B., & Sahoo, S. P. (2022). Prediction of link evolution using community detection in social network. *Computing, 104*(5), 1–22. doi:10.100700607-021-01035-4

Kumari, A., Sahoo, B., Behera, R. K., Misra, S., & Sharma, M. M. (2021). Evaluation of Integrated Frameworks for Optimizing QoS in Serverless Computing. *International Conference on Computational Science and Its Applications,* 277–288. 10.1007/978-3-030-87007-2_20

Kumari, S., Chaudhry, S. A., Wu, F., Li, X., Farash, M. S., & Khan, M. K. (2015). An improved smart card based authentication scheme for session initiation protocol. *Peer-to-Peer Networking and Applications, 10*(1), 92–105. doi:10.100712083-015-0409-0

Kumar, P. M., & Gandhi, U. D. (2018). A novel three-tier Internet of Things architecture with machine learning algorithm for early detection of heart diseases. *Computers & Electrical Engineering, 65,* 222–235.

Kumar, S., & Dutta, A. (2016). Performance analysis of spatial domain digital watermarking techniques. *Proceedings of the 2016 IEEE International conference on information communication and embedded systems (ICICES),* 1–4. 10.1109/ICICES.2016.7518910

Kumar, S., & Singh, B. K. (2018). A Review of Digital Watermarking in HealthCare Domain. *Proceedings of the 3rd International Conference on Computational Systems and Information Technology for Sustainable Solutions (CSITSS),* 156–159. 10.1109/CSITSS.2018.8768733

Kumar, S., Singh, B. K., & Yadav, M. (2020). A Recent survey on multimedia and database watermarking. *Multimedia Tools and Applications, 79*(27), 20149–20197. doi:10.100711042-020-08881-y

Lades, M., Vorbruggen, J. C., Buhmann, J., Lange, J., Malsburg, C. V. D., Wurtz, R. P., & Konen, W. (1993). Distortion invariant object recognition in the dynamic link architecture. *IEEE Transactions on Computers, 42*(3), 300–311. doi:10.1109/12.210173

Lai, D. Y. (2011, January 1). *Intelligent online risk-based authentication using Bayesian network model.* http://dspace.library.uvic.ca/handle/1828/3290

Lakhan, A., Khoso, F. H., Arain, A. A., & Kanwar, K. (2021). Serverless based functions aware framework for healthcare application. *International Journal (Toronto, Ont.), 9.*

Lanitis, A., Taylor, C. J., & Cootes, T. F. (1997). Automatic interpretation and coding of face images using flexible models. *IEEE Transactions on Pattern Analysis and Machine Intelligence, 19*(7), 743–756. doi:10.1109/34.598231

Larney, S., Peacock, A., Leung, J., College, S., Hickman, M., & Vickerman, P. (2017). Global, regional, and country-level coverage of interventions to prevent and manage HIV and hepatitis C among people who inject drugs: A systematic review. *The Lancet. Global Health, 5*(12), e1208–e1220. doi:10.1016/S2214-109X(17)30373-X PMID:29074410

Larsen, J. R., Martin, M. R., Martin, J. D., Kuhn, P., & Hicks, J. B. (2020). Modeling the Onset of Symptoms of CO-VID-19. *Frontiers in Public Health*, *8*, 473.

Laskar & Hemachandran. (2013). Digital image watermarking techniques and its Applications. *International Journal of Engineering Research & Technology (Ahmedabad)*, *2*(3), 1–8.

Latif, S. (2017). How 5g wireless (and concomitant technologies) will revolutionize healthcare? *Future Internet*, *9*(4), 93.

Lauenborg, J., Grarup, N., Damm, P., Borch, J. K., Jørgensen, T., Pedersen, O., & Hansen, T. (2009). Common type 2 diabetes risk gene variants associate with gestational diabetes. *J Clin Endocrinol Metab, 94*(1), 145-50.

Law, P. K. (2020). COVID-19 pandemic: Its origin, implications and treatments. *Open Journal of Regenerative Medicine*, *9*(02), 43–64. doi:10.4236/ojrm.2020.92006

Lee, C. F., Shen, J. J., Chen, Z. R., & Agrawal, S. (2019). Self-Embedding Authentication Watermarking with Effective Tampered Location Detection and High-Quality Image Recovery. *Sensors (Basel)*, *19*(10), 1–18. doi:10.339019102267 PMID:31100886

Lee, C.-F., Shen, J.-J., & Chen, Z.-R. (2018). A Survey of Watermarking-Based Authentication for Digital Image. *Proceedings of the 3rd International Conference on Computer and Communication Systems*, 207–211. 10.1109/CCOMS.2018.8463259

Lee, T. S. (1996). Image representation using 2D Gabor wavelets. *IEEE Transactions on Pattern Analysis and Machine Intelligence*, *18*(10), 959–971. doi:10.1109/34.541406

Lemheney, A. J. (2016). Developing virtual reality simulations for office-based medical emergencies. *Journal of Virtual Worlds Research*, *9*(1).

Lennon, M. R., Bouamrane, M. M., Devlin, A. M., O'connor, S., O'donnell, C., Chetty, U., Agbakoba, R., Bikker, A., Grieve, E., Finch, T., Watson, N., Wyke, S., & Mair, F. S. (2017). Readiness for delivering digital health at scale: Lessons from a longitudinal qualitative evaluation of a national digital health innovation program in the United Kingdom. *Journal of Medical Internet Research*, *19*(2), e6900. doi:10.2196/jmir.6900 PMID:28209558

Lenzini, G., Bargh, M. S., & Hulsebosch, B. (2008). Trust-enhanced security in location-based adaptive authentication. *Electronic Notes in Theoretical Computer Science*, *197*(2), 105–119. doi:10.1016/j.entcs.2007.12.020

Li, F. (2022). GAN-Based Spatial Image Steganography with Cross Feedback Mechanism. *Signal Processing, 190*. doi:10.1016/j.sigpro.2021.108341

Li, L. (2021). Adversarial Batch Image Steganography against CNN-Based Pooled Steganalysis. *Signal Processing, 181*. . doi:10.1016/j.sigpro.2020.107920

Li, Q. (2021). Image Steganography Based on Style Transfer and Quaternion Exponent Moments. *Applied Soft Computing, 110*. . doi:10.1016/j.asoc.2021.107618

Li, S., Ashok, A., Zhang, Y., Xu, C., Lindqvist, J., & Gruteser, M. (2016, March). Whose move is it anyway? Authenticating smart wearable devices using unique head movement patterns. *2016 IEEE International Conference on Pervasive Computing and Communications (PerCom)*. http://dx.doi.org/10.1109/percom.2016.7456514

Libbrecht, M. W., & Noble, W. S. (2015). Machine learning applications in genetics and genomics. *Nature Reviews. Genetics*, *16*(6), 321–332. doi:10.1038/nrg3920 PMID:25948244

Li, C.-Y., & Hsu, C.-T. (2008). Image retrieval with relevance feedback based on graph-theoretic region correspondence estimation. *IEEE Transactions on Multimedia*, *10*(3), 447–456.

Li, F., Clarke, N., Papadaki, M., & Dowland, P. (2013). Active authentication for mobile devices utilisingbehaviour profiling. *International Journal of Information Security*, *13*(3), 229–244. doi:10.100710207-013-0209-6

Li, J., Cai, J., Khan, F., Rehman, A. U., Balasubramaniam, V., Sun, J., & Venu, P. (2020). A Secured Framework for SDN-Based Edge Computing in IoT-Enabled Healthcare System. *IEEE Access: Practical Innovations, Open Solutions*, *8*, 135479–135490. doi:10.1109/ACCESS.2020.3011503

Li, J., Dai, J., Issakhov, A., Almojil, S. F., & Souri, A. (2021). Towards decision support systems for energy management in the smart industry and Internet of Things. *Computers & Industrial Engineering*, *161*, 107671. doi:10.1016/j.cie.2021.107671

Li, M., Wang, X., Gao, K., & Zhang, S. (2017). A Survey on Information Diffusion in Online Social Networks. *Models and Methods. Information*, *8*, 118.

Lin, A., Foroozan, R., Carrier, D., & Yen, M. T. (2004). Diagnosis of metastatic carcinoma to the cavernous sinus by computed tomograpy–guided fine-needle aspiration. *American Journal of Ophthalmology*, *138*(5), 864–866. doi:10.1016/j.ajo.2004.05.036 PMID:15531326

Li, Q., Guo, N. N., Han, Z. Y., Zhang, Y. B., Qi, S. X., Xu, Y. G., ... Liu, Y. Y. (2012). Application of an autoregressive integrated moving average model for predicting the incidence of hemorrhagic fever with renal syndrome. *The American Journal of Tropical Medicine and Hygiene*, *87*(2), 364.

Li, Q., Wang, X., Wang, X., Ma, B., Wang, C., Xian, Y., & Shi, Y. (2020). A Novel Grayscale Image Steganography Scheme Based on Chaos Encryption and Generative Adversarial Networks. *IEEE Access: Practical Innovations, Open Solutions*, *8*, 168166–168176. doi:10.1109/ACCESS.2020.3021103

Liu, C. (2004). Gabor-based kernel pca with fractional power polynomial models for face recognition. *IEEE Transactions on Pattern Analysis and Machine Intelligence*, *26*(5), 572–581. doi:10.1109/TPAMI.2004.1273927 PMID:15460279

Liu, C.-K., Hsu, C.-Y., Yang, F.-Y., Wu, J., Kuo, K., & Lai, P. (2017). Population health management outcomes obtained through a hospital-based and telehealth informatics-enabled telecare service. *2017 IEEE Biomedical Circuits and Systems Conference (BioCAS)*. 10.1109/BIOCAS.2017.8325127

Liu, J., Ke, Y., Zhang, Z., Lei, Y., Li, J., Zhang, M., & Yang, X. (2020). Recent Advances of Image Steganography With Generative Adversarial Networks. *IEEE Access: Practical Innovations, Open Solutions*, *8*, 60575–60597. doi:10.1109/ACCESS.2020.2983175

Liu, J., & Liu, Y. (2018). Application of computer molecular simulation technology and artificial intelligence in drug development. *Technol. Innov. Appl.*, *2*, 46–47.

Liu, K., & Kehtarnavaz, N. (2013). Real-time robust vision-based hand gesture recognition using stereo images. *Journal of Real-Time Image Processing*, *11*(1), 201–209. doi:10.100711554-013-0333-6

Liu, L. (2016). Smart homes and home health monitoring technologies for older adults: A systematic review. *International Journal of Medical Informatics*, *91*, 44–59.

Liu, Q., Liu, X., Jiang, B., & Yang, W. (2011). Forecasting incidence of hemorrhagic fever with renal syndrome in China using ARIMA model. *BMC Infectious Diseases*, *11*(1), 1–7.

Liu, S., Pan, Z., & Song, H. (2017). Digital image watermarking method based on DCT and fractal encoding. *IET Image Processing*, *11*(10), 815–821. doi:10.1049/iet-ipr.2016.0862

Liu, X., Zhang, J., Wang, H., Gong, X., & Cheng, Y. (2014). A Novel Text Watermarking Algorithm Based on Graphic Watermarking Framework. *Proceedings of the Ninth International Conference on Broadband and Wireless Computing, Communication and Applications*, 84–88. 10.1109/BWCCA.2014.49

Liu, X., Zhang, R., & Liu, Q. (2017). A temporal credential-based mutual authentication with multiple-password scheme for wireless sensor networks. *PLoS One*, *12*(1), e0170657. doi:10.1371/journal.pone.0170657 PMID:28135288

Liu, Z. L., Anderson, T. D., & Cruz, J. M. (2012). Consumer environmental awareness and competition in two-stage supply chains. *European Journal of Operational Research*, *218*(3), 602–613. doi:10.1016/j.ejor.2011.11.027

Liu, Z., Bonazzi, R., & Pigneur, Y. (2016). Privacy-based adaptive context-aware authentication system for personal mobile devices. J. *Mobile Multimedia*, *12*(1&2), 159–180.

Liu, Z., Guo, C., & Wang, B. (2020). A physically secure, lightweight three-factor and anonymous user authentication protocol for iot. *IEEE Access: Practical Innovations, Open Solutions*, *8*, 195914–195928. doi:10.1109/ACCESS.2020.3034219

Li, X., Ma, S., & Yang, G. (2017). Synthesis of Difference Patterns for Monopulse Antennas by an Improved Cuckoo Search Algorithm. *IEEE Antennas and Wireless Propagation Letters*, *16*, 141–144. doi:10.1109/LAWP.2016.2640998

Li, X., Niu, J., Khurram Khan, M., & Liao, J. (2013). An enhanced smart card based remote user password authentication scheme. *Journal of Network and Computer Applications*, *36*(5), 1365–1371. doi:10.1016/j.jnca.2013.02.034

Li, Z., Sun, Q., Lian, Y., & Giusto, D. D. (2005). A secure image-based authentication scheme for mobile devices. In *Lecture Notes in Computer Science* (pp. 751–760). Springer Berlin Heidelberg. doi:10.1007/11538356_78

Lo'ai, A. T., Mehmood, R., Benkhlifa, E., & Song, H. (2016). Mobile cloud computing model and big data analysis for healthcare applications. *IEEE Access: Practical Innovations, Open Solutions*, *4*, 6171–6180. doi:10.1109/ACCESS.2016.2613278

Lopez-Hernandez, Martinez-Gonzalez, Hernandez-Reyes, Palacios-Luengas, & Vazquez-Medina. (2020). A Steganography Method Using Neural Networks. *IEEE Latin America Transactions*, *18*(3), 495-506. doi:10.1109/TLA.2020.9082720

Lu & Li. (2020). Survey on lie group machine learning. *Big Data Mining and Analytics*, *3*(4), 235-258. . doi:10.26599/BDMA.2020.9020011

Lu, Xue, Yeung, Liu, Huang, & Shi. (2021). Secure Halftone Image Steganography Based on Pixel Density Transition. *IEEE Transactions on Dependable and Secure Computing*, *18*(3), 1137-1149. doi:10.1109/TDSC.2019.2933621

Lucangeli, L., D'Angelantonio, E., Camomilla, V., & Pallotti, A. (2021, June). SISTINE: Sensorized Socks for Telemonitoring of Vascular Disease Patients. In *2021 IEEE International Workshop on Metrology for Industry 4.0 & IoT (MetroInd4. 0&IoT)* (pp. 192-197). IEEE.

Luo, F. (2018). An improved particle swarm optimization algorithm based on adaptive weight for task scheduling in cloud computing. *Proceedings of the 2nd International Conference on Computer Science and Application Engineering*.

Lu, & Sinnott. (2020). *Security and privacy solutions for smart healthcare systems*. Innovation in Health Informatics A Smart Healthcare Primer Next Gen Tech Driven Personalized Med&Smart Healthcare.

Magoulas, G. D., & Prentza, A. (1999, July). Machine learning in medical applications. In *Advanced course on artificial intelligence* (pp. 300–307). Springer.

Mahata, G. C., & Goswami, A. (2009a). A fuzzy replenishment policy for deteriorating items with ramp type demand rate under inflation. *International Journal of Operational Research*, *5*(3), 328–348. doi:10.1504/IJOR.2009.025200

Mahfoodh, H., Aleid, K., Bahzad, A., Matar, S., Shubbar, Z. S., & Mattar, E. (2021). Sustaining Work Continuity through Hybrid Work Environments: Tracking Systems. *2021 International Conference on Innovation and Intelligence for Informatics, Computing, and Technologies, 3ICT 2021*, 677–684. 10.1109/3ICT53449.2021.9581371

Mahmoudi, F., Shanbehzadeh, J., Moghadam, A. M. E., & Zadeh, S. H. (2003). Image retrieval based on shape similarity by edge orientation autocorrelogram. *Pattern Recognition, 36*(8), 1725–1736. doi:10.1016/S0031-3203(03)00010-4

Mahmud, R., Ramamohanarao, K., & Buyya, R. (2018). Latency-aware application module management for fog computing environments. *ACM Transactions on Internet Technology, 19*(1), 1–21. doi:10.1145/3186592

Mahmud, R., Srirama, S. N., Ramamohanarao, K., & Buyya, R. (2019). Quality of Experience (QoE)-aware placement of applications in Fog computing environments. *Journal of Parallel and Distributed Computing, 132*, 190–203. doi:10.1016/j.jpdc.2018.03.004

Majeed, A., & Rauf, I. (2020). Graph Theory: A Comprehensive Survey about Graph Theory Applications in Computer Science and Social Networks. *Inventions, 5*, 10. doi:10.3390/inventions5010010

Makinde, O. D., & Mutuku, W. N. (2014). Hydromagnetic thermal boundary layer of nanofluids over a convectively heated at plate with viscous dissipation and Ohmic heating. *Universitatea Politecnica Bucuresti Scientific Bulletin Series A, 76*(2), 181–192.

Malawski, M., Gajek, A., Zima, A., Balis, B., & Figiela, K. (2020). Serverless execution of scientific workflows: Experiments with hyperflow, aws lambda and google cloud functions. *Future Generation Computer Systems, 110*, 502–514. doi:10.1016/j.future.2017.10.029

Mallapragada, P. K., Jin, R., Jain, A. K., & Liu, Y. (2009, November). SemiBoost: Boosting for Semi-Supervised Learning. *IEEE Transactions on Pattern Analysis and Machine Intelligence, 31*(11), 2000–2014. doi:10.1109/TPAMI.2008.235 PMID:19762927

Malmberg, F., Lindblad, J., Sladoje, N., & Nyström, I. (2010). A graph-based framework for sub-pixel image segmentation. *Theoretical Computer Science*. Advance online publication. doi:10.1016/j.tcs.2010.11.030

Manivannan, M., & Suseendran, G. (2017). A Review of Watermarking Requirements, Techniques, Documents, Human Perception and Applications for Medical Images. *International Journal of Innovative Research in Applied Sciences and Engineering, 1*(2), 58–65. doi:10.29027/IJIRASE.v1.i2.2017.58-65

Mansour, R. F., Amraoui, A. E., Nouaouri, I., Diaz, V. G., Gupta, D., & Kumar, S. (2021). Artificial Intelligence and Internet of Things Enabled Disease Diagnosis Model for Smart Healthcare Systems. *IEEE Access: Practical Innovations, Open Solutions, 9*, 45137–45146. doi:10.1109/ACCESS.2021.3066365

Manvi, S. S., & Shyam, G. K. (2014). Resource management for Infrastructure as a Service (IaaS) in cloud computing: A survey. *Journal of Network and Computer Applications, 41*, 424–440. doi:10.1016/j.jnca.2013.10.004

Mapetu, J. P. B., Chen, Z., & Kong, L. (2019). Low-time complexity and low-cost binary particle swarm optimization algorithm for task scheduling and load balancing in cloud computing. *Applied Intelligence, 49*(9), 3308–3330.

Mareli, M., & Twala, B. (2018). An adaptive Cuckoo search algorithm for optimisation. *Applied Computing and Informatics, 14*(2), 107-115.

Marini, F., & Walczak, B. (2015). Particle swarm optimization (PSO). A tutorial. *Chemometrics and Intelligent Laboratory Systems, 149*, 153–165.

Marnada, P., Raharjo, T., Hardian, B., & Prasetyo, A. (2021). Agile project management challenge in handling scope and change: A systematic literature review. *Procedia Computer Science, 197*, 290–300. doi:10.1016/j.procs.2021.12.143

Martin, J. L., Varilly, H., Cohn, J., & Wightwick, G. R. (2010). Preface: Technologies for a smarter planet. *IBM Journal of Research and Development*, *54*(4), 1–2. doi:10.1147/JRD.2010.2051498

Martinovic, I., Rasmussen, K., Roeschlin, M., & Tsudik, G. (2017). Authentication using pulse-response biometrics. *Communications of the ACM*, *60*(2), 108–115. doi:10.1145/3023359

Mashud, A. H. M. M., Pervin, M., Mishra, U., & Daryanto, Y. (2021). A sustainable inventory model with controllable carbon emissions in green-warehouse farms. *Journal of Cleaner Production*, *298*(126777), 1–15. doi:10.1016/j.jclepro.2021.126777

Matas, J., Jonsson, K., & Kittler, J. (1999). Fast face localisation and verification. *Image and Vision Computing*, *17*(8), 575–581. doi:10.1016/S0262-8856(98)00176-0

Matchev, K. T., Matcheva, K., & Roman, A. (2022). *Unsupervised Machine Learning for Exploratory Data Analysis of Exoplanet Transmission Spectra*. https://arxiv.org/abs/2201.02696

Mavrovouniotis, M., Li, C., & Yang, S. (2017). A survey of swarm intelligence for dynamic optimization: Algorithms and applications. *Swarm and Evolutionary Computation*, *33*, 1–17. doi:10.1016/j.swevo.2016.12.005

Max-dependency, C. (2005). *Feature Selection Based on Mutual Information*. Academic Press.

McGrath, G., & Brenner, P. R. (2017). Serverless computing: Design, implementation, and performance. *2017 IEEE 37th International Conference on Distributed Computing Systems Workshops (ICDCSW)*, 405–410. 10.1109/ICDCSW.2017.36

McGrath, J. L. (2018). Using virtual reality simulation environments to assess competence for emergency medicine learners. *Academic Emergency Medicine*, *25*(2), 186–195.

MD.ai. (2021). *MD.ai annotator project*. https://public.md.ai/annotator/project/aGq4k6NW

MD.ai. (2021). *Python client library*. https://github.com/mdai/mdai-client-py

Mehran, N., Kimovski, D., & Prodan, R. (2019, October). MAPO: a multi-objective model for IoT application placement in a fog environment. In *Proceedings of the 9th International Conference on the Internet of Things* (pp. 1-8). 10.1145/3365871.3365892

Mell, P., & Grance, T. (2011). *The NIST definition of cloud computing*. Academic Press.

Merav, C., Eyal, C., Sigal, F., Zamir, H., Uri, N., & Eshel, B.J. (2012). Artificial Neural Networks Based Controller for Glucose Monitoring during Clamp Test. *PLOS ONE*. https://journals.plos.org/plosone/article?id=10.1371/journal.pone.0044587

Miltiadis, Visvizi, Sarirete, & Chui. (2021). Preface: Artificial intelligence and big data analytics for smart healthcare: A digital transformation of healthcare primer. *Artificial Intelligence and Big Data Analytics for Smart Healthcare*.

Minh, Q. T., Nguyen, D. T., Van Le, A., Nguyen, H. D., & Truong, A. (2017, November). Toward service placement on fog computing landscape. In *2017 4th NAFOSTED conference on information and computer science* (pp. 291-296). IEEE. 10.1109/NAFOSTED.2017.8108080

Mirzaei, Sidi, Keasar, & Crivelli. (2019). Purely Structural Protein Scoring Functions Using Support Vector Machine and Ensemble Learning. *IEEE/ACM Transactions on Computational Biology and Bioinformatics*, *16*(5), 1515-1523. . doi:10.1109/TCBB.2016.2602269

Misbahuddin, M., Bindhumadhava, B. S., &Dheeptha, B. (2017, August). Design of a risk based authentication system using machine learning techniques. *2017 IEEE SmartWorld, Ubiquitous Intelligence & Computing, Advanced & Trusted Computed, Scalable Computing & Communications, Cloud & Big Data Computing, Internet of People and Smart City Innovation (SmartWorld/SCALCOM/UIC/ATC/CBDCom/IOP/SCI)*. http://dx.doi.org/ doi:10.1109/uic-atc.2017.8397628

Mishra, A., Rajpal, A., & Bala, R. (2018). Bi-directional extreme learning machine for semi-blind watermarking of compressed images. *Journal of Information Security and Applications, 38*, 71–84. doi:10.1016/j.jisa.2017.11.008

Mishra, A., Basumallick, S., Lu, A., Chiu, H., Shah, M. A., Shukla, Y., & Tiwari, A. (2021). The healthier healthcare management models for COVID-19. *Journal of Infection and Public Health, 14*(7), 927–937. doi:10.1016/j.jiph.2021.05.014 PMID:34119847

Mishra, A., & Chakraborty, B. (2018). AD8232 based smart healthcare system using internet of things (IoT). *International Journal of Engineering Research & Technology (Ahmedabad), 7*(4), 13–16.

Mishra, A., Singh, C., Dwivedi, A., Singh, D., & Biswal, A. K. (2021, October). Network Forensics: An approach towards detecting Cyber Crime. In *2021 International Conference in Advances in Power, Signal, and Information Technology (APSIT)* (pp. 1-6). IEEE.

Mishra, K. N., & Chakraborty, C. (2020). A novel approach towards using big data and IoT for improving the efficiency of m-health systems. In *Advanced computational intelligence techniques for virtual reality in healthcare* (pp. 123–139). Springer. doi:10.1007/978-3-030-35252-3_7

Mishra, R. B. (1975). Optimum production lot size model for a system with deteriorating inventory. *International Journal of Production Research, 13*(5), 495–505. doi:10.1080/00207547508943019

Mishra, U., Wu, J. Z., Tsao, Y. C., & Tsend, M. L. (2020b). Sustainable inventory system with controllable non-instantaneous deterioration and environmental emission rates. *Journal of Cleaner Production, 244*(118807), 1–29. doi:10.1016/j.jclepro.2019.118807

Mistry, C., Stelea, B., Kumar, V., & Pasquier, T. (n.d.). *Demonstrating the Practicality of Unikernels to Build a Serverless Platform at the Edge*. Academic Press.

Mitra, R., & Ganiga, R. (2019). A novel approach to sensor implementation for healthcare systems using internet of things. *International Journal of Electrical & Computer Engineering, 9*(6).

Mitushi, S., & Sunita, V. (2020). Diabetes Prediction using Machine Learning Techniques. *International Journal of Engineering Research & Technology*. https://www.ijert.org/diabetes-prediction-using-machine-learning-techniques

Moeinaddini, E., & Ghasemkhani, R. (2015). A novel image watermarking scheme using blocks coefficient in DHT domain. *Proceedings of the International Symposium on Artificial Intelligence and Signal Processing (AISP)*, 159–164. 10.1109/AISP.2015.7123512

Mohammad, T., & Bijan, R. (2015). Importance of Data Mining in Healthcare: A Survey. *Proceedings of the IEEE/ACM International Conference on Advances in Social Networks Analysis and Mining*, 1057–1062. 10.1145/2808797.2809367

Mohan, A., Sane, H., Doshi, K., Edupuganti, S., Nayak, N., & Sukhomlinov, V. (2019). Agile cold starts for scalable serverless. *11th USENIX Workshop on Hot Topics in Cloud Computing (HotCloud 19)*.

Mohan, S., Thirumalai, C., & Srivastava, G. (2019). Effective heart disease prediction using hybrid machine learning techniques. *IEEE Access: Practical Innovations, Open Solutions, 7*, 81542–81554.

Mokdad, Ford, Bowman, Nelson, Engelgau, & Vinicor. (2000). Diabetes trends in the U.S.: 1990-1998. *Diabetes Care 1, 23*(9), 1278–1283. doi:10.2337/diacare.23.9.1278

Moodley, S., Schoenhagen, P., Gillinov, A. M., Mihaljevic, T., Flamm, S. D., Griffin, B. P., & Desai, M. Y. (2013). Preoperative multidetector computed tomograpy angiography for planning of minimally invasive robotic mitral valve surgery: Impact on decision making. *The Journal of Thoracic and Cardiovascular Surgery*, *146*(2), 262–268. doi:10.1016/j.jtcvs.2012.06.052 PMID:22841167

Moon, M. J. (2020). Fighting COVID-19 with agility, transparency, and participation: Wicked policy problems and new governance challenges. *Public Administration Review*, *80*(4), 651–656. doi:10.1111/puar.13214 PMID:32836434

Moore, D. (1987). Classification and regression trees. *Cytometry*, *8*(5), 534–535. doi:10.1002/cyto.990080516

Moosazadeh, M., & Ekbatanifard, G. (2019). A new DCT-based robust image watermarking method using teaching-learning-based optimization. *Journal of Information Security and Applications*, *47*, 28–38. doi:10.1016/j.jisa.2019.04.001

Moradi, G., Farnia, M., Shokoohi, M., Shahbazi, M., Moazen, B., & Rahmani, K. (2015). A qualitative study in Iran explored methadone maintenance treatment programs in prisons from the perspective of medical and non-medical prison staff. *International Journal of Health Policy and Management*, *4*(9), 583–589. doi:10.15171/ijhpm.2015.60 PMID:26340487

Mordor-intelligence. (2021). *Impact of global covid 19 and smart healthcare Healthcare Facilities Management Market | Growth, Trends, COVID-19 Impact, and Forecasts (2022 - 27).* mordorintelligence.com

Moshe, P., Tadej, B., Eran, A., Olga, K., Natasa, B., Shahar, M., Torben, B., Magdalena, A.S., Ido, M., Revital, N., & Thomas, D. (n.d.). Nocturnal Glucose Control with an Artificial Pancreas at a Diabetes Camp. *The New England Journal of Medicine*. https://www.nejm.org/doi/10.1056/NEJMoa1206881#article_citing_articles

Mostafa Rushdi, A. (2021). Machine learning approaches for thermal updraft prediction in wind solar tower systems. *Renewable Energy*, *177*, 1001–1013. doi:10.1016/j.renene.2021.06.033

Muhammad, G., Alshehri, F., Karray, F., Saddik, A. E., Alsulaiman, M., & Falk, T. H. (2021). A comprehensive survey on multimodal medical signals fusion for smart healthcare systems. *Information Fusion*, *76*, 355–375. doi:10.1016/j.inffus.2021.06.007

Muhammad, K., Khan, S., Kumar, N., Del Ser, J., & Mirjalili, S. (2020). Vision-based personalized Wireless Capsule Endoscopy for smart healthcare: Taxonomy, literature review, opportunities and challenges. *Future Generation Computer Systems*, *113*, 266–280. doi:10.1016/j.future.2020.06.048

Muhammed, T. (2018). UbeHealth: A personalized ubiquitous cloud and edge-enabled networked healthcare system for smart cities. *IEEE Access: Practical Innovations, Open Solutions*, *6*, 32258–32285.

Mu, J., Xiong, R., Fan, X., Liu, D., Wu, F., & Gao, W. (2020). Graph-Based Non-Convex Low-Rank Regularization for Image Compression Artifact Reduction. *IEEE Transactions on Image Processing*, *29*, 5374–5385. doi:10.1109/TIP.2020.2975931 PMID:32149688

Mukherjee, S. (2021). Pencil Shell Matrix Based Image Steganography with Elevated Embedding Capacity. *Journal of Information Security and Applications, 62.* . doi:10.1016/j.jisa.2021.102955

Mukherjee, T., Wickersham, J., Desai, M., Pillai, V., Kamarulzaman, A., & Altice, F. (2016). Factors associated with interest in receiving prison-based methadone maintenance therapy in Malaysia. *Drug and Alcohol Dependence*, *164*, 120–127. doi:10.1016/j.drugalcdep.2016.04.037 PMID:27207155

Mulligan, D. (2020). *Results tracker app and deployment on EKS.* Elastic Kubernetes Service.

Murmuria, R., Stavrou, A., Barbará, D., & Fleck, D. (2015). Continuous authentication on mobile devices using power consumption, touch gestures and physical movement of users. In Research in Attacks, Intrusions, and Defenses (pp. 405–424). Springer International Publishing. doi:10.1007/978-3-319-26362-5_19

Mustafa, A., & Rahimi, A. M. (2021). Automated Machine Learning for Healthcare and Clinical Notes Analysis. *Computers, 2021*(10), 24. doi:10.3390/computers10020024

Mustafa, S., Nazir, B., Hayat, A., Madani, S. A., & ... (2015). Resource management in cloud computing: Taxonomy, prospects, and challenges. *Computers & Electrical Engineering, 47*, 186–203. doi:10.1016/j.compeleceng.2015.07.021

Muteeh, A., Sardaraz, M., & Tahir, M. (2021). MrLBA: Multi-resource load balancing algorithm for cloud computing using ant colony optimization. *Cluster Computing*, 1–11.

Mutlag, A. A., Abd Ghani, M. K., Arunkumar, N., Mohammed, M. A., & Mohd, O. (2019). Enabling technologies for fog computing in healthcare IoT systems. *Future Generation Computer Systems, 90*, 62–78. doi:10.1016/j.future.2018.07.049

Nadeem, S., & Haq, R. U. (2014). Effect of thermal radiation for magnetohydrodynamic boundary layer flow of a nanofluid past a stretching sheet with convective boundary conditions. *Journal of Computational and Theoretical Nanoscience, 11*(1), 32–40. doi:10.1166/jctn.2014.3313

Nagavelli, U., Samanta, D., & Chakraborty, P. (2022). Machine Learning Technology-Based Heart Disease Detection Models. *Journal of Healthcare Engineering, 2022*, 2022. doi:10.1155/2022/7351061 PMID:35265303

Nambiar, A. R., Reddy, N., & Dutta, D. (2017). Connected health: opportunities and challenges. *IEEE International Conference on Big Data*, 1658-1662.

Naramgari, S., & Sulochana, C. (2016). Dual solutions of radiative MHD nanofluid flow over an exponentially stretching sheet with heat generation/absorption. *Applied Nanoscience, 6*(1), 131–139. doi:10.100713204-015-0420-z

Naranjo, P. G. V., Pooranian, Z., Shojafar, M., Conti, M., & Buyya, R. (2019). FOCAN: A Fog-supported smart city network architecture for management of applications in the Internet of Everything environments. *Journal of Parallel and Distributed Computing, 132*, 274–283. doi:10.1016/j.jpdc.2018.07.003

Naseem, I., Togneri, R., & Bennamoun, M. (2010). Linear Regression for Face Recognition. *IEEE Transactions on Pattern Analysis and Machine Intelligence, 32*(11), 2106–2112. doi:10.1109/TPAMI.2010.128 PMID:20603520

Nasr, Islam, Shehata, Karray, & Quintana. (2021). Smart Healthcare in the Age of AI: Recent Advances, Challenges, and Future Prospects. In *Computers and Society*. Cornell University.

Navin, K., Mukesh Krishnan, M. B., Lavanya, S., & Shanthini, A. (2017). A mobile health based smart hybrid epidemic surveillance system to support epidemic control programme in public health informatics. *2017 International Conference on IoT and Application (ICIOT)*. 10.1109/ICIOTA.2017.8073606

Nefian, A. V., & Hayes, M. H. (1998). Hidden Markow models for face recognition. *Proceedings of the 1998 IEEE International Conference on Acoustics, Speech and Signal Processing*, 2721-2724.

Ness, M. M., Saylor, J., Di Fusco, L. A., & Evans, K. (2021). Healthcare providers' challenges during the coronavirus disease (COVID-19) pandemic: A qualitative approach. *Nursing & Health Sciences*.

Neverova, N., Wolf, C., Lacey, G., Fridman, L., Chandra, D., Barbello, B., & Taylor, G. (2016). Learning human identity from motion patterns. *IEEE Access: Practical Innovations, Open Solutions, 4*, 1810–1820. doi:10.1109/ACCESS.2016.2557846

Nikolic, M., Tuba, E., & Tuba, M. (2016). Edge detection in medical ultrasound images using adjusted canny edge detection algorithm. *Proceedings of the 2016 24th Telecommunications Forum (TELFOR)*, 1–4. 10.1109/TELFOR.2016.7818878

Noghrehabadadi, A., Ghalambaz, M., & Ghanbarzadeh, A. (2012). Heat transfer of magnetohydrodynamic viscous nanofluids over an isothermal stretching sheet. *Journal of Thermophysics and Heat Transfer, 26*(4), 686–689. doi:10.2514/1.T3866

Olekh, T. M., Vlasenko, O. V., Kolesnikova, K., & Lukianov, D. (2013). *Markov's model in Project Management Communications in Organizational and Technscal System.* Unpublished. doi:10.13140/rg.2.1.5015.0484

Ometov, A., Bezzateev, S., Mäkitalo, N., Andreev, S., Mikkonen, T., & Koucheryavy, Y. (2018). Multi-Factor authentication: A survey. *Cryptography, 2*(1), 1. doi:10.3390/cryptography2010001

Ophir, G., Maayan, F., Hayit, G., Patrick, D. B., Huangqi, Z., Wenbin, J., Adam, B., & Eliot, S. (2020). *Rapid AI development cycle for the coronavirus (COVID-19) pandemic: Initial results for automated detection & patient monitoring using deep learning CT image analysis.* arXiv preprint arXiv:2003.05037

Ornoy, A. (2011). Prenatal origin of obesity and their complications: Gestational diabetes, maternal overweight and the paradoxical effects of fetal growth restriction and macrosomia. *Reproductive Toxicology (Elmsford, N.Y.), 32*(2), 205–212.

Osman, H., & Baki, M. F. (2018). A Cuckoo Search Algorithm to Solve Transfer Line Balancing Problems With Different Cutting Conditions. *IEEE Transactions on Engineering Management, 65*(3), 505–518. doi:10.1109/TEM.2018.2797223

Outlier - an overview | ScienceDirect Topics. (n.d.). Retrieved April 13, 2022, from https://www.sciencedirect.com/topics/computer-science/outlier

Pal, D., Triyason, T., & Padungweang, P. (2018). Big data in smart-cities: Current research and challenges. *Indonesian Journal of Electrical Engineering and Informatics, 6*(4), 351–360.

Panda, N., & Majhi, S. K. (2019). How effective is spotted hyena optimizer for training multilayer perceptrons. *Int J Recent Technol Eng*, 4915-4927.

Pan, L., & Bangay, S. (2014, October). Generating repudiable, memorizable, and privacy preserving security questions using the propp theory of narrative. *2014 International Conference on Cyber-Enabled Distributed Computing and Knowledge Discovery.* 10.1109/CyberC.2014.20

Partha, M. K., Murthy, P. V. S. N., & Rajasekhar, G. P. (2005). Effect of viscous dissipation on the mixed convection heat transfer from an exponentially stretching surface. *Heat and Mass Transfer, 41*(4), 360–366. doi:10.100700231-004-0552-2

Patel, D., Patra, M. K., & Sahoo, B. (2020). GWO Based task allocation for load balancing in containerized cloud. In *2020 International Conference on Inventive Computation Technologies (ICICT)*, pp. 655-659. IEEE.

Patel, A. R. (2017). Vitality of robotics in healthcare industry: an Internet of Things (IoT) perspective. In *Internet of Things and Big Data Technologies for Next Generation Healthcare* (pp. 91–109). Springer.

Patra, M. K., Sahoo, S., Sahoo, B., & Turuk, A. K. (2021). Cloud-Edge Centric Service Provisioning in Smart City Using Internet of Things. In *Advances in Parallel & Distributed Processing, and Applications* (pp. 619–631). Springer.

Patro, R., Acharya, M., Nayak, M. M., & Patnaik, S. (2017). A fuzzy imperfect quality inventory model with proportionate discount under learning effect. *International Journal of Intelligent Enterprise, 4*(4), 303–327. doi:10.1504/IJIE.2017.089211

Patro, R., Acharya, M., Nayak, M. M., & Patnaik, S. (2017). A fuzzy inventory model with time dependent weibull deterioration, quadratic demand and partial backlogging. *International Journal of Management and Decision Making, 16*(3), 243–279. doi:10.1504/IJMDM.2017.085636

Pattanaik, B. (2021). Contrasting the Performance Metrics of Discrete Transformations on Digital Image Steganography Using Artificial Intelligence. *Materials Today: Proceedings.* . doi:10.1016/j.matpr.2020.12.076

Paul, L. C., & Sumam, A. A. (2012). Face Recognition Using Principal Component Analysis Method. *International Journal of Advanced Research in Computer Engineering and Technology, 1*, 135–139.

Pavel, M., Jimison, H. B., Korhonen, I., Gordon, C. M., & Saranummi, N. (2015). Behavioral Informatics and Computational Modeling in Support of Proactive health Management and care. *IEEE Transactions on Biomedical Engineering*, *62*(12), 2763–2775. doi:10.1109/TBME.2015.2484286 PMID:26441408

Pazhaniraja, N., Paul, P. V., Roja, G., Shanmugapriya, K., & Sonali, B. (2017, March). A study on recent bio-inspired optimization algorithms. In *2017 Fourth International Conference on Signal Processing, Communication and Networking (ICSCN)* (pp. 1-6). IEEE. 10.1109/ICSCN.2017.8085674

Perera, C., Jayaraman, P. P., Zaslavsky, A., Christen, P., & Georgakopoulos, D. (2014, January). Mosden: An internet of things middleware for resource constrained mobile devices. In *2014 47Th hawaii international conference on system sciences* (pp. 1053-1062). IEEE.

Perkins, D. (1975). A Definition of Caricature and Caricature and Recognition. *Studies In Visual Communications*, *2*(1), 1–24. doi:10.1525/var.1975.2.1.1

Petsas, T., Tsirantonakis, G., Athanasopoulos, E., & Ioannidis, S. (2015, April 21). Two-factor authentication: Is the world ready? *Proceedings of the Eighth European Workshop on System Security*. 10.1145/2751323.2751327

Pham, D., & Karaboga, D. (2012). *Intelligent optimisation techniques: genetic algorithms, tabu search, simulated annealing and neural networks*. Springer Science & Business Media.

Phillips, P. J., Wechsler, H., Huang, J., & Rauss, P. (1998). The FERET database and evaluation procedure for face-recognition algorithms. *Image and Vision Computing*, *16*(5), 295–306. doi:10.1016/S0262-8856(97)00070-X

Pico-Valencia, P., Holgado-Terriza, J. A., & Quiñónez-Ku, X. (2020). A Brief Survey of the Main internet Based Approaches. An Outlook from the internet of Things Perspective. *2020 3rd International Conference on Information and Computer Technologies (ICICT)*. 10.1109/ICICT50521.2020.00091

Piri, J., Mohapatra, P., Singh, D., Samanta, D., Singh, D., Kaur, M., & Lee, H.-N. (2022). Mining and Interpretation of Critical Aspects of Infant Health Status Using Multi-Objective Evolutionary Feature Selection Approaches. *IEEE Access: Practical Innovations, Open Solutions*, *10*, 32622–32638. doi:10.1109/ACCESS.2022.3161154

Piva, A., Bartolini, F., & Barni, M. (2002). Managing copyright in open networks. *IEEE Transactions on Internet Computing*, *6*(3), 18–26. doi:10.1109/MIC.2002.1003126

Podilchuk, C. I., & Delp, E. J. (2001). Digital watermarking: Algorithms and applications. *IEEE Signal Processing Magazine*, *18*(4), 33–46. doi:10.1109/79.939835

Ponnivalavan, K., & Pathinathan, T. (2015). Intuitionistic pentagonal fuzzy number. *Journal of Engineering and Applied Sciences (Asian Research Publishing Network)*, *10*(12), 5446–5450.

Popović, K., & Hocenski, Ž. (2010). Cloud computing security issues and challenges. *The 33rd international convention mipro*, 344–349.

Pramanik, S. (2020). Application of Bi-Orthogonal Wavelet Transform and Genetic Algorithm in Image Steganography. *Multimedia Tools and Applications*, *79*(25), 17463–82. . doi:10.1007/s11042-020-08676-1

Pramanik, M. I. (2017). Smart health: Big data enabled health paradigm within smart cities. *Expert Systems with Applications*, *87*, 370–383.

Pranav, P., & Chirag, P. (2013, December). Various Graphs and Their Applications in Real World. *International Journal of Engineering Research & Technology (Ahmedabad)*, *2*(12).

Premarathne, U. S., Khalil, I., & Atiquzzaman, M. (2015). Location-dependent disclosure risk based decision support framework for persistent authentication in pervasive computing applications. *Computer Networks*, *88*, 161–177. doi:10.1016/j.comnet.2015.06.002

Preuveneers, D., & Joosen, W. (2015, April 13). SmartAuth. *Proceedings of the 30th Annual ACM Symposium on Applied Computing*. 10.1145/2695664.2695908

Priya, C. V. L., & Raj, N. R. N. (2017). Digital watermarking scheme for image authentication. *Proceedings of the 2017 IEEE International Conference on Communication and Signal Processing (ICCSP)*, 2026–2030. 10.1109/ICCSP.2017.8286758

Pustokhina, I. V. (2022). Blockchain-Based Secure Data Sharing Scheme Using Image Steganography and Encryption Techniques for Telemedicine Applications. In Wearable Telemedicine Technology for the Healthcare Industry. Academic Press. doi:10.1016/B978-0-323-85854-0.00009-5

Qasim, A. F., Meziane, F., & Aspin, R. (2017). Digital watermarking: Applicability for developing trust in medical imaging workflows state of the art review. *Future Generation Computer Systems*, *27*, 45–60. doi:10.1016/j.cosrev.2017.11.003

Qi, B. (2020). A Novel Haze Image Steganography Method via Cover-Source Switching. *Journal of Visual Communication and Image Representation*, *70*. . doi:10.1016/j.jvcir.2020.102814

Quan, Z., Kaiyang, Q., Yamei, L., Dehui, Y., Ying, J., & Hua, T. (2018). Predicting Diabetes Mellitus With Machine Learning Techniques. *Frontiers in Genetics*, *9*, 515. https://www.ncbi.nlm.nih.gov/pmc/articles/PMC6232260/

Raghavendra Rao, A., & Samanta, D. (2022). *A Real-Time Approach with Deep Learning for Pandemic Management. Στο Healthcare Informatics for Fighting COVID-19 and Future Epidemics*. Springer.

Rahmani, A. M. (2018). Exploiting smart e-Health gateways at the edge of healthcare Internet-of-Things: A fog computing approach. *Future Generation Computer Systems*, *78*, 641–658.

Rahnama, B., Elci, A., & Celik, S. (2010). Securing RFID-based authentication systems using ParseKey+. *Proceedings of the 3rd International Conference on Security of Information and Networks - SIN '10*. 10.1145/1854099.1854142

Rajan, M. A., Girish Chandra, M., & Lokanatha, C. (2008). Concepts of Graph Theory Relevant to Ad-hoc Networks. *International Journal of Computers, Communications & Control*, *3*, 465–469.

Rajan, R. A. (2018). Serverless architecture-a revolution in cloud computing. *2018 Tenth International Conference on Advanced Computing (ICoAC)*, 88–93. 10.1109/ICoAC44903.2018.8939081

Raju, C. S. K., Sandeep, N., Sugunamma, V., Babu, M. J., & Reddy, J. R. (2016). Heat and mass transfer in magneto-hydrodynamic casson fluid over an exponentially permeable stretching surface, *Engineering Science and Technology. International Journal (Toronto, Ont.)*, *19*(1), 45–52.

Ramakrishnan, A., Tombal, J., Preuveneers, D., & Berbers, Y. (2015, December 11). PRISM. *Proceedings of the 13th International Conference on Advances in Mobile Computing and Multimedia*. 10.1145/2837126.2837157

Ramprasad, R., Batra, R., Pilania, G., Mannodi-Kanakkithodi, A., & Kim, C. (2017). Machine learning in materials informatics: recent applications and prospects. *NPJ Computational Materials*, *3*(1), 1-13.

Rao, A. S., Vardhan, B. V., & Shaik, H. (2021). Role of Exploratory Data Analysis in Data Science. *Proceedings of the 6th International Conference on Communication and Electronics Systems, ICCES 2021*, 1457–1461. 10.1109/ICCES51350.2021.9488986

Rathi, Rajput, Mishra, Grover, Tiwari, Jaiswal, & Hossain. (2021). An edge AI-enabled IoT healthcare monitoring system for smart cities. *Computers & Electrical Engineering*, *96*(B).

Rausch, T., Rashed, A., & Dustdar, S. (2021). Optimized container scheduling for data-intensive serverless edge computing. *Future Generation Computer Systems, 114*, 259–271. doi:10.1016/j.future.2020.07.017

Rautray, R., & Balabantaray, R. C. (2018). An evolutionary framework for multi document summarization using Cuckoo search approach: MDSCSA. *Applied Computing and Informatics, 14*(2), 134-144.

Rautray, R., Balabantaray, R. C., Dash, R., & Dash, R. (2019). CSMDSE-Cuckoo Search Based Multi Document Summary Extractor: Cuckoo Search Based Summary Extractor. *International Journal of Cognitive Informatics and Natural Intelligence, 13*(4), 56–70. doi:10.4018/IJCINI.2019100103

Ray, A., & Chaudhuri, A. K. (2021). Smart healthcare disease diagnosis and patient management: Innovation, improvement and skill development. *Machine Learning with Applications, 3*, 100011. doi:10.1016/j.mlwa.2020.100011

Ray, A., & Roy, S. (2020). Recent trends in image watermarking techniques for copyright protection: A survey. *International Journal of Multimedia Information Retrieval, 9*(4), 249–270. doi:10.100713735-020-00197-9

Ray, P. P., Dash, D., & De, D. (2019). Edge computing for Internet of Things: A survey, e-healthcare case study and future direction. *Journal of Network and Computer Applications, 140*, 1–22. doi:10.1016/j.jnca.2019.05.005

Reamaroon, N., Sjoding, M. W., Lin, K., Iwashyna, T. J., & Najarian, K. (2019, January). Accounting for Label Uncertainty in Machine Learning for Detection of Acute Respiratory Distress Syndrome. *IEEE Journal of Biomedical and Health Informatics, 23*(1), 407–415. doi:10.1109/JBHI.2018.2810820 PMID:29994592

Reddi, R., & Jasmina, B. (2016). Screening and Diagnosis of Gestational Diabetes Mellitus, Where Do We Stand. *Journal of Clinical and Diagnostic Research : JCDR, 10*(4), QE01–QE04.

Redfern, J. (2017). Smart health and innovation: Facilitating health-related behaviour change. *The Proceedings of the Nutrition Society, 76*(3), 328–332.

Regan, G. (2019). A serverless architecture for wireless body area network applications. *Model-Based Safety and Assessment: 6th International Symposium, IMBSA 2019, Thessaloniki, Greece, October 16–18, 2019 Proceedings, 11842*, 239.

Ren, Y., Wen, P., Liu, H., Zheng, Z., Chen, Y., Huang, P., & Li, H. (2021, May 10). Proximity-Echo: Secure two factor authentication using active sound sensing. *IEEE INFOCOM 2021 - IEEE Conference on Computer Communications.* http://dx.doi.org/10.1109/infocom42981.2021.9488866

Reshma, V. K. (2020). Optimized Support Vector Neural Network and Contourlet Transform for Image Steganography. *Evolutionary Intelligence.* . doi:10.1007/s12065-020-00387-8

Ribeiro de Mello, E., Silva Wangham, M., Bristot Loli, S., da Silva, C. E., Cavalcanti da Silva, G., de Chaves, S. A., & Bristot Loli, B. (2020). Multi-factor authentication for shibboleth identity providers. *Journal of Internet Services and Applications, 11*(1), 8. Advance online publication. doi:10.118613174-020-00128-1

Ribeiro, O., Gomes, L., & Vale, Z. (2021, April). IoT-Based Human Fall Detection Solution Using Morlet Wavelet. In *Sustainable Smart Cities and Territories International Conference* (pp. 14-25). Springer.

Rimal, B. P., Choi, E., & Lumb, I. (2009). A taxonomy and survey of cloud computing systems. *2009 Fifth International Joint Conference on INC, IMS and IDC*, 44–51. 10.1109/NCM.2009.218

Ristov, S., Pedratscher, S., & Fahringer, T. (2021). AFCL: An Abstract Function Choreography Language for serverless workflow specification. *Future Generation Computer Systems, 114*, 368–382. doi:10.1016/j.future.2020.08.012

Ritchie, J., Lewis, J., Nicholls, C. M., & Ormston, R. (2014). *Qualitative research practises a guide for social science students and researchers.* Sage.

Riva, O., Qin, C., Strauss, K., & Lymberopoulos, D. (2012). Progressive authentication: deciding when to authenticate on mobile phones. In *21st USENIX Security Symposium (USENIX Security 12)* (pp. 301-316). USENIX.

Rivera, E., Tengana, L., Solano, J., Castelblanco, A., López, C., & Ochoa, M. (2020, November 9). Risk-based authentication based on network latency profiling. *Proceedings of the 13th ACM Workshop on Artificial Intelligence and Security*. 10.1145/3411508.3421377

Robert, S., & Tracey, K. (2020). Design Thinking in Software and AI Projects. doi:10.1007/978-1-4842-6153-8

Robinson, C. (2017). Disclosure of personal data in ecommerce: A cross-national comparison of Estonia and the United States. *Telematics and Informatics*, *34*(2), 569–582. doi:10.1016/j.tele.2016.09.006

Rocha, C. C., Lima, J. C. D., Dantas, M. A. R., & Augustin, I. (2011, June). A2BeST: An adaptive authentication service based on mobile user's behavior and spatio-temporal context. *2011 IEEE Symposium on Computers and Communications (ISCC)*. 10.1109/ISCC.2011.5983933

Rosenblatt, F. (1958). The perceptron: A probabilistic model for information storage and organization in the brain. *Psychological Review*, *6*(6), 386–408. doi:10.1037/h0042519 PMID:13602029

Rushdi, M. A., Rushdi, A. A., Dief, T. N., Halawa, A. M., Yoshida, S., & Schmehl, R. (2020, May 09). Power prediction of airborne wind energy systems using multivariate machine learning. *Energies*, *13*(9), 2367. doi:10.3390/en13092367

Rustad, S. (2021). Inverted LSB Image Steganography Using Adaptive Pattern to Improve Imperceptibility. *Journal of King Saud University - Computer and Information Sciences*. . doi:10.1016/j.jksuci.2020.12.017

Saab, M. M. (2021). Nursing students' views of using virtual reality in healthcare: A qualitative study. *Journal of Clinical Nursing*.

Saad, A. H. S., Mohamed, M. S., & Hafez, E. H. (2021). Coverless Image Steganography Based on Optical Mark Recognition and Machine Learning. *IEEE Access: Practical Innovations, Open Solutions*, *9*, 16522–16531. doi:10.1109/ACCESS.2021.3050737

Sabeti, V. (2022). An Adaptive Image Steganography Method Based on Integer Wavelet Transform Using Genetic Algorithm. *Computers & Electrical Engineering, 99*. . doi:10.1016/j.compeleceng.2022.107809

Sahoo, S., Acharya, M., & Nayak. M.M. (2019). A three rates of EOQ/EPQ model for instantaneous deteriorating items involving fuzzy parameter under shortages. *International Journal of Innovative Technology and Exploring Engineering, 8*(8S2), 405-418.

Sahoo, S., & Acharya, M. (2021). *An inventory model for seasonal deteriorating items with price dependent demand and preservation technology investment in crisp and fuzzy environments. Recent Trends in Applied Mathematics*. Springer Verlag.

Sahoo, S., Acharya, M., & Nayak, M. M. (2020a). Application of Preservation Technology and Disposal Costs for Instantaneous Deteriorating Seasonal Products under Crisp and Fuzzy Environments. *International Journal of Advanced Science and Technology*, *29*(8s), 392–405.

Sahoo, S., Acharya, M., & Nayak, M. M. (2020b). A Cloudy Fuzzy Inventory Model for Deteriorating Items with Price Dependent Demand. *TEST Engineering and Management*, *83*, 6090–6097.

Sahoo, S., Parveen, S., & Panda, J. (2007). The present and future of nanotechnology in human health care. *Nanomedicine; Nanotechnology, Biology, and Medicine*, *3*(1), 20–31.

Sahu, A. K. (2021). Multi-Directional Block Based PVD and Modulus Function Image Steganography to Avoid FOBP and IEP. *Journal of Information Security and Applications, 58.* . doi:10.1016/j.jisa.2021.102808

Saini, L. K., & Shrivastava, V. (2014). A Survey of Digital Watermarking Techniques and its Applications. *International Journal of Computer Science Trends and Technology, 2*(3), 70–73.

Sairamya, N. J., Susmitha, L., George, S. T., & Subathra, M. S. P. (2019). Hybrid Approach for Classification of Electroencephalographic Signals Using Time–Frequency Images With Wavelets and Texture Features. In Intelligent Data Analysis for Biomedical Applications (pp. 253-273). Academic Press.

Salahuddin, M. A., Al-Fuqaha, A., Guizani, M., Shuaib, K., & Sallabi, F. (2018). *Softwarization of internet of things infrastructure for secure and smart healthcare.* arXiv preprint arXiv:1805.11011.

Salembier, P., & Garrido, L. (2000). Binary Partition Tree as an Efficient Representation for Image Processing, Segmentation, and Information Retrieval. *IEEE Transactions on Image Processing, 9*, 561–576.

Salembier, P., Liesegang, S., & López-Martínez, C. (2019, May). Ship Detection in SAR Images Based on Maxtree Representation and Graph Signal Processing. *IEEE Transactions on Geoscience and Remote Sensing, 57*(5), 2709–2724. doi:10.1109/TGRS.2018.2876603

Salhi, A. l., Kardouchi, M., & Belacel, N. (2012). Fast and efficient face recognition system using random forest and histograms of oriented gradients. *Proceedings of the International Conference of Biometrics Special Interest (BIOSIG) Group*, 1-12.

Saltz, J. S., & Grady, N. W. (2017). The ambiguity of data science team roles and the need for a data science workforce framework. *Proceedings - 2017 IEEE International Conference on Big Data, Big Data 2017*, 2355–2361. 10.1109/BigData.2017.8258190

Samanta, D., Karthikeyan, M. P., Agarwal, D., Biswas, A., Acharyya, A., & Banerjee, A. (2022). Trends in terahertz biomedical applications. *Generation, Detection and Processing of Terahertz Signals*, 285–299.

Samanta, D., Dutta, S., Galety, M. G., & Pramanik, S. (2022). *A Novel Approach for Web Mining Taxonomy for High-Performance Computing. Στο Cyber Intelligence and Information Retrieval.* Springer.

Samanta, D., Karthikeyan, M. P., Banerjee, A., & Inokawa, H. (2021). Tunable graphene nanopatch antenna design for on-chip integrated terahertz detector arrays with potential application in cancer imaging. *Nanomedicine (London), 16*(12), 1035–1047.

Samantaray, M., Biswal, A. K., Singh, D., Samanta, D., Karuppiah, M., & Joseph, N. P. (2021, December). Optical Character Recognition (OCR) based Vehicle's License Plate Recognition System Using Python and OpenCV. In *2021 5th International Conference on Electronics, Communication and Aerospace Technology (ICECA)* (pp. 849-853). IEEE.

Sanchez, V., & Hernández-Cabronero, M. (2018, October). Graph-Based Rate Control in Pathology Imaging with Lossless Region of Interest Coding. *IEEE Transactions on Medical Imaging, 37*(10), 2211–2223. doi:10.1109/TMI.2018.2824819 PMID:29993629

Sankaran, A., Malhotra, A., Mittal, A., Vatsa, M., & Singh, R. (2015, September). On smartphone camera based fingerphoto authentication. *2015 IEEE 7th International Conference on Biometrics Theory, Applications and Systems (BTAS).* http://dx.doi.org/10.1109/btas.2015.7358782

Sarangi, S. K., Panda, R., Das, P. K., & Abraham, A. (2018). Design of optimal high pass and band stop FIR filters using adaptive Cuckoo search algorithm. *Engineering Applications of Artificial Intelligence, 70*, 67–80. doi:10.1016/j.engappai.2018.01.005

Saritha, K., Devi, B. M., Kurni, M., Samanta, D., & Joseph, N. P. (2022). *Controlling Node Failure Localization in Data Networks Using Probing Mechanisms. Στο Micro-Electronics and Telecommunication Engineering.* Springer.

Sarker, I. H., Hoque, M. M., Uddin, M. K., & Tawfeeq, A. (2021). Mobile Data Science and Intelligent Apps: Concepts, AI-Based Modeling and Research Directions. *Mobile Networks and Applications*, 26(1), 285–303. doi:10.100711036-020-01650-z

Sarosh, P., Parah, S. A., Bhat, G. M., & Muhammad, K. (2021). A Security Management Framework for Big Data in Smart Healthcare. *Big Data Research*, 25, 100225. doi:10.1016/j.bdr.2021.100225

Sato, W., Fujimura, T., Kochiyama, T., & Suzuki, N. (2013). Relationships among facial mimicry, emotional experience, and emotion recognition. *PLoS One*, 8(3), 1–8. doi:10.1371/journal.pone.0057889 PMID:23536774

Saurez, E., Hong, K., Lillethun, D., Ramachandran, U., & Ottenwälder, B. (2016, June). Incremental deployment and migration of geo-distributed situation awareness applications in the fog. In *Proceedings of the 10th ACM International Conference on Distributed and Event-based Systems* (pp. 258-269). 10.1145/2933267.2933317

Savakar, D. G., & Ghuli, A. (2019). Robust invisible digital image watermarking using hybrid scheme. *Arabian Journal for Science and Engineering*, 44(4), 3995–4008. doi:10.100713369-019-03751-8

Sawyer, W. G., Hamilton, M. A., Fregly, B. J., & Banks, S. A. (2003). Temperature modeling in a total knee joint replacement using patient-specific kinematics. *Tribology Letters*, 15(4), 343–351. doi:10.1023/B:TRIL.0000003057.60259.71

Schad, J., Dittrich, J., & Quiané-Ruiz, J.-A. (2010). Runtime measurements in the cloud: Observing, analyzing, and reducing variance. *Proceedings of the VLDB Endowment International Conference on Very Large Data Bases*, 3(1-2), 460–471. doi:10.14778/1920841.1920902

Schwaber, K. (1997). SCRUM Development Process. *Business Object Design and Implementation,* 117–134. doi:10.1007/978-1-4471-0947-1_11

Schwid, H. A. (1999). Use of a computerized advanced cardiac life support simulator improves retention of advanced cardiac life support guidelines better than a textbook review. *Critical Care Medicine*, 27(4), 821–824.

Scott, J. A. (1988). The computation of temperature rises in the human eye induced by infrared radiation. *Physics in Medicine and Biology*, 33(2), 243–257. doi:10.1088/0031-9155/33/2/004 PMID:3362967

Sepczuk, M., & Kotulski, Z. (2018). A new risk-based authentication management model oriented on user's experience. *Computers & Security*, 73, 17–33. doi:10.1016/j.cose.2017.10.002

Sert, O. C., Şahin, S. D., Özyer, T., & Alhajj, R. (2019). Analysis and prediction in sparse and high dimensional text data: The case of Dow Jones stock market. *Physica A*, 123752.

Sewak, M., & Singh, S. (2018). Winning in the era of serverless computing and function as a service. *2018 3rd International Conference for Convergence in Technology (I2CT)*, 1–5. 10.1109/I2CT.2018.8529465

Shackelford, A. (2015). CloudFront and DNS Management. In Beginning Amazon Web Services with Node. In JS (pp. 93–120). Springer.

Shafiei, H., Khonsari, A., & Mousavi, P. (2019). *Serverless computing: A survey of opportunities, challenges and applications.* arXiv preprint arXiv:1911.01296.

Shahid & Kumar. (2018). Digital Video Watermarking: Issues and Challenges. *International Journal of Advanced Research in Computer Engineering and Technology*, 7(4), 400–405.

Shah, N. H., & Cardenas-Barron, L. E. (2015). Retailer's decision for ordering and credit policies for deteriorating items when a supplier offers order-linked credit period or cash discount. *Applied Mathematics and Computation, 259*(15), 569–578. doi:10.1016/j.amc.2015.03.010

Shahrad, M., Balkind, J., & Wentzlaff, D. (2019). Architectural implications of function-as-a-service computing. *Proceedings of the 52nd Annual IEEE/ACM International Symposium on Microarchitecture*, 1063–1075. 10.1145/3352460.3358296

Shah, S. A., Ren, A., Fan, D., Zhang, Z., Zhao, N., Yang, X., Luo, M., Wang, W., Hu, F., Rehman, M., Badarneh, O., & Abbasi, Q. H. (2018). Internet of things for sensing: A case study in the healthcare system. *Applied Sciences (Basel, Switzerland), 8*(4), 508. doi:10.3390/app8040508

Shah, S. W. A., & Kanhere, S. (2018). Wi-Auth: WiFi based Second Factor User Authentication. *Proceedings of the 14th EAI International Conference on Mobile and Ubiquitous Systems: Computing, Networking and Services.* 10.4108/eai.7-11-2017.2274992

Shahzad, S. K., Ahmed, D., Naqvi, M. R., Mushtaq, M. T., Iqbal, M. W., & Munir, F. (2021). Ontology Driven Smart Health Service Integration. *Computer Methods and Programs in Biomedicine, 207*, 106146. doi:10.1016/j.cmpb.2021.106146 PMID:34020375

Sharifzadeh, M., Aloraini, M., & Schonfeld, D. (2020). Adaptive Batch Size Image Merging Steganography and Quantized Gaussian Image Steganography. *IEEE Transactions on Information Forensics and Security, 15*, 867–879. doi:10.1109/TIFS.2019.2929441

Sharma & Batra. (2021). An Enhanced Huffman-PSO Based Image Optimization Algorithm for Image Steganography. *Genetic Programming and Evolvable Machines, 22*(2), 189–205. . doi:10.1007/s10710-020-09396-z

Sharma, H. (2021). Multi-Image Steganography and Authentication Using Crypto-Stego Techniques. *Multimedia Tools and Applications, 80*(19), 29067–93. doi:10.1007/s11042-021-11068-8

Sharma, V. K. (2022). Hilbert Quantum Image Scrambling and Graph Signal Processing-Based Image Steganography. *Multimedia Tools and Applications.* . doi:10.1007/s11042-022-12426-w

Sharma, D. K. (2021). The aspect of vast data management problem in healthcare sector and implementation of cloud computing technique. *Materials Today: Proceedings.*

Sharma, G., & Kalra, S. (2018). A lightweight multi-factor secure smart card based remote user authentication scheme for cloud-IoT applications. *Journal of Information Security and Applications, 42*, 95–106. doi:10.1016/j.jisa.2018.08.003

Sharma, N., Sharma, P., Irwin, D., & Shenoy, P. (2011). Predicting solar generation from weather forecasts using machine learning. *2011 IEEE International Conference on Smart Grid Communications (SmartGridComm)*, 528-533. 10.1109/SmartGridComm.2011.6102379

Sharma, R. R., Kumar, M., Maheshwari, S., & Ray, K. P. (2020). EVDHM-ARIMA-based time series forecasting model and its application for COVID-19 cases. *IEEE Transactions on Instrumentation and Measurement, 70*, 1–10.

Sharmila, D., & Uthayakumar, R. (2016). An Inventory model with three rates of production rate understock and time dependent demand for time varying deterioration rate with shortages. International Journal of Advanced Engineering. *Management Science, 2*(9), 1595–1602.

Shashikiran, B. S. (2021). Minimal Block Knight's Tour and Edge with LSB Pixel Replacement Based Encrypted Image Steganography. *SN Computer Science, 2*(3), 139. . doi:10.1007/s42979-021-00542-7

Shehab, M., Khader, A. T., & Al-Betar, M. A. (2017). A survey on applications and variants of the cuckoo search algorithm. *Applied Soft Computing, 61*, 1041–1059. doi:10.1016/j.asoc.2017.02.034

Sherekar, S., Thakare, V., & Jain, S. (2008). Role of Digital Watermark in e-governance and ecommerce. *International Journal of Computer Science and Network Security*, *8*(1), 257–261.

Shi, E., Niu, Y., Jakobsson, M., & Chow, R. (2011). Implicit authentication through learning user behavior. In *Lecture Notes in Computer Science* (pp. 99–113). Springer Berlin Heidelberg. doi:10.1007/978-3-642-18178-8_9

Shi, J., & Malik, J. (2000). Normalized cuts and image segmentation. *IEEE Transactions on Pattern Analysis and Machine Intelligence*, *22*, 888–905.

Shnain, A. H., & Shaheed, S. H. (2019). User authentication by secured graphical password implementation in problems e-commerce. *Journal of Computational and Theoretical Nanoscience*, *16*(5), 2327–2332. doi:10.1166/jctn.2019.7894

Shone, N., Dobbins, C., Hurst, W., & Shi, Q. (2015, October). Digital memories based mobile user authentication for iot. *2015 IEEE International Conference on Computer and Information Technology; Ubiquitous Computing and Communications; Dependable, Autonomic and Secure Computing; Pervasive Intelligence and Computing*. http://dx.doi.org/10.1109/cit/iucc/dasc/picom.2015.270

Shrinivas, Vetrivel, Santhakumaran, & Elango. (2010). Applications of graph theory in computer science an overview. *International Journal of Engineering Science and Technology*, 2.

Shukla, D., Tiwari, N., & Dubey, D. (2016). Survey on digital watermarking techniques. International Journal of Signal Processing. *Image Processing and Pattern Recognition*, *9*(1), 239–244. doi:10.14257/ijsip.2016.9.1.23

Shukla, S., Hassan, M. F., Khan, M. K., Jung, L. T., & Awang, A. (2019). An analytical model to minimize the latency in healthcare internet-of-things in fog computing environment. *PLoS One*, *14*(11), e0224934. doi:10.1371/journal.pone.0224934 PMID:31721807

Siddiqui, G. F., Iqbal, M. Z., Saleem, K., Saeed, Z., Ahmed, A., Hameed, I. A., & Khan, M. F. (2020). A Dynamic Three-Bit Image Steganography Algorithm for Medical and e-Healthcare Systems. *IEEE Access: Practical Innovations, Open Solutions*, *8*, 181893–181903. doi:10.1109/ACCESS.2020.3028315

Sim, R., Mori, G., & Rekleitis, Y. (2009). Second and Third Canadian Conferences on Computer and Robot Vision. *Image and Vision Computing*, *27*(1-2), 1–2. doi:10.1016/j.imavis.2008.09.002

Singh & Chandha. (2013). A Survey of Digital Watermarking Techniques, Applications and Attacks. *International Journal of Engineering and Innovative Technology*, *2*(9), 165–175.

Singh, C., Gaba, N. S., Kaur, M., & Kaur, B. (2019). Comparison of different CI/CD tools integrated with cloud platform. *2019 9th International Conference on Cloud Computing, Data Science & Engineering (Confluence)*, 7–12. 10.1109/CONFLUENCE.2019.8776985

Singh, D., Prusty, S. K., Sarangi, S. S., Sahoo, S., & Biswal, A. K. (2020). *Anxiety, Psychological Effects and Prevention during COVID-19 in India*. Academic Press.

Singh, A. K., Kumar, B., Singh, G., & Mohan, A. (2017). *Medical Image Watermarking: Techniques and Applications. Multimedia Systems and Applications*. Springer. doi:10.1007/978-3-319-57699-2

Singhal, A., Singh, P., Lall, B., & Joshi, S. D. (2020). Modeling and prediction of COVID-19 pandemic using Gaussian mixture model. *Chaos, Solitons, and Fractals*, *138*, 110023.

Singh, D., Bhanipati, J., Biswal, A. K., Samanta, D., Joshi, S., Shukla, P. K., & Nuagah, S. J. (2021). Approach for Collision Minimization and Enhancement of Power Allocation in WSNs. *Journal of Sensors*.

Singh, D., Biswal, A. K., Samanta, D., Singh, D., & Lee, H. N. (2022). Juice Jacking: Security Issues and Improvements in USB Technology. *Sustainability*, *14*(2), 939.

Singh, D., Febbo, P. G., Ross, K., Jackson, D. G., Manola, J., Ladd, C., Tamayo, P., Renshaw, A. A., D'Amico, A. V., Richie, J. P., Lander, E. S., Loda, M., Kantoff, P. W., Golub, T. R., & Sellers, W. R. (2002). Gene Expression Correlates of Clinical Prostate Cancer Behavior. *Cancer Cell*, *1*(2), 203–209. doi:10.1016/S1535-6108(02)00030-2 PMID:12086878

Singh, G. (2017). A review of secure medical image watermarking. *Proceedings of the IEEE International Conference on Power, Control, Signals and Instrumentation Engineering (ICPCSI)*, 3105–3109. 10.1109/ICPCSI.2017.8392297

Singh, P., & Chadha, R. S. (2013). A survey of digital watermarking techniques, applications and attacks. *International Journal of Engineering and Innovative Technology*, *2*(9), 165–175.

Singh, R. K., Rani, M., Bhagavathula, A. S., Sah, R., Rodriguez-Morales, A. J., Kalita, H., ... Kumar, P. (2020). Prediction of the COVID-19 pandemic for the top 15 affected countries: Advanced autoregressive integrated moving average (ARIMA) model. *JMIR Public Health and Surveillance*, *6*(2), e19115.

Singla, K., Arora, R., & Kaushal, S. (2021). An approach towards IoT-based healthcare management system. In *Proceedings of the sixth international conference on mathematics and computing* (pp. 345-356). Springer.

Sivasubramanian, N., & Konganathan, G. (2020). A novel semi fragile watermarking technique for tamper detection and recovery using IWT and DCT. *Computing*, *102*(6), 1365–1384. doi:10.100700607-020-00797-7

Sivasubramanian, S. (2012). Amazon dynamoDB: a seamlessly scalable non-relational database service. *Proceedings of the 2012 ACM SIGMOD International Conference on Management of Data*, 729–730. 10.1145/2213836.2213945

Skouri, K., Konstantaras, I., Papachristos, S., & Ganas, I. (2009). Inventory models with ramp type demand rate, partial backlogging and Weibull deterioration rate. *European Journal of Operational Research*, *192*(1), 79–92. doi:10.1016/j.ejor.2007.09.003

Slowik, A., & Kwasnicka, H. (2018). Nature Inspired Methods and Their Industry Applications—Swarm Intelligence Algorithms. *IEEE Transactions on Industrial Informatics*, *14*(3), 1004–1015. doi:10.1109/TII.2017.2786782

Sodhi, K. S., & Lal, M. (2013). Comparative Analysis of PCA-based Face Recognition System using different Distance Classifiers. *International Journal of Application or Innovation in Engineering & Management.*, *2*, 341–348.

Soebiyanto, R. P., Adimi, F., & Kiang, R. K. (2010). Modeling and predicting seasonal influenza transmission in warm regions using climatological parameters. *PLoS One*, *5*(3), e9450.

Solano, J., Camacho, L., Correa, A., Deiro, C., Vargas, J., & Ochoa, M. (2019). Risk-Based static authentication in web applications with behavioral biometrics and session context analytics. In *Lecture Notes in Computer Science* (pp. 3–23). Springer International Publishing. doi:10.1007/978-3-030-29729-9_1

Solano, J., Camacho, L., Correa, A., Deiro, C., Vargas, J., & Ochoa, M. (2020). Combining behavioral biometrics and session context analytics to enhance risk-based static authentication in web applications. *International Journal of Information Security*, *20*(2), 181–197. doi:10.100710207-020-00510-x

Song, C., Sudirman, S., Merabti, M., & Llewellyn-Jones, D. (2010). Analysis of digital image watermark attacks. *Proceedings of the 7th IEEE Consumer Communications and Networking Conference*, 1–5. 10.1109/CCNC.2010.5421631

Song, R. (2010). Advanced smart card based password authentication protocol. *Computer Standards & Interfaces*, *32*(5–6), 321–325. doi:10.1016/j.csi.2010.03.008

Soni, A. N. (2018). Smart Devices Using Internet of Things for Health Monitoring. *International Journal of Innovative Research in Science, Engineering and Technology, 7*(5), 6355–6361.

Sonune, S., Kalbande, D., Yeole, A., & Oak, S. (2017). Issues in IoT healthcare platforms: a critical study and review. *IEEE International Conference on Intelligent Computing and Control (I2C2).* 10.1109/I2C2.2017.8321898

Sood, Kaur, Sharma, Mehmuda, & Kumar. (2018). IoT enabled Smart Wearable device – Sukoon. *2018 Fourteenth International Conference on Information Processing (ICINPRO).*

Sookhak, M., Jabbarpour, M. R., Safa, N. S., & Yu, F. R. (2021). Blockchain and smart contract for access control in healthcare: A survey, issues and challenges, and open issues. *Journal of Network and Computer Applications, 178,* 102950. doi:10.1016/j.jnca.2020.102950

Sowmya, S. (2021). Protection of Data using Image Watermarking Technique. *Global Transitions Proceedings, 2*(2), 386–391. doi:10.1016/j.gltp.2021.08.035

Spooren, J., Preuveneers, D., & Joosen, W. (2015, April 21). Mobile device fingerprinting considered harmful for risk-based authentication. *Proceedings of the Eighth European Workshop on System Security.* 10.1145/2751323.2751329

Sravanthi, K. (2014). Applications of Graph Labeling in Communication Networks. *Oriental Journal of Computer Science and Technology, 7*(1), 139–145.

Sreenivasan, K. R., Havlicek, M., & Deshpande, G. (2014). Nonparametric hemodynamic deconvolution of FMRI using homomorphic filtering. *IEEE Transactions on Medical Imaging, 34*(5), 1155–1163. doi:10.1109/TMI.2014.2379914 PMID:25531878

Sriram, T. V., Rao, M. V., Narayana, G. S., Kaladhar, D. S. V. G. K., & Vital, T. P. R. (2013). Intelligent Parkinson disease prediction using machine learning algorithms. *International Journal of Engineering and Innovative Technology, 3*(3), 1568–1572.

Strauss, A. T., Martinez, D. A., Garcia-Arce, A., Taylor, S., Mateja, C., Fabri, P. J., & Zayas-Castro, J. L. (2015). A user needs assessment to inform health information exchange design and implementation. *BMC Medical Informatics and Decision Making, 15*(1), 1–11. doi:10.118612911-015-0207-x PMID:26459258

Subashini, V. J., Poornachandra, S., & Ramakrishnan, M. (2013). A fragile watermarking technique for fingerprint protection. *Proceedings of the IEEE Recent Advances in Intelligent Computational Systems (RAICS),* 322–326. 10.1109/RAICS.2013.6745495

Subramaniam, S., Majumder, S., Faisal, A. I., & Deen, M. J. (2022). Insole-Based Systems for Health Monitoring: Current Solutions and Research Challenges. *Sensors (Basel), 22*(2), 438.

Subramanian, N., Cheheb, I., Elharrouss, O., Al-Maadeed, S., & Bouridane, A. (2021). End-to-End Image Steganography Using Deep Convolutional Autoencoders. *IEEE Access: Practical Innovations, Open Solutions, 9,* 135585–135593. doi:10.1109/ACCESS.2021.3113953

Subramanian, N., Elharrouss, O., Al-Maadeed, S., & Bouridane, A. (2021). Image Steganography: A Review of the Recent Advances. *IEEE Access: Practical Innovations, Open Solutions, 9,* 23409–23423. doi:10.1109/ACCESS.2021.3053998

Subramaniyaswamy, V. (2019). An ontology-driven personalized food recommendation in IoT-based healthcare system. *The Journal of Supercomputing, 75*(6), 3184–3216.

Sujay, S. N., Reddy, H. S. M., & Ravi, J. (2017). Face recognition using extended LBP features and multilayer SVM classifier. Proceedings International Conference on Electrical, Electronics, Communication, Computer, and Optimization Techniques, 713-716.

Sukumar, A. (2021). Robust Image Steganography Approach Based on RIWT-Laplacian Pyramid and Histogram Shifting Using Deep Learning. *Multimedia Systems, 27*(4), 651–66. . doi:10.1007/s00530-020-00665-6

Sun, H.-M., Chen, Y.-H., Fang, C.-C., & Chang, S.-Y. (2012). PassMap. *Proceedings of the 7th ACM Symposium on Information, Computer and Communications Security - ASIACCS '12.* http://dx.doi.org/10.1145/2414456.2414513

Sun, G., Liu, Y., Chen, Z., Liang, S., Wang, A., & Zhang, Y. (2018). Radiation Beam Pattern Synthesis of Concentric Circular Antenna Arrays Using Hybrid Approach Based on Cuckoo Search. *IEEE Transactions on Antennas and Propagation, 66*(9), 4563–4576. doi:10.1109/TAP.2018.2846771

Sun, G., Liu, Y., Li, J., Zhang, Y., & Wang, A. (2017). Sidelobe reduction of large-scale antenna array for 5G beamforming via hierarchical cuckoo search. *Electronics Letters, 53*(16), 1158–1160. doi:10.1049/el.2016.4768

Sun, J., Zhang, R., Zhang, J., & Zhang, Y. (2014, October). TouchIn: Sightless two-factor authentication on multi-touch mobile devices. *2014 IEEE Conference on Communications and Network Security.* 10.1109/CNS.2014.6997513

Suresh, S., Lal, S., Chen, C., & Celik, T. (2018). Multispectral Satellite Image Denoising via Adaptive Cuckoo Search-Based Wiener Filter. *IEEE Transactions on Geoscience and Remote Sensing, 56*(8), 4334–4345. doi:10.1109/TGRS.2018.2815281

Suresh, S., Lal, S., Reddy, C. S., & Kiran, M. S. (2017). A novel adaptive cuckoo search algorithm for contrast enhancement of satellite images. *IEEE Journal of Selected Topics in Applied Earth Observations and Remote Sensing, 10*(8), 3665–3676. doi:10.1109/JSTARS.2017.2699200

Su, W., Ni, J., Hu, X., & Fridrich, J. (2021, March). Image Steganography With Symmetric Embedding Using Gaussian Markov Random Field Model. *IEEE Transactions on Circuits and Systems for Video Technology, 31*(3), 1001–1015. doi:10.1109/TCSVT.2020.3001122

Sweety, B. E., Srimathi, H., & Bagavandas, M. (2019). A Survey Of Machine Learning Algorithms In Health Care. *International Journal of Scientific & Technology Research, 8*(11).

Syta, E., Kurkovsky, S., & Casano, B. (2010). RFID-Based authentication middleware for mobile devices. *2010 43rd Hawaii International Conference on System Sciences.* http://dx.doi.org/10.1109/hicss.2010.320

Taha, T. B., Ngadiran, R., & Ehkan, P. (2018). Adaptive image watermarking algorithm based on an efficient perceptual mapping model. *IEEE Access: Practical Innovations, Open Solutions, 6,* 66254–66267. doi:10.1109/ACCESS.2018.2878456

Taher, B. H., Liu, H., Abedi, F., Lu, H., Yassin, A. A., & Mohammed, A. J. (2021). A secure and lightweight three-factor remote user authentication protocol for future iot applications. *Journal of Sensors, 2021,* 1–18. doi:10.1155/2021/8871204

Taiwo, O., & Ezugwu, A. E. (2020). Smart healthcare support for remote patient monitoring during covid-19 quarantine. *Informatics in Medicine Unlocked, 20,* 100428. doi:10.1016/j.imu.2020.100428 PMID:32953970

Takada, T., & Hattori, Y. (2020, September 28). Giving motivation for using secure credentials through user authentication by game. *Proceedings of the International Conference on Advanced Visual Interfaces.* 10.1145/3399715.3399950

Taleizadeh, A. A., Hazarkhani, B., & Moon, I. (2020). Joint pricing and inventory decisions with carbon emission considerations, partial backordering and planned discounts. *Annals of Operations Research, 290*(3), 95–113. doi:10.100710479-018-2968-y

Tan, L. (2020). Steganalysis of Homogeneous-Representation Based Steganography for High Dynamic Range Images. *Multimedia Tools and Applications, 79*(27), 20079–105. . doi:10.1007/s11042-019-08257-x

Taneja, M., & Davy, A. (2017, May). Resource aware placement of IoT application modules in Fog-Cloud Computing Paradigm. In *2017 IFIP/IEEE Symposium on Integrated Network and Service Management (IM)* (pp. 1222-1228). IEEE. 10.23919/INM.2017.7987464

Tang, Z., Yap, P.-T., & Shen, D. (2019, August). A New Image Similarity Metric for Improving Deformation Consistency in Graph-Based Groupwise Image Registration. *IEEE Transactions on Biomedical Engineering, 66*(8), 2192–2199. doi:10.1109/TBME.2018.2885436 PMID:30530309

Tanna, M., & Singh, H. (2018). *Serverless Web Applications with React and Firebase: Develop real-time applications for web and mobile platforms.* Packt Publishing Ltd.

Tao, H., Chongmin, L., Mohamad Zain, J., & Abdalla, A. N. (2014). Robust Image Watermarking Theories and Techniques: A Review. *Journal of Applied Research and Technology, 12*(1), 122–138. doi:10.1016/S1665-6423(14)71612-8

Tavares, J. M. R. S., Dutta, P., Dutta, S., & Samanta, D. (2022). Cyber Intelligence and Information Retrieval. In *Proceedings of CIIR 2021.* Springer.

Tavousi, F., Azizi, S., & Ghaderzadeh, A. (2021). A fuzzy approach for optimal placement of IoT applications in fog-cloud computing. *Cluster Computing*, 1–18.

Thapa, M., Sandeep, D., & Meenakshi, A. (2011). Digital Image Watermarking Technique Based on Different Attacks. *International Journal of Advanced Computer Science and Applications, 2*(4), 14–19. doi:10.14569/IJACSA.2011.020402

The LesSS Company B.V. (2016). LeSS Framework. *LeSS,* 1–2. https://less.works/less/framework/index.html

Theodoridis, S., & Koutroumbas, K. (2009). Feature Selection. *Pattern Recognition*, 261–322. doi:10.1016/B978-1-59749-272-0.50007-4

Thirunavukkarasu, G. S., Champion, B., Horan, B., Seyedmahmoudian, M., & Stojcevski, A. (2018). Iot-based system health management infrastructure as a service. *Proceedings of the 2018 International Conference on Cloud Computing and Internet of Things*, 55–61. 10.1145/3291064.3291070

Thomas, K., Pullman, J., Yeo, K., Raghunathan, A., Kelley, P. G., Invernizzi, L., Benko, B., Pietraszek, T., Patel, S., Boneh, D., & Bursztein, E. (2019). Protecting accounts from credential stuffing with password breach alerting. In *28th USENIX Security Symposium (USENIX Security 19)* (pp. 1556–1571). USENIX Association.

Thorpe, J., MacRae, B., & Salehi-Abari, A. (2013). Usability and security evaluation of GeoPass. *Proceedings of the Ninth Symposium on Usable Privacy and Security - SOUPS '13*. 10.1145/2501604.2501618

Tian, S., Yang, W., Grange, J. M. L., Wang, P., Huang, W., & Ye, Z. (2019). Smart healthcare: Making medical care more intelligent. *Global Health Journal, 3*(3), 62–65. doi:10.1016/j.glohj.2019.07.001

Tiwari & Sharmila. (2017). Digital Watermarking Applications, Parameter Measures and Techniques. *International Journal of Computer Science and Network Security, 17*(3), 184–194.

Tiwari, S., Ahmed, W., & Sarkar, B. (2019). Sustainable ordering policies for non-instantaneous deteriorating items under carbon emission and multi-trade-credit-polices. *Journal of Cleaner Production, 240*(118183), 1–19.

Tiwari, S., Cardenas-Barron, L. E., Khanna, A., & Jaggi, C. K. (2016). Impact of trade credit and inflation on retailer's ordering policies for non-instantaneous deteriorating items in a two-warehouse environment. *International Journal of Production Economics, 176*, 154–169. doi:10.1016/j.ijpe.2016.03.016

Ti, Z., Deng, X. W., & Yang, H. (2020). Wake modeling of wind turbines using machine learning. *Applied Energy, 257*, 114025. doi:10.1016/j.apenergy.2019.114025

Tomar, A., & Gupta, N. (2020). Prediction for the spread of COVID-19 in India and effectiveness of preventive measures. *The Science of the Total Environment, 728*, 138762.

Tong, L., Li, Y., & Gao, W. (2016, April). A hierarchical edge cloud architecture for mobile computing. In *IEEE INFO-COM 2016-The 35th Annual IEEE International Conference on Computer Communications* (pp. 1-9). IEEE. 10.1109/INFOCOM.2016.7524340

Tosuni, B. (2015). Graph Theory in Computer Science - An Overview. *International Journal of Academic Research and Reflection, 3*(4).

Traore, I., Woungang, I., Obaidat, M. S., Nakkabi, Y., & Lai, I. (2012, November). Combining mouse and keystroke dynamics biometrics for risk-based authentication in web environments. *2012 Fourth International Conference on Digital Home*. 10.1109/ICDH.2012.59

Traore, I., Woungang, I., Obaidat, M. S., Nakkabi, Y., & Lai, I. (2013). Online risk-based authentication using behavioral biometrics. *Multimedia Tools and Applications, 71*(2), 575–605. doi:10.100711042-013-1518-5

Treiber, N. A., Heinermann, J., & Kramer, O. (2016). Wind power prediction with machine learning. In *Computational Sustainability* (pp. 13–29). Springer. doi:10.1007/978-3-319-31858-5_2

Tripathi, A., Shukla, S., & Arora, D. (2018). A hybrid optimization approach for load balancing in cloud computing. In *Advances in Computer and Computational Sciences* (pp. 197–206). Springer. doi:10.1007/978-981-10-3773-3_19

Tripathi, G., Ahad, M. A., & Paiva, S. (2020). S2HS-A blockchain based approach for smart healthcare system. In *Healthcare*. Elsevier.

Tripathi, V., & Shakeel, F. (2017, December). Monitoring health care system using internet of things-an immaculate pairing. In *2017 International Conference on Next Generation Computing and Information Systems (ICNGCIS)* (pp. 153-158). IEEE.

Tsai, W. T., Sun, X., & Balasooriya, J. (2010, April). Service-oriented cloud computing architecture. In *2010 seventh international conference on information technology: New generations* (pp. 684-689). IEEE. 10.1109/ITNG.2010.214

Tse, D., Chow, C. K., Ly, T. P., Tong, C. Y., & Tam, K. W. (2018). The challenges of big data governance in healthcare. *17th IEEE International Conference on Trust, Security and Privacy in Computing and Communications*, New York, NY. 10.1109/TrustCom/BigDataSE.2018.00240

Tukey, J. W. (1977a). *Exploratory Data Analysis*. doi:10.1007/978-1-4419-7976-6

Tukey, J. W. (1977b). Exploratory Data Analysis by John W. Tukey. In *Biometrics* (Vol. 33, p. 768). https://www.jstor.org/stable/2529486

Tulin, O., Muhammed, T., Eylul, A. Y., Ulas, B. B., Ozal, Y., & Acharya, R. (2020). *Automated detection of COVID-19 cases using deep neural networks with X-ray images*. Computers in Biology and Medicine Journal.

Tuli, S., Basumatary, N., Gill, S. S., Kahani, M., Arya, R. C., Wander, G. S., & Buyya, R. (2020). HealthFog: An ensemble deep learning based Smart Healthcare System for Automatic Diagnosis of Heart Diseases in integrated IoT and fog computing environments. *Future Generation Computer Systems, 104*, 187–200. doi:10.1016/j.future.2019.10.043

Uchechukwu, A., Li, K., &Shen, Y. (2014). Energy consumption in cloud computing data centers. *International Journal of Cloud Computing and Services Science (IJ-CLOSER), 3*(3), 31-48.

Ullah, H., Gopalakrishnan Nair, N., Moore, A., Nugent, C., Muschamp, P., & Cuevas, M. (2019). 5G Communication: An Overview of Vehicle-to-Everything, Drones, and Healthcare Use-Cases. *IEEE Access: Practical Innovations, Open Solutions, 7*, 37251–37268. doi:10.1109/ACCESS.2019.2905347

Umar, M. S., & Rafiq, M. Q. (2012, March). Select-to-Spawn: A novel recognition-based graphical user authentication scheme. *2012 IEEE International Conference on Signal Processing, Computing and Control*. 10.1109/ISPCC.2012.6224382

Upadhyay & Dhapola. (2015). Embedded Systems And its Application in Medical Field. *Emerging Trends in Computer Science and Information, 3*.

Uthra, G., Thangavelu, K., & Shunmugapriya S. (2017). Ranking generalized intuitionistic pentagonal fuzzy number by centroidal approach. *International Journal of Mathematics and Its Applications, 5*(4),589-593.

Vaidya, P., & PVSSR, C. M. (2017). A robust semi-blind watermarking for color images based on multiple decompositions. *Multimedia Tools and Applications, 76*(24), 25623–25656. doi:10.100711042-017-4355-0

Vaishya, R., Javaid, M., Khan, I. H., & Haleem, A. (2020). Artificial Intelligence (AI) applications for COVID-19 pandemic. *Diabetes & Metabolic Syndrome, 14*(4), 337–339. doi:10.1016/j.dsx.2020.04.012 PMID:32305024

Vassaux, B., Nguyen, P., Baudry, S., Bas, P., & Chassery, J. (2002). Scrambling technique for video object watermarking resisting to mpeg-4. *Proceedings of the Video/Image Processing and Multimedia Communications 4th EURASIP-IEEE Region 8 International Symposium on VIPromCom*, 239–244. 10.1109/VIPROM.2002.1026662

Velasquez, K., Abreu, D. P., Curado, M., & Monteiro, E. (2017). Service placement for latency reduction in the internet of things. *Annales des Télécommunications, 72*(1-2), 105–115. doi:10.100712243-016-0524-9

Verbeeck, N., Caprioli, R. M., & van de Plas, R. (2020). Unsupervised machine learning for exploratory data analysis in imaging mass spectrometry. *Mass Spectrometry Reviews, 39*(3), 245–291. doi:10.1002/mas.21602 PMID:31602691

Verma, P., Sood, S. K., & Kalra, S. (2018). Cloud-centric IoT based student healthcare monitoring framework. *Journal of Ambient Intelligence and Humanized Computing, 9*(5), 1293–1309.

Verma, V. S., & Jha, R. K. (2015). An Overview of Robust Digital Image Watermarking. *IETE Technical Review, 32*(6), 479–496. doi:10.1080/02564602.2015.1042927

Vijayalakshmi, A., Jose, D. V., & Unnisa, S. (2021). Wearable Sensors for Pervasive and Personalized Health Care. In *IoT in Healthcare and Ambient Assisted Living* (pp. 123–143). Springer.

Vijayan, T., & Kumaran, M. (2008). Inventory model with a mixture of back-orders and lost sales under fuzzy cost. *European Journal of Operational Research, 189*(1), 105–119. doi:10.1016/j.ejor.2007.05.049

Voyant, C., Notton, G., Kalogirou, S., Nivet, M. L., Paoli, C., Motte, F., & Fouilloy, A. (2017). Machine learning methods for solar radiation forecasting: A review. *Renewable Energy, 105*, 569–582. doi:10.1016/j.renene.2016.12.095

Vuong, Q. H., Ho, M. T., Vuong, T. T., La, V. P., Ho, M. T., Nghiem, K. C., Tran, B. X., Giang, H. H., Giang, T. V., Latkin, C., Nguyen, H. K. T., Ho, C. S. H., & Ho, R. C. M. (2019). Artificial Intelligence vs. Natural Stupidity: Evaluating AI Readiness for the Vietnamese Medical Information System. *Journal of Clinical Medicine, 8*(2), 168. doi:10.3390/jcm8020168 PMID:30717268

Wadhera, S., Kamra, D., Rajpal, A., Jain, A., & Jain, V. (2021). A Comprehensive Review on Digital Image Watermarking. *Proceedings of the WCNC-2021: Workshop on Computer Networks & Communications*, 126–140.

Wang, L., & Wong, A. (2020). *Covid-net: A tailored deep convolutional neural network design for detection of covid-19 cases from chest radiography images*. arXiv preprint arXiv:200309871

Wang. (2020). GuardHealth: Blockchain empowered secure data management and Graph Convolutional Network enabled anomaly detection in smart healthcare. *Journal of Parallel and Distributed Computing, 142*(August), 1–12.

Wang, B., & Ma, M. (2012). A smart card based efficient and secured multi-server authentication scheme. *Wireless Personal Communications, 68*(2), 361–378. doi:10.100711277-011-0456-7

Wang, C. Y. (1989). Free Convection on a Vertical Stretching Surface. *ZAMM. Journal of Applied Mathematics and Mechanics, 69*(11), 418–420.

Wang, C., Wang, D., Xu, G., & Guo, Y. (2017). A lightweight password-based authentication protocol using smart card. *International Journal of Communication Systems, 30*(16), e3336. doi:10.1002/dac.3336

Wangping, J., Ke, H., Yang, S., Wenzhe, C., Shengshu, W., Shanshan, Y., ... Yao, H. (2020). Extended SIR prediction of the epidemics trend of COVID-19 in Italy and compared with Hunan, China. *Frontiers in medicine, 7*, 169.

Wang, W., Huang, H., Xiao, F., Li, Q., Xue, L., & Jiang, J. (2021). Computation-transferable authenticated key agreement protocol for smart healthcare. *Journal of Systems Architecture, 118*, 102215. doi:10.1016/j.sysarc.2021.102215

Wasay, A., Athanassoulis, M., & Idreos, S. (2015). Queriosity: Automated Data Exploration; Queriosity: Automated Data Exploration. *2015 IEEE International Congress on Big Data.* 10.1109/BigDataCongress.2015.116

Wazirali, R., Ahmad, R., Al-Amayreh, A., Al-Madi, M., & Khalifeh, A. (2021). Secure Watermarking Schemes and Their Approaches in the IoT Technology: An Overview. *Electronics (Basel), 10*(14), 1–28. doi:10.3390/electronics10141744

Wei, J., & Yu, Y. (2018). An effective hybrid cuckoo search algorithm for unknown parameters and time delays estimation of chaotic systems. *IEEE Access: Practical Innovations, Open Solutions, 6*, 6560–6571. doi:10.1109/ACCESS.2017.2738006

Wenchao, X., & Yilin, B. (2017). Medical Health Big Data Classification Based on KNN Classification Algorithm. *IEEE Access: Practical Innovations, Open Solutions.* Advance online publication. doi:10.1109/ACCESS.2019.2955754

White, G., Cabrera, C., Palade, A., & Clarke, S. (2018, November). Augmented reality in IoT. In *International Conference on Service-Oriented Computing* (pp. 149-160). Springer.

Wiederhold, B. K. (2014). Special issue on virtual reality and pain. Cyberpsychology Behavior and Social Networking, 17(6).

Wiederhold, B. K., & Wiederhold, M. D. (2005). *Virtual reality therapy for anxiety disorders: Advances in evaluation and treatment.* American Psychological Association.

Wiefling, S., Dürmuth, M., & Lo Iacono, L. (2020, December 7). More than just good passwords? A study on usability and security perceptions of risk-based authentication. *Annual Computer Security Applications Conference.* 10.1145/3427228.3427243

Wiefling, S., Lo Iacono, L., & Dürmuth, M. (2019). Is this really you? An empirical study on risk-based authentication applied in the wild. In *ICT Systems Security and Privacy Protection* (pp. 134–148). Springer International Publishing. doi:10.1007/978-3-030-22312-0_10

Wiefling, S., Patil, T., Dürmuth, M., & Lo Iacono, L. (2020). Evaluation of risk-based re-authentication methods. In *ICT Systems Security and Privacy Protection* (pp. 280–294). Springer International Publishing. doi:10.1007/978-3-030-58201-2_19

Wiefling, S., Tolsdorf, J., & Lo Iacono, L. (2021). Privacy Considerations for Risk-Based Authentication Systems. In *2021 International Workshop on Privacy Engineering* (pp. 315–322). IEEE.

Williams, P. A., & McCauley, V. (2016). *Always connected: the security challenges of the healthcare internet of things.* 3rd IEEE World Forum on the Internet of Things, Reston, VA.

Williams, C., Mostashari, F., Mertz, K., Hogin, E., & Atwal, P. (2012). From the office of the national coordinator: The strategy for advancing the exchange of health information. *Health Affairs, 31*(3), 527–536.

Wiskott, L. (1999). The role of topographical constraints in face recognition. *Pattern Recognition Letters, 20*(1), 89–96. doi:10.1016/S0167-8655(98)00122-6

Wiskott, L., Fellous, J. M., Krüger, N., & Malsburg, C. V. D. (1997). Face recognition by elastic bunch graph matching. *Proceedings of International Conference on Image Processing held at Santa Barbara during*, 129-132. 10.1109/ICIP.1997.647401

Wu, N., Green, B., Ben, X., & O'Banion, S. (2020). *Deep transformer models for time series forecasting: The influenza prevalence case.* arXiv preprint arXiv:2001.08317.

Wu, F., Wu, T., & Yuce, M. R. (2019). An internet-of-things (IoT) network system for connected safety and health monitoring applications. *Sensors (Basel), 19*(1), 21. doi:10.339019010021 PMID:30577646

Wu, T. (2017). An autonomous wireless body area network implementation towards IoT connected healthcare applications. *IEEE Access: Practical Innovations, Open Solutions, 5*, 11413–11422.

Wu, T.-S., Lee, M.-L., Lin, H.-Y., & Wang, C.-Y. (2013). Shoulder-surfing-proof graphical password authentication scheme. *International Journal of Information Security, 13*(3), 245–254. doi:10.100710207-013-0216-7

Wu, W., An, S. Y., Guan, P., Huang, D. S., & Zhou, B. S. (2019). Time series analysis of human brucellosis in mainland China by using Elman and Jordan recurrent neural networks. *BMC Infectious Diseases, 19*(1), 1–11.

Wu, X. (2018). Mixed reality technology launches in orthopedic surgery for comprehensive preoperative management of complicated cervical fractures. *Surgical Innovation, 25*(4), 421–422.

Xiao, Q., Li, C., Tang, Y., & Chen, X. (2021, April). Energy Efficiency Modeling for Configuration-Dependent Machining via Machine Learning: A Comparative Study. *IEEE Transactions on Automation Science and Engineering, 18*(2), 717–730. doi:10.1109/TASE.2019.2961714

Xia, Z., Yuan, C., Lv, R., Sun, X., Xiong, N. N., & Shi, Y.-Q. (2020). A novel weber local binary descriptor for fingerprint liveness detection. *IEEE Transactions on Systems, Man, and Cybernetics. Systems, 50*(4), 1526–1536. doi:10.1109/TSMC.2018.2874281

Xie, P. (2014). *Facial movement based human user authentication.* Iowa State University. http://dx.doi.org/ doi:10.31274/etd-180810-3817

Xiong, J., Xiong, J., & Claramunt, C. (2014). A spatial entropy-based approach to improve mobile risk-based authentication. *Proceedings of the 1st ACM SIGSPATIAL International Workshop on Privacy in Geographic Information Collection and Analysis - GeoPrivacy '14.* 10.1145/2675682.2676400

Xu & Uberbacher. (1997). 2D image segmentation using minimum spanning trees. *Image and Vision Computing, 15*, 47-57.

Xu, Q., & Deng, W. (2008). Adaptively weighted 2DPCA based on local feature for face recognition. *Fourth International Conference on Natural Computation*, 76-79.

Yaman, M. A., Subasi, A., & Rattay, F. (2018). Comparison of Random Subspace and Voting Ensemble Machine Learning Methods for Face Recognition. *Symmetry, 10*(11), 1–19. doi:10.3390ym10110651

Yang, Li, & Xie. (2015, March). MotionAuth: Motion-based authentication for wrist worn smart devices. *2015 IEEE International Conference on Pervasive Computing and Communication Workshops (PerCom Workshops)*. http://dx.doi.org/ doi:10.1109/percomw.2015.7134097

Yang, Hsu, & Wu. (2021). A hybrid multiple-criteria decision portfolio with the resource constraints model of a smart healthcare management system for public medical centers. *Socio-Economic Planning Sciences*, 101073.

Yang, X.-S., & Deb, S. (2014). Cuckoo search: Recent advances and applications. *Neural Computing & Applications*, *24*(1), 169–174. doi:10.100700521-013-1367-1

Yang, Y., Liu, X., & Deng, R. H. (2017). Lightweight break-glass access control system for healthcare Internet-of-Things. *IEEE Transactions on Industrial Informatics*, *14*(8), 3610–3617.

Yang, Y., Zhang, H., & Chen, X. (2020). Coronavirus pandemic and tourism: Dynamic stochastic general equilibrium modeling of infectious disease outbreak. *Annals of Tourism Research*, *83*, 102913.

Yang, Z., Zeng, Z., Wang, K., Wong, S. S., Liang, W., Zanin, M., ... He, J. (2020). Modified SEIR and AI prediction of the epidemics trend of COVID-19 in China under public health interventions. *Journal of Thoracic Disease*, *12*(3), 165.

Yaqoob, I. (2021). Blockchain for healthcare data management: Opportunities, challenges, and future recommendations. *Neural Computing & Applications*, 1–16.

Yempally, S., Singh, S. K., & Velliangiri, S. (2021, October). Review of an IoT-based Remote Patient Health Monitoring System. In 2021 Smart Technologies, Communication and Robotics (STCR) (pp. 1-5). IEEE.

Yeole, A. S., & Kalbande, D. R. (2016, March). Use of Internet of Things (IoT) in healthcare: A survey. In *Proceedings of the ACM Symposium on Women in Research 2016* (pp. 71-76). 10.1145/2909067.2909079

Yicheng, F., Huangqi, Z., Jicheng, X., Minjie, L., Lingjun, Y., Peipei, P., & Wenbin, J. (2020). Sensitivity of chest CT for COVID-19: Comparison to RT-PCR. *Radiology*, 200–432. PMID:32073353

Yildirim, M. (2021). Steganography-Based Voice Hiding in Medical Images of COVID-19 Patients. *Nonlinear Dynamics*, *105*(3), 2677–2692. doi:10.1007/s11071-021-06700-z

Yin, Akmandor, Mosenia, & Jha. (2018). *Smart Healthcare, now*. Academic Press.

Younge, A. J., Von Laszewski, G., Wang, L., Lopez-Alarcon, S., & Carithers, W. (2010). Efficient resource management for cloud computing environments. *International conference on green computing*, 357–364. 10.1109/GREEN-COMP.2010.5598294

Zahoor, E., Munir, K., Perrin, O., & Godart, C. (2013). An event-based approach for declarative, integrated and self-healing web service composition. *International Journal of Services Computing*, *1*, 13-24.

Zeadally, S., & Bello, O. (2019). Harnessing the power of internet of things based connectivity to improve healthcare. Internet of Things. doi:10.1016/j.iot.2019.100074

Zeadally, S., Isaac, J. T., & Baig, Z. (2016). Security attacks and solutions in electronic health (e-health) systems. *Journal of Medical Systems*, *40*(12), 1–12. doi:10.100710916-016-0597-z PMID:27730389

Zeinab, K. A. M., & Elmustafa, S. A. A. (2017). Internet of things applications, challenges and related future technologies. *World Scientific News*, *2*(67), 126–148.

Zeroual, A., Harrou, F., Dairi, A., & Sun, Y. (2020). Deep learning methods for forecasting COVID-19 time-Series data: A Comparative study. *Chaos, Solitons, and Fractals*, *140*, 110121.

Zhang, Y., Qin, H., & Kong, T. (2010). A novel robust text watermarking for word document. *Proceedings of the 3rd International Congress on Image and Signal Processing*, 38–42. 10.1109/CISP.2010.5648007

Zhang. (2019). *Gradient Descent based Optimization algorithms for Deep Learning Models training*. Academic Press.

Zhang, Fu, & Ni, Liu, & Yang. (2020). A generative method for steganography by cover synthesis with auxiliary semantics. *Tsinghua Science and Technology*, 25(4), 516–527. doi:10.26599/TST.2019.9010027

Zhang, G., Kou, L., Zhang, L., Liu, C., Da, Q., & Sun, J. (2017). A New Digital Watermarking Method for Data Integrity Protection in the Perception Layer of IoT. *Security and Communication Networks*, 2017, 1–12. doi:10.1155/2017/3126010

Zhang, H., Zhang, X., Wang, Y., Qian, X., & Wang, Y. (2018). Extended cuckoo search-based kernel correlation filter for abrupt motion tracking. *IET Computer Vision*, 12(6), 763–769. doi:10.1049/iet-cvi.2017.0554

Zhang, J., Tan, X., Wang, X., Yan, A., & Qin, Z. (2018). T2FA: Transparent two-factor authentication. *IEEE Access: Practical Innovations, Open Solutions*, 6, 32677–32686. doi:10.1109/ACCESS.2018.2844548

Zhang, J., Zhao, X., He, X., & Zhang, H. (2022). Improving the Robustness of JPEG Steganography With Robustness Cost. *IEEE Signal Processing Letters*, 29, 164–168. doi:10.1109/LSP.2021.3129419

Zhang, M., Zhu, Y., Zhang, C., & Liu, J. (2019). Video processing with serverless computing: a measurement study. *Proceedings of the 29th ACM Workshop on Network and Operating Systems Support for Digital Audio and Video*, 61–66. 10.1145/3304112.3325608

Zhang, T., Yang, J., Zhao, D., & Ge, X. (2007). Linear local tangent space alignment and application to face recognition. *Neurocomputing*, 70(7-9), 1547–1553. doi:10.1016/j.neucom.2006.11.007

Zhang, X., Yao, L., Kanhere, S. S., Liu, Y., Gu, T., & Chen, K. (2018). MindID. *Proceedings of the ACM on Interactive, Mobile, Wearable and Ubiquitous Technologies*, 2(3), 1–23. doi:10.1145/3264959

Zhang, Y., Luo, X., Guo, Y., Qin, C., & Liu, F. (2020, August). Multiple Robustness Enhancements for Image Adaptive Steganography in Lossy Channels. *IEEE Transactions on Circuits and Systems for Video Technology*, 30(8), 2750–2764. doi:10.1109/TCSVT.2019.2923980

Zhao, J., Liu, S., Zhou, M., Guo, X., & Qi, L. (2018). Modified cuckoo search algorithm to solve economic power dispatch optimization problems. *IEEE/CAA Journal of Automatica Sinica*, 5(4), 794-806.

Zhao, J., Liu, S., Zhou, M., Guo, X., & Qi, L. (2018). An Improved Binary Cuckoo Search Algorithm for Solving Unit Commitment Problems: Methodological Description. *IEEE Access: Practical Innovations, Open Solutions*, 6, 43535–43545. doi:10.1109/ACCESS.2018.2861319

Zheng, N., Bai, K., Huang, H., & Wang, H. (2014, October). You are how you touch: User verification on smartphones via tapping behaviors. *2014 IEEE 22nd International Conference on Network Protocols*. http://dx.doi.org/10.1109/icnp.2014.43

Zhong, Kanhere, & Chou. (2017, March). VeinDeep: Smartphone unlock using vein patterns. *2017 IEEE International Conference on Pervasive Computing and Communications (PerCom)*. http://dx.doi.org/10.1109/percom.2017.7917845

Zhou, B., Lohokare, J., Gao, R., & Ye, F. (2018, October 15). EchoPrint. *Proceedings of the 24th Annual International Conference on Mobile Computing and Networking*. 10.1145/3241539.3241575

Zhou, J., Zhai, L., & Pantelous, A. A. (2020). Market segmentation using high-dimensional sparse consumers data. *Expert Systems with Applications*, 145, 113136. doi:10.1016/j.eswa.2019.113136

Zhou, L., Feng, G., Shen, L., & Zhang, X. (2020). On Security Enhancement of Steganography via Generative Adversarial Image. *IEEE Signal Processing Letters*, *27*, 166–170. doi:10.1109/LSP.2019.2963180

Zhou, S. K., Chellappa, R., & Zhao, W. (2006). Unconstrained face recognition. *Neurocomputing*, *45*, 478–493.

Zhu, X., Yu, S., & Pei, Q. (2016, December). QuickAuth: Two-Factor quick authentication based on ambient sound. *2016 IEEE Global Communications Conference (GLOBECOM)*. 10.1109/GLOCOM.2016.7842192

Zimmerman, H. J. (1978). Fuzzy programming and linear programming with several objective functions. *Fuzzy Sets and Systems*, *1*(1), 45–55. doi:10.1016/0165-0114(78)90031-3

Zimmermann, H. J. (1996). *Fuzzy Set Theory and Its Applications*. Kluwer Academic Publishers. doi:10.1007/978-94-015-8702-0

Zupan, J. (1994). Introduction to artificial neural network (ANN) methods: What they are and how to use them. *Acta Chimica Slovenica*, *41*, 327–327.

About the Contributors

Debabrata Samanta is presently working as Assistant Professor, Department of Computer Science, CHRIST (Deemed to be University), Bangalore, India. He obtained his Bachelors in Physics (Honors), from Calcutta University; Kolkata, India. He obtained his MCA, from the Academy of Technology, under WBUT, West Bengal. He obtained his PhD in Computer Science and Engg. from National Institute of Technology, Durgapur, India, in the area of SAR Image Processing. He is keenly interested in Interdisciplinary Research & Development and has experience spanning fields of SAR Image Analysis, Video surveillance, Heuristic algorithm for Image Classification, Deep Learning Framework for Detection and Classification, Blockchain, Statistical Modelling, Wireless Adhoc Network, Natural Language Processing, V2I Communication. He has successfully completed six Consultancy Projects. He has received funding 8,110 USD under Open Access, Publication fund. He has received funding under International Travel Support Scheme in 2019 for attending conference in Thailand. He has received Travel Grant for speaker in Conference, Seminar etc for two years from July, 2019. He is the owner of 21 Patents (3 Design Indian Patent and 2 Australian patent Granted, 16 Indian Patents published) and 2 copyright. He has authored and coauthored over 195 research papers in international journal (SCI/SCIE/ESCI/Scopus) and conferences including IEEE, Springer and Elsevier Conference proceeding. He has received "Scholastic Award" at 2nd International conference on Computer Science and IT application, CSIT-2011, Delhi, India. He is a co-author of 13 books and the co-editor of 11 books, available for sale on Amazon and Flipkart. He has presented various papers at International conferences and received Best Paper awards. He has author and co-authored of 08 Book Chapters. He also serves as acquisition editor for Springer, Wiley, CRC, Scrivener Publishing LLC, Beverly, USA. and Elsevier. He is a Professional IEEE Member, an Associate Life Member of Computer Society Of India (CSI) and a Life Member of Indian Society for Technical Education (ISTE). He is a Convener, Keynote speaker, Session chair, Co-chair, Publicity chair, Publication chair, Advisory Board, Technical Program Committee members in many prestigious International and National conferences. He was invited speaker at several Institutions.

Debabrata Singh received the Ph.D. degree in computer science and engineering from the Siksha 'O' Anusandhan (SOA) Deemed to be University, Bhubaneswar, Odisha, India. He is currently working as an Associate Professor with the Department of Computer Application, ITER, SOA Deemed to be University. He is keenly interested in interdisciplinary research and development and has experience spanning fields of WSN, bioinformatics, wireless ad hoc networks, network security, cloud computing, cloud native applications, and the IoT applications. In his past 15 years of teaching experience, he has authored or coauthored over 73 research papers in international journal (SCI/SCIE/ESCI/Scopus) and conferences, including IEEE, Springer, and Elsevier conference proceeding. He also serves as an acquisition editorial/reviewing board member in reputed journals. He has received the "Bentham Ambassador" Award in 2019 and the Best Outstanding Researcher Award 2020 from the Kamarajar Institute of Education and Research (KIER).

* * *

Milu Acharya is Professor in the Department of Mathematics, Institute of Technical Education and Research, Siksha 'O' Anusandhan University, Bhubaneswar Odisha. She completed her Post graduation in Mathematics in 1992, MPhil in 1994 and received her PhD in 1997 in Complex Analysis from Utkal University, Bhubaneswar, Odisha. She has guided 12 students to complete their PhDs. She has nearly 60 publications in national and international journals. She has more than 27 years of teaching experience in teaching students from MTech, MCA and BTech courses. Her field of research includes complex analysis, numerical analysis, operations research, fluid dynamics and fuzzy optimisation theory.

Shreeya Bajpai is second year student of Bachelor of Computer Science at Christ (Deemed-to-be) University, India. Her research topic is algorithms.

Anil Kumar Biswal is currently pursing PhD in Computer Science and Engineering from ITER, Siksha 'O' Anusandhan (Deemed to be University). He has also an extensive record of teaching for the past 7 years and his research interests include Wireless Sensor Networks, Cloud Computing and IoT. He has worked on various research projects that solve some social related issues like traffic with street light monitoring process, drowsiness detection system, designing women safety App, etc.

Subhashree Choudhury (Senior Member, IEEE) was born in Odisha, India, in 1987. She graduated from Biju Patnaik University of Technology (BPUT), Odisha in Electrical Engineering in the year 2009, obtained Master's Degree from Siksha 'O' Anusandhan University in Electrical Engineering in 2012 and Ph. D from Siksha O Anusandhan (Deemed to be University) in 2017 in the area of Power System Operation and Control. From 2009 to 2010, she was a Lecturer with SMIT, BPUT, Odisha. From 2012 to 2018, she was an Assistant Professor with Department of Electrical and Electronics Engineering, Siksha 'O' Anusandhan (Deemed to University), Bhubaneswar, India. Since 2018, she has been working as Associate Professor with Department of Electrical and Electronics Engineering, Siksha 'O' Anusandhan (Deemed to University), Bhubaneswar, India. She has published more than 50 papers in various International Journals and Conference proceedings and has authored 6 book chapters. She has acted as a reviewer of Sustainable Cities and Society-Elsevier, International Journal of Control- Taylor & Francis, Journal of Franklin Institute-Elsevier, IET Control Theory and Applications, ISA Transactions-Elsevier, LNEE Springer Book Series and many IEEE conferences. Her research interests include microgrid control, Renewable energy and energy storage integration to microgrids, soft computing, evolutionary computing techniques, and its application to power system planning, operation and control.

Rajshree Dahal is research scholar of Department of Mathematics, CHRIST University, Bangalore. She is fascinated to do research in the field of Graph Theory. She published two research papers on application of Graph Theory in real world.

K. Renuka Devi completed her Bachelor of Engineering during 2018 and Master of Engineering in Computer Science during 2020 from Dr. Mahalingam College of Engineering and Technology, Pollachi, India. She is currently working as an Assistant Professor in the department of Information Technology at Dr. Mahalingam College of Engineering and Technology, Pollachi, India. She is a member of ACM since 2018. Her main research work focuses on Data and Web Mining, Image processing.

Sunita Vikrant Dhavale, BE, ME, PhD (CSE), C|EH, is currently working as Assistant Professor in Department of Computer Engineering, Defense Institute of Advanced Technology (DIAT), Pune. Her research area includes cyber security, artificial intelligence, image/audio/video security, bio metric, deep learning. She is EC-Council's Certified Ethical Hacker (CEH-v9). She has authored two books and more than 30 papers in reputed international journals and conference proceedings.She is member of various professional bodies including IEEE, ACM, ISACA,IETE, IAENG. She is recipient of 1) NVIDIA Hardware Research Grant - TITAN V GPU for Jan 2019, 2) IETE-M N Saha Memorial Award -2016, 3) Outstanding Women Achiever Award for Engineering Category by VENUS International Women Awards (VIWA-2016), 4) Top performer in Four Week online FDP titled "FDP301x: Mentoring Educators in Educational Technology", organized by Pandit Madan Mohan Malaviya National Mission for Teachers and Teaching (PMMMNMTT), MHRD, GoI, IIT Bombay, May 2018 5) Top performer in Four Week AICTE approved online FDP by IIT Bombay on - Use of ICT in Education for Online and Blended Learning, May 2016.

Mamata Garnayak is currently working as an Assistant Professor in Computer Science and Engineering department at Centurion University of Technology and Management, Bhubaneswar, Odisha, India. She has 15 years of working experience in various engineering colleges. She recently submitted her thesis in Recommender Systemat Kalinga Institute of Industrial Technology (Deemed to be University) Bhubaneswar, Odisha, India. Her research area includes Artificial Intelligence and Machine Learning.

Ritwika Das Gupta is a final year student of Department of Computer Science, CHRIST University.

Balasamy K. received the B.Tech. degree in Information Technology Engineering in 2006 from the Anna University, Chennai, and the M.E. degree in Computer Science and Engineering in 2009 from the Anna University of Technology, Coimbatore. He is an Assistant Professor in the Department of Artificial Intelligence and Data Science in Bannari Amman Institute of Technology, India. He is the Life Member of ISTE. His areas of interest include database management, image processing, cloud computing.

Rita Komalasari is a Researcher at the University of YARSI Indonesia. She is interested in A Social-Ecological Model (SEM) to manage Methadone programmes in prisons.

Vivin Krishnan received his M.Tech degree in Software Engineering from CUSAT, Kochi, India. He has been working with IBM India Software Labs (ISL), Bangalore since 2007. He presently leads the MobileFirst Platform product development in ISL. He is currently pursuing his Ph.D from CHRIST (Deemed to be University), Bangalore, India. His research interests include Zero Trust architecture, Risk-based authentication, Cloud security.

Ankit Kumar is working as an Assistant Professor, Department of Computer Engineering & Applications. His research Area in Wireless Sensor Networks. He has published multiple papers in Taylor and Francis's different journals related to Networks. His articles are published in 54 International Journals, 11 National Journals. He has received 8 patents. His work has been profiled broadly, such as in Information Security, Cloud Computing Image Processing, Neural Network, and Network. His research interests include Computer Network Information security, Computational Model, Compiler Design, and Data Structure. He is a Reviewer and Editor of many reputed journals.

Senbagavalli M. has received a bachelor's degree in Information Technology from Periyar University in 2004, a Master's degree in Computer Science and Engineering from Anna University in the year 2009, and a Ph.D. in Computer Science and Engineering from Anna University, Chennai in the year 2017. At present, she has been working as an Associate Professor in the Department of Information Technology at Alliance University—Bangalore since May 2018. Her research interests include data mining, sentiment analysis, deep learning, data science, and networks. She has published some patents and papers in national and international journals. She serves on the Editorial Boards of the International Journal of Research Review in Engineering and Management and the Journal of Trading, Economics, and Business, and she reviews for Springer Nature.

Jyothi Mandala obtained her doctorate from Acharya Nagarjuna University, Guntur, Andhra Pradesh. M.Tech (CSE) from JNTU- Kakinada, B.Tech (IT) from JNTU-Hyderabad. She is currently working as Assistant Professor in the Department of Computer Science and Engineering, CHRIST (Deemed to be) University, Kengeri Campus, Bangalore, Karnataka, India. She is having more than 16 years of Academic experience. She has many publications in reputed journals and guided UG, PG and PhD Students. She has 1 National and 2 American Society patents. She got best faculty award for Computer Graphics in college level. Her research areas are Information Security, Data Privacy, Data Mining .To share her expertise knowledge in various subjects to the students and enthusiastic learners, she started a YouTube channel JYOTHI MANDALA, now the YouTube channel has 7000+ subscribers with 1 Million+ views.

Arup Kumar Mohanty received his B.Tech. degree in Information Technology from College of Engineering and Technology, Odisha, India, in 2006; the M.Tech. degree in Computer Science and Informatics from Siksha 'O' Anusandhan Deemed to be University in 2013 and Ph.D from Siksha 'O' Anusandhan(Deemed to be University) in the year 2021. He is an assistant professor with the department of CSIT, Siksha 'O' Anusandhan (Deemed to be University), Bhubaneswar, India. He has published more than 5 papers in various International Journals and Conference proceedings His research area includes soft computing, computational finance, evolutionary computing and data mining.

Sagarika Mohanty is a PhD student in the Department of Computer Science and Engineering, National Institute of Technology, Rourkela, India. Her research interest includes software defined networking, fog computing and network optimization.

Ramesh Chandra Poonia received the Ph.D. degree in computer science from Banasthali University, Banasthali, India, in July 2013. Recently, he completed his Postdoctoral Fellowship at the CPS Laboratory, Department of ICT and Natural Sciences, Norwegian University of Science and Technology, Ålesund, Norway. He is working as an Associate Professor at the Department of Computer Science, CHRIST

(Deemed to be University), Bengaluru, India. He has published more than 82 research articles in refereed journals and international conferences and several edited books and conference proceedings. His research interests include sustainable technologies, cyber-physical systems, and intelligent algorithms for autonomous systems.

Ganeshan R. is Assistant Professor senior grade 2 in the School of Computer Science and Engineering of VIT-Bhopal University. He is having experience in different colleges and University. He was completed his doctorate degree in Anna University in the field of Information and Communication Engineering with specialization of Computer Science and Engineering. The research area includes Network Security and Forensics, Ethical Hacking, and Cyber Security. He has published various research papers which are indexed by Scopus and SCI journals. He is having various Professional Society membership cards like CSI, IAEng, SDIWC and ICSES.

Linesh Raja is currently working as Assistant Professor at Manipal University Jaipur. He earned a Ph.D. in computer science from Jaipur National University, India Before that he has completed his Master's and Bachelor's degree from Birla Institute of Technology, India. Dr. Linesh has published several research papers in the field of wireless communication, mobile networks security and internet of things in various reputed national and international journals. He has chaired various sessions of international conferences. He has edited the Handbook of Research on Smart Farming Technologies for Sustainable Development, IGI Global. At the same time he is also acting as a guest editor of various reputed journal publishing house, such as Taylor & Francis, Inderscience and Bentham Science.

Rasmita Rautray received her BTech. in CSE degree from BPUT University, India in 2003, M.Tech degree (in Computer Sc. & Engg.) in 2006 from the Utkal Patnaik University and completed her Ph.D (in Computer Sc.) under Siksha 'O' Anusandhan University in the 2017. She is currently working as Associate Professor in the Department of Computer Science and Engineering at Institute of Technical Education and Research (I.T.E.R.), Faculty of Engineering under Siksha 'O' Anusandhan University. She has more than 14 years of academic experience. Her major research Interests includes Data mining, Soft computing and Information Retrieval to name a few.

Sreeja S. is currently working as Assistant Professor in Department of Computer Science, CHRIST (Deemed to be University) Bangalore. Her area of interests in research includes but not limited to Information Security, Authentication, Bio-molecular Computing, DNA Cryptography, and Public Key Cryptography. She has published her research work in peer-reviewed journals including ELSEVIER, INDERSCIENCE and in proceedings of renowned International conferences by IEEE, SPRINGER, and ACM. She also received IEEE best thesis award (second) for her Ph.D. thesis during graduate congress GraTE '7' 2019. She also served as a reviewer for prestigious IEEE Conferences, Session chair and Publications Co-Chair for IEEE PhD Colloquium on Ethically Driven Innovation & Technology for Society 2019 and 2020.She is an active IEEE ComSoc Excom member.

Manju Bargavi S. K. is currently working as a Professor in School of CS & IT, Jain (Deemed-to-be University) Bangalore, Karnataka, India. She has blended the wide experience of 17 years in teaching and research in the field of Computer Science. She has published several international journals, patents and books related to the Computer Science and Engineering. She serves on the reviewer on many international journals related in Data Science, Network and Artificial Intelligence. Her area of research is Ad hoc Networks, Security, IoT and AI.

Sipra Sahoo is currently working as an Associate Professor with Department of Computer Science and Engineering, Siksha 'O' Anusandhan (Deemed to University), Bhubaneswar, India. She was born in 1984 in Odisha,India. She graduated from Biju Patnaik University of Technology (BPUT), Odisha in Information Technology in the year 2005, obtained Master's degree from Utkal University in the year 2008 and Ph.D from Utkal Universiy in the year 2020. She has published more than 15 papers in various International Journals and Conference proceedings. Her research area includes soft computing, recommender system, evolutionary computing and data mining.

Swagatika Sahoo is a research scholar in the department Mathematics, Siksha 'O' Anusandhan Deemed to be University, Bhubaneswar. She completed her M.Sc. in 2010 and M.Phil. in 2012. Her current area of research is Fuzzy Optimization theory and Operations research.

Daniya T. received her B.Tech degree in Information Technology from Anna University, Chennai, India and M.Tech degree from MS University, India, in 2009 and 2011 respectively. She is currently doing Ph.D degree in Computer Science and Engineering at Sathyabama Institute of Science and Technology Chennai, India. She is currently working as an Assistant Professor with the Department of Information Technology, GMR Institute of Technology, Rajam, Andhra Pradesh India. Her research interest is Artificial Intelligence, Machine Learning and Deep Learning. She Published 15 research articles in various journals and conferences.

Apurv Taunk is currently working at Capgemini India as a Senior Analyst. He was born on 30/03/1998. He has completed his B.Tech in Computer Science & Engineering in the year 2020 from Institute of Technical Education and Research, Siksha O Anusandhan (Deemed to be University) University, Jagmohannager, Bhubaneswar, Odisha, India. His research interests include Machine Learning & Recommender systems. He has one Scopus Indexed paper in his credit till date.

Index

A

AdaBoost 338-340, 346, 350

adaptive authentication 154, 164-167, 170-172, 174, 176

AI 1-10, 55-57, 59, 80, 93, 110-113, 115-120, 143-146, 148-149, 151-153, 182, 194, 202, 204, 211, 270-271, 279-280, 305-306, 339, 343, 393, 395, 397, 402, 406, 419, 421, 435

Amazon Lambda 203

Application of Big Data 52

application placement 383, 385-386, 389-390, 397-399, 401-402, 404, 406

Arduino-Uno 247

Artificial Intelligence 1, 5-10, 29-30, 54-56, 59, 66, 68, 81-83, 106, 110-113, 115-116, 118-120, 144, 148-149, 152-153, 170, 176, 181-182, 184, 200-202, 244, 261-263, 270, 276, 279-280, 302-303, 305, 336, 353, 356, 421

artificial neural network (ANN) 21, 180-181, 184, 202

B

big data 4, 9-10, 52-55, 68, 72, 76-78, 80-84, 115, 118, 175, 200, 223, 259, 261-263, 267-269, 276-278, 305, 324, 339, 352, 406, 438

Binary Conversion 228

Binary Cuckoo Search 12, 18, 31

BMI 279, 281, 284, 289, 293-294, 303, 339, 341, 343

Body Area Sensor 393

Buongiorno Model 325

C

carbon emission 121-123, 129, 132, 142

chronic disease 115, 248, 279, 339, 351

classification 3-4, 12, 18-19, 21-23, 26, 28, 81, 86, 89-90, 96, 117, 143-147, 151-152, 201, 258, 267, 282, 300, 305, 314, 340, 346, 348, 351, 357, 359-360, 362-366, 371-372

Clinical Data 6, 86

cloud computing 53-55, 63, 80-84, 165, 172, 204-205, 209-210, 223-227, 261-263, 270-272, 274-276, 339, 384-386, 388, 397, 403, 405-408

COVID-19 5, 10, 59-60, 143-147, 149, 151-153, 180-183, 199-202, 211, 216, 246, 248, 259, 267, 352, 384, 406-407, 435

cuckoo search 12-19, 26-31

D

Decoding 228, 233, 236

Deep Learning 1, 55, 66, 116-117, 143-144, 146-147, 152-153, 181, 199, 202, 246, 258, 302-303, 306, 337, 351-352, 404, 408

Design Thinking 143, 145, 148, 151-153

diabetes 29, 67, 202, 279-282, 290, 301-304, 338-341, 345-346, 350-351

Dimensionality Reduction 12, 49, 340

disease 1, 7, 10, 55-56, 58-59, 63, 66, 68, 81, 83, 113, 115-119, 143, 152, 180-183, 199-202, 217, 221, 247-248, 251, 258, 263, 267-269, 279-281, 338-339, 351-352, 384-385, 407

Dynamo DB 203, 218

E

Ecological 374

edge computing 4, 9, 209, 226, 243, 261-262, 271-272, 275-277, 384, 389-390, 392, 407

Encoding 5, 106, 228, 235, 294, 296-297

ERR 160, 353, 368

e-verification 86

Evolutionary approach 12

Exploratory Data Analysis 284-285, 297, 306-308, 310-311, 313-316, 323-324

F

FACE RECOGNIZATION 353, 360
FAR 353, 367
Fast Healthcare Interoperability Resources 219, 222
Fog computing 84, 224, 272, 383-390, 401, 404, 406-408
FRR 353, 367-368
function as a service 203-205, 207-208, 215, 217-218, 227

G

gestational diabetes 279-280, 301, 303-304, 339
glucose levels 114, 279
green technology investment 121, 123, 132, 134, 139-140
Grey Wolf Optimization (GWO) 180, 401

H

health records 57, 66, 70, 112, 120, 268-269, 279, 339
healthcare 1-5, 9-11, 28, 52-58, 60-70, 74-75, 80-86, 96-99, 104-106, 110-120, 144, 154, 163, 180-181, 200, 203-205, 209-223, 226, 244, 247-249, 251, 257-278, 301-304, 339-340, 350, 352, 378, 380, 383-386, 389-395, 397, 401-408
healthcare systems 1-2, 5, 10, 81-83, 110, 113, 118-120, 203, 219, 259, 261, 263-264, 266-268, 271-272, 277
HIPAA 9, 203, 212, 214, 265, 277
human centric AI 143, 145, 151

I

Image Steganography 104, 228, 242-246
Internet of Medical Things 54, 261-264, 266, 271-272, 275-277
Internet of Things (IoT) 62, 83, 110, 112-113, 154, 247, 258, 260, 383-384
Intuitionistic fuzzy number 123-125

L

Least Significant Bit Algorithm 228

M

Machine Learning (ML) 1, 3-4, 10, 28, 54-57, 63, 68, 75, 83, 115-119, 144, 158, 164-168, 175, 180-182, 187, 199-202, 204, 211, 223-224, 245, 262-263,

267, 276, 279, 302-304, 306, 309, 314, 320, 323-324, 327-328, 331, 335-340, 342, 345-346, 348, 350-353, 356-357, 369-371, 373, 409-410
machine learning algorithm 83, 166, 168, 267
Magnetohydrodynamics 325
medical services 1, 5, 8-9, 54-55, 72, 76, 112, 248, 277
methadone program 374, 377, 379-380
microarray data 12, 28
multi-factor authentication 154-155, 162-164, 168-169, 172-173, 175-176

N

naive Bayes 166, 279, 338-339, 346, 349-350
nanofluid 325-328, 334-336

O

OS Virtualization 261
Own Ware-house 121

P

Particle Swarm Optimization (PSO) 180, 201, 401
Patient controlling 247
policy alternatives 374
problem-solving 32, 308, 416
project management 409-410, 412, 430, 437-438
Python 146, 149, 153, 183, 187, 206-207, 215, 230-232, 259, 312, 341-343

Q

quality of service (QoS) 383

R

random forest 3, 338-340, 346-347, 349-350, 353, 364-366, 372-373
recognition systems 32, 354, 371
Rented Ware-house 121
resource allocation 224, 389
risk score 154, 164-169
risk-based authentication 154-155, 163-170, 174, 176-179

S

scalability 53, 77, 204, 206, 212, 221, 270, 385, 409
Scrum 409, 415-416, 422-434, 436-438
serverless computing 203-205, 208, 210-211, 218, 223-227, 384, 404-405

shortest path 313, 409, 416-420

shortest paths graphs 32

smart city 4, 9, 52-53, 70, 76, 80, 82, 173, 175, 257, 277, 384-385, 405-407

smart health 2, 4, 10, 52-56, 59, 61, 70-72, 75-80, 84, 166, 216, 258, 339

smart healthcare 4-5, 9-11, 52-55, 58, 61, 63-69, 74, 80-81, 83-84, 257-259, 261-267, 269, 271-278, 303, 383-385, 404, 406, 408

Smart Healthcare Application 383

spanning trees 32, 39-40, 51

stretching sheet 325-326, 335-336

supervised learning 116, 306, 309, 331, 363

SVM 4, 6, 8, 12, 15, 18, 21, 23, 167, 338-339, 346, 350, 353, 362-365, 372-373

T

transformation 10, 44, 52-53, 82, 90, 94-95, 114, 183, 211, 309, 316, 321, 409, 430, 435-436

TSR 353, 368

Two-ware House 121

U

Ubiquitous Health (U-Health) care 247

Unsupervised Learning 306, 351

V

viscous dissipation 325, 327, 334, 336

W

watermarking methodology 87, 89, 101-104

Weibull distribution deterioration 122, 140

X

XGBoot 338

X-ray 143-147, 149, 152-153, 220

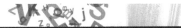
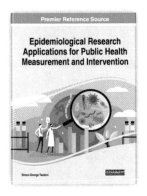
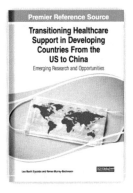
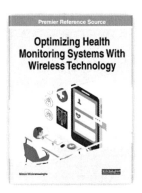
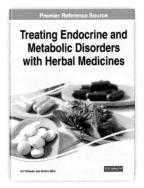
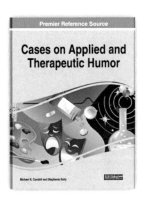
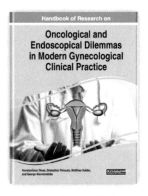
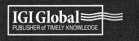

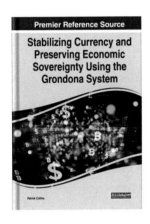
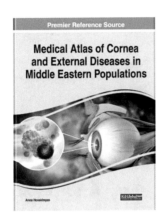
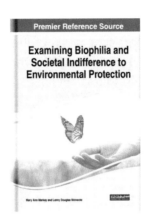
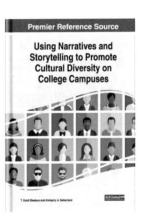

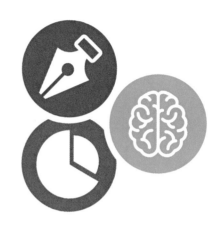

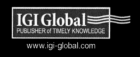

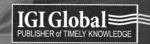

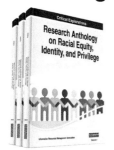
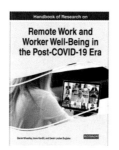
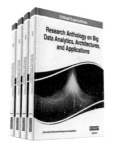
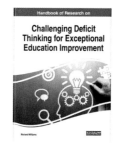

Printed in the United States
by Baker & Taylor Publisher Services